RADIOGRAPHIC PATHOLOGY

for TECHNOLOGISTS

SEVENTH EDITION

RADIOGRAPHIC PATHOLOGY

for TECHNOLOGISTS

NINA KOWALCZYK, PhD, RT(R)(CT)(QM), FASRT, FAEIRS
The Ohio State University
Columbus, Ohio

ELSEVIER

ELSEVIER

3251 Riverport Lane
St. Louis, Missouri 63043

RADIOGRAPHIC PATHOLOGY FOR TECHNOLOGISTS,
SEVENTH EDITION

ISBN: 978-0-323-41632-0

Notices

Previous editions copyrighted 2014, 2009, 2004, 1998, 1994, and 1988.

International Standard Book Number: 978-0-323-41632-0

Executive Content Strategist: Sonya Seigafuse
Senior Content Development Manager: Laurie Gower
Associate Content Development Specialist: Elizabeth Kilgore
Publishing Services Manager: Julie Eddy
Senior Project Manager: Marquita Parker
Design Direction: Patrick Ferguson

Printed in the United States of America

Last digit is the print number: 9 8 7 6 5 4

Working together
to grow libraries in
developing countries

www.elsevier.com • www.bookaid.org

Contributors

Emilee Berger Palmer, BSRT(R)(CT)
Imaging Specialist
OhioHealth
Columbus, Ohio

Tricia Leggett, DHEd, RT(R)(QM)
Bowerston, Ohio

Beth McCarthy, BS, RT(R) (CV)
Research Specialist
Cardiovascular Medicine
The Ohio State University Wexner Medical Center
Columbus, Ohio

Delaney McGuirt, BS, RT(R)(MR)
MRI Catheterization Technologist
National Institutes of Health
Bethesda, Maryland
*Contributing in her personal capacity

Heidi Nichols, RRA, RT(R)(CT)
Diagnostic Imaging Program Director
Northcentral Technical College
Wausau, Wisconsin

Leslie Partridge, MS, RRA, RT(R)
The Ohio State University Wexner Medical Center
Columbus, Ohio

Reviewers

Elaine Beaudoin, MS, RT(R)
Clinical Coordinator, Radiologic Technology
Niagara County Community College
Sanborn, New York

Chris Beaudry, MEd, ARRT(R)(M)(CT)
Program Coordinator, Radiologic Sciences
Yakima Valley Community College
Yakima, Washington

Patricia M. Davis, BS, RT(R)(MR), ARRT
Medical Imaging/Technology Coordinator, Clinical
   Assistant Professor
Indiana University Kokomo
Kokomo, Indiana

Nicole B. Dhanraj, PhD, RT(R)(CT)(MR)
Guam Memorial Hospital, Radiology
Tamuning, Guam

Bradford W. Gildon, MA, BSRT, RT(R)
Assistant Professor, Medical Imaging and Radiation
   Sciences
University of Oklahoma Health Sciences Center
College of Allied Health
Oklahoma City, Oklahoma

**Kerry Greene-Donnelly, MBA, RT(R)(M)(CT)
(QM)**
Assistant Professor/Clinical Coordinator-CT
Medical Imaging Sciences Program
Upstate Medical University
Syracuse, New York

Kristi Klein, MSEd, RT(R)(M)(CT)
Radiography Program Director
Madison Area Technical College
Madison, Wisconsin

Nancy Lamouroux, BS, RT(R)
Clinical Coordinator/Instructor, Radiologic Science
Kilgore College
Kilgore, Texas

Cynthia A. Meyers, MSRT(R)
Program Director, Radiologic Technology
Niagara County Community College
Sanborn, New York

Sandra E. Moore, MA, RT(R)(M)
Radiography Program Director
The Johns Hopkins Hospital
Baltimore, Maryland

April H. Pait, BS, RT(R)(M)
Team Leader of Imaging Centralized Scheduling,
   Radiology
Cone Health
Greensboro, North Carolina

Preface

The seventh edition of *Radiographic Pathology for Technologists* has been thoroughly updated and revised to offer students and radiologic science and imaging professionals information on the pathologic appearance of common diseases in a variety of diagnostic imaging modalities. It also presents basic information on the pathologic process, signs and symptoms, diagnosis, and prognosis of the various diseases.

The seventh edition includes the latest information concerning recent advances in genetic mapping, biomarkers, and up-to-date imaging modalities used in daily practice. The authors have attempted to present this material in a succinct, but reasonably complete, fashion to meet the needs of professionals in various imaging specialties. With each new edition, the authors have also reviewed the scope of the material covered in the text to provide the reader with a relevant and broad base of knowledge.

New to this Edition

- Full color design to enhance the understanding of content, as well as improved anatomic and pathologic images.
- Almost 100 new illustrations have been added or updated to complement new, updated, or expanded material.
- Updated content to reflect the latest ACR Appropriateness criteria and ASRT curriculum guidelines
- Chapters 5, 6, & 7 have been significantly updated to reflect diagnostic imaging modalities most commonly used in the diagnosis and treatment of pathologies of the abdomen, GI, hepatobiliary, and GU systems.
- Several new terms have been added to the glossary, and other definitions have been expanded or updated.

Learning Enhancements

- Each chapter includes a list of learning objectives, an outline, and key terms.
- Chapter content is followed by a summary and multiple-choice and short answer review questions, which can be used by the reader to assess acquired knowledge or by the instructor to stimulate discussion.
- Bold print has been used to focus the reader's attention on the key terms in each chapter, which are defined in the glossary at the end of the book along with other relevant terms.

Using the Book

The presentation of the seventh edition presumes that the reader has some background in human anatomy and physiology, imaging procedures, and medical and imaging terminology. The reader may build on this knowledge by assimilating information presented in this text.

To facilitate a working knowledge of the principles of radiologic pathology, study materials presented in the seventh edition remain sophisticated enough to be true to the complexity of the subject, yet simple and concise enough to permit comprehension by all readers. For student radiographers, sonographers, radiation therapists, and nuclear medicine technologists, this text is best used in conjunction with formal instruction from a qualified instructor. The practicing imaging professional may use this book as a self-teaching instrument to broaden and reinforce existing knowledge of the subject matter and also as a means to acquaint himself or herself with changing concepts and new material. The book can serve as a resource for continuing education because it provides an extensive range of information.

Ancillaries

Evolve Resources

Evolve is an interactive learning environment designed to work in coordination with *Radiographic Pathology for Technologists*. Included on the Evolve website are a test bank in Exam View containing approximately 400 questions, an electronic images collection consisting of images from the textbook, PowerPoint presentations per chapter, and the answers to the multiple-choice review questions in this book. Instructors may use Evolve to provide an Internet-based course component that reinforces and expands the concepts presented in class. Evolve may be used to publish the class syllabus, outlines, and lecture notes; set up "virtual office hours" and e-mail communication; share important dates and information through the online class calendar; and encourage student participation through chat rooms and discussion boards. Evolve also allows instructors to post examinations and manage their grade books online. For more information, visit http://evolve.elsevier.com/Kowalczyk/pathology/ or contact an Elsevier sales representative.

Acknowledgments

As I reflect on this current revision, I spent some time reviewing the first edition which was published in 1988. It is unbelievable that this was almost 30 years ago, but when I compare the issues I am amazed at the growth of imaging within the practice of medicine. The radiologic and imaging sciences touch every aspect of current medical care from prevention to diagnosis through treatment. Our professions have changed significantly in parallel with the growth of technology allowing us to play a very critical role in the health and wellbeing of individuals across the globe! Mapping the genome has also had a significant impact of how we categorize, track, and treat pathologic conditions. We have made great strides in oncology, cardiopulmonary disease, and are moving head on into the realms of neuroscience to solve mysteries of the human brain. Organ transplantation is also now a commonly accepted procedure allowing millions of people to live longer and healthier lives. I am also so proud of how the radiologic and imaging professions have embraced the new technologies to keep our professions on the forefront of innovation while also ensuring the importance of advocating for our patients and families, especially in terms of radiation safety and quality imaging. I hope educators, students, and radiologic and imaging professionals continue to find this textbook to be a credible resource in their daily practice.

As always, I could not have completed the seventh edition of this text without a great team of contributors, many of whom are new to this edition. I would like to thank my son, Nick, for his support; my graduates for their inspiration; and my colleagues within the radiologic sciences for their encouragement. I also want to thank the editorial team at Elsevier who worked diligently to keep me on track throughout the revision process.

The images in this book come from a variety of fine organizations that are to be thanked for graciously allowing us to use their material. They include the American College of Radiology, as well as The Ohio State University Wexner Medical Center, OhioHealth, Nationwide Children's Hospital, all located in Columbus, Ohio and Northcentral Technical College in Wausau, Wisconsin.

Nina Kowalczyk

Contents

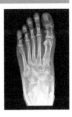
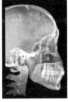
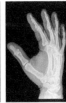

CHAPTER 1

Introduction to Pathology

ⓔ http://evolve.elsevier.com/Kowalczyk/pathology/

Introduction

Pathology is the study of disease. Many types of disease exist, and many conditions can be readily demonstrated by imaging studies. Image-guided interventional procedures and therapeutic protocols are often utilized in the management of disease. Therefore it is critical for radiologic professionals to have a thorough understanding of basic pathologic processes. This foundation begins with a working knowledge of common pathologic terms, an understanding of the effect and prevention of disease on U.S. health care expenditures, and the role of genetics in the individualized treatment of different pathologic processes. It is also important to understand the role of the Centers for Disease Control and Prevention (CDC) in terms of tracking, monitoring, and reporting trends in health and aging. This information is captured and reported by the National Center for Health Statistics (NCHS).

This chapter serves as a brief introduction to terms associated with pathology, recent health trends, and a review of cellular biology and genetics.

Pathologic Terms

Any abnormal disturbance of the function or structure of the human body as a result of some type of injury is called a **disease.** After injury, **pathogenesis** occurs. *Pathogenesis* refers to the sequence of events producing cellular changes that ultimately lead to observable changes known as **manifestations.** These manifestations may be displayed in a variety of fashions. A **symptom** refers to the patient's perception of the disease. Symptoms are subjective, and only the patient can identify these manifestations. For example, a headache is considered a symptom. A **sign** is an objective manifestation that is detected by the physician during examination. Fever, swelling, and skin rash are

all considered signs. A group of signs and symptoms that characterizes a specific abnormal disturbance is a **syndrome.** For example, respiratory distress syndrome is a common disorder in premature infants. However, some disease processes, especially in the early stages, do not produce symptoms and are termed **asymptomatic.**

Etiology is the study of the cause of a disease. Common agents that cause diseases include viruses, bacteria, trauma, heat, chemical agents, and poor nutrition. At the molecular level, a genetic abnormality of a single protein may also serve as the etiologic basis for some diseases. Proper infection control practices are important in a health care environment to prevent hospital-acquired **nosocomial** disease. Staphylococcal infection that follows hip replacement surgery is an example of a nosocomial disease, that is, one acquired from the environment. The cause of the disease, in this case, could be poor infection control practices. **Iatrogenic** reactions are adverse responses to medical treatment itself (e.g., a collapsed lung that occurs in response to a complication that arises during arterial line placement). If no causative factor can be identified, a disease is termed **idiopathic.**

The length of time over which the disease is displayed may vary. **Acute** diseases usually have a quick onset and last for a short period, whereas **chronic** diseases may manifest more slowly and last for a very long time. An example of an acute disease is pneumonia, and multiple sclerosis is considered a chronic condition. An acute illness may be followed by lasting effects termed **sequelae,** which is a condition that is caused by a previously acquired disease. For example, a stroke, or cerebrovascular accident, resulting in long-term neurologic deficits. Similarly, chronic illnesses often manifest in acute episodes, for example, an individual diagnosed with diabetes mellitus experiencing hypoglycemia or hyperglycemia.

Two additional terms refer to the identification and outcome of a disease. A **diagnosis** is the identification of a disease an individual is believed to have, and the predicted course and outcome of the disease is called a **prognosis.**

The structure of cells or tissue is termed **morphology.** Pathologic conditions may cause morphologic changes that alter normal body tissues in a variety of ways. Sometimes, the disease process is destructive, decreasing the normal density of a tissue. This occurs when tissue composition is altered by a decrease in the atomic number of the tissue, the compactness of the cells, or by changes in tissue thickness; for example, atrophy from limited use. Such disease processes are radiographically classified as *subtractive, lytic,* or *destructive* and require a decrease in the exposure technique. Conversely, some pathologic conditions cause an increase in the normal density of a tissue, resulting in a higher atomic number or increased compactness of cells. These are classified as *additive* or *sclerotic* disease processes and require an increase in the exposure technique. It is important for the radiographer to know common pathologic conditions that require an alteration of the exposure technique so that high-quality radiographs can be obtained to assist in the diagnosis and treatment of the disease.

Government agencies compile statistics annually with regard to the incidence, or rate of occurrence, of disease. **Epidemiology** is the investigation of disease in large groups. Health care epidemiology is grounded in the belief of distributions of health states. For example,

good health, disease, disability, or death. These distributions are not random within a population and are influenced by multiple factors, including biologic, social, and environmental factors. Health care epidemiologists conduct research primarily by working with medical statistics, data associations, and large cohort studies. The **prevalence** of a given disease refers to the number of cases found in a given population. The **incidence** of disease refers to the number of new cases found in a given period. Diseases of high prevalence in an area where a given causative organism is commonly found are said to be *endemic* to that area. For example, histoplasmosis is a fungal disease of the respiratory system endemic to the Ohio and Mississippi River valleys. It is not uncommon to see a relatively high prevalence of this disease in these areas. However, its appearance in great numbers in the western United States could represent an epidemic. An epidemic is defined as the rapid wide spread occurrence of a disease to a large number of people in a given population.

Monitoring Disease Trends

Over the past century, life expectancy in the United States has continued to increase. The majority of children born at the beginning of the twenty-first century are expected to live well into their seventh decade (Fig. 1.1). In 2013, life expectancy was 78.8 years. Over the past 100 years, the principal causes of death have shifted from acute infections to chronic diseases. These changes have occurred as a result of biomedical and

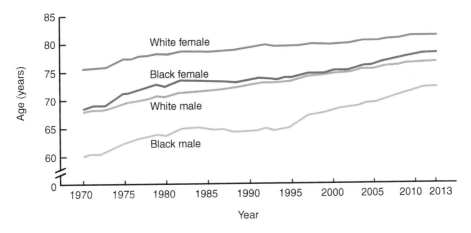

FIG. 1.1 Life expectancy by race and sex: United States 1970 to 2013. Available at http://www.cdc.gov/nchs/data/nvsr/nvsr64/nvsr64_02.pdf

pharmaceutical advances, public health initiatives, and social changes (Fig. 1.2). Experts disagree about the trend of increased life expectancy continuing into the twenty-first century. Some believe that increased knowledge of disease etiology and continued development of medical technology in combination with screening, early intervention, and treatment of disease could have positive results. However, many experts express concern about the quality of life of older adults. In other words, the possibility of older adults spending their added years in declining health and lingering illness, instead of being active and productive, is a concern.

The **mortality rate** is the average number of deaths caused by a particular disease in a population. Death certificates are collected by each state, forwarded to the NCHS, and subsequently processed and published as information on mortality statistics and trends. The NCHS and the U.S. Department of Health and Human Services (USDHHS) monitor and report mortality rates in terms of leading causes of death according to gender, race, age, and specific causes of death such as heart disease or malignant neoplasia. Trends in these mortality patterns are identified by age, gender, and ethnic origin and tracked to help identify necessary interventions. For instance, the age-adjusted death rate for heart disease has steadily decreased for both women and men in the United States. This trend demonstrates a 30% to 40% decline

over the past 20 years; resulting, in part, from health education and changes in lifestyle behaviors. Because mortality information is gathered from death certificates, changes in the descriptions and coding of "cause of death" and the amount of information forwarded to the NCHS may alter these statistics. For instance, there were changes in the way deaths were recorded and ranked in terms of the leading causes of death occurring between 1998 and 1999. Since 1999, mortality data and cause-of-death statistics have been gathered and classified according to the *Tenth Revision, International Classification of Diseases* (ICD-10), and in 2007 additional ICD-10 codes were added to clarify the underlying causes of death.

Chronic diseases continue to be the leading causes of death in the United States for adults age 45 years and older. Heart disease and malignant neoplasia remained the top two causes of deaths in 2013 for both males and females, responsible collectively for 46% of all deaths. The third, fourth, and fifth top causes of death in 2013 were lower respiratory disease, unintentional injuries as a result of accidents, and cerebrovascular disease. Alzheimer disease continues to increase and was ranked as the sixth leading cause of death in 2013. Emphasis has been placed on reducing the deaths associated with these chronic diseases, and slight decline was noted through 2013. The decrease in deaths as a result of heart disease may be clearly attributed to advances in the prevention and treatment

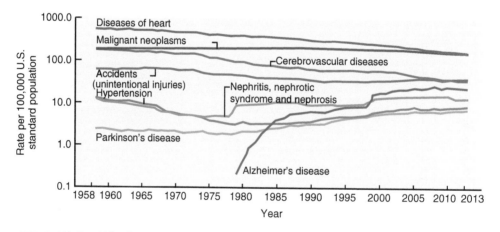

FIG. 1.2 National Vital Statistics Report of the age-adjusted death rates for selected leading causes of death in the United States from 1958 to 2013. Available at http://www.cdc.gov/nchs/data/nvsr/nvsr64/nvsr64_02.pdf

of cardiac disease. An increased understanding of the genetics of cancer is certainly responsible for better screening and individualized treatment for many types of neoplastic disease. Advances in diagnostic and therapeutic radiologic procedures have also played a role in the reduction of deaths associated with these chronic diseases.

As the mortality rate for heart disease and cancer have declined, increases have been noted in Alzheimer disease and diabetes mellitus. Among children and young adults (age 1–44 years), injury remains the leading cause of death.

Mortality rates from any specific cause may fluctuate from year to year, so trends are monitored over a 3-year period. These data are used to evaluate the health status of U.S. citizens and identify segments of the population at greatest risk for specific diseases and injuries. Current data are available on the NCHS website and may be accessed at www.cdc.gov/.

The incidence of sickness sufficient to interfere with an individual's normal daily routine is referred to as the **morbidity rate.** The CDC is also responsible for trending morbidity rates in the United States. States must submit death certificates to the NCHS, making it fairly easy to obtain accurate data about the mortality rate of a specific population. It is more difficult to obtain accurate data about the morbidity rate. This information comes primarily from physicians and other health care workers reporting morbidity statistics and information to the various governmental and private agencies.

Health Care Resources

Health care delivery in the United States has two fundamental and diverse functions, with one area focused on healthy lifestyle for prevention and the second area focusing on restoration of health after a disease has occurred. Improvements in health care interventions such as technology, electronic communications, and pharmaceuticals have greatly contributed to a shift from inpatient services to outpatient services (Fig. 1.3). Ambulatory care centers range from hospital outpatient and emergency departments to physicians' offices. In response to this shift, emphasis has been placed on increasing the number of physician generalists, including family practitioners, internal medicine physicians, and pediatricians. Inpatient admissions and hospital length of stay have remained fairly consistent over the past 10 years; however, emergency department visits have continued to steadily increase since the late 1990s, with many emergency departments reporting admissions exceeding their capacity (Fig. 1.4).

The rate of growth in U.S. health expenditures is staggering, and they cover a wide range of categories (Fig. 1.5). In 2014 U.S. health spending accounted for 17.5% of the gross domestic product, a larger share than in any other major industrialized country, with U.S. health care expenditures totaling 3.0 trillion (Table 1.1). The 2014 increase is a result of the Affordable Care Act which allows Americans improved access, affordability, and quality in health care. This act was signed into law March 2010. Regulation of private

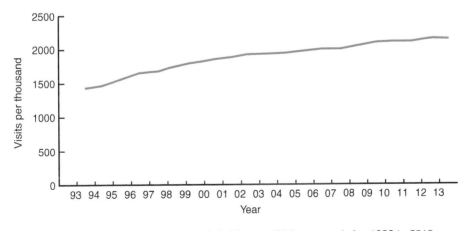

FIG. 1.3 Number of outpatient hospital visits per 1000 persons during 1993 to 2013.

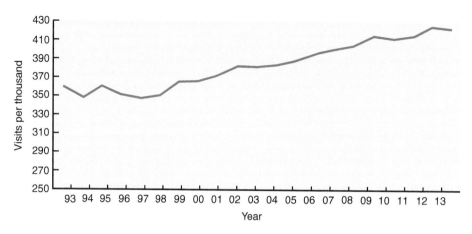

FIG. 1.4 Number of emergency department visits per 1000 persons during 1993 to 2003.

Health Care Expenditures Projected for 2016–2025

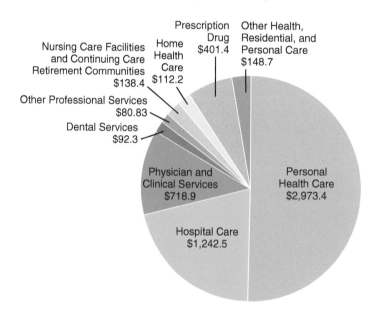

National Health Expenditure Data, Projected. CMS.gov. U.S. Centers for Medicare and Medicaid Services. Baltimore, MD. March 21, 2017.
https://www.cms.gov/research-statistics-data-and-systems/statistics-trends-and-reports/nationalhealthexpenddata/nationalhealthaccountsprojected.html

FIG. 1.5 Health care expenditures projected for 2016-2025 ($ in billions).

health insurance companies and establishment of a Health Insurance Marketplace are among the benefits of this new legislation. The major sources of funding for health care include Medicare, funded by the federal government for older adults and disabled individuals; Medicaid, funded by federal and state governments for the poor; and privately funded health care plans. However, private insurance and out-of-pocket spending on health care in 2013 was $9.523 per person. The insured rate is projected to increase as a result of the Affordable Care Act with a projected 8.4 million individuals gaining coverage in 2014 (Fig. 1.6). At the time of publishing this text, portions of the Affordable Care Act have been repealed, and the program is in transition. The diagnosis and treatment of cancer and other chronic diseases consume enormous financial and other resources in health care. Therefore emphasis on wellness and disease prevention must continue to reduce these costs. Studies have shown that it is much more cost-effective to provide preventive care than to wait until a disease has progressed.

TABLE 1.1
National Total Health Expenditures* from 1980 to 2024

Year	Total Expenditures (Billions)
1980	$255,658
1990	$724,277
2000	$1,377,972
2005	$2,034,816
2010	$2,604,131
2015	$3,243,542
2020	$4,273,810
2024	$5,425,069

*Years 2020 to 2024 are projections.
Centers for Medicare & Medicaid Services (CMS) National Health Expenditure Data, 2014 available at https://www.cms.gov/Research-Statistics-Data-and-Systems/Statistics-Trends-and-Reports/NationalHealthExpendData/NationalHealthAccountsProjected.html

Human Genetic Technology

The Human Genome Project was a 13-year (1990–2003) project coordinated by the U.S. Department of Energy and the National Institutes of Health. The goals of the project were to identify the 30,000 genes in the human deoxyribonucleic acid (DNA); to determine the sequences of the three billion chemical base pairs that make up human DNA; to electronically store the data; to improve tools for data analysis; and to address ethical, legal, and social issues that arose from the project.

With the exception of reproductive (germ) cells, each cell in the human body contains 22 pairs of autosomal chromosomes, two sex chromosomes (XX or XY), and the small chromosome found in each mitochondria within the cell. Collectively, this is known as a genome. The genome contains between 50,000 to 100,000 genes that are located on approximately three billion base pairs of DNA and forms the basic unit of genetics. Genetics play a significant role in the diagnosis, monitoring, and treatment of disease; thus, it is imperative that radiologic science professionals have a basic understanding of the role of genetics and genetic markers in the development and treatment of disease.

The genome project resulted in the identification of thousands of DNA sequence landmarks and the development of two types of gene maps (Fig. 1.7). Physical maps are used to determine the physical location of a particular gene on a specific chromosome. Genetic maps are used to assign the distance between the genetic markers, that is, mapping or linking DNA

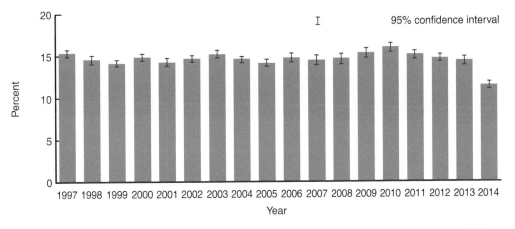

FIG. 1.6 Percentage of persons of all ages without health insurance coverage, United States, 1997 to 2014.

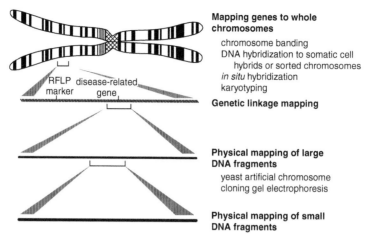

Mapping genes to whole chromosomes
    chromosome banding
    DNA hybridization to somatic cell
        hybrids or sorted chromosomes
    in situ hybridization
    karyotyping
Genetic linkage mapping

Physical mapping of large DNA fragments
    yeast artificial chromosome
    cloning gel electrophoresis

Physical mapping of small DNA fragments

©1992 by BSCS & The American Medical Association.

FIG. 1.7 Mapping genes to whole chromosomes at different levels of resolution.

fragments to a specific chromosome. Genetic linkage maps are useful in tracking inheritance of traits and diseases that are transmitted from parent to child because genetic markers that are in proximity increase the probability that the genes will be inherited together.

As more information was discovered through the Human Genome Project, researchers determined that the genome sequence was 99.9% identical for all humans, leaving only a small percentage of variation among people. However, this 0.1% variation greatly affects an individual's predisposition to certain diseases and his or her response to drugs and toxins. Researchers were able to identify common DNA pattern sequences and common patterns of genetic variations of single DNA bases, termed **single-nucleotide polymorphisms** (SNPs). This led to the development of haplotype mapping, often referred to as the *Hap Map*. A **haplotype** comprises closely linked SNPs on a single chromosome, and it is a very important resource in identifying specific DNA sequences affecting disease, response to pharmaceuticals, and response to environmental factors.

This continued research has led to improved diagnosis of disease, earlier detection of genetic predispositions to disease, gene therapy, newborn screening, customized pharmaceutical applications, DNA fingerprinting, and DNA forensics. This serves as the basis for the current emphasis on individualized medicine, as no two patients are the same. It also has resulted in the ability to predict the development of certain diseases, thus allowing earlier intervention. Additional information about the National Human Genome Institute can be found at www.genome.gov.

Altered Cellular Biology

To protect themselves and avoid injury, cells adapt by altering the genes responsible for their function and differentiation in response to their environment. When a cell is injured and unable to maintain homeostasis, it can respond in several ways. It may adapt and recover from the injury, or it may die as a result of the injury (Fig. 1.8). Many cells adapt by altering their pattern of growth, as demonstrated in Fig. 1.9. **Atrophy** is a generalized decrease in cell size. An example of atrophy is when muscle cells decrease in size after the loss of innervation (supply of nerves to a part) and use. **Hypertrophy** is a generalized increase in cell size. If the aortic valve is diseased, then the left ventricle enlarges because of the increased muscle mass needed to pump blood into the aorta. **Hyperplasia** is an increase in the number of cells in a tissue as a result of excessive proliferation. An estrogen-secreting ovarian tumor causing endometrial epithelial cells to multiply is an example of hyperplasia. **Metaplasia** is the conversion of one cell type into another that is not normal for that tissue (Table 1.2). The epithelial cells in the respiratory tract of a smoker undergo metaplasia as a response to the chronic irritation from the chemicals in the smoke.

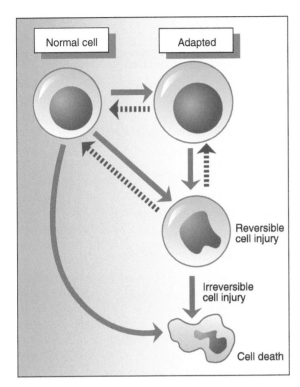

FIG. 1.8 Cellular injury and responses of normal adapted and reversibly injured cells and cell death.

Dysplasia refers to abnormal changes occurring in mature cells. Individual cells within a tissue vary in size, shape, and color, and they are often nonfunctional. Dysplastic adaptations are considered precancerous and are most commonly associated with neoplasms within the reproductive system and the respiratory tract.

Disease Classifications

Diseases are grouped into several broad categories. Those in the same category may not necessarily be closely related, but groupings such as those discussed in the following sections tend to produce lesions that are similar in morphology—that is, their form and structure. Pathologies discussed in this text are generally grouped into the following classifications:

- Congenital and hereditary
- Inflammatory
- Degenerative
- Metabolic
- Traumatic
- Neoplastic

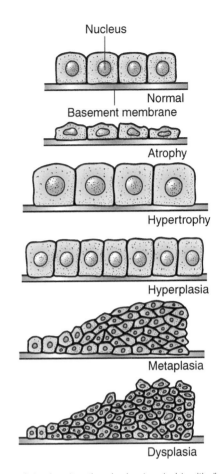

FIG. 1.9 Adaptive alterations in simple cuboid epithelial cells.

TABLE 1.2
Altered Cellular Biology

Cell State	Description
Anaplasia	Absence of tumor cell differentiation, loss of cellular organization
Dysplasia	Abnormal changes in mature cells; also termed *atypical hyperplasia*
Metaplasia	Abnormal transformation of a specific differentiated cell into a differentiated cell of another type

Congenital and Hereditary Disease

Diseases present at birth and resulting from genetic or environmental factors are termed **congenital**. It is estimated that 2% to 3% of all live births have one or more congenital abnormalities, although some of these may not be visible until a year or so after birth. A major category of congenital disease is caused by abnormalities in the number and distribution of chromosomes. In somatic cells chromosomes exist in the nucleus of each cell in pairs, with one member from the male parent and the other from the female parent. In humans, chromosomes are normally composed of 22 pairs of autosomes (those other than the sex chromosomes) and one pair of sex chromosomes. Down syndrome is a congenital condition caused by an error in autosomal mitosis that leads to an extra chromosome 21, so the affected individual has 47 chromosomes rather than the normal 46.

Hereditary diseases are caused by developmental disorders genetically transmitted from either parent to a child through abnormalities of individual genes in chromosomes and are derived from ancestors. For example, hemophilia is a well-known hereditary disease in which proper blood clotting is absent. A genetic abnormality present on the sex chromosome is a sex-linked inheritance; an abnormality on one of the other 22 chromosomes is an autosomal inheritance. The inherited disease may be *dominant* (transmitted by a single gene from either parent) or *recessive* (transmitted by both parents to an offspring). Amniocentesis, a standard procedure typically guided by sonography, is used prenatally to assess the presence of certain hereditary disorders.

A congenital defect is not necessarily hereditary because it may have been acquired in utero. Intrauterine injury during a critical point in development may have been caused by maternal infection, radiation, or drug use. Abnormalities of this type occur sporadically and cannot generally be recognized before birth. However, their likelihood is greatly lessened by following proper precautions against infection, avoiding radiation (particularly during the early term of pregnancy), and avoiding drugs or agents not specifically recognized by a physician as safe for use during pregnancy.

Inflammatory Disease

An **inflammatory** disease results from the body's reaction to a localized injurious agent. Types of inflammatory diseases include infective, toxic, and allergic diseases. An infective disease results from invasion by microorganisms such as viruses, bacteria, or fungi.

Viruses consist of a protein coat surrounding a genome of either ribonucleic acid (RNA) or DNA, without an organized cell structure. They are classified by the type of viral genome and are not capable of replicating outside of a living cell. Bacteria are unicellular organisms that lack an organized nucleus. They tend to colonize on environmental surfaces and are extremely adaptable, which allows them to become resistant to antibiotics over time. Fungi are microorganisms that can form complex structures containing organelles and may grow as mold or yeast. For instance, pneumonia is a type of inflammatory disease that may result from a viral, bacterial, or fungal infection. Toxic diseases are caused by poisoning of biologic substances, and allergic diseases are an overreaction of the body's own defenses.

Some diseases in this classification are considered autoimmune disorders. Under normal conditions, antibodies are formed in response to foreign antigens. In certain diseases, however, they form against and injure the patient's own tissues. These are known as **autoantibodies,** and diseases associated with them are termed **autoimmune disorders.** Rheumatoid arthritis is an example of an autoimmune disorder.

An inflammatory reaction (*i.e.,* inflammation) is a generalized pathologic process that is nonspecific to the agent causing the injury. The body's purpose in creating an inflammatory reaction is to localize the injurious agent and prepare for subsequent repair and healing of the injured tissues. Substances released from the damaged tissues may cause both local and systemic effects (Fig. 1.10). Those effects seen local to the injury include capillary dilatation to allow fluids and leukocytes, specifically, to infiltrate into the area of damage. Cellular necrosis (death) is common in acute inflammation, and the leukocytes serve to remove dead material through phagocytosis (the ingestion of other cells or particles). The characteristics of such acute inflammation include heat, redness of skin, swelling, pain, and some loss of function as the body tends to protect the injured part. If the inflammatory process is significant, systemic effects such as an elevation of body temperature become evident.

Chronic inflammation differs from the acute stage in that damage caused by an injurious agent may not necessarily result in tissue death. In fact, necrosis is relatively uncommon in cases of chronic inflammation. It differs also in the duration of the inflammation, with

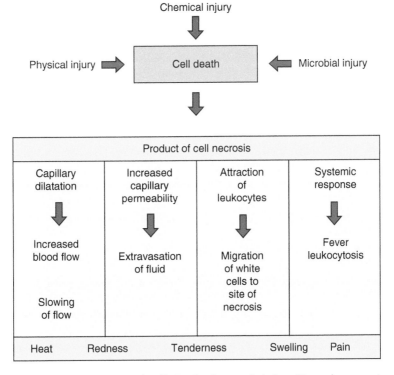

FIG. 1.10 Local and systemic effects of cell necrosis induced by various agents.

chronic conditions lasting for long periods, such as the presence of neuropathy resulting in an individual with chronic diabetes mellitus.

The repair of tissues damaged by an inflammatory process attempts to return the body to normal. Tissue regeneration is the process by which damaged tissues are replaced by new tissues that are essentially identical to those that have been lost. Although this is the most desirable type of repair, tissues vary in their ability to replace themselves. Damaged nerve cells, for example, are not likely to readily regenerate. Fibrous connective tissue repair is the alternative to regeneration, but it is less desirable because it leads to scarring and fibrosis. Damaged tissues are replaced by a scar and lack the structure and function of the original tissue.

Debridement (removal of dead cells and materials) is an essential component of the healing process. It may be accomplished both at the cellular level and through human intervention, as in the case of burns or removal of foreign objects such as pieces of glass. The repair process begins with the migration of adjacent cells into the injured area and replication of the cells via mitosis to fill the void in the tissue. This new growth includes capillaries, fibroblasts, collagen, and elastic fibers. Remodeling of the new tissue, the last phase in the healing process, occurs in response to normal use of the tissue. For instance, remodeling of the bone after a skeletal fracture may take months, but the results often return the injured bone to its original contour.

Infection refers to an inflammatory process caused by a disease-causing organism. Under favorable conditions, the invading pathogenic agent multiplies and causes injurious effects. Generally, localized infection is accompanied by inflammation, but inflammation may occur without infection. Virulence refers to the ease with which an organism can cause disease. An organism with high virulence is likely to produce progressive disease in susceptible persons; one with low virulence produces disease only in highly susceptible persons under favorable conditions. A variety of factors such as the presence of dead tissue or blockage of normal body passages may predispose an individual to bacterial infection.

Degenerative Disease

Degenerative diseases are caused by deterioration of the body. Although they are usually associated with the aging process, some degenerative conditions may exist in younger patients. For instance, an individual may develop a degenerative disease following a traumatic injury, regardless of age.

The process of aging results from the gradual maturation of physiologic processes that reach a peak and then gradually fade (i.e., degenerate) to a point at which the body can no longer survive. Heredity, diet, and environmental factors are known to affect the rate of aging. Over time, the functional abilities of tissues decrease because either their cell numbers are reduced or the function of each individual cell declines, with both typically participating in pathologies resulting from aging. Atherosclerosis, osteoporosis, and osteoarthritis are three diseases commonly associated with the aging process. Each is discussed later in this text.

Metabolic Disease

Metabolism is the sum of all physical and chemical processes in the body. Diseases caused by a disturbance of the normal physiologic function of the body are classified as metabolic diseases. These include endocrine disorders such as diabetes mellitus and hyperparathyroidism and disturbances of fluid and electrolyte balance.

Endocrine glands secrete their products (hormones) into the bloodstream to regulate various metabolic functions. The major endocrine glands include the pituitary, thyroid, parathyroid, adrenal glands, pancreatic islets, ovaries, and testes. An endocrine disorder may consist of hypersecretion, which causes an overactivity of the target organ, or hyposecretion, which results in underactivity. The clinical effects of an endocrine disturbance depend on the degree of dysfunction as well as the age and sex of the individual.

Dehydration is the most common disturbance of fluid balance. It is caused by insufficient intake of water or excessive loss of it. Electrolytes are mineral salts (most commonly sodium and potassium) that are dissolved in the body's water. They may be depleted because of vomiting, diarrhea, or use of *diuretics* (substances that promote the excretion of salt and water). Disturbance of either fluid balance or electrolyte balance upsets *homeostasis,* the body's normal internal resting state.

Traumatic Disease

Another general classification of diseases is **traumatic** diseases. These diseases may result from mechanical forces such as crushing or twisting of a body part or from the effects of ionizing radiation on the human body. In addition, disorders resulting from extreme hot or cold temperatures, for example, burns and frostbite, are also classified as traumatic.

Trauma may injure a bone, resulting in *fractures,* which are covered extensively in Chapter 12. It may also injure soft tissues. A *wound* is an injury of soft parts associated with rupture of the skin. Traumatic injuries may damage soft tissues even if the skin is not broken. Bleeding into the tissue spaces as a result of capillary rupture is known as a *bruise* or a *contusion.*

Neoplastic Disease

Neoplastic disease results in new, abnormal tissue growth. Normally, growing and maturing cells are subject to mechanisms that direct cell proliferation and cell differentiation, controlling their growth rate. *Proliferation* refers to cell division, and *differentiation* refers to the process of cellular specialization. When this control mechanism goes awry because of mutations within the chromosomes of the cell (genetic instability), an overgrowth of cells develops and results in a neoplasm. Cells are classified as either differentiated or undifferentiated, depending on the resemblance of the new cells to the original cells in the host organ or site. If the differences are small, the growth is termed *differentiated* and has a low probability for malignancy. If the cells within the neoplasm exhibit atypical characteristics, they are termed *poorly differentiated* or *undifferentiated* and have a higher probability of malignancy. Neoplastic cells are similar to normal cells in that they include both parenchymal and supporting tissues. In neoplastic disease, parenchymal cell proliferation and differentiation are altered, and because the parenchymal tissue is the functional tissue of the cell, it must receive adequate blood supply to survive. Classification of the neoplasm depends on the type of altered parenchymal cells, that is, tissue type of the tumor (Table 1.3).

Neoplasms originate from mutations within the genetic code (Box 1.1), which may silence the genes, *tumor-suppressor genes,* or cause them to become overactive, *oncogenes* (Fig. 1.11). This abnormal growth of cells leads to the formation of either a benign tumor or a malignant

TABLE 1.3
Tissue Types and Tumors*

Connective Tissue	Benign Tumors	Malignant Tumors
Adult fibrous tissue	Fibroma	Fibrosarcoma
Fat	Lipoma	Liposarcoma
Cartilage	Chondroma	Chondrosarcoma
Bone	Osteoma	Osteosarcoma
Connective tissue (fibrous)	Fibrous histiocytoma	Malignant fibrous histiocytoma
Endothelium & Mesothelium	**Benign Tumors**	**Malignant Tumors**
Blood vessels	Hemangioma, hemaniopericytoma	Hemangiosarcoma, angiosarcoma
Lymph vessels	Lymphangioma	Lymphagniosarcoma
Mesothelium		Mesothelioma
Hemopoietic cells	Preleukemias, myeloproliferative disorders	Leukemia (various types)
Lymphoid tissue	Plasmacytosis	Plasmacytoma, multiple myeloma, Hodgkin lymphoma, Non-Hodgkin lymphoma
Muscle	**Benign Tumors**	**Malignant Tumors**
Smooth muscle	Leiomyoma	Leiosarcoma
Striated muscle	Rhabdomyoma	Rhabdomyosarcoma
Epithelial Tissue	Benign Tumors	Malignant Tumors
Stratified squamous	Papilloma, seborrheic keratosis, some adnexal tumors	Squamous cell carcinoma, epidermoid carcinoma, some malignant adnexal tumors
Glandular epithelium	Adenoma, hepatic adenoma, renal tubular adenoma, bile duct adenoma	Adenocarcinoma, hepatoma, hepatocellular carcinoma, renal cell carcinoma, hypernephroma, cholangiocarcinoma
Transitional epithelium	Transitional cell papilloma	Transitional cell carcinoma
Placenta	Hydatidiform mole	Choriocarcinoma
Testis		Seminoma, embryonal cell carcinoma
Neural	**Benign Tumors**	**Malignant Tumors**
Glial cells		Glioma (grades I-III), glioblastoma multiform Nerve cells (grade IV)
Nerve cells	Ganglioneuroma	Neuroblastoma, medulloblastoma
Meninges	Meningioma	Malignant meningioma
Nerve sheath	Schwannoma, neurilemmoma, neurofibroma	Malignant meningioma, malignant schwannoma, neurofibrosarcoma

*This list is intended to provide only an introduction to tumor nomenclature.
Modified from SEER Training Modules, *Tumor List*. U. S. National Institutes of Health, National Cancer Institute. 23 March 2017 <https://training.seer.cancer.gov/disease/categories/tumors.html>.

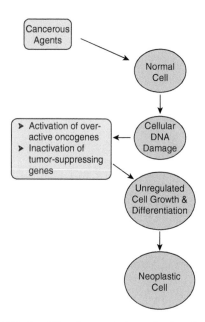

FIG. 1.11 Development of neoplastic cells.

tumor (a neoplasm). A **benign neoplasm** is composed of well-differentiated cells with uncontrolled growth. Thus a benign neoplasm remains localized and is generally noninvasive. A **malignant neoplasm** exhibits the loss of control of both cell proliferation and cell differentiation, which changes its functional capabilities. Malignant neoplasms grow at a faster rate compared with benign neoplasms and tend to spread and invade other tissues. Malignant neoplasms may be solid tumors confined to a specific organ or tissue, or they may be hematologic in nature, affecting the blood and lymph systems.

Sometimes, it is difficult to classify abnormal cells as either benign or malignant because they may exhibit characteristics of both types. Thus the abnormal growth is graded, depending on the composition of particular cells.

The spread of malignant cancer cells resulting in a secondary tumor distant from the primary lesion is termed *metastasis.* **Metastatic spread** may occur in a variety of ways. If the cancerous cells invade the circulatory system, they may be spread via blood vessels, and this process is termed **hematogenous spread.** The cells may spread via the lymphatic system, and this is termed **lymphatic spread.** The lymph node into which the primary neoplasm drains is termed the *sentinel node.* If the cancerous cells spread into surrounding tissue by virtue of proximity, it is termed **invasion.** However, if the cancerous cells travel to a distant site or organ system, it is termed **seeding.** Certain types of cancer occur more often as metastases rather than originating in a given organ.

Lesion is a term used to describe the many types of cellular change that may occur in response to disease. Some lesions may be visible immediately; others may be detectable initially only through diagnostic means such as laboratory testing. *Cancer* is a general term often used to denote various types of malignant neoplasms. Note that the terms *cancer* and *carcinoma* are not synonymous. A **carcinoma** is one type of cancer and is derived from epithelial tissue. Adenocarcinoma of the colon is an example of a type of carcinoma. Other cancers include **sarcoma,** which arises from connective tissue (*e.g,* fibrosarcoma); **leukemia,** which arises from blood cells; and **lymphoma,** which arises from lymphatic cells. Both benign and malignant tumors are also named according to the tissue type of origin (see Table 1.3). In the case of a benign neoplasm, the suffix "oma" is added to the word root, for instance, *adenoma.* Malignant neoplasms are named by adding the name of the tissue type to the word root, for instance, *adenocarcinoma.* Medical imaging plays a major role in the diagnosis and staging of a variety of neoplastic diseases. The primary diagnostic and staging methods include imaging procedures such as computed tomography (CT), magnetic resonance imaging (MRI), positron emission tomography (PET), single photon emission computed tomography (SPECT), radiography, and ultrasonography. Other diagnostic methods include endoscopic procedures, identification of tumor markers in blood, clinical laboratory tests of cells and tissues, and gene profiling. Treatment modalities often include radiation therapy in combination with surgery, chemotherapy, hormone or antihormone therapy, immunotherapy using biologic response modifiers such as interferons and interleukins, and targeted drug therapies. The choice of a modality or a combination of modalities depends on many factors, including the type of cancer, its location and stage, and the treating oncologist. The goal of treatment may be curative, allowing the patient to remain free of disease for 5 years or more, or palliative, which is designed to relieve pain when a cure is not possible and to improve the quality of life.

Staging and Grading Cancer

Decisions regarding the appropriate treatment of malignant tumors and in determining prognosis and end results are guided by classifications that stage and grade the disease. Although several clinical classifications of cancer exist, the TNM (tumor–node–metastasis) system emerged in the 1950s and is now considered a recognized standard and is endorsed by the American Joint Committee on Cancer (AJCC). The AJCC is cosponsored by several prominent health organizations, including the American Cancer Society and the American College of Radiology.

The TNM system is based on the premise that cancers of similar histology or origin are similar in their patterns of growth or extension. The "T" refers to the size of the untreated primary cancer or tumor. As the size increases, lymph node involvement (N) occurs, eventually leading to distant metastases (M). The addition of numbers to these three letters indicates the extent of malignancy and the progressive increase in size or involvement of the tumor. For example, T0 indicates that no evidence of a primary tumor exists, whereas T1, T2, T3, and T4 indicate an increasing size or extension. Lack of regional lymph node metastasis is indicated by N0, and N1, N2, and N3 indicate increasing involvement of regional lymph nodes. Finally, M0 indicates no distant metastasis, and M1 indicates the presence of distant metastasis.

Neoplastic cells are examined histologically, and these growths are graded according to their degree of differentiation based on a scale of I (well differentiated) to IV (poorly differentiated). The combination of tumor classification and grading serves as a shorthand notation for the description of the clinical extent of a given malignant tumor. It facilitates treatment planning, provides an indication of prognosis, assists in evaluating treatment results, facilitates information exchange among treatment centers, and allows unambiguous categorization of malignancies to aid in the continuing investigation of cancer.

Summary

Technologic advances in the field of radiology have, without a doubt, done much to relieve human suffering, but medical imaging alone cannot provide a definitive diagnosis. Medical imaging must be used in conjunction with other diagnostic and therapeutic modalities to provide the best treatment for each specific disease process. The following chapters provide the student radiographer with a better understanding of the disease processes of the various physiologic systems. This information should help students analyze and critique each radiograph to ensure that it provides optimal information to assist physicians in their diagnosis.

Review Questions

1. The prediction of the course and end of a disease and an outlook based on that prediction best define its:
   a. Diagnosis
   b. Etiology
   c. Prognosis
   d. Syndrome

2. A compression fracture of the lumbar spine that results from steroid treatments for pain reduction of arthritis would be an example of _____ disease.
   a. Degenerative
   b. Iatrogenic
   c. Idiopathic
   d. Traumatic

3. A disease such as Tay-Sachs syndrome that is transmitted genetically is termed:
   a. Congenital
   b. Hereditary
   c. Metabolic
   d. Neoplastic

4. Sickness sufficient to interfere with one's normal daily routine refers to its:
   a. Etiology
   b. Morbidity
   c. Mortality
   d. Pathogenesis

5. Which of the following would be considered a symptom of a disease process?
   a. Bloody stool
   b. Nausea
   c. Skin rash
   d. Swelling
6. A disease that manifests slowly and is present for a long period is said to be:
   a. Acute
   b. Asymptomatic
   c. Chronic
   d. Congenital
7. Which of the following disease classifications is usually associated with the normal aging process?
   a. Congenital
   b. Degenerative
   c. Inflammatory
   d. Metabolic
8. If 4000 cases of a given disease are found in a given population, the _____ of the disease is defined.
   a. Incidence
   b. Morphology
   c. Metabolism
   d. Prevalence
9. The relative ease with which an organism can overcome normal bodily defenses refers to its:
   a. Infection
   b. Necrosis
   c. Pestilence
   d. Virulence
10. A neoplastic growth is evaluated to determine its degree of histologic differentiation. This is termed:
    a. Grading
    b. Metastasis
    c. Morphology
    d. Staging
11. Generalized increase in cell size refers to:
    a. Hypertrophy
    b. Atrophy
    c. Metaplasia
    d. Hyperplasia
12. Which of the following terms refers to abnormal changes of mature cells?
    a. Hypertrophy
    b. Dysplasia
    c. Metaplasia
    d. Hyperplasia
13. Explain the concept of neoplastic disease. Are all neoplasms cancer?
14. What is the difference between mortality and morbidity rate? How is each important to the practice of medicine and to public health agencies?
15. Differentiate between an acute and chronic illness. Give two examples of each.

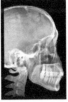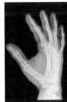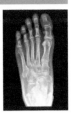

CHAPTER 2

Skeletal System

ⓔ http://evolve.elsevier.com/Kowalczyk/pathology/

Craniosynostosis
Craniotubular dysplasias
Developmental
    dysplasia of the hip
    (DDH)
Diaphysis
Diploë
Endochondroma
Epiphysis
Escherichia coli
Ewing sarcoma
Exostoses
Ganglion
Giant cell tumors
Gouty arthritis
Hyperostosis frontalis
    interna
Involucrum
Juvenile rheumatoid
    arthritis (JRA)

Medullary canal
Metaphysis
Osteoarthritis
Osteoblastoma
Osteoblasts
Osteochondroma
Osteoclastomas
Osteoclasts
Osteogenesis
    imperfecta (OI)
Osteoid osteoma
Osteoma
Osteomyelitis
Osteopetrosis
Osteophytes
Osteosarcoma
Polydactyly
Pott disease
Psoriatic arthritis

Reiter syndrome
Rheumatoid arthritis
    (RA)
Scoliosis
Sequestrum
Simple unicameral bone
    cyst
Spina bifida
Spondylolisthesis
Spondylolysis
Staphylococcus aureus
Syndactyly
Tendonitis
Tenosynovitis
Trabeculae
Trabecular pattern
Transitional vertebra
Tuberculosis
Whiplash

Anatomy and Physiology

The skeletal system is composed of 206 separate bones and is responsible for body support, protection, movement, and blood cell production. It contains more than 98% of the body's total calcium and up to 75% of its total phosphorus. The system is commonly divided into the axial skeleton, which contains 80 bones, and the appendicular skeleton (Fig. 2.1), which contains 126 bones. Bone is a type of connective tissue, but it differs from other connective tissue because of its matrix of calcium phosphate. The construction of this matrix further classifies bone tissue as either compact/cortical (dense) or cancellous (spongy) (Fig. 2.2).

The outer portion of bone is composed of **compact bone,** and the inner portion, termed the **medullary canal,** is made up of **cancellous bone.** Bone marrow is located within the medullary canal and is interspersed between the **trabeculae.** This intricate, web-like bony structure is visible on a properly exposed radiograph of the skeletal system and is often referred to as the **trabecular pattern.** The term **diploë** is specific to the cancellous bone located within the skull which separates the inner and outer layers of the compact bone. The red bone marrow is responsible for the production of bone erythrocytes and leukocytes. In a normal adult, red bone marrow is found primarily in the bones of the trunk. At the approximate age of 20 years, the majority of the red bone marrow is replaced by yellow bone marrow composed mainly of fat.

Osteoblasts are the bone-forming cells that line the medullary canal and are interspersed throughout the periosteum. They are responsible for bone growth and thickening, ossification, and regeneration. **Osteoclasts** are specialized cells that break down bone to enlarge the medullary canal and allow for bone growth. This production and breakdown of bone play an important role in serum calcium and phosphorus equilibrium. Certain metabolic disease processes may alter the percentage of calcium, resulting in either hypocalcemia or hypercalcemia.

The bones of the skeletal system may also be classified according to their shape to include long, short, flat, and irregular bones. The **diaphysis** of a long bone refers to the shaft portion and is the primary site

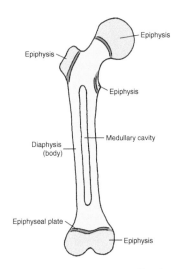

FIG. 2.3 Endochondral ossification.

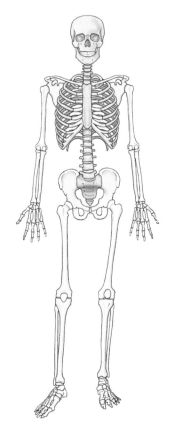

FIG. 2.1 Axial skeleton and appendicular skeleton.

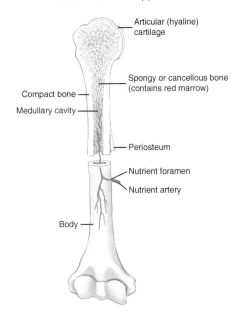

Articular (hyaline) cartilage

Spongy or cancellous bone (contains red marrow)

Compact bone

Medullary cavity

Periosteum

Nutrient foramen

Nutrient artery

Body

FIG. 2.2 Bone composition.

of ossification, whereas the **epiphysis** refers to the expanded end portion and is the secondary site of ossification (Fig. 2.3). The **metaphysis** refers to the growth zone between the epiphysis and the diaphysis. It is the area of greatest metabolic activity in a bone. A cartilaginous growth plate is located between the metaphysis and the epiphysis in the bone of a growing child. Radiographically, these growth areas appear radiolucent. As the body matures, this cartilage calcifies and is no longer radiographically visible in the adult.

The periosteum is a fibrous membrane that encloses all of the bone except the joint surfaces and is crucial to supplying blood to the underlying bone. Osteoblasts located within the periosteum increase bone thickness relative to individual activities. The more physical stress a bone is under, the more thickly the compact portion develops; therefore, it is common medical practice to allow patients with healing fractures of the hip or femur to bear weight on the injured bone, which helps shorten the healing period. Disuse atrophy occurs when a bone is not allowed to bear weight and results in significant decalcification and thinning of the bone (Fig. 2.4).

The 206 bones of the body are connected to one another by one of three types of joints: (1) *Fibrous (synarthrodial) joints* form firm, immovable joints such as the sutures of the skull; (2) *cartilaginous (amphiarthrodial) joints* such as those found between the vertebral bodies are

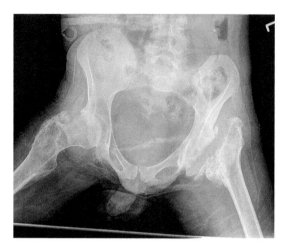

FIG. 2.4 Radiography demonstrating muscle atrophy and bone thinning as a result of a lack of weight-bearing activity.

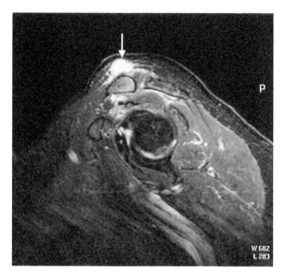

FIG. 2.5 Magnetic resonance imaging scan (short-τ inversion recovery sequences) showing a subcutaneous cyst on the scapula.

slightly movable; (3) *synovial (diarthrodial) joints* such as the knee are freely movable. The ends of the bones composing a synovial joint are lined with articular cartilage and are held together by ligaments. The joint capsules are lined by a synovial membrane responsible for the secretion of synovia, a lubricating fluid containing mucin, albumin, fat, and mineral salts. The joint capsule also contains a rich nerve supply making them sensitive to stretching.

Imaging Considerations

Radiography

In examining a skeletal radiograph, it is important to begin by properly orienting the image receptor and recognizing the radiographic projection. The radiographic exposure technique selected is very important in achieving a proper diagnosis. Proper technique is achieved when the soft tissues and bony structures of interest are both adequately penetrated and the trabecular pattern is visible. Any motion of the part in question impairs the visibility of the detail present.

Soft tissue areas often hold clues to the diagnosis and are examined by the interpreting physician. Any signs of muscle atrophy, soft tissue swelling, calcifications, opaque foreign bodies, or the presence of gas may indicate disease. Analysis of the configuration of the bone and its relationship to other bones serves to detect or exclude fractures, dislocations, congenital anomalies, or acquired deformities.

The interface between cortical (compact) bone and soft tissue is also important. Any periosteal new bone formation seen may be a response to trauma, tumors, or infection. Juxtaarticular erosions are often seen in cases of arthritis. Cortical resorption may be demonstrated as smudgy, irregular loss of the cortical margin. In addition, the internal bone structure is important and should be examined for abnormally altered texture, alterations in the amount of mineralization, or foci of destruction. Careful consideration of all areas mentioned assists the physician in arriving at the correct diagnosis.

Magnetic Resonance Imaging

Magnetic resonance imaging (MRI) is an important modality used in imaging of skeletal pathology, particularly in providing soft tissue detail because of its superior contrast resolution. It is considered the modality of choice for detection and staging of soft tissue tumors involving the extremities. It is also extremely useful in evaluation of joints, particularly the knee and the shoulder (Fig. 2.5). Newer imaging techniques and improved equipment allow MRI to detect a greater number of musculoskeletal subtleties with higher-resolution imaging (Fig. 2.6). Sometimes these subtleties mimic bone pain but involve soft tissues instead, which is an important distinction. Bone marrow imaging done with MRI is superior to other modalities in visualizing subtle

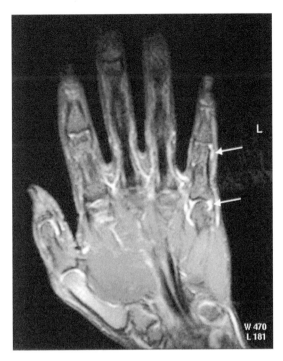

FIG. 2.6 Magnetic resonance imaging scan (short-τ inversion recovery sequences) showing synovitis of the metacarpophalangeal and interphalangeal joints.

abnormalities within the musculoskeletal system. Also, MRI may play a larger role in trauma medicine, particularly with the refinement of open-bore and short-bore technologies.

Computed Tomography

Computed tomography (CT) is an important tool in skeletal imaging because with newer technology the examination can be performed quickly and noninvasively, even in cases of trauma. CT has the ability to define the presence and extent of fractures or dislocations, to assess abnormalities in joints and associated soft tissues, and to help diagnose spinal disorders (Fig. 2.7). Cortical bone gives no signal in MRI, but CT provides ready visualization of bone details and is often used as a follow-up to conventional radiographic imaging for improved detail. Bone tumors, in particular, are now usually imaged with spiral or helical CT because of its excellent ability to display bone margins and trabecular patterns and to assess both bone and soft tissue involvement of tumors. Although CT results in greater contrast resolution compared with radiography, much

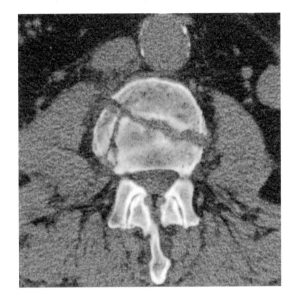

FIG. 2.7 Computed tomography scan demonstrating a burst fracture of the third lumbar vertebra.

of the role for imaging other related soft tissues has been usurped by MRI. Quantitative computed tomography (QCT) is also used in evaluating bone mass loss, especially within the vertebral bodies of the spine. In fact, research has demonstrated QCT to have a greater diagnostic sensitivity than dual x-ray absorptiometry (DXA).

Nuclear Medicine Procedures

Nuclear medicine retains an advantage not offered by either MRI or CT in skeletal imaging: the ability to look at the entire body at one time in a convenient fashion (Fig. 2.8). It provides decision making as to whether any pathology shown is an old injury or a new problem, with activity indicating that the bone involved is affected by some new process. In addition, the bone scan is still the standard of care for examination of metastatic processes because it demonstrates metabolic reaction of the bone to the disease process and is more sensitive than comparative radiographic studies. This is also true in many other traumatic or inflammatory diseases of the skeletal system. However, the utilization of positron emission tomography (PET) scanning in skeletal pathologies has started to increase, particularly the use of 18F-NaF (2-deoxy-2-[18F] fluoro-D-glucose). Although primarily used in diagnosing and staging of metastatic disease, it may be appropriate in certain individuals with back

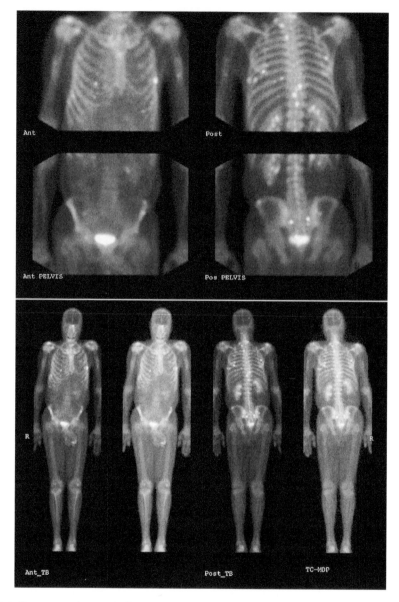

FIG. 2.8 Bone scan demonstrating metastatic disease throughout the ribs, thoracic vertebrae, and pelvis resulting from carcinoid disease.

pain, to confirm child abuse (especially rib fractures) following abnormal radiographs, and for the diagnosis of osteomyelitis, trauma, inflammatory and degenerative arthritis, avascular necrosis, osteonecrosis of the mandible, condylar hyperplasia, metabolic bone disease, Paget disease, bone graft viability, complications of the prosthetic joints, and reflex sympathetic dystrophy.

Congenital and Hereditary Diseases

Osteogenesis Imperfecta

Osteogenesis imperfecta (OI), sometimes referred to as *brittle bone disease,* is a serious and rather rare heritable or congenital disease affecting the skeletal system.

OI is most commonly an autosomal dominant defect. The eight recognized types are classified as type I to type VIII, with type I being the mildest and type VIII the most severe. Prenatal testing of cultured skin fibroblasts (CSF) helps diagnose types II, III, and IV. It is caused by mutations in the two structural genes that encode the α_1- and α_2-peptides of type I collagen, the main collagen of bone, tendon, and skin. The specific mutations occur in the *COL1A1, COL1A2, CRTAP,* and *LEPRE1* genes. Thus deficient and imperfect formation of osseous tissue, skin, sclera, inner ear, and teeth is noted in individuals with this disease. The two main clinical groups of OI are based on the age of onset and the severity of the disease. (1) *Osteogenesis imperfecta congenita* is present at birth. Infants with this disease usually have multiple fractures at birth that heal only to give way to new fractures. This results in limb deformities and dwarfism and may lead to death. (2) In *osteogenesis imperfecta tarda*, fractures might not appear for some years after birth and then generally stop once adulthood is reached (Fig. 2.9). In some cases, however, a hearing disorder persists because of otosclerosis, which is the formation of abnormal connective tissue around the auditory ossicles. Radiographic evaluation will demonstrate multiple fractures in various stages of healing and a general decrease in bone mass. The bone cortex is thin and porous, and the trabeculae are thin, delicate, and widely separated.

Achondroplasia

The most common inherited disorder affecting the skeletal system is **achondroplasia,** which results in bone deformity and dwarfism. It occurs in 1 in 15,000 to 40,000 newborns. It is caused by an autosomal dominant gene (*FGFR3*) at the 4p chromosome location, and this gene does not skip generations. Individuals with this gene have about a 50% chance of transmitting it to their children. Because of a disturbance in endochondral bone formation, the cartilage located in the epiphyses of the long bones does not convert to bone in the normal manner, impairing the longitudinal growth of the bones. Thus patients with this type of osteochondrodysplasia have a normal trunk size and shortened extremities (Fig. 2.10, A). In some instances, ultrasonography may be used for prenatal diagnosis of achondroplasia. An adult with achondroplasia is usually no more than 4 feet in height, with lower extremities usually less than half the normal length. Additional clinical

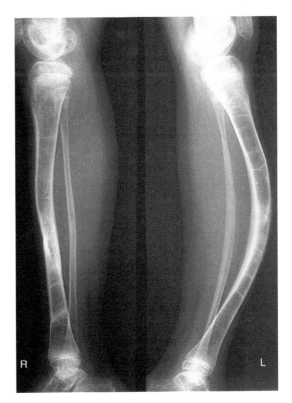

FIG. 2.9 Tibia–fibula radiograph demonstrating bowed lower extremities resulting from osteogenesis imperfecta tarda. This condition was recognized shortly after the child began to walk.

manifestations of this disorder include extreme lumbar spine lordosis, spinal stenosis, bowed legs (genu varum), a bulky forehead with midface hypoplasia (see Fig. 2.10, B), and a narrowing of the foramen magnum within the skull, which causes neural compression. Occasionally, orthopedic surgery may be necessary in the management of complications associated with achondroplasia. The Ilizarov procedure has also been used in an attempt to lengthen the shortened limbs. This procedure was perfected by Dr. Gavriil Ilizarov and has been used for over 30 years. It consists of a corticotomy of the limb, followed by attachment of an Ilizarov fixator, which consists of two circular frames that surround the limb, wires, and rods. By using this method, bones may be made to grow at a rate of approximately 1 mm per day. Most recently, clinical trials have involved growth hormone (GH) injections in the treatment of children with achondroplasia, beginning at an early age, generally between the ages of 1 to 6 years. Conclusive results

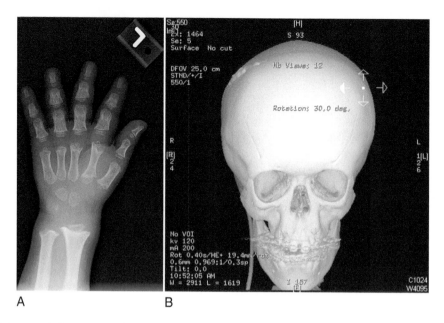

A   B

FIG. 2.10 A, Bone age radiograph of a 3-year-old demonstrating an abnormal flared appearance of the metaphyses and shortened, broad phalanges consistent with achondroplasia. B, Three-dimensional reconstruction of computed tomography scan demonstrating midface hypoplasia typical of achondroplasia.

cannot be determined until the children in the current study reach their adult heights. Early research indicates that introduction of GH may have an adverse effect on the cardiovascular system. In addition, these patients may receive genetic and social counseling.

Bone age radiographic studies, left hand to include distal radius, may be used to monitor patients with GH deficiency. These images are analyzed to compare the chronologic age with the radiographic bone age by using one of two methods: (1) the atlas matching method, which was established by Greulich and Pyle (GP) in the 1950s; or (2) the point scoring system of Tanner and Whitehouse, which was developed in the 1960s. A new digital atlas was developed by Vicente Gilsanz and Osman Ratibin in 2005. The images of the new GR atlas are much more precise and have a better quality than those of the older GP atlas.

Osteopetrosis

Osteopetrosis and *marble bone* are terms used to characterize a variety of disorders involving an increase in bone density and defective bone contour, often referred to as *skeletal modeling*. These pathologies involve mutations at the *CLCN7* gene. The spectrum of osteopetrosis includes (1) infantile malignant *CLCN7*-related autosomal recessive osteopetrosis (ARO), which has its onset in infancy; (2) intermediate autosomal osteopetrosis (IAO), which develops in childhood; and (3) autosomal dominant osteopetrosis type II (ADOII), which occurs in late childhood or adolescence. In osteopetrosis, bones are abnormally heavy and compact but nevertheless brittle. The disorders characterizing osteopetrosis include osteosclerosis, craniotubular (affecting the cranium and tubular long bones) dysplasias, and craniotubular hyperostosis. It is important for the technologist to be aware that both the osteosclerotic and craniotubular hyperostotic disorders require an increase in exposure factors to adequately penetrate the bony anatomy because of abnormal bone density (Fig. 2.11). In some cases, adequate radiographic density may never be achieved. All bones are affected, but the most significant changes occur in the long bones of the extremities, vertebrae, pelvis, and base of the skull. Radiographs demonstrate an increase in the density and thickness of the cortex and an increase in the number and size of trabeculae, with a marked reduction of the marrow space.

Albers-Schönberg disease is a fairly common form of osteosclerotic osteopetrosis. This autosomal dominant, delayed, benign skeletal anomaly involves increased bone density in conjunction with fairly normal bone contour. In fact, many patients with Albers-Schönberg disease are asymptomatic, and it is often discovered after radiographing the patient for an unrelated problem. Although this is a hereditary disorder, the bone sclerosis is not radiographically visible at birth.

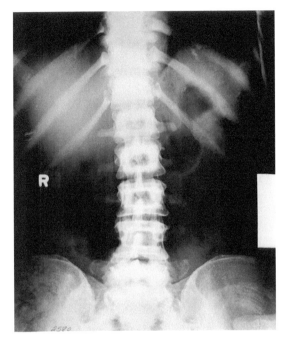

FIG. 2.11 Anteroposterior lumbar spine radiograph demonstrating uniform sclerosis of the bone associated with osteopetrosis.

As the individual ages, radiographic manifestations of the osteopetrosis become visible, especially in the region of the cranium and spine; however, the general health of the individual is unimpaired.

Craniotubular dysplasias are a group of rare autosomal recessive or dominant hereditary diseases, which mainly result in abnormal or defective bone contour of the cranium and long bones. They are generally caused by a defect in the osteoclast. Radiographs are useful in demonstrating this alteration in contour, scleroses, and changes within the cortical bone. Craniotubular hyperostosis includes a variety of fairly rare hereditary diseases, causing both an increase in bone density and abnormal bone modeling. Both of these craniotubular anomalies manifest in childhood. Although these disorders do not normally impair the individual's general health, bony overgrowth may entrap cranial nerves, resulting in some dysfunction such as facial palsy or deafness.

Hand and Foot Malformations

A variety of abnormalities of the fingers and toes may occur during fetal development but can be surgically corrected at birth. Failure of the fingers or toes to separate is called **syndactyly** and causes the physical appearance of webbed digits (Fig. 2.12). It is also associated with Apert syndrome, which is a genetic syndrome involving mutations of the *FGFR2* gene. Apert syndrome is also responsible for craniosynostosis. **Polydactyly** (Fig. 2.13) refers to the presence of extra digits, and treatment includes surgical intervention and therapy.

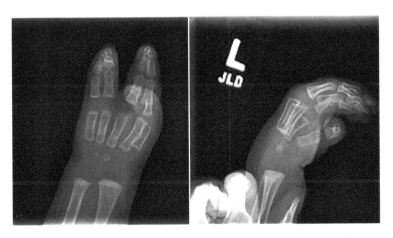

FIG. 2.12 Hand radiograph of an infant demonstrating acrosyndactyly.

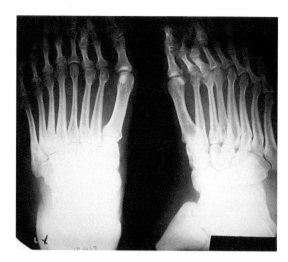

FIG. 2.13 Foot radiograph demonstrating additional digits associated with familial polydactyly.

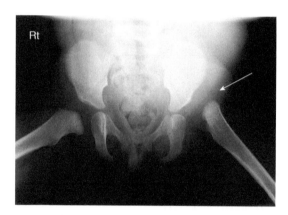

FIG. 2.14 Frog leg lateral projection of the pelvis of an infant demonstrating congenital dislocation of the left hip.

Clubfoot (talipes) is a congenital malformation of the foot that prevents normal weight bearing. The foot is most commonly turned inward at the ankle. This congenital malformation is more common in males than in females and may occur bilaterally. It is generally corrected by casting or splinting the foot in the correct anatomic position.

Developmental Dysplasia of the Hip

A malformation of the acetabulum often results in developmental dysplasia of the hip (DDH). Because the acetabulum does not form completely, the head of the femur is displaced superiorly and posteriorly (Fig. 2.14). Often, the ligaments and tendons responsible for proper placement of the femoral head are also affected. DDH may be unilateral or bilateral and occurs more frequently in females than in males. Other risk factors include a breech position in utero, being the first child, or low levels of amniotic fluid. DDH affects approximately 1 in 1000 births and may be associated with cerebral palsy, myelomeningocele, arthrogryposis, and Larsen syndrome. Larsen syndrome is a mutation of the *FLNB* gene affecting the production of filament B protein. Sonography may be used to diagnose this anomaly early in life through visualization of the cartilaginous structures of the hip. Conventional radiographs of the hip are often difficult to interpret in the neonate. Radiographic measurements of the anteroposterior (AP) pelvis are obtained and compared with standardized lines. This anomaly should be treated early with immobilization through casting or splinting the affected hip to allow the acetabulum to grow and form a normal joint. If left untreated, this anomaly may result in uneven limb length, hip muscle weakness, and an uneven gait.

Vertebral Anomalies

Scoliosis refers to an abnormal lateral curvature of the spine (Fig. 2.15). Structural scoliosis is associated with vertebral rotation. The lateral curves are usually convex to the right in the thoracic region and to the left in the lumbar region of the spine. Up to 80% of all structural scoliosis cases are idiopathic, although factors such as connective tissue disease and diet have been implicated. Scoliosis does not generally become visually apparent until adolescence. It tends to affect females more frequently than males and may cause numerous complications, including cardiopulmonary complications, degenerative spinal arthritis, and fatigue and joint dysfunction syndromes. Nonstructural scoliosis, in which the primary issue is not vertebral rotation, usually results from unequal leg lengths or compensatory postural changes affected by chronic pain elsewhere in the body.

Radiography is important in the diagnosis and treatment of scoliosis. Initial evaluation requires initial AP or posteroanterior (PA) and lateral standing radiographs and follow-up radiographs on a fairly routine basis. Radiologists use one of several methods to measure the spine's curvature, so consistent quality from one examination to another is important. Effective radiation protection techniques are vital because of the large size of

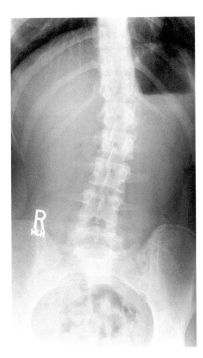

FIG. 2.15 Anteroposterior lumbar spine radiograph demonstrating congenital scoliosis.

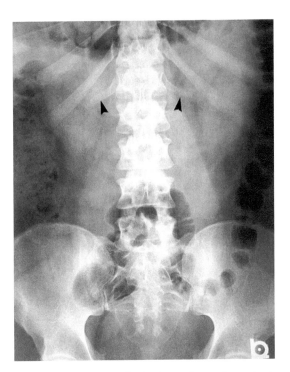

FIG. 2.16 Anteroposterior lumbar spine radiograph demonstrating bilateral lumbar ribs.

the exposure field, the young age of the patient, and the frequency of the examinations. Special attention is necessary in shielding the breasts of young female patients during radiographic examination throughout the treatment process. The PA projection should be obtained whenever possible because it significantly reduces the radiation dose to the breast area. Scoliosis may be corrected by placing the individual in a brace or body cast in patients with curves of 25 to 35 degrees. Surgical treatment with spinal fusion is prescribed for curves greater than 40 degrees.

A **transitional vertebra** is one that takes on the characteristics of both vertebrae on each side of a major division of the spine. Most frequently, such vertebrae occur at the junction between the thoracic and lumbar spine or at the junction between the lumbar spine and the sacrum. The first lumbar vertebra and the seventh cervical vertebra may have rudimentary ribs articulating with the transverse processes (Fig. 2.16). A cervical rib most commonly occurs at C7 and may exert pressure on the brachial nerve plexus or the subclavian artery, requiring surgical removal of the rib.

Spina bifida is an incomplete closure of the vertebral canal that is particularly common in the lumbosacral area (Fig. 2.17). Often, such patients have no visible abnormality or neurologic deficit, but failure of fusion of the two laminae is visible radiographically (spina bifida occulta). In more severe cases, the spinal cord or nerve root may be involved, which results in varying degrees of paralysis. Treatment of spina bifida is determined on the basis of the extent of the anomaly and requires the services of a variety of physicians.

Cranial Anomalies

The premature or early closure of any of the cranial sutures is called **craniosynostosis.** This congenital anomaly causes an overgrowth of the unfused sutures to accommodate brain growth, which alters the shape of the head (Fig. 2.18). It is often associated with Apert syndrome, a genetic disorder that is caused by a mutation of the *FGFR2* gene on chromosome 10. Although this defect may be corrected with surgery, brain damage may occur.

Anencephaly is a congenital abnormality in which the brain and cranial vault do not form (Fig. 2.19). In most cases, only the facial bones are formed. This abnormality

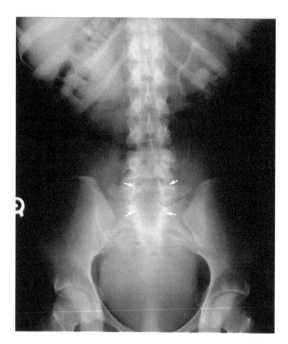

FIG. 2.17 Abdominal radiograph of a patient with spina bifida occulta of the lower lumbar vertebrae.

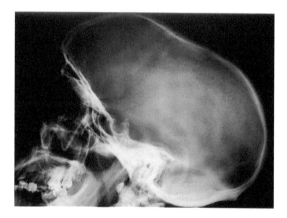

FIG. 2.18 Lateral skull radiograph demonstrating premature closure of the sagittal suture. This results in dolichocephaly and prominent convolutional markings caused by the increased intracranial pressure.

results in death shortly after birth and may be diagnosed before birth by ultrasonography. Anencephaly is a neural tube defect and its cause is unknown. It is suspected that anencephaly may be caused by a combination of multiple genetic (*MTHFR* gene) and environmental factors such as deficiency of folate, diabetes mellitus, exposure to high heat in early pregnancy, or use of certain antiseizure medications during pregnancy.

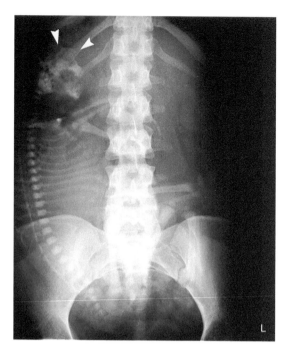

FIG. 2.19 Abdominal radiograph of a pregnant woman carrying a fetus with anencephaly. Note the absence of the cerebral cranial bones.

Inflammatory Diseases

Osteomyelitis

Osteomyelitis is an infection of the bone and bone marrow caused by a pathogenic microorganism spread via the bloodstream (hematogenous), from an infection within a contiguous site, or through direct introduction of the microorganism (Fig. 2.20). Signs and symptoms may include dull pain, heat in the affected area, and an intermittent low-grade fever. Generally, hematogenous osteomyelitis develops at the ends of the long bones. The distal femur, proximal tibia, humerus, and radius are most commonly affected in children and the vertebrae in adults. Infants and children are more commonly affected by acute hematogenous osteomyelitis because of increased vascularity and the rapid growth of their long bones. In addition, children often have a lowered resistance to the pathogenic organism, most commonly *Staphylococcus aureus.* Infection may be spread to the marrow space via the nutrient artery from an infection of the skin, ear, or pharynx. In infants, hematogenous osteomyelitis may also be caused by group B streptococci and *Escherichia coli.* In adults, hematogenous osteomyelitis is commonly

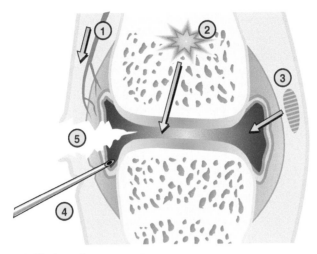

1. The hematogenous route
2. Dissemination from osteomyelitis
3. Spread from adjacent soft tissue infection
4. Diagnostic or therapeutic procedures
5. Penetration damage by puncturing or cutting

FIG. 2.20 Routes of infection to the joint.

secondary to bacteremia caused by genitourinary tract, soft tissue, or respiratory infections. As in children, *S. aureus* and streptococci are the pathogenic microorganisms primarily responsible for the infections.

Osteomyelitis resulting from contiguous infections is often associated with burns, sinus disease, periodontal infection, soft tissue infection, or skin ulcers resulting from peripheral vascular disease. Pathogenic microorganisms may also be directly introduced to bones by penetrating wounds, open fractures, fractures treated with internal fixation devices, or prosthetic replacements.

No specific bone changes may be demonstrated radiographically in the very early stage of infection. But the infection spreads rapidly, with the acute stage of osteomyelitis characterized by the formation of an abscess, leading to an inflammatory reaction within the bone that causes a rise in internal bone pressure. Osteomyelitis may be diagnosed with evidence of an elevated erythrocyte sedimentation rate (ESR) or cross-reactive protein (CRP) level; however, normal laboratory values should not exclude this diagnosis. Because of the constriction of the periosteum, blood vessels compress and thrombose, leading to bone necrosis within 24 to 48 hours. Unfortunately, not until about 10 to 14 days later is new periosteal bone repair radiographically evident

to indicate the presence of the disease. Therefore it is imperative that the condition be recognized clinically and treated with antibiotics and local drainage.

Initially, radiography may demonstrate soft tissue swelling in the area around the affected bone. MRI demonstrates water-like signal characteristics. Follow-up radiography may be performed 10 to 14 days after medical treatment to aid in the diagnosis.

With the effective use of antibiotics, osteomyelitis seldom passes the acute stage. When it does, treatment with antibiotics in combination with surgical drainage of pus from under the periosteum often results in a complete cure of the bone lesion in a majority of cases. Chronic osteomyelitis, however, is characterized by extensive bone destruction with irregular, sclerotic reactions throughout the bone (Fig. 2.21). A sequestrum is dead, devascularized bone that appears very dense. An involucrum is a shell of new supporting bone laid down by the periosteum around the sequestrum. An accurate diagnosis is extremely important to distinguish osteomyelitis from a neoplastic bone disease.

Radiography is not a very sensitive means of diagnosing the condition because a 30% to 50% loss of bone calcium is required before the destructive changes of osteomyelitis are radiographically visible. Nuclear medicine bone

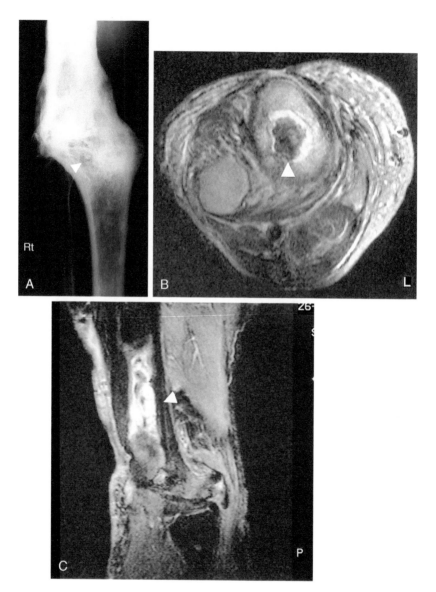

FIG. 2.21 A, Chronic osteomyelitis demonstrated in a knee with prior fusion. An involucrum surrounded by fluid densities is seen in the middle of a large intramedullary cavity approximately 3 cm above the fusion site. B, The involucrum demonstrated on a sagittal magnetic resonance imaging (MRI) scan from the same patient. C, The sequestrum demonstrated on an axial MRI image from the same patient, appearing as very dense bone as a result of devascularization.

scan studies and MRI are much more sensitive in detecting acute osteomyelitis; however, nuclear medicine bone scans are not as useful for secondary osteomyelitis.

Tuberculosis

Tuberculosis of the bone is a chronic inflammatory disease caused by *Mycobacterium tuberculosis*. It is usually more advanced and often left untreated for a longer period compared with pulmonary tuberculosis. It most commonly affects the hip, knee, and spine. Radiographically, the ends of the long bones display a "worm-eaten" appearance, with the disease slowly destroying the epiphyses, spreading to the articular cartilage, and, in some cases, infecting the joint space (Fig. 2.22).

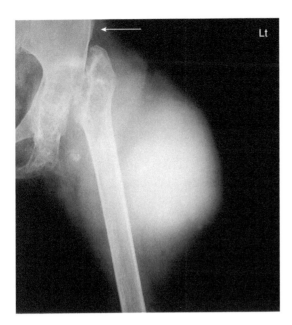

FIG. 2.22 Hip radiograph of a 47-year-old man with extensive destruction of the femoral head and neck caused by tuberculosis of the hip with a cold abscess.

Tuberculosis of the spine is also called **Pott disease.** Recognized in ancient times, it has been described in Egyptian mummies dating back to 3000 BC. It destroys the spine, causing softening and eventual collapse of the vertebrae, which results in paravertebral abscess formation and exerts abnormal pressure on the spinal cord.

Arthropathies

Arthropathy, a collective term used to denote disorders of the joints, includes, but is not limited to, arthritis, bursitis, tendonitis, and tenosynovitis. Joint inflammation is known as **arthritis** and may be caused by a variety of etiologic factors. For many years, osteoarthritis was believed to be a noninflammatory type of arthritis; however, current research has indicated that all types of arthritis involve inflammation of joints. An accurate clinical history is of extreme importance because different types of arthritis are characterized by specific features. For example, it is important to identify the number of joints involved, the location of the joints involved, and the presence of any other disease process. Some types of arthritis involve several joints, but others involve only one joint. In addition, certain types of arthritis have a preference for specific joints while sparing others. Finally, some types of arthritis are associated with specific disease processes caused by a host of factors such as bacteria or autoimmune response.

Arthritis may be further classified as *acute* and *chronic*; the most common forms are chronic and disabling.

Infectious Arthritis

Infectious arthritis, or septic arthritis, is caused by a variety of factors including *S. aureus,* streptococci, and *Neisseria gonorrheae.* The infectious agents may enter the joint through a break in skin, via extension from an adjacent infection such as osteomyelitis or an infected wound, or as a result of bacteremia. Common clinical symptoms of an acute bacterial infectious arthritis are rapid onset of pain, redness and swelling of the affected joint, which is often accompanied by fever. Diagnosis is generally made by analysis of blood and synovial fluid from the infected area. Some of the laboratory tests that may be requested include a culture, gram stain, ESR (or sed rate), or CRP following aspiration of the joint. Infectious arthritis usually responds rapidly to antibiotic therapy. Early radiographic changes demonstrate soft tissue swelling and joint effusions, with joint space narrowing that is visible only approximately 2 weeks after the infection. Radiographs obtained during the healing stage demonstrate recalcification and sclerosis, which often result in joint ankylosis.

Psoriatic arthritis is an inflammatory arthritis associated with psoriasis of the skin and involves a rheumatoid-like destructive process that predominantly affects the distal interphalangeal (DIP) joints of the hands and feet. It may cause asymmetric destruction of digits. Radiographic findings characteristic of psoriatic arthritis include bony ankylosis of the interphalangeal (IP) joints of the hands and feet and resorption of the terminal tufts of the distal phalanges. A distinctive radiographic difference between psoriatic arthritis and **rheumatoid arthritis (RA)** is that in psoriatic arthritis bone density is usually preserved.

Rheumatoid Arthritis

Rheumatoid arthritis (RA) is a chronic autoimmune disease that may fluctuate in severity. It is triggered by exposure of an immunogenetically susceptible host to an arthritogenic antigen and is characterized by chronic inflammation and overgrowth of the synovial tissues, most often in the extremities. RA develops slowly, and as synovial tissues proliferate, they progressively destroy cartilage, bone, and supporting structures. Genetic factors are also believed to predispose an individual to RA. An analysis of blood chemistry identifies the presence of an autoantibody against γ-globulin, also known as the *serologic rheumatoid factor* (RF). It usually occurs between the ages of 30 and 40

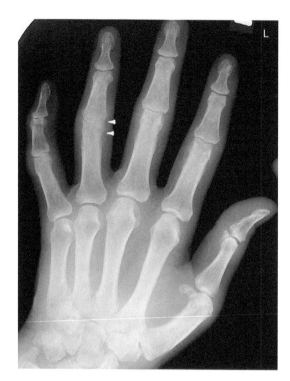

FIG. 2.23 Hand radiograph demonstrating soft tissue joint swelling associated with early rheumatoid arthritis.

(Fig. 2.25). New advancements in disease-modifying antirheumatic drugs (DMARD) such as methotrexate and the availability of new biologic agents have enhanced the success of the management of RA. Diagnosis of RA in adults was originally based on the 1987 revised classification criteria of the American College of Radiology (ACR); however, in 2010, a new set of criteria was developed by the ACR and EULAR (European Leagues Against Rheumatism). These new criteria present a specific approach for identifying patients earlier in the disease process so that intervening treatment may begin sooner. The 2010 criteria indicating the presence of RA are as follows:

- Confirmed presence of synovitis in at least one joint
- Absence of an alternative diagnosis that better explains the synovitis
- Achievement of a total score of 6 or greater (of a possible 10) from the individual scores in the following four domains:
- Number and site of involved joints (score range 0–5)
- Serologic abnormality (score range 0–3)
- Elevated acute-phase response (score 0–1)
- Symptom duration (2 levels, range 0–1)

Juvenile rheumatoid arthritis (JRA), also known as Still disease, affects children under age 16 years and is similar to the adult form of RA. However, differences in the pattern of involvement and prognosis do exist. Generally, fibrosis and proliferation are less than in the adult form. It is estimated that JRA affects nearly 100,000 children in the United States. Symptoms include pain, swelling, and stiffness of the affected joint with periods of activity or exacerbations and remissions of the disease process. The majority of children have long periods of remission without significant joint damage. The prognosis is generally good, with fewer than 20% having progressive destructive disease.

The ACR criterion for the diagnosis of JRA differs from that of adult RA. JRA is indicated if (1) the child is younger than 16 years at the onset of the disease, (2) symptoms of arthritis (swelling or effusion) are present in one or more joints for at least 6 weeks, and (3) the onset can be assigned to one of three JRA onset types: (a) pauciarticular, (b) polyarticular, and (c) systemic. Pauciarticular JRA is the most common form and it is more common in females than in males. It affects four or fewer joints, most commonly the knee, ankle, and elbow joints. Polyarticular RA affects five or more joints, generally those in the hands, feet, and weight-bearing joints. Systemic JRA is the least common form of RA in children and it can affect many areas of the body, including joints and internal organs.

years and is three times more common in women than in men. In the United States, approximately 2.5 million adults are affected by RA. Symptoms include pain, swelling, and stiffness of the affected joint, with periods of activity or exacerbations and remissions of the disease process.

Although any joint may be involved, RA typically begins in the peripheral joints, particularly in the small bones of hands and feet and in the knee. The radiographic changes seen early in this disease are soft tissue swelling and osteoporosis of the affected bones (Fig. 2.23). As the disease progresses, cortical erosion with joint space narrowing occurs because of the overgrowth of synovial tissue into the articular spaces. This severe damage makes the joint unstable and leads to deformity caused by displacement of the bones in the joint. The late changes of this condition may be quite severe, resulting in bone and cartilage destruction and subluxation or dislocation of the involved joint (Fig. 2.24). Eventually, the joints become ankylosed (fused), which necessitates surgical intervention. Surgical procedures such as synovium excision, dislocation corrections, joint reconstructions, and prosthetic joint replacements may be performed to improve joint function

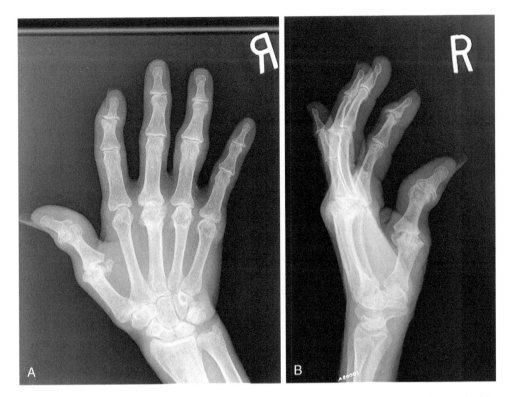

FIG. 2.24 Posteroanterior A, and lateral B, hand images demonstrating advanced rheumatoid arthritis with subluxation of the first metacarpophalangeal joint.

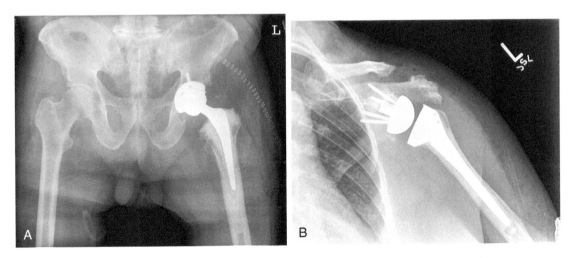

FIG. 2.25 A, Radiograph of an anteroposterior pelvis demonstrating proper placement of a prosthetic hip replacement. B, Radiograph of an oblique shoulder demonstrating proper placement of a prosthetic shoulder replacement.

Reiter syndrome is a variant of rheumatoid arthritis occurring most commonly in young males. It has been associated with bacterial infections of the gastrointestinal (GI) and genitourinary systems by organisms such as *Chlamydia trachomatis*, *Shigella*, *Salmonella*, *Yersinia*, or *Campylobacter*.

The sacroiliac joints, heels (calcanei), and toes are generally affected in this syndrome, sometimes referred to as "lover's heel." Although the radiographic appearance may mimic RA, Reiter syndrome affects the feet instead of hands. It is characterized by asymmetric involvement of the joints of the lower extremities, ill-defined erosions of bone with adjacent areas of proliferation, and a tendency to produce heterotrophic bone.

Nuclear medicine bone scans are helpful in diagnosing early stage Reiter syndrome in the sacroiliac joints, and the disease may be imaged before any findings are visible on a conventional radiograph. The preferred treatment is nonsteroidal antiinflammatory drugs (NSAIDs).

Ankylosing Spondylitis

Ankylosing spondylitis (Marie-Strümpell disease) is a progressive form of arthritis, mainly involving the spine; in this disease, joints and articulations become ankylosed, especially the sacroiliac joints. It tends to affect men between the ages of 20 and 40 years and is believed to have a genetic predisposition because it is 20 times more common in the first-degree relatives of individuals known to have this disorder. Most commonly, an individual will report low back pain of varying intensities, often nocturnal in nature and associated with morning stiffness. Other early signs and symptoms include low-grade fever, fatigue, weight loss, and anemia. Early radiographic changes demonstrate bilateral narrowing and fuzziness of the sacroiliac joints. Eventually, the sacroiliac joints become obliterated, and the condition progresses up the spine. Later radiographic changes show calcification of the bones of the spine and ossification of the vertebral ligaments. The articular cartilage is destroyed, and fibrous adhesions develop. These adhesions lead to bone fusion and calcification of the annulus fibrosis of the intervertebral disks as well as the anterior and lateral spinal ligaments. The spine becomes a rigid block of bone, giving the condition its characteristic nickname "bamboo spine" (Fig. 2.26). In addition to radiographic indications, blood serum analysis is used in

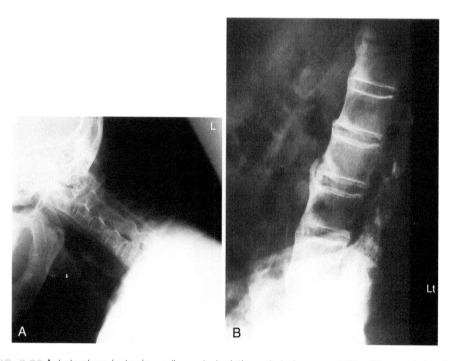

FIG. 2.26 A, Lateral cervical spine radiograph depicting ankylosing spondylitis with granulation tissue beneath the anterior longitudinal ligament destroying the corners of the contiguous vertebra. B, Lateral lumbar spine radiograph of a 64-year-old man with ankylosing spondylitis. Note the fusion of the vertebrae into a solid block of bone.

the diagnosis of ankylosing spondylitis. The human leukocyte antigen B27 (HLA-B27) test may be ordered individually or as part of a group of tests that includes rheumatoid factor (RF), ESR, or CRP. It is treated with NSAIDs, cyclooxygenase 2 (COX-2) inhibitors, therapeutic exercise, and postural training.

Osteoarthritis

The most common type of arthritis is **osteoarthritis**, also known as *degenerative joint disease* (DJD). It affects men and women equally, although patients are usually asymptomatic until they are in their 50s. Osteoarthritis is a disease of cartilage and is classified as *primary* or *secondary*. Primary osteoarthritis may be inflammatory or erosive and destructive, resulting from a noninflammatory deterioration of the joint cartilage that occurs with normal wear and tear. In some cases, individuals may have a genetic predisposition for developing osteoarthritis. Secondary osteoarthritis occurs as a result of bone stress associated with trauma, congenital anomalies, or other diseases that alter the hyaline cartilage and surrounding tissue. Osteoarthritis generally affects the large, primary weight-bearing joints of the body such as the hip, where it is particularly disabling, or the knees and ankles (Fig. 2.27). Osteoarthritis may also affect the interphalangeal joints of the fingers. Osteoarthritis of the fingers, which is thought to be hereditary, affects women, especially after menopause, more than it affects men. With this condition, fingers become enlarged and often develop bony knobs termed *Heberden nodes* and *Bouchard nodes*. Osteoarthritis of the fingers is most often managed with medications, splints, and heat treatments.

In joints affected by this disease, articular cartilage degenerates and is gradually worn away, exposing underlying bone. Radiographically, this loss of articular cartilage appears as a narrowing of the joint space. An overgrowth of articular cartilage occurs on the peripheral surfaces of the joint and often calcifies, which results in **osteophytes** or bone spurs that are radiographically visible (Fig. 2.28). In terms of radiographic diagnosis, the formation of osteophytes is indicative of osteoarthritis and helps distinguish it from other types of arthritis.

Clinically, an individual with osteoarthritis experiences pain and progressive stiffening of the affected joint. Methods of halting its gradual progression are few; it is second only to cardiovascular disease in causing long-term disability. Treatment consists of the use of medications such as NSAIDs, COX-2 inhibitors, and acetaminophen. Exercise is one of the best treatments to decrease pain, increase flexibility, and help with weight control. The use of corticosteroid injections, walking aids, rest, and heat treatment may also be incorporated in the treatment regimen. Surgery may be used to resurface or reposition bones or remove loose pieces of bone or cartilage; in cases of severe pain, surgical prosthetic joint replacement provides great relief and allows return of joint mobility.

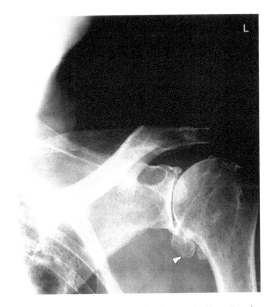

FIG. 2.28 Shoulder radiograph demonstrating the formation of an osteophyte at the inferior lip of the glenoid labrum caused by primary osteoarthritis.

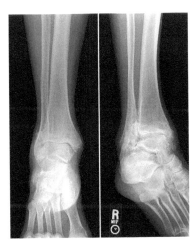

FIG. 2.27 Anteroposterior and oblique ankle radiographs demonstrating osteoarthritis.

Gouty Arthritis

Gouty arthritis (Gout) is an inherited metabolic disorder in which excess amounts of uric acid are produced and deposited in the joint and adjacent bone. The condition occurs more frequently in men and most commonly affects the metatarsophalangeal joint of the great toe. It is characterized by acute attacks with intervals of remission. This disease may occur in patients placed on long-term diuretics, for instance, to treat congestive heart failure.

The crystallization of uric acid within the joint causes an acute inflammatory reaction. Large masses of these sodium urate crystalline deposits in joints and other sites are called *tophi*. Bone changes include erosion (Fig. 2.29) with overhanging edges. One long-term complication of gout is the formation of radiolucent kidney stones caused by increased excretion of uric acid by the kidneys. Treatment of gout consists of medications either to promote excretion of uric acid by the kidneys or to inhibit the production of uric acid within the body.

Inflammation of Associated Joint Structures

The specialized connective tissues that attach muscle to bone are called *tendons*. Tendons are enclosed in a synovial sheath. **Tendonitis** is inflammation of a tendon, and inflammation of the tendon and the sheath is a condition known as **tenosynovitis** (Fig. 2.30). Tenosynovitis may spread to the associated tendon, resulting in tendonitis. Chronic tendonitis may also cause the formation of calcium deposits in either the affected tendon or an associated sheath. Such calcium deposits that form in the shoulder joint as a result of chronic trauma often cause rotator cuff tears, which can be detected by shoulder radiographs, shoulder arthrogram studies, and MRI examinations of the shoulder (Fig. 2.31). Bursae, which are sacs lined with a synovial membrane, are found in locations where tendons pass over bony prominences. If the bursa becomes inflamed, it is called **bursitis**. Inflammation of these associated structures may be caused by acute or chronic trauma (e.g., "housemaid's knee"), acute or chronic infection, inflammatory arthritis, gout, and, rarely, infection by pyogenic or tuberculous organisms. These inflammatory conditions are characterized by pain, localized tenderness, and limited motion of the involved joint. In cases of chronic bursitis, the walls of the bursa become thickened, and calcium deposits may be radiographically visible within the bursa. Common areas for bursitis are the shoulder, elbow, knee (prepatellar), and greater trochanter of the hip.

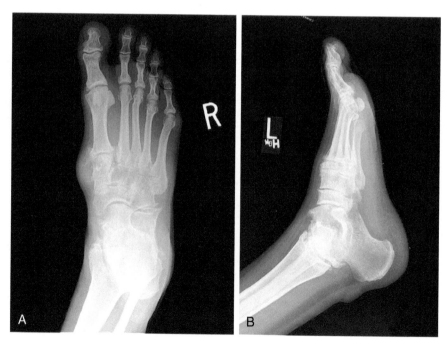

FIG. 2.29 Posteroanterior A, and lateral, B, foot radiographs demonstrating erosion of the tarsal bones from gout.

Common medical treatment of bursitis and tendonitis includes NSAIDs in combination with analgesics. In severe cases, aspiration of any accumulated fluid and corticosteroid injections may be included in the treatment. Surgical intervention is necessary when tendons or bursae ossify, especially in conjunction with rotator cuff tears. A **ganglion** is a cystic swelling that develops in connection with a tendon sheath (Fig. 2.32). Ganglions commonly occur in the back part of the wrist joint, but they can occur in any joint space. Ganglion cysts are

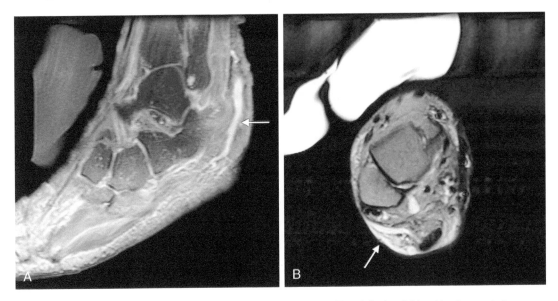

FIG. 2.30 Magnetic resonance imaging scans (A, sagittal; B, axial) of a right ankle demonstrate tenosynovitis involving the posterior tibialis muscle following a strain injury.

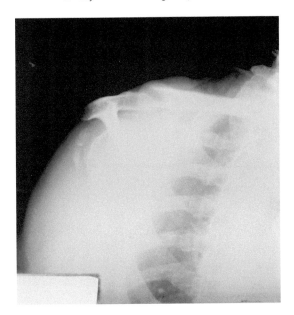

FIG. 2.31 Calcific tendonitis of the left shoulder resulting from rotator cuff disease. The radiograph demonstrates radiopaque calcium deposits within the shoulder joint.

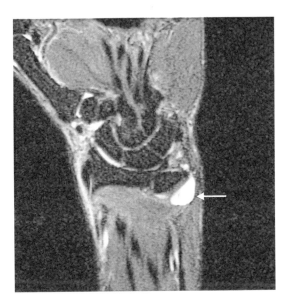

FIG. 2.32 Coronal magnetic resonance image of the wrist demonstrating a cystic lesion on the volar aspect of the wrist along the ulnar side.

treated with simple aspiration, aspiration with corticosteroid injection, or surgical excision, if symptomatic.

Vertebral Column

The causes of vertebral column injuries include direct trauma, hyperextension–flexion injuries, osteoporosis, and metastatic destruction. **Whiplash** is a broad term that encompasses soft tissue neck injuries from a variety of causes and is discussed further in Chapter 12.

Radiographic indications of spinal column injuries include the interruption of smooth, continuous lines formed by the vertebrae stacked one on another and may result from hyperextension or hyperflexion injuries (Figs. 2.33 and 2.34). *Anterospondylolisthesis* refers to the anterior slipping of the body of the vertebra (Fig. 2.35), and *retrospondylolisthesis* refers to the posterior slipping of the vertebral body. Anterospondylolisthesis is also known as **spondylolisthesis.** The patient with this condition may have

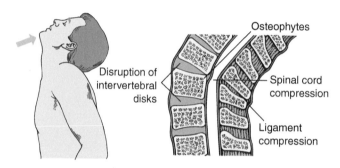

FIG. 2.33 Hyperextension injuries of the spine. Hyperextension may result in fracture or nonfracture injuries with spinal cord damage.

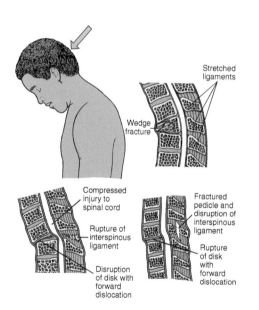

FIG. 2.34 Hyperflexion injury of the spine. Hyperflexion produces subluxation of vertebrae, which compromises the central canal and compresses spinal cord parenchyma or vascular structures.

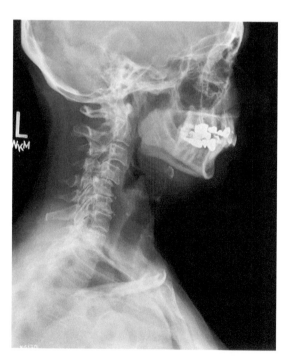

FIG. 2.35 Lateral spine radiograph demonstrating anterospondylolisthesis of the cervical spine.

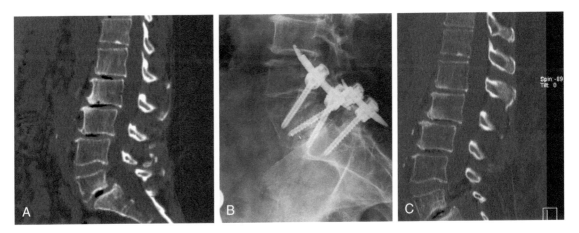

FIG. 2.36 A, Sagittal reconstruction of lumbar spine demonstrating spondylolisthesis before surgical intervention. B, L5-S1 lateral radiograph after surgical fusion for spondylolisthesis. C, Sagittal reconstruction of lumbar spine demonstrating spondylolisthesis after surgical intervention.

symptoms identical to those of a herniated disk. Approximately 90% of such slippage commonly occurs at the L5-S1 junction and is best detected on a lateral projection. Conservative medical management (e.g., rest, chiropractic manipulative therapy) is the preferred choice for treatment before surgical fusion. Surgical intervention (Fig. 2.36) depends on the degree of slippage and is classified as grade I to IV, with grade I being the least severe and grade IV the most severe.

The vertebral bodies may also lose some height, or the interspace may narrow. Perhaps the most common condition of the vertebral column is generalized back pain, typically in the lumbar area. Such back pain may not always result from bone involvement. Disk disease may cause muscle spasm with referred pain throughout the back. Finally, back pain may be secondary to referred pain from the hip. Conventional radiography is the most common imaging modality used to assess low back pain because it can demonstrate vertebral fractures and subluxation, **spondylolysis,** or erosion of vertebral bodies. However, they are of little value in the evaluation of disk pathologies.

A cleft, or breaking down of the body of a vertebra between the superior and inferior articular processes (pars interarticularis), results in spondylolysis. Typically, this occurs in the arch of the fifth lumbar vertebra as a result of developmental or congenital anomaly rather than acute trauma. It appears radiographically as a

TABLE 2.1
Anatomic Components of the Scotty Dog

Dog Part	Anatomic Component
Eye	Pedicle
Nose	Transverse process
Ear	Superior articular process
Foreleg	Inferior articular process
Neck	Pars interarticularis
Body	Lamina

"collar" or "broken neck" on the "Scotty dog" (Table 2.1) and is demonstrated on an oblique projection of the lumbar spine (Fig. 2.37).

Myelography performed in combination with CT (Fig. 2.38) enables evaluation of bone detail; however, it is still an invasive procedure. MRI provides a noninvasive alternative to CT myelography. MRI demonstrates the spine in multiple planes and is unsurpassed in its ability to demonstrate the spinal cord, nerve roots, subarachnoid and epidural spaces, vertebral disks, and the paraspinal tissues (Fig. 2.39). MRI does have limitations, such as patient compliance and contraindications for performing MRI examination such as pacemakers, aneurysm clips, and so on. In cases of vertebral fracture, CT is the modality of choice for demonstrating bone anatomy.

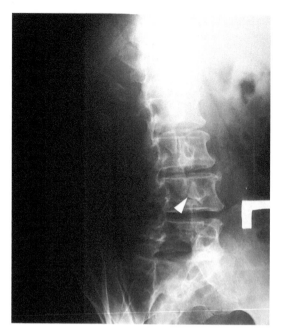

FIG. 2.37 Oblique radiograph of the lumbar spine demonstrating spondylolysis of the fourth and fifth lumbar spines on the left side. Note the break in the "Scotty dog's neck."

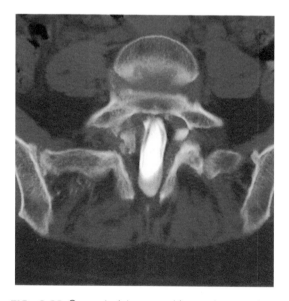

FIG. 2.38 Computed tomographic myelogram demonstrating the subarachnoid space and intervertebral disks.

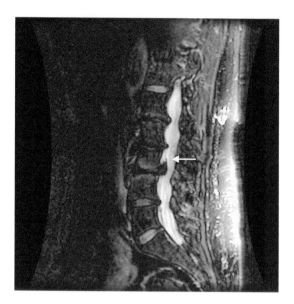

FIG. 2.39 Magnetic resonance image of the lumbar spine reconstructed in a sagittal plane demonstrating the spinal cord, subarachnoid space, and intervertebral disks.

Neoplastic Diseases

Many varieties of bone tumors are seen in patients of all ages; however, primary bone tumors are more common in children than in adults, and metastatic bone lesions far outnumber the incidence of primary bone neoplasms in the adult. The most common benign tumors are osteoma, osteochondroma, and giant cell tumor. The primary malignant bone tumors are osteosarcoma, Ewing tumor, and multiple myeloma.

The diagnosis of a bone abnormality is often made radiographically on the basis of the patient's age, the pattern of bone destruction, the location of the tumor, and the tumor's position within the bone. In terms of age, benign tumors most often occur within the first three decades of life; a bone tumor in older adults is likely to be malignant. The pattern of bone destruction in benign lesions is expansion of bone and sharp, sclerotic margins. Malignant neoplasms often infiltrate, permeate, and destroy anatomic margins. The location of a tumor is also important. For example, half of all osteosarcomas appear in the distal femoral or proximal tibial metaphysis. Similarly, **chondrosarcomas** tend to involve the trunk, shoulder girdle, and proximal long bones.

Alkaline phosphatase, osteonectin, osteocalcin, and collagen are used as potential bone tissue markers; however, these proteins may be difficult to distinguish if the origin is the bone matrix or from collagenous mimics, which are found in bone neoplasms. For this reason, they may not be helpful as genetic markers.

Radiographic studies contribute greatly to the diagnosis and management of patients with bone tumors. Radiographs are used to disclose the lesions and show the growth characteristics that assist in determining their benign or malignant nature. In conjunction with CT, plain radiographs identify malignant growth patterns and the proper site for biopsy. Sometimes, seemingly unrelated examinations such as a barium enema or chest radiography may be ordered by the physician to rule out distant metastases.

CT plays a key role in the primary diagnosis and continued evaluation of neoplasms of the skeletal system because of its ability to produce images with excellent soft tissue and contrast resolution. Sectional images of the area of interest provide physicians with the exact location and extent of the specific tumor, allowing the surgeon to identify the optimal surgical procedure and possibly limiting the surgical resection of the affected bone as well as assisting in the postsurgical management of the disease process. CT is also commonly used to assist during bone biopsy procedures.

As mentioned earlier in this chapter, radionuclide bone scans are helpful in assessing neoplastic diseases because the bone scan reflects the metabolic reaction of bone to the neoplastic disease process. Nuclear medicine procedures may also be performed during the initial stages of treatment planning to identify possible metastatic involvement of other anatomic sites.

Because cortical bone does not produce a signal, MRI provides the unique ability to clearly demonstrate fat and bone marrow because of their high water content. This information is helpful in differentiating between normal bone marrow and tumor tissue in the assessment of many neoplastic diseases of the skeletal system.

It is important to note that many neoplastic lesions may have similar radiographic appearances or are difficult to differentiate with imaging procedures alone. Therefore the final diagnosis must include a biopsy of the abnormality. Some biopsies may be performed under CT, MRI, or fluoroscopic guidance, whereas

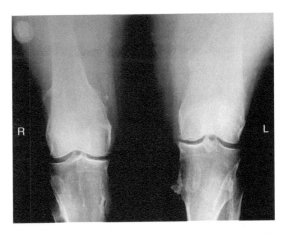

FIG. 2.40 Bilateral anteroposterior knee radiographs demonstrating osteochondroma with exostoses within the knee joint.

others must be performed surgically to obtain sufficient tissue for analysis. Histopathologic diagnosis is required for a definitive diagnosis.

A staging system for both benign and malignant bone tumors was developed by Enneking in 1980. Arabic numerals are used for benign lesions (1, 2, 3) and Roman numerals (I, II, III) for malignant lesions. For benign lesions, three stages exist: (1) stage 1, which includes benign, inactive tumors; (2) stage 2, in which the bone tumor is benign but active; and (3) stage 3, which includes aggressive benign lesions with bone destruction, soft tissue extensions, or pathologic fractures. Malignant bone lesions need to be staged after biopsy and histologic analysis have been done. Staging for malignant skeletal lesions includes histologic grade (low G1 or high G2), local extent of tumor (intracompartmental T1 or extracompartmental T2), and presence or absence of metastatic disease. The classification examples of IA, IB, IIA, IIB, III, and so on are assigned on the basis of the tumor characteristics, lymph node involvement, metastasis, and grade of the neoplasm.

Osteochondroma (Exostosis)

The most common benign bone tumor is **osteochondroma** (Fig. 2.40), which is three times more common in men than in women. An osteochondroma arises from the growth zone between the epiphysis and diaphysis of long bones, also called *metaphysis*. Most commonly, it involves the lower femur or upper tibia and is capped by growing

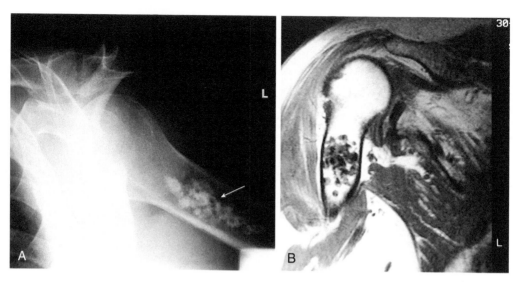

FIG. 2.41 A, Conventional shoulder radiograph in a 66-year-old man demonstrates calcification in the proximal diaphysis of the right humerus. B, Follow-up magnetic resonance image demonstrates an intramedullary lesion without breakthrough of the cortex, consistent with an endochondroma.

cartilage attached to the skeleton by a bony stalk. The cortex of an osteochondroma blends with normal bone, and the growth tends to protrude up and away from the nearest joint, most commonly the knee. **Exostoses** or excessive bone growth may appear as singular or multiple lesions and are normally diagnosed in childhood or adolescence. Multiple hereditary exostoses (MHE) indicate a hereditary disorder and usually appear at an earlier age than compared with the single-lesion osteochondroma. MHE have been linked to mutations in the following genes: *EXT1* on chromosome 8q23-q24, *EXT2* on chromosome 11p11-p12, and *EXT3* on the short arm of chromosome 19. It is theorized that the *EXT* genes also have the function of tumor suppression. In addition, MHE may transform to malignant neoplasms such as chondrosarcoma. Many times, osteochondromas are asymptomatic unless the affected long bone is traumatized, which results in a pathologic fracture of the diseased bone. An osteochondroma has an osteosclerotic or osteoblastic radiologic appearance. CT and MRI are used in initial differentiation between an osteochondroma and a malignant lesion.

Osteoma

An **osteoma** is a less frequent benign growth most commonly located in the skull. These lesions are composed of very dense, well-circumscribed, normal bone tissue that usually projects into the orbits or paranasal sinuses. They are generally slow-growing tumors of little significance unless they cause obstruction, impinge on the brain or eye, or interfere with the oral cavity. A term associated with osteoma of the skull is **hyperostosis frontalis interna.**

Endochondroma

An **endochondroma** is a slow-growing benign tumor composed of hyaline cartilage and is hypothesized to be a result of incomplete endochondral ossification. It grows in the marrow space and most commonly affects the small bones of the hands and feet of individuals between the ages of 30 and 40 years. These benign tumors do not invade surrounding tissue as they grow; however, they do expand the cortical bone, causing thinning. Radiographically, endochondromas appear as radiolucent lesions containing small, stippled calcifications (Fig. 2.41). They are well-circumscribed and appear as a "bubbly" lesion of the bone. The erosion of the cortex may cause pain and swelling and increase the incidence of pathologic fractures. Multiple growths, termed *enchondromatosis* (Ollier disease), may also occur in childhood and, like multiple osteochondromas, may undergo malignant transformation with a risk of 25% to 30%. CT and MRI are useful in distinguishing endochondromas from chondrosarcomas.

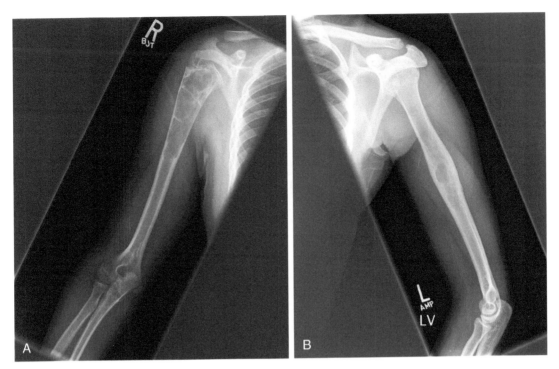

FIG. 2.42 A, Anteroposterior (AP) projection demonstrating multiple well-circumscribed radiolucencies in the proximal humerus consistent with a simple unicameral bone cyst. B, AP humerus radiograph demonstrating a well-circumscribed radiolucency midshaft consistent with a simple unicameral bone cyst.

Simple Unicameral Bone Cyst

A **simple unicameral bone cyst** (UBC) is a wall of fibrous tissue filled with fluid. These frequently occur in the long bones of children, most commonly in the humerus and proximal femur. Eighty percent of all simple bone cysts occur between 3 and 14 years of age and twice as often in boys as in girls. The cyst is usually first noticed when the patient reports pain, caused by increased tumor growth or as a result of a pathologic fracture.

Radiographically, UBCs appear radiolucent with well-defined margins from normal bone surrounding the lesion (Fig. 2.42). Occasionally, the cyst may be surrounded by a thin rim of sclerotic bone. Small cysts tend to heal and obliterate themselves; larger cysts require surgical intervention. The benign bone cyst is treated by surgical excision and packing with bone chips to obtain complete healing. Percutaneous steroid injection into the lesion is another form of treatment that was introduced in the 1970s, and it is inexpensive and has a decreased morbidity rate compared with surgical intervention.

Aneurysmal Bone Cyst

An **aneurysmal bone cyst** (ABC) is an idiopathic condition and not a true neoplasm. These cysts generally occur in the metaphysis of long bones in individuals under the age of 20 years and consist of numerous blood-filled arteriovenous communications. Vertebral lesions usually occur in the lumbar region and account for 15% to 20% of aneurysmal bone cysts. Following the Human Genome project, it has been discovered that this bone cyst is most likely caused by translocation of 17p13 and overactivity of the oncogene *USP6* (ubiquitin-specific protease). These are slow-growing lesions, and the most common symptoms are pain and swelling at the site of the cyst. This cystic growth causes a thinning of the cortex that is apparent radiographically and as a well-circumscribed lesion associated with soft tissue extension and periosteal bulging.

A bone scan demonstrates peripheral uptake with a centralized decreased uptake. Angiography shows persistent accumulation of contrast media throughout the cyst. CT and MRI may also be used for imaging ABCs. CT better delineates the cyst in the vertebral column, and MRI shows fluid levels or the presence of a soft tissue mass. The most common treatment of an ABC is surgical removal of the lesion and subsequent bone grafting; however, radiation therapy may be used for treatment in some areas in the vertebral region where surgical removal is difficult. Caution is used with radiation therapy because of the risk of postradiation malignancies.

Osteoid Osteoma and Osteoblastoma

Other common benign tumors of the skeletal system are osteoid osteoma and osteoblastoma. Although similar in histologic features, they differ in size, origin, and symptoms. Osteoid osteomas are less than 2 cm in dimension, whereas osteoblastomas are larger. Osteoblastomas more frequently involve the spine, and pain may not be present. Furthermore, they are not associated with a marked bone reaction or new bone production and are classified radiographically as osteolytic lesions. Osteoblastomas have a higher recurrence rate compared with osteoid osteomas and, in rare cases, may undergo malignant transformation to osteogenic sarcoma.

Osteoid osteomas occur twice as often in men as in women and almost always develop before the age of 30 years. It has been discovered that genetic markers include an elevated amount of E2 but may also include F2 alpha, 6-keto-F1 alpha, and thromboxane B2. Osteoid osteomas are most commonly found in the femur, tibia, or spine of the young adult. They arise within the cortical bone and erode underlying bone tissue, resulting in a lytic lesion called a *nidus*. The area of erosion is surrounded by a zone of dense, sclerotic bone, making the radiographic appearance of osteoid osteomas very distinctive (Fig. 2.43). The radiographic appearance of an osteoid osteoma demonstrates a well-circumscribed, small radiolucent area containing a dense center (nidus). The radiolucent area is surrounded by very dense, sclerotic bone. The nidus is composed of osteoid or newly formed bone; thus this tumor is classified as an osteosclerotic lesion. CT scans with 1- to 2-mm cuts are of great value in identifying, localizing, and providing biopsy guidance in the diagnosis of osteoid osteomas

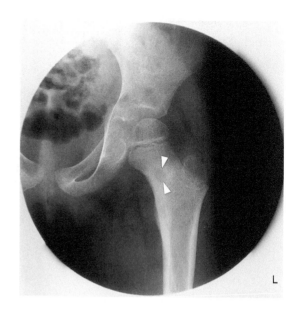

FIG. 2.43 Anteroposterior hip radiograph of a 7-year-old girl who complained of a 2-month history of pain. The radiograph demonstrates an osteoid osteoma as evidenced by the well-defined defect in the cortical area of the femoral neck.

(Fig. 2.44). MRI is also a common modality used to assist in the diagnosis (Fig. 2.45). The erosion of surrounding tissue and the presence of prostaglandin and nerve fibers in the nidus cause extreme pain, often at night, and the pain is readily relieved by NSAIDs. CT-guided laser ablation and surgical removal are common treatments for these benign lesions.

Giant Cell Tumor (Osteoclastoma)

Giant cell tumors (GCTs) are characterized by the presence of numerous, multinucleated osteoclastic giant cells. GCTs of the tendon sheath are the second most common benign soft tissue lesions of the hand and wrist. Unlike the previously mentioned neoplastic diseases, GCTs may be either benign or malignant. Approximately 50% of osteoclastomas are benign, 35% to 50% recur after surgical excision, and 15% are aggressively malignant from the beginning. This neoplasm affects women more often than men and is found in individuals between the ages of 20 and 30 years. Anatomically, this disease tends to affect the ends or epiphyses of long bones, especially the lower femur, the upper tibia, and the lower radius. It begins in the medullary canal and expands outward, producing a club-like

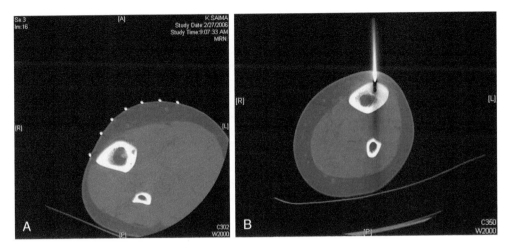

FIG. 2.44 Axial computed tomography (CT) scan demonstrating an osteoid osteoma A, in preparation for CT-guided needle biopsy B.

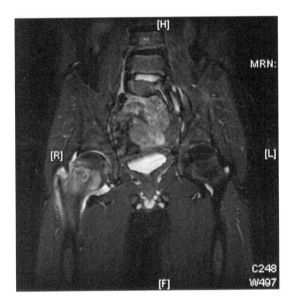

FIG. 2.45 Coronal magnetic resonance images demonstrating an osteoid osteoma in the right femoral neck.

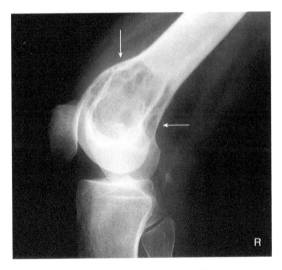

FIG. 2.46 Lateral knee radiograph of a 30-year-old man who complained of a painful knee for approximately 2 months. The radiograph demonstrates a benign osteoclastoma of the knee.

deformity of the end of the long bone. In addition, soft tissue extensions may be present, but the GCT does not involve the joint space.

Clinical signs and symptoms of a GCT are nonspecific and include pain, tenderness, an occasional palpable mass, and an occasional pathologic fracture. Because this is an osteoclastic disease process, bone and cartilage formation generally do not occur in these lesions; therefore, the radiographer must decrease exposure factors

to avoid overpenetration of the affected bone. Radiographically, a GCT is a mass of osteolytic or cystic areas surrounded by a thin shell of bone, giving it the classic "soap bubble" appearance (Fig. 2.46). CT and MRI are also excellent modalities to image this neoplastic disease. GCTs are usually located in the epiphysis, producing erosion and thinning of the cortical bone without new bone growth. Treatment of an osteoclastoma consists of cryosurgery, surgical excision of the lesion, and bone grafting. The surgical site in the patient should be closely monitored radiographically and at regular intervals.

Osteosarcoma (Osteogenic Sarcoma)

Except for myeloma, the most common primary malignancy of the skeleton is **osteosarcoma,** which arises from osteoblasts. The cause of osteosarcoma is linked genetically to deletion of genetic material on chromosome 13 and the oncogene *src*. Genetic instability is essential for the development of sarcomas. Patients with osteosarcoma frequently lose function of the proteins p53 and RB1, which are tumor suppressors and protect the genome from acquiring mutations that may lead to malignancy. Of osteosarcomas, 50% involve the proteins p53, RB, and MDM2, which may be utilized as genetic markers. Genetic syndromes associated with osteosarcoma include Li-Fraumeni, Rothmund-Thomson, and Werner syndromes. Li-Fraumeni syndrome is associated with mutation of the tumor suppressor gene *p53;* Rothmund-Thomson syndrome involves mutation of the *RECQL4* gene; and Werner syndrome, also referred to as *adult progeria,* may involve environmental factors such as exposure to radiation. This neoplasm is most frequently found in the metaphyses of long bones, with approximately 50% affecting the knee. Osteosarcoma may occur at any age, but 75% occur in patients younger than 20 years old. It is occasionally seen in older individuals with Paget disease or after high-level radiation exposure to bone, and the tumors are known as *postradiation sarcomas.* Clinically, the patient may have pain and swelling.

Osteosarcoma is a highly aggressive bone-forming neoplasm which is believed to originate in mesenchymal stem cells and/or osteoblastic precursor cells (Fig. 2.47). As the tumor grows from the metaphysis, it lifts the periosteum from the cortical bone and lays down spicules of new bone radiating out from the origin, which gives the radiographic appearance of a sunray or sunburst. This appearance results from the radiopaque and radiolucent changes within the newly created space between the cortex of the metaphysis and the displaced periosteum and is termed a *periosteal reaction.* In some cases, a soft tissue mass that is not enclosed in bone may form as the neoplasm breaks through the cortex lifting the periosteum. MRI is an excellent modality for demonstrating this soft tissue extension (Fig. 2.48). Radiographic

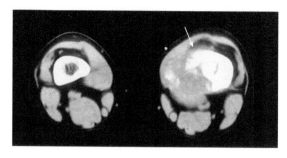

FIG. 2.47 Magnetic resonance image of the left femur is helpful in determining the medullary extension of the osteosarcoma.

findings (Fig. 2.49) vary greatly in appearance because some osteosarcoma tumors produce very little osteoid tissue and contain no calcifications, whereas others are densely opaque. 18F-Fluorodeoxyglucose positron emission tomography (FDG-PET) is the most frequently used imaging modality for assessing osteosarcoma, but its role in sarcoma analysis is not well delineated because of limited reimbursement. The most significant advantage is the simultaneous evaluation of bone and soft tissues with quantitative metabolic data. Accurate diagnosis must be made through biopsy of the questionable lesion. Blood serum analysis often shows elevated serum alkaline phosphatase as a result of the osteoblastic activity.

Osteosarcoma is a highly malignant disease with a poor prognosis because lung metastasis almost always occurs via the bloodstream. This metastatic lung disease may appear as multiple, rounded, calcified shadows within the lung fields on a conventional chest radiograph. If the chest radiograph is clear, high-resolution CT of the chest often demonstrates micrometastases, which are commonly present in the lungs before the primary osteosarcoma is discovered. Secondary growths or spread to other bones is very rare with osteosarcoma. In the past, treatment of osteosarcoma included amputation of the limb followed by chemotherapy. Today, most physicians place the patient on preoperative chemotherapy after the initial diagnosis is confirmed by bone biopsy. After initial chemotherapy, the patient undergoes limb salvage via a tumor resection with implantation of a cadaver allograft, vascularized grafts, or prostheses. This is followed by postsurgical chemotherapy involving high doses of methotrexate. This change in the management of osteosarcoma has increased 5-year survival rates from 20% to over 80%.

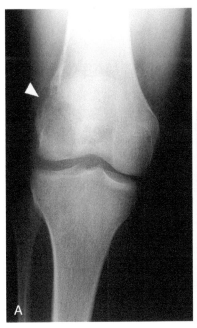

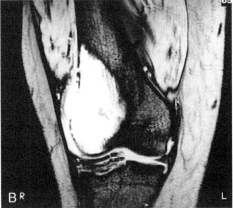

FIG. 2.48 A, Anteroposterior radiograph of the right knee demonstrates a tumor in the distal lateral femoral condyle. Interruption of the cortex and reactive sclerotic bone changes raise suspicion of metastatic disease or primary malignancy. B, Follow-up magnetic resonance image of the knee reveals an osteosarcoma that has replaced the distal femoral condyle.

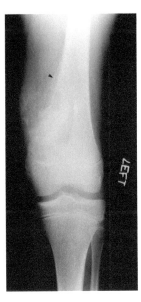

FIG. 2.49 Posteroanterior projection of the knee of a 14-year-old boy with painful swelling above the left knee. The radiograph demonstrates cortical destruction along the posteromedial margin of the distal femur consistent with an osteosarcoma of the left femur.

Ewing Sarcoma

Another primary malignant bone tumor is **Ewing sarcoma.** This neoplasm occurs at a younger age than any other primary malignant bone neoplasm, usually between the ages of 5 and 15 years, and rarely after age 30 years. It is also more common in boys than in girls and shows a predilection for Caucasians, with African Americans rarely affected.

Unlike osteosarcoma, Ewing sarcoma arises from the medullary canal and involves bone more diffusely, giving rise to uniform thickening of bone. These lesions tend to be very extensive, often involving the entire shaft of a long bone. Also, unlike osteogenic sarcoma, Ewing sarcoma does not begin at the end of a long bone. It does, however, tend to affect the extremities and the pelvis. Although Ewing sarcoma is a fairly rare disease, it is extremely malignant. Clinical symptoms are nonspecific and include pain and tenderness of the affected area. Radiography, CT, and MRI are essential in establishing the diagnosis and identifying the extent of the disease. The lesions undergo a combination of bone formation in the early stages and destruction in the later stages, with new bone being formed on the surface (Fig. 2.50). This process often gives a classic onionskin or laminated appearance radiographically. Diagnosis is made by biopsy with the identification of an 11:22 chromosomal translocation within the tumor cells. Affirmation of this lesion is completed by immunohistochemistry or polymerase chain reaction (PCR) analysis, which demonstrates the presence of the *EWS-FLI1* fusion gene. The *EWS* gene is located on chromosome 22 and the *FLI-1* gene is located on chromosome 11. Cytologic analysis demonstrates characteristic blue, round cell histology. Multidrug preoperative and postoperative chemotherapy, in combination with radiation therapy or surgical resection, has proven effective in improving the prognosis from a 60% 5-year survival rate to an 80% 5-year survival rate. Treatments based on newer research include the use of monoclonal antibodies, myeloablation therapy, or a combination of chemotherapy and hemopoietic stem cell transplantation.

Chondrosarcoma

A chondrosarcoma is a malignant tumor of cartilaginous origin and is composed of atypical cartilage. It is only half as common as osteosarcoma; approximately 10% of all malignant tumors of the skeletal system are

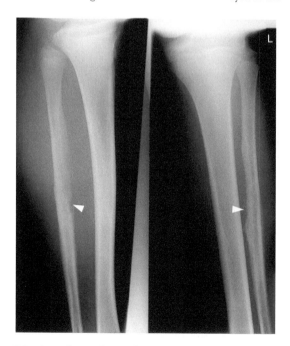

FIG. 2.50 Lower leg radiographs of a 12-year-old boy complaining of left leg pain demonstrate Ewing sarcoma of the tibia, as indicated by the lytic defect in the proximal diaphysis of the fibula.

chondrosarcomas. Common locations for chondrosarcoma are the pelvis, shoulder, and ribs. Men are three times more likely than women to develop chondrosarcoma, and it is more common in older adults. As mentioned earlier in this chapter, benign exostoses and multiple endochondromas may be transformed into chondrosarcomas. However, this type of change accounts for only about 10% of cases, with approximately 90% of chondrosarcomas arising afresh without prior cartilaginous lesions. Chondrosarcomas may be bulky, and they tend to destroy the bone as they extend through the cortex into surrounding soft tissue. These lesions have the ability to implant or seed into surrounding soft tissue, so careful excision is necessary. Radiographically, a chondrosarcoma shows irregular or circular radiolucencies in combination with granular areas of calcification. These tumors cause destruction and penetration of the cortex and extension into surrounding soft tissue. Often, the actual tumor may be larger than its radiographic appearance. Neither radiation therapy nor chemotherapy is particularly effective in the treatment of chondrosarcomas. Major surgery such as amputation or chest resection is often the treatment of choice, leading to a 5-year survival rate of approximately 40%.

Metastases from Other Sites

Virtually any type of cancer may metastasize to bone; metastatic disease from carcinomas is the most common malignant tumor of the skeleton, with secondary bone tumors of any origin far outnumbering primary bone tumors. Patients with skeletal metastases are usually older than 40 years. Principal signs and symptoms are pain and pathologic fracture.

The bones of the skeletal system that contain red bone marrow are the major bones affected by the metastatic disease because of their abundant vascularization. These include flat bones (such as the ribs, sternum, pelvis, and skull), the vertebrae, and the upper ends of the femora (Fig. 2.51) and humeri. The spine is the most common site for metastasis to occur, accounting for approximately 40% of all metastatic lesions. Radionuclide bone scans are more accurate than conventional radiography in the detection of metastasis because 3% to 5% bone destruction produces a "hot spot." Metastatic bone lesions appear as multiple, irregularly distributed areas of increased uptake that do not correspond to a single anatomic structure (Fig. 2.52). Bone scans are extremely helpful when assessing metastatic breast cancer because approximately 20% of women with breast cancer have a solitary area of increased activity, often without pain, in the site of the metastatic tumor. Radiographically, signs of bone metastasis include alteration of bone density and architecture. These may be osteolytic, osteoblastic, or mixed. Osteolytic metastases account for 75% of all metastatic lesions, and to be visible radiographically, the lesions must be greater than 1 cm in diameter with a loss of about 30% to 50% of bone density. CT is often employed, especially for imaging the spine, to clear up discrepancies in which a bone scan may indicate metastatic disease that cannot be confirmed by plain radiographic analysis. MRI may also be used to differentiate between tumor tissue and normal bone marrow. Recently whole body FDG-PET, whole body MRI, MRI-PET, and CT-PET have been advocated for imaging metastatic disease.

Certain characteristics help distinguish between a primary malignant neoplasm and a secondary one. Periosteal response is much more common with primary malignant tumors. Soft tissue masses are common in primary tumors and rare in metastases. Lesions longer than 10 cm often represent a primary malignant tumor; most metastatic tumors range between 2 and 4 cm in length. Tumors that expand bone are primary in nature, with rare exceptions. Most primary tumors are solitary, whereas metastatic lesions are usually multiple. Definitive diagnosis is obtained through biopsy.

The most common primary sites for metastatic bone cancer are the breast, lung, prostate, kidney, thyroid, and bowel, with the tumor spreading via proximity (direct extension), the bloodstream, or the lymphatic system. Treatment of metastatic disease is based on the primary disease, but radiation therapy in combination with either chemotherapy or hormone therapy is commonly used to manage such patients. Bone scans and PET scans are used to monitor the progress of therapy; a reduction in uptake on serial scans is a positive sign.

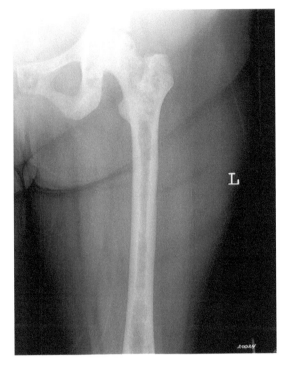

FIG. 2.51 Anteroposterior hip radiograph demonstrating metastatic disease from a primary breast cancer.

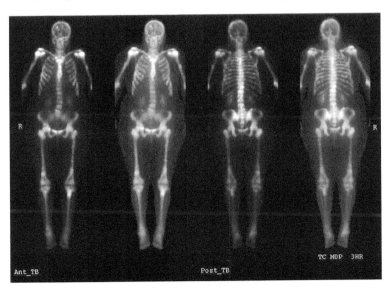

FIG. 2.52 Bone scan of the patient in Fig. 2.46 demonstrating multiple areas of metastatic disease.

Pathologic Summary of the Skeletal System

Pathology	Imaging Modality of Choice
Osteogenesis imperfecta	Radiography
Achondroplasia	Radiography
Osteopetrosis	Radiography
Anencephaly	Ultrasonography
Osteomyelitis	MRI, nuclear medicine, radiographs
Tuberculosis	Radiography
Infectious arthritis	Radiography
Psoriatic arthritis	Radiography
Reiter syndrome	Nuclear medicine, radiography
Rheumatoid arthritis	Radiography
Ankylosing spondylitis	Radiography
Osteoarthritis	Radiography
Joint structures	MRI
Gouty arthritis	Radiography
Osteochondroma	Radiography, MRI
Osteoma	Radiography, MRI
Endochondroma	Radiography, MRI
Unicameral bone cyst	Radiography, MRI
Aneurysmal bone cyst	CT, MRI
Osteoid osteoma	CT
Osteoblastoma	Radiography, MRI
Giant cell tumor	Radiography, MRI
Osteosarcoma	Radiography, MRI
Ewing sarcoma	Radiography, MRI
Chondrosarcoma	Radiography, MRI
Bone metastases from other sites	MRI, CT, FDG-PET

CT, Computed tomography; *MRI,* magnetic resonance imaging; *FDG-PET,* 18F-fluorodeoxyglucose positron emission tomography.

Review Questions

1. Specialized cells responsible for the formation of bone are termed:
   a. Chondroblasts
   b. Osteoblasts
   c. Osteoclasts
   d. Both b and c

2. A freely movable joint is classified as:
   a. Amphiarthrodial
   b. Diarthrodial
   c. Synarthrodial
   d. Triarthrodial

3. Bone marrow is located anatomically within the:
   a. Cortex
   b. Medullary canal
   c. Periosteum
   d. Trabeculae

4. The end portion of a long bone is referred to as the:
   a. Epiphysis
   b. Diaphysis
   c. Diploë
   d. Metaphysis

5. One of the most common primary malignant tumors of the skeleton that arises from osteoblasts is:
    a. Giant cell tumor
    b. Osteoid osteoma
    c. Osteosarcoma
    d. Osteochondroma

6. The most common inherited disorder that results in dwarfism is:
    a. Achondroplasia
    b. Albers-Schönberg disease
    c. Osteogenesis
    d. Spina bifida imperfecta

7. A variant of rheumatoid arthritis associated with bacterial infections by organisms such as *Chlamydia trachomatis* or *Campylobacter* is:
    a. Juvenile arthritis
    b. Psoriatic arthritis
    c. Osteoarthritis
    d. Reiter syndrome

8. The formation of extra digits is termed:
    a. Adactyly
    b. Polydactyly
    c. Syndactyly
    d. Talipes

9. An abnormal lateral curvature of the spine is referred to as:
    a. Ankylosing spondylitis
    b. Scoliosis
    c. Spondylolisthesis
    d. Spondylolysis

10. Osteomyelitis is a disease of the skeletal system that is:
    a. Arthritic
    b. Congenital
    c. Inflammatory
    d. Neoplastic

11. Osteoarthritis affects the weight-bearing joints within the body and may be treated with:
    a. Exercise
    b. Medication
    c. Surgery
    d. All of the above

12. The type of arthritis believed to be an autoimmune disease is:
    a. Bursitis
    b. Gout
    c. Osteoarthritis
    d. Rheumatoid arthritis

13. Which of the following neoplastic diseases affects children more frequently than adults?
    a. Chondrosarcoma
    b. Ewing sarcoma
    c. Osteochondroma
    d. Osteoclastoma

14. The most common benign bone tumor is:
    a. Endochondroma
    b. Osteoid osteoma
    c. Osteoma
    d. Osteochondroma

15. All of the following are malignant neoplasms of the skeletal system except:
    a. Chondrosarcoma
    b. Ewing sarcoma
    c. Osteosarcoma
    d. Osteoma

16. A 60-year-old patient who was discharged from the hospital after knee replacement surgery continued to complain of generalized pain in the area of the knee for several days. If you were this patient's physician, what imaging test might you order, and why?

17. A 35-year-old woman visits her family physician with complaints of swelling that comes and goes in her hands. What might be the initial suspicion, and what diagnostic procedure(s) might be ordered?

18. How may CT and MRI be used to complement skeletal radiography in the diagnosis and treatment of osteosarcoma?

19. A male construction worker sees his physician because of lower back pain. What are two possible causes that are unrelated to the bony vertebral column?

20. In diagnosing bone tumors, what are some of the characteristics taken into consideration?

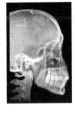
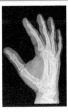
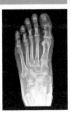

CHAPTER 3

Respiratory System

e http://evolve.elsevier.com/Kowalczyk/pathology/

Anatomy and Physiology

The respiratory system is responsible for two major functions. **Ventilation** involves the movement of air in and out of the lungs, and **diffusion** relates to the gas exchange between the lungs and the circulatory system. This system is usually subdivided into the upper respiratory tract—the nose, mouth, pharynx, and larynx—and the lower respiratory tract—the trachea, bronchi, alveoli, and lungs (Fig. 3.1). The thoracic cavity consists of the right and left pleural cavities and the mediastinum. The parietal pleura lines the thoracic cavity, and the visceral pleura adheres directly to lung tissue.

Anatomically, the mediastinum is divided into the anterior, middle, and posterior portions. The anterior mediastinum contains the thyroid and thymus glands. The middle mediastinum contains the heart and great vessels, esophagus, and trachea. The posterior mediastinum contains the descending aorta and the spine.

The anatomic bony structures of the thorax provide support and protection, and assist in both inspiration and expiration. These bony structures include the ribs, sternum, and thoracic vertebrae.

The paranasal sinuses are lined with respiratory epithelium and communicate with the nasal cavities, hence their inclusion in this chapter. The maxillary and ethmoid sinuses are the only paranasal sinuses present at birth. The frontal sinuses generally develop shortly after birth and are fully developed by the age of 10 years. The sphenoid sinus begins to develop

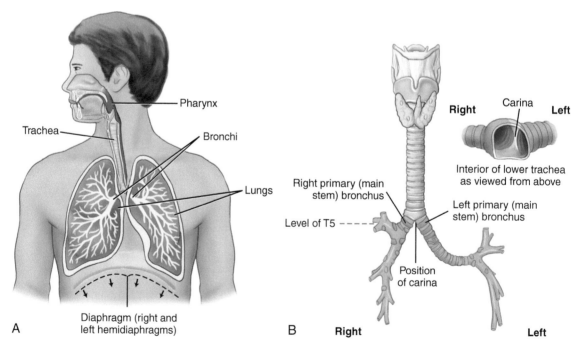

FIG. 3.1 A, The respiratory system. B, The trachea and its bifurcation at the carina.

around the age of 2 or 3 years and is fully developed by late adolescence.

Imaging Considerations

Radiography

The most frequently performed examination in any radiology department is chest radiography. Although this examination may seem routine, chest radiography provides important information about soft tissues, bones, the pleura, the mediastinum, and lung tissue.

Exposure Factor Conditions

Correct exposure factor selection is critical because an incorrect exposure factor may obscure or appear to create pathologic findings. This is particularly true for serial mobile radiographs because the interpreting physician relies heavily on consistent exposure conditions to analyze the change in pathology after treatment. Institutions may record exposure techniques for mobile chest images so that different technologists can use similar exposure factors to maintain consistency among the radiographs. Photostimulable phosphor–computed tomography (CT) imaging plates and direct readout (DR) image receptors are commonly used for mobile chest radiography to eliminate exposure repeats caused by the inadequacy or inconsistency of technical factors. Although accurate technical selection is important when using digital radiography systems to ensure that an appropriate exposure indicator is obtained, both systems offer wider latitude of error over conventional film or screen systems because of a wider dynamic range.

Some sources describe pathologies, including those in the chest, as *additive*, that is, they are harder than normal to penetrate or *subtractive* (destructive), that is, they are easier than normal to penetrate. In the respiratory system, any condition that adds fluid or tissue to the normally aerated chest (e.g., pneumonia) requires an increase in technical factors to afford proper penetration and exposure. Similarly, any condition that increases the aeration of the chest (e.g., emphysema) reduces the amount of radiation required for proper exposure to be achieved. Most experts agree that when chest radiography is performed using a digital imaging system, the radiographer must use his or her knowledge of pathologic conditions and specific image receptor characteristics to assess whether a change in milliampere second

(mAs) or kilovoltage peak (kVp) is required to adjust the radiographic exposure. The kilovoltage range should be chosen based on the energy level necessary to penetrate the part of interest, keeping in mind the presence of additive or subtractive pathologies.

The use of automatic exposure control (AEC) in chest radiography facilitates consistent radiographic exposures but requires careful analysis of the clinical history and conscious thought about the type of disease present and its location to ensure truly optimal diagnostic-quality radiographs. Activation of the sensor, for example, over an area of significant aeration or consolidation (tissue or fluid accumulation) may result in excessive or insufficient exposure, respectively. Although the image may look fine during the initial visual examination, care must be taken to always utilize an exposure indicator to assess proper technique selection. Experience with AEC, combined with careful thought in selecting the proper sensor, eliminates these mistakes.

Position and Projection

Patient position and projection are also critical exposure conditions that may distort the final image. *Position* refers to the arrangement of the patient's body (e.g., erect, supine, recumbent), and *projection* refers to the path of the x-ray beam (e.g., anteroposterior [AP], i.e., entering through the body's anterior surface and exiting the posterior surface). The standard projections for chest radiography are the erect posteroanterior (PA) and left lateral (Fig. 3.2). Each of these serves to place the heart closer to the film because the heart lies in the anterior part of the chest and mostly to the left side. When combined with a standard 72-inch source-to-image distance (SID), magnification of the heart is minimized.

Chest Radiography

On a normal erect PA chest image, the costophrenic and cardiophrenic angles are demonstrated, with the right hemidiaphragm appearing 1 to 2 cm higher than the left because of the position of the liver. When a patient is radiographed in the recumbent position, the lower lung fields may be obscured because of abdominal pressure raising the level of the diaphragm (Fig. 3.3).

Other projections of the thorax are used less frequently than the erect PA and left lateral projections. The AP projection is the method of choice for mobile radiography when the patient is too ill to tolerate a

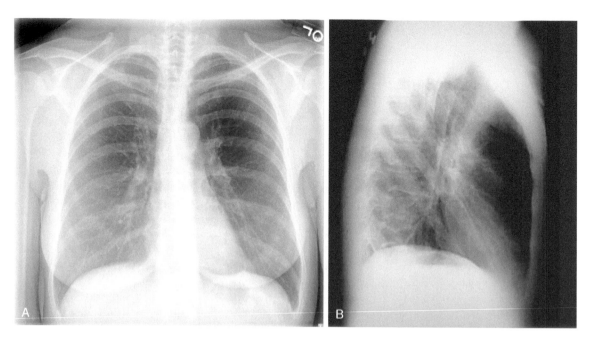

FIG. 3.2 A, Normal erect posteroanterior chest. B, Normal erect lateral chest.

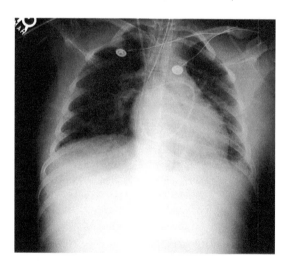

FIG. 3.3 Recumbent anteroposterior chest demonstrating obscuring of the lower lung fields.

visit to the department and assume an erect position. As much as possible, it is important that mobile chest radiographs be taken with the patient sitting in bed in the erect position to demonstrate any air–fluid levels present. Maintenance of the beam perpendicular to the plane of the image receptor is essential to avoid any foreshortening of the heart. Furthermore, use of the 72-inch SID is very important for mobile radiography

to minimize magnification of the heart, which is located farther from the image receptor in the AP projection. To improve image quality, many institutions commonly employ a short dimension grid when using a digital imaging system.

The AP and PA projections of the patient lying in the lateral decubitus position are useful under specific conditions such as diagnosing free air in the pleural space or pleural fluid. For example, for a right lateral decubitus chest radiograph, the patient lies on his or her right side. In this position, any fluid present tends to layer out along the edge of the lung field on the dependent side, which enhances its visibility, whereas the free air rises toward the left side.

For evaluation of the standard PA chest radiograph, the size and radiolucency of both lungs should be compared. Criteria for adequate inspiration and penetration of chest radiographs vary from institution to institution; however, a rule of thumb is that adequate inspiration should provide visualization of 10 posterior ribs within the lung field. In addition, all thoracic vertebrae and intervertebral disk spaces should be faintly visible through the mediastinum on an adequately penetrated chest radiograph. The average movement of the lungs and diaphragm between inspiration and expiration is approximately 3 cm (Fig. 3.4).

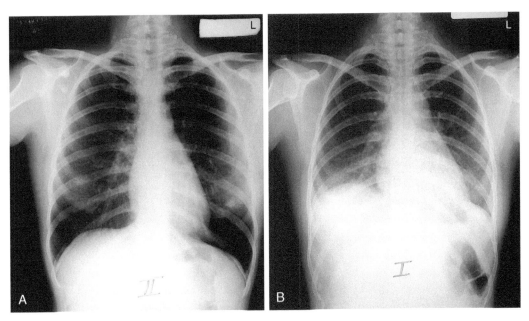

FIG. 3.4 A, Normal appearance of chest during inspiration. B, Expiration film on the same patient demonstrates elevation of the diaphragm and a heart that is more transverse and appears larger.

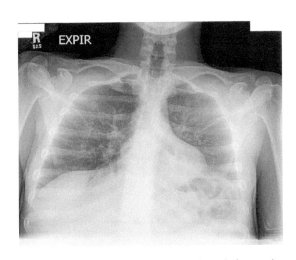

FIG. 3.5 Lordotic chest radiograph taken during expiration to demonstrate a possible pneumothorax.

Oblique projections of the thorax are useful in separating superimposed structures such as the sternum, esophagus, and thoracic spine. A lordotic chest radiograph is useful in demonstrating the apical regions of the lung, which are normally obscured by bony structures on the standard PA projection (Fig. 3.5). Certain diseases such as tuberculosis (TB) have a predilection for the apices.

Soft Tissues of the Chest

Various soft tissue densities are present on chest radiographs. They may vary with patient age, sex, and pathologic conditions. The pectoral muscles are normally demonstrated overlying and extending beyond the lung fields. Radiographs of both men and women demonstrate breast shadows in the midchest region (Fig. 3.6). These shadows are normally homogeneous in appearance, and female breasts may obscure the costophrenic angles. Elevation of the breasts may be necessary to better demonstrate the bases of the lungs. Surgical removal of one or both breasts is also evident on chest radiographs; breast prostheses, which appear as well-defined, circular, radiopaque densities, are also evident. Nipple shadows may be visible at the level of the fourth or fifth anterior rib spaces and may occasionally mimic nodules or masses in the chest. These soft tissue structures may be differentiated with nipple markers or oblique projections of the chest.

Bony Structures of the Chest

The ribs, sternum, and thoracic spine enclose the thoracic cavity. These structures assist the technologist in the assessment of the technical adequacy of chest radiographs. Congenital anomalies of the ribs may be demonstrated (Fig. 3.7), as well as calcified costal cartilages. This calcification

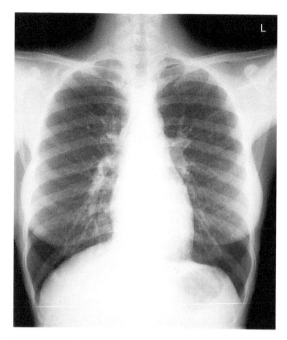

Breast shadows are readily recognizable on the normal posteroanterior chest radiograph.

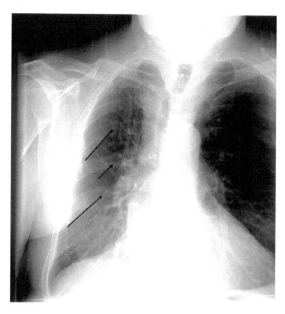

Right-sided rib fractures (*arrows*) in combination with a right clavicular fracture.

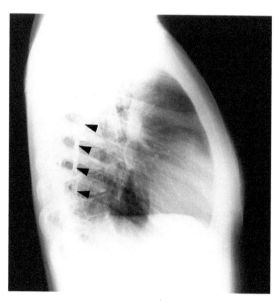

Congenital intrathoracic rib seen as curving, tubular density in the posterior thorax. Usually these ribs are attached at one or both ends of a posterior rib and lie extrapleurally inside the thoracic cage.

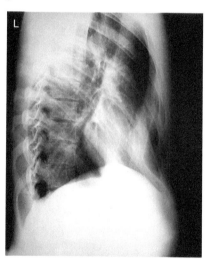

Lateral projection of the chest demonstrating pectus excavatum, including compression of the heart toward the spine.

generally occurs in patients in their late 20s and beyond. Rib fractures may be seen (Fig. 3.8), sometimes with an accompanying pneumothorax. A depressed sternum (pectus excavatum) may also be demonstrated, possibly displacing the heart (Fig. 3.9). The thoracic spine may be assessed for scoliosis, which may affect the chest cavity, and kyphosis or compression fractures of the vertebrae.

Mediastinum

The mediastinum contains all thoracic organs except the lungs. The heart occupies a large portion of the mediastinum, and the shape of the heart varies with age, degree of respiration, and patient position. Other organs contained within the mediastinum include the thyroid and thymus glands and nervous and lymphatic tissues (Fig. 3.10).

Radiographically, the mediastinum is divided into three sections: (1) The anterior mediastinal masses generally arise from the thyroid gland, thymus gland, or lymphatic tissue; (2) the middle mediastinal masses are commonly lymphatic tissue; and (3) the posterior mediastinal masses usually arise from nervous or bony tissue.

In infants, the mediastinum appears wide because the thymus is normally large in a healthy infant. In frontal projections, it may extend beyond the heart borders and caudally to the diaphragm, and in a lateral projection, it may fill the anterior portion of the mediastinum, which is normally radiolucent later in life. This radiographic appearance is readily visible in both PA and lateral views and is referred to as the "sail sign" because of its characteristic appearance (Fig. 3.11). Diagnosis is difficult because the width of the upper mediastinum varies greatly with the phase of respiration. A crying child may present an opportune moment for the technologist to make an exposure, but the resultant Valsalva maneuver adds to the distortion of the thymus. The Valsalva maneuver increases both the intrathoracic pressure and the intraabdominal pressure by asking the patient to inhale deeply and hold the breath to force the diaphragm and chest muscles against a closed glottis. True mediastinal masses are rare in infants and generally represent congenital malformations or neoplasms. In the mediastinum of older adults, the aorta dilates, and the aortic knob becomes much more visible.

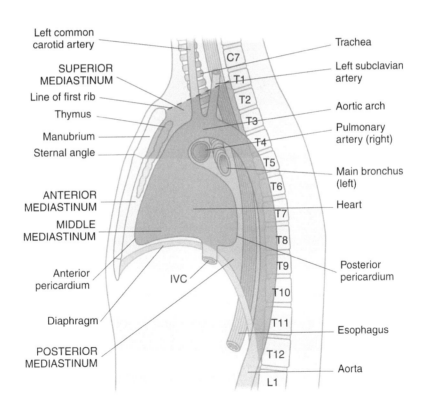

FIG. 3.10 Sagittal view of the mediastinum.

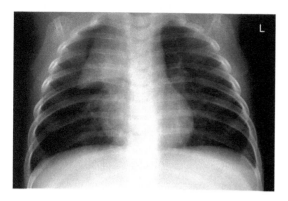

FIG. 3.11 Normal enlargement of the thymus in a 3-month-old infant demonstrates the "sail sign," evidenced by the uniform density increase in the right upper lung area.

Mediastinal emphysema (pneumomediastinum) occurs when there has been a disruption in the esophagus or airway and air is trapped in the mediastinum (Fig. 3.12). It may result from chest trauma, endoscopy, or violent vomiting. When unaccompanied by a pneumothorax, spontaneous mediastinal emphysema is usually self-limiting, subsiding in a few days without complication. Air in the mediastinum from rupture of the esophagus (usually from vomiting) or a major bronchus (usually from trauma) is more serious and requires prompt diagnosis and surgical intervention. An esophagogram may be performed with a water-soluble contrast agent to verify that a leak has not occurred.

When the pneumomediastinum is extensive, air may pass from the mediastinum into the subcutaneous

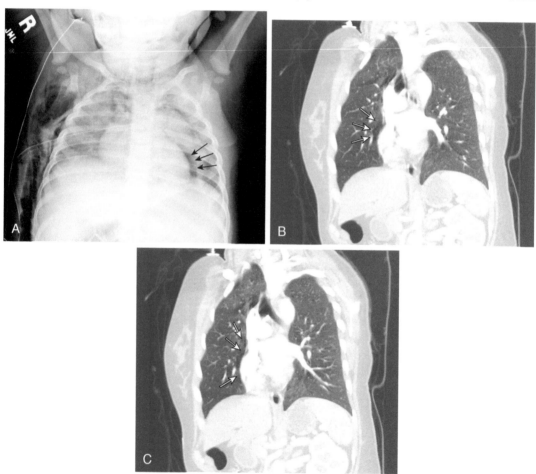

FIG. 3.12 A, Portable pediatric anteroposterior chest radiograph demonstrating a pneumomediastinum; B and C, Oblique coronal chest computed tomography scan demonstrating a pneumomediastinum around the heart.

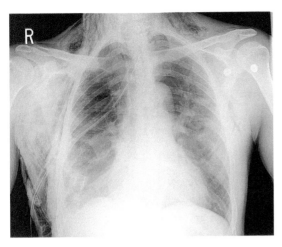

FIG. 3.13 Significant subcutaneous emphysema seen throughout the thorax, especially extending along the right border of the chest.

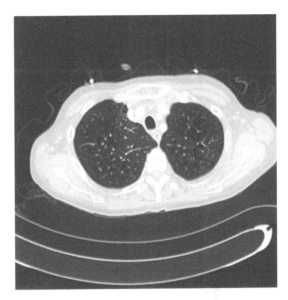

FIG. 3.14 High-resolution computed tomography scan of a normal chest.

tissues of the chest or neck, resulting in **subcutaneous emphysema** (Fig. 3.13). Diagnosis of this may be made by feeling air bubbles in the skin of the chest or neck.

Glandular enlargements of the thyroid gland are demonstrated by a displacement or narrowing of the trachea. The thyroid gland is usually located superior to the lung apices, but an ectopic thyroid gland may also displace the trachea. Clinical manifestations of an ectopic thyroid gland are often absent, and the mass may be discovered accidentally when chest radiography is performed for some other purpose.

In some instances, a routine chest radiograph may be requested upon admission to the hospital, but for stable patients, this must be based on specific clinical indications such as a need for cardiac monitoring or the presence of extrathoracic disease. Although many institutions routinely obtain mobile chest radiographs for all patients in the intensive care unit, recent research indicates that the diagnostic and therapeutic value of routine chest radiography is low in this population. On the basis of current evidence, the American College of Radiology (ACR) suggests that routine mobile chest radiography indications include, but are not limited to, patients with acute cardiopulmonary conditions, monitoring and/or life-support devices, those who are critically or medically unstable, and those of old age or with a clinical condition

preventing transport to the imaging department. In cases involving the placement of an endotracheal tube, central venous line, arterial line, and chest tubes, radiographs should only routinely be obtained upon placement of the device. Follow-up chest radiography should not be routine for these patients and should be performed based on appropriate clinical indications.

Computed Tomography

Volumetric CT offers the advantage of imaging the entire chest with one breath hold, which allows for better evaluation of the chest, especially the diaphragm area. Advances in CT software allowing for high-resolution, thin-slice thicknesses ranging from 1 mm to 1.5 mm (Fig. 3.14) and faster scan times, in combination with dynamic scanning (Fig. 3.15), have greatly enhanced the role of CT in chest imaging. CT is the method of choice for evaluation of pulmonary adenopathy. Standard radiography is only about 50% sensitive to chest disease, typically displaying advanced pathologic conditions. The excellent specificity of CT, however, may be a problem because most people have granulomatous disease, which is often benign. A rule of thumb for evaluating the character of a visualized nodule relates to its size: those less than 1 cm in size are usually benign, and those larger than 1 cm may be malignant. Also, the presence of calcium within a nodule is a reasonable

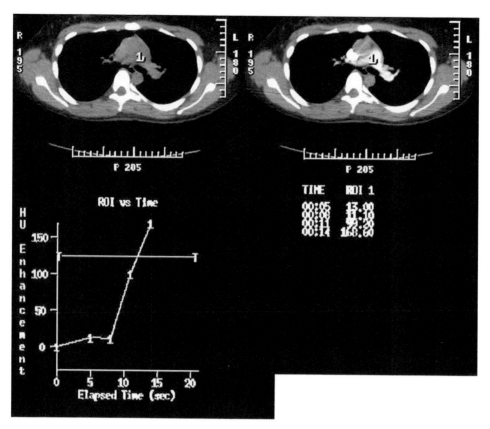

FIG. 3.15 Contrast-enhanced computed tomography (CT) of the chest using CT software to track the bolus of intravenous contrast media.

indication of benignancy, particularly in the middle of the lesion or diffusely within the nodule, but eccentric calcification may indicate malignancy.

CT is also sensitive in detecting emboli within the thoracic vessels (Fig. 3.16). In fact, the current standard of care when a pulmonary embolus is suspected is a computed tomographic angiogram (CTA) of the chest with contrast.

Chest CT is also indicated in the clinical staging of small cell lung carcinomas and in the detection of metastatic disease of the chest. Percutaneous transthoracic needle aspiration is commonly performed under CT guidance. Needle aspirations are performed to obtain cytologic specimens from lesions within the lungs (Fig. 3.17), pleural space, and mediastinum. Following the biopsy, chest radiographs may be obtained to check for a possible pneumothorax or hemorrhage.

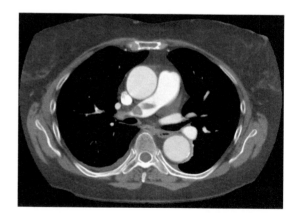

FIG. 3.16 Computed tomography scan of the lung demonstrating a massive embolism within the main pulmonary artery branches and smaller bronchial vessels.

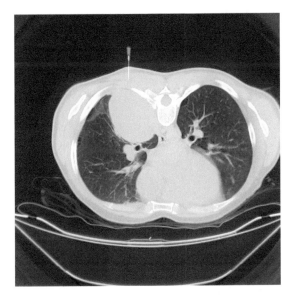

FIG. 3.17 Computed tomography–assisted core biopsy of a large right lung mass.

Nuclear Medicine Procedures

Perfusion and ventilation scans, as performed in nuclear medicine, are useful in evaluating chest disease, particularly in the case of obstructive disease and in cases of suspected pulmonary emboli when a CTA is contraindicated. Injection of a radionuclide into the venous system for a perfusion causes it to become trapped in the pulmonary circulation, allowing for γ-camera visualization of its distribution. In a ventilation scan, the patient inhales a radioactive gas (such as xenon) and holds their breath while an image is taken of the gas distribution throughout the lungs (Fig. 3.18).

Positron emission tomography (PET) captures information regarding metabolic activity. The primary imaging agent used in PET of the lungs is fluorodeoxyglucose (FDG), making it useful in distinguishing benign from malignant lesions within the chest because it has the capability of imaging an increase in glucose uptake from neoplastic cells. FDG whole body PET is useful in the evaluation of solitary pulmonary nodules and in the staging of bronchogenic carcinoma (Fig. 3.19).

Single photon emission computed tomography (SPECT) is used to analyze function of internal organs. This nuclear medicine imaging test, which is similar to a PET scan, requires a radiotracer to be introduced into

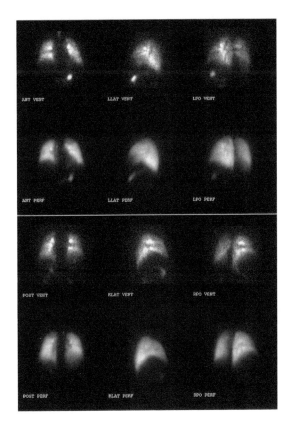

FIG. 3.18 Example of a nuclear medicine perfusion and ventilation scan performed to evaluate a possible pulmonary embolism.

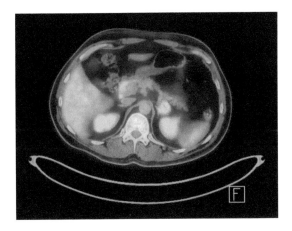

FIG. 3.19 Axial positron emission tomography and computed tomography of the abdomen used for staging bronchogenic carcinoma (same as Fig. 3.53, A).

the body. Recent research demonstrates SPECT scanning is helpful in the diagnosis of pulmonary emboli (PE) and in the evaluation of patients with chronic obstructive pulmonary disease (COPD). This imaging modality will likely continue to evolve over time as additional uses are determined.

Chest Tubes, Vascular Access Lines, and Catheters

A variety of tubes, lines, and catheters can be placed in relation to particular parts of the respiratory system. It is important for the technologist to be familiar with each of these and exercise great caution in attempting patient movement with any in place. It is best to have assistance from another technologist or nursing personnel to ensure that the lines and tubes are free of any obstructions before patient movement occurs. Furthermore, the technologist who is unsure whether the patient is allowed to sit erect should always ask the patient's nurse. The x-ray tube, image receptor, and exposure technique should be established before the patient is moved. Patients in critical care units often can be erect for only a short period because of the instability of their blood pressure. Finally, it is necessary to cover cassettes

with a plastic bag to limit infection transfer and keep the cold cassette surface from touching the patient's back.

An endotracheal (ET) tube is a large plastic tube inserted through the patient's nose or mouth into the trachea. It helps to manage the patient's airway, allows for frequent suctioning, and allows for mechanical ventilation. Its proper position is below the vocal cords and above the carina (Fig. 3.20). Movement of a patient with an ET tube should be done with great caution because inadvertent displacement or extubation may leave the patient without a patent airway.

A chest tube is a large plastic tube inserted through the chest wall between the ribs. It allows drainage of air (e.g., pneumothorax) or fluid (e.g., pleural effusion or hemothorax) from the thoracic cavity (Fig. 3.21) and allows the lungs to inflate to help the patient breathe normally. Those placed lower on the chest wall are usually for fluid drainage; those placed higher are usually for air removal. After open heart surgery, a chest tube may be placed in the mediastinum for proper fluid drainage. Its location is midline, just below the sternum. The collection device attached to the chest tube must be kept below the level of the chest to allow for proper drainage. The amount of time a chest tube remains in the thorax is dependent on the amount of deflation of the lung.

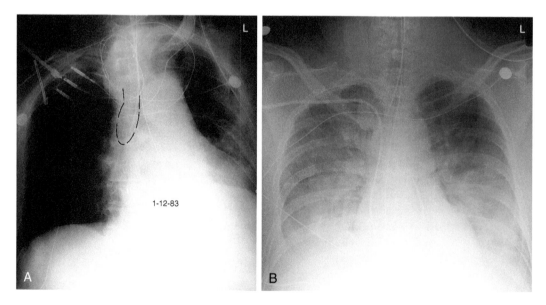

FIG. 3.20 A, Incorrect endotracheal (ET) tube placement creates a shift of the heart and mediastinum to the left with loss of air volume in the left lung. The ET tube tip lies in the proximal right main stem bronchus, inferior to the carina. B, Correct placement of the ET tube demonstrating balanced lung ventilation.

Central venous pressure (CVP) lines are usually inserted via the subclavian vein, but they may also be placed through the jugular vein, antecubital vein, or femoral vein. Proper insertion places the tip of the CVP catheter in the distal superior vena cava (SVC) just above the right atrium (Fig. 3.22). This catheter

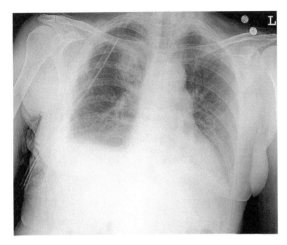

FIG. 3.21 Portable chest radiograph demonstrating proper chest tube placement in the right lung near the apex.

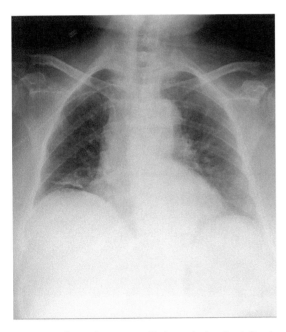

FIG. 3.22 Central venous catheter entering the left subclavian vein is positioned with the tip properly placed in the distal superior vena cava.

provides an alternative injection site to compensate for loss of peripheral infusion sites or to allow for infusion of massive volumes of fluids. In addition, it allows for measurement of CVP, which indicates the patient's fluid status and provides information about the function of the heart's right side. However, pulmonary artery catheters have largely supplanted the use of CVP lines for these purposes because they provide even greater accuracy in measurements. Chest radiographs are generally requested following the insertion of a CVP line to check for proper placement and the presence of a pneumothorax or hemothorax. Improperly placed catheters may result in cardiac arrhythmias.

A pulmonary artery catheter (Swan-Ganz catheter) is usually inserted via the subclavian vein, but other injection sites include the antecubital vein, jugular vein, and femoral vein. It is a multilumen catheter that serves to evaluate cardiac function. The pulmonary artery catheter measures pulmonary wedge pressure, reflecting left atrial pressure. It does not enter the heart's left side but is positioned in the pulmonary artery (Fig. 3.23). Inflation of the balloon at the tip of the catheter allows the tube to float into a smaller pulmonary artery capillary. Diagnosis and management of heart failure resulting from myocardial infarction and cardiogenic shock represent the most common use of the catheter.

Access catheters such as a Hickman catheter or a Port-a-Cath are usually inserted via the subclavian vein. Hickman catheters are open to the outside of the body with the tip of the catheter placed in the SVC. Port access devices are placed under the skin, just below the clavicle (Fig. 3.24). Because these devices are not open to the outside, a port access device is less likely to become infected and requires little maintenance. Access catheters allow multiple tapping for injection of various agents, typically chemotherapeutics. Patients in whom these catheters are used typically have poor peripheral venous access because of the toxic effects of chemotherapeutic drugs. Location in the subclavian vein provides ready access to the venous circulation and its blood flow return to the heart.

An intraaortic balloon pump (IABP) catheter is a specialized device typically inserted during surgery or percutaneously at the bedside in critical care units. A 40-mL balloon at the distal end of the catheter allows for inflation and deflation by a pump that is synchronized to the patient's cardiac cycle to provide mechanical support of the left ventricle. These devices reduce the workload of

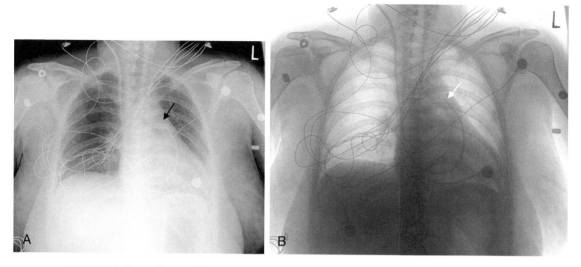

FIG. 3.23 A, Swan-Ganz catheter placement from the right interjugular vein (IJ) with the tip in the proximal right pulmonary artery. B, Inverted image of the same patient.

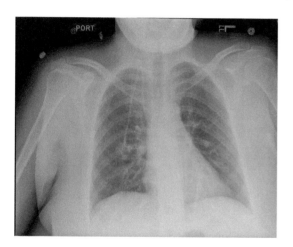

FIG. 3.24 Portable anteroposterior chest radiograph demonstrating the placement of a double port.

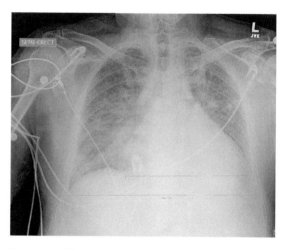

FIG. 3.25 Portable anteroposterior chest radiograph demonstrating an intraaortic pump placement.

the heart and help improve systemic blood flow, including increased blood supply to the cardiac muscle. The balloon is placed in the descending aorta below the subclavian artery and above the renal arteries (Fig. 3.25). Particular caution should be used in moving affected patients because movement may cause the balloon to float downward, possibly blocking the lower circulation.

Ventricular pacing electrodes may be placed for temporary or permanent purposes. Temporary pacing electrodes are inserted via the antecubital vein into the right ventricle. They provide electrical pacing of

the heart in patients experiencing a very slow heart rate (i.e., bradycardia) as a result of misfiring of the heart's electrical system. Also, patients who have had open heart surgery may have these electrodes placed directly on the heart's surface and brought externally beneath the sternum at midline as a temporary precaution against heart arrhythmia problems. Permanent electrodes are used for permanent heart pacing needs. The pacemaker generator is inserted under the skin, below the right clavicle, with the electrodes placed into the right ventricle (Fig. 3.26).

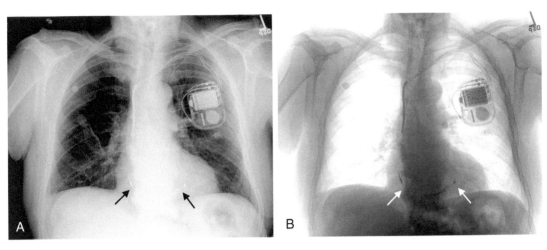

FIG. 3.26 A, Portable chest radiograph taken after pacemaker insertion demonstrating proper placement of lead wires. B, Inverted image of the same patient.

Respiratory Failure

Respiratory failure is a term used to describe a lack of respiratory function or a lack of oxygen and carbon dioxide exchange. This may occur at two levels: (1) within the lungs (intrapulmonary gas exchange) or (2) as a result of impaired breathing (inability to move air into and out of the lungs). This may occur following acute trauma to the chest or as a result of an acute or chronic lung disease. When ventilation is normal, carbon dioxide (CO_2) is removed from the lungs to maintain metabolic homeostasis at the cellular level, thus ensuring that the partial pressure of CO_2 (P_{CO_2}) in arterial blood is approximately 40 mm Hg. When P_{CO_2} levels are above 40 mm Hg, this signals that the CO_2 is not being removed properly, which denotes hypoventilation that can cause hypoxemia and hypercapnia. **Hypoxemia** denotes low oxygen levels within arterial blood and results from a failure of the gas exchange function. Common causes include toxic gas or smoke inhalation, COPD, atelectasis, severe pneumonia, high altitudes, hypoventilation, or impaired diffusion (a physical separation of gas and blood) resulting from pulmonary edema or an acute lung injury. In cases of congenital heart defects, hypoxemia may also be caused by shunting of blood from the right side to the left side of the heart without passing through the lungs. The term **hypercapnia** refers to failure of ventilation resulting in the inability to move air into and out of the lungs, with consequent increased blood CO_2 content. Hypercapnic or hypotoxic respiratory failure may be caused by upper airway obstruction, insufficient respiratory drive, respiratory muscle fatigue or paralysis, or a dysfunction of the central nervous system (CNS) resulting in a defective ventilatory pump. Individuals in respiratory failure usually exhibit tachypnea, tachycardia, irregular or gasping breathing patterns, and paradoxical abdominal motion. If the hypoxemia is acute, it may cause cardiac arrhythmias and alteration of consciousness ranging from confusion to coma.

Arterial blood gas (ABG) measurement is the primary method for diagnosing respiratory failure and for determining the severity of the failure. An arterial oxygen level (P_{O_2}) less than 60 mm Hg, an arterial P_{CO_2} greater than 45 mm Hg, or both are indicative of respiratory failure. Chest radiographs are often obtained to help identify the cause of respiratory failure. The treatment of respiratory failure includes establishing a patent airway, administration of bronchodilating drugs, and controlled oxygen therapy with the use of specialized, nonventilator masks termed *continuous positive airway pressure* (CPAP) and *bilevel positive airway pressure* (BiPAP) devices. Individuals may also be intubated and placed on a mechanical positive pressure ventilator (PPV). Care must also be taken to maintain cardiac output and to assist the failing circulation secondary to cardiac dysfunction.

Congenital and Hereditary Diseases

Cystic Fibrosis

Cystic fibrosis is a generalized disorder resulting from a genetic defect transmitted as an autosomal recessive gene that affects the function of exocrine glands. The recessive gene responsible for the development of cystic fibrosis has been localized to 250,000 base pairs of genomic deoxyribonucleic acid (DNA) on chromosome 7q. Mutations to this cystic fibrosis transmembrane regulator (*CFTR*) gene make the epithelial membrane impermeable to the chlorine ion, which leads to an increase in the absorption of sodium and water from the bronchi to blood, thus lowering the water content within the mucociliary portion of the respiratory epithelium. This dehydration of the mucous layer leads to an accumulation of viscous secretions that obstruct the airway. Cystic fibrosis involves many organs in addition to the respiratory system, and nearly all exocrine glands are affected in varying distribution and degree of severity. These glands and other organs affected include the salivary glands, small bowel, pancreas, biliary tract, female cervix, and male genital system. In the respiratory system, evidence suggests that the lungs are histologically normal at birth. Pulmonary damage is initiated by gradually increasing secretions as a result of hypertrophy of the bronchial glands, leading to obstruction of the bronchial system. The resultant plugging promotes staphylococcal infection, followed by more tissue damage, and atelectasis (collapse of lung tissue) and emphysema. Once the cycle is in motion, it is difficult to stop.

The signs and symptoms of cystic fibrosis usually include a chronic cough and wheezing associated with recurrent or chronic pulmonary infections. The cough is often accompanied by sputum, gagging, vomiting, and disturbed sleep. Barrel-chest deformity, clubbing of fingers, and cyanosis occur as the disease progresses. In adolescents and adults, pulmonary complications associated with cystic fibrosis include pneumothorax, hemoptysis, and right-sided heart failure secondary to pulmonary hypertension.

Despite increasing life spans to the age of 30 years or older, CF remains the most common lethal genetic disease in white children. Its diagnosis rests largely on a medical history of a sibling with cystic fibrosis, laboratory findings indicating elevated sodium and chloride

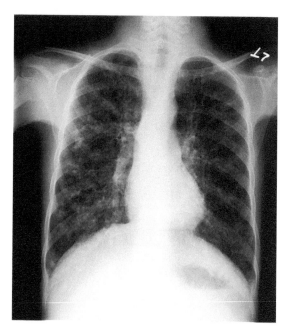

FIG. 3.27 Increased lung volume resulting from generalized obstructive disease and air trapping, which is characteristic of cystic fibrosis, as seen in this 9-year-old boy. Also seen are areas of irregular aeration with cystic and nodular densities.

levels in sweat, and genetic testing for *CFTR* gene mutations. Chest radiography aids in the diagnosis of cystic fibrosis. Radiographs taken over a period of years demonstrate gradually worsening structural abnormalities. Early changes of bronchial thickening and hyperinflation (Fig. 3.27) progress to extensive bronchiectasis, cyst formation, lobar atelectasis, scarring, pulmonary artery and right ventricular enlargement, and overinflation of the lung and chest wall. Conventional sinus radiography and CT studies of the paranasal sinuses demonstrate persistent opacification of the paranasal sinuses.

The prognosis associated with cystic fibrosis is determined by the degree of pulmonary involvement and varies greatly. However, respiratory failure resulting from deterioration of the lungs is inevitable and eventually leads to death in the 40s. Treatment methods include antimicrobial drugs to combat infection, bronchodilators administered through inhalers, respiratory physical therapy, and in some cases, a lung transplant may be performed in patients with end-stage lung disease. At this time, gene therapy is not available for cystic fibrosis.

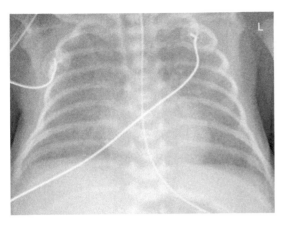

FIG. 3.28 Respiratory distress syndrome in a preterm infant. Note the "ground glass" appearance of the lungs, especially in the right perihilar area.

Respiratory Distress Syndrome

Also known as hyaline membrane disease, **respiratory distress syndrome** (RDS) is a disorder affecting premature infants or those born at less than a 37-week gestation. Incomplete maturation of the type II alveolar cells within the surfactant-producing system causes unstable alveoli, the structures in which gas exchanges occur in the lungs. Infants are particularly in need of a low surface tension in the alveoli, and surfactant (an agent that lowers surface tension) provides this. Its deficiency results in alveolar collapse with widespread atelectasis. RDS occurs more frequently in premature, white, male infants. It also occurs in premature infants of mothers with diabetes mellitus because insulin may inhibit the production of surfactant. When an increased risk is assumed before birth, corticosteroid drugs may be administered to the mother before delivery.

The signs of RDS include rapid and labored breathing within the first 24 hours after delivery with the atelectasis and respiratory failure progressively worsening. Because of the rigid lung structure, resistance develops in the pulmonary circulatory system. This may result in the development of patent ductus arteriosus, which allows blood to be shunted between the ventricles of the heart. In severe cases, respiratory and metabolic acidosis may develop because blood passing through the lungs is not adequately oxygenated and its CO_2 is inadequately eliminated.

Chest radiography demonstrates severe atelectasis with an air-bronchogram sign, characterized by bronchi surrounded by nonaerated alveoli (Fig. 3.28). This is a life-threatening condition, but if the infant's ventilation is adequately supported, surfactant production should begin within a few days. Treatment consists of maintenance of a proper thermal environment and satisfactory levels of tissue oxygenation, which is monitored frequently via ABG measurements. In some instances, pulmonary surfactant may be introduced intratracheally to reduce the severity of the disease. Once the surfactant is present, RDS will resolve in 4 or 5 days.

Inflammatory Diseases

Pneumonias

Pneumonia is the most frequent type of lung infection, resulting in an inflammation of the lung (pneumonitis) and compromised pulmonary function. Pneumonia ranks eighth among the leading causes of death in the United States and is the most common lethal nosocomial infection. The main causes of pneumoniae are bacteria, viruses, and mycoplasmas. In adults, bacteria such as *Streptococcus pneumoniae* (*Pneumococcus*), *Staphylococcus aureus*, *Haemophilus, H. influenzae*, and *Legionella pneumophila* are the most common causes of typical pneumonia. *Chlamydia pneumoniae* and *Mycoplasma pneumoniae* are common causes of atypical pneumonias in adolescents and young adults. Atypical pneumonias present less obvious radiographic signs compared with typical bacterial pneumonias. Viral pathogens such as the influenza virus, parainfluenza virus, adenovirus, and respiratory syncytial virus may cause pneumonias. In addition, fungal pneumonias may result from *Pneumocystis carinii*, especially in individuals with compromised immune systems.

The inflammation may affect the entire lobe of a lung (lobar pneumonia), a segment of a lung (segmental pneumonia), the bronchi and associated alveoli (bronchopneumonia), or interstitial lung tissue (interstitial pneumonia). Chest radiography is important in determining the location of the inflammation, with the pneumonias appearing as soft, patchy, ill-defined alveolar infiltrates or pulmonary densities. Alveolar infiltration results when the alveolar air spaces are filled with fluid or cells. Symptoms associated with pneumonia include a cough, fever, and sputum production, usually developing over days. Individuals with pneumonia often exhibit tachypnea, and during physical evaluation, crackles may be heard in conjunction with bronchial breath sounds.

Pneumococcal (lobar) **pneumonia** is the most common bacterial pneumonia because this type of

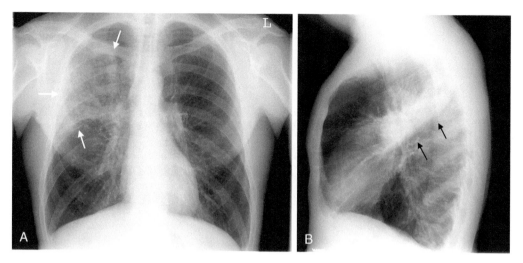

FIG. 3.29 Posteroanterior, A, and lateral, B, chest radiographs demonstrating pneumococcal pneumonia infiltrates in the upper lobe of the right lung. Note that the lateral projection clearly demonstrates the segment of the lobe affected, and the posteroanterior projection shows a faint outline of the air-filled bronchi.

bacteria is often present in healthy throats. This infection is generally preceded by an upper respiratory infection. When the body defenses are weakened, the bacteria multiply, work their way into the lungs, and inflame the alveoli. This disease is usually accompanied by chills, cough, and fever. Pneumococcal pneumonia generally affects the alveoli of an entire lobe of a lung, without affecting the bronchi themselves (Fig. 3.29). Chest radiography demonstrates collection of fluid in one or more lobes, with the lateral view serving to identify the degree of segmental involvement. Pleural fluid may often be seen in lateral decubitus projections of the chest. Antibiotics—based on Gram stain laboratory results, patient age, and epidemiology—and bed rest are the treatment for pneumococcal pneumonia, which usually resolves in approximately 1 week. Immunization with the polysaccharide pneumococcal vaccine is recommended in children under 2 years of age and in older adults, especially residents of nursing homes and extended care facilities.

Staphylococcal pneumonia occurs sporadically except during epidemics of influenza, when secondary infection with staphylococci is common. It is severe and may be fatal, especially in infants. A pneumatocele (a thin-walled, air-containing cyst) is the characteristic radiographic lesion and is more typically seen in children. These may enlarge and form abscesses in the

later stages of the disease. Another characteristic sign is the spread of patchy areas localized in and around the bronchi (Fig. 3.30). Drug therapy with particular chemotherapeutic agents is the treatment of choice.

Legionnaires' disease is the name given to a severe bacterial pneumonia that became known after it caused the deaths of four people attending an American Legion convention in Philadelphia in 1976. The causative bacterium (*L. pneumophila*) was unknown at the time of the 1976 outbreak, and its explosive effects attracted significant attention. *L. pneumophila* thrives in warm, moist places and may be transmitted through heating and cooling systems. According to the Centers for Disease Control and Prevention (CDC), approximately 8000 to 18,000 people in the United States are hospitalized and treated annually. Clinically, patients complain of malaise, muscular aches, chest pain with a nonproductive cough, and occasional vomiting and diarrhea. Outbreaks of this disease occur in large buildings such as hotels and hospitals, most frequently in late summer to early fall. *L. pneumophila* tends to affect middle-aged men more frequently than it does other groups of individuals. Risk factors include smoking, alcohol abuse, and immunosuppression from corticosteroids. Its radiographic appearance is similar to those of other bacterial pneumonias, with patchy infiltrates

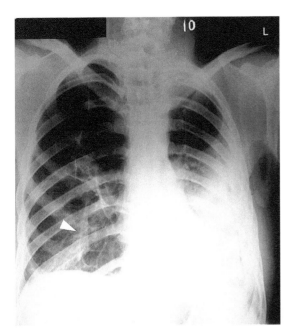

FIG. 3.30 Staphylococcal pneumonia in a 20-year-old man, indicated by multiple large pneumatoceles in the right lung and consolidation of the left lower lobe of the lung. An empyema in the lower left lung was later drained surgically.

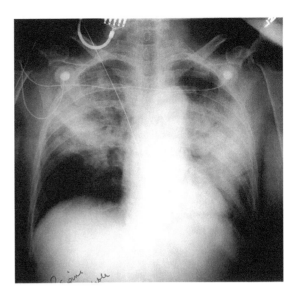

FIG. 3.31 Legionnaires' disease in a 55-year-old woman, showing rounded opacities in the upper half of the right lung and lower two thirds of the left lung.

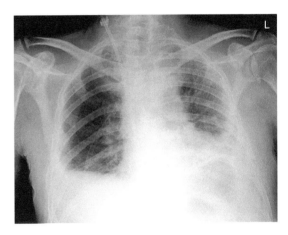

FIG. 3.32 Aspiration pneumonia caused by aspiration of gastric contents.

throughout the lungs (Fig. 3.31). Diagnosis is made by one of four methods. The two more common methods include culturing the *L. pneumophila* organism from sputum or bronchoscopy brushings and performing urinary antigen assays. Direct fluorescent antibody stain of exudate or serology using the indirect fluorescent antibody assay may also detect the presence of this disease, but both of these diagnostic methods require a high level of technical expertise. Treatment consists primarily of antibiotic administration (erythromycin or azithromycin) and oxygen therapy.

Mycoplasma pneumonia is caused by mycoplasmas, the smallest group of living organisms. They have characteristics of both bacteria and viruses. Because they do not have a typical bacterial cell wall, some confusion existed in the scientific community with regard to their classification. Currently, they are classified as "bacteria-like." *Mycoplasma* pneumonia is most common among older children and young adults. Radiographically, this disease appears as a fine reticular pattern in a segmental distribution, followed by patchy areas of air space consolidation. In severe cases, the radiographic appearance may mimic TB. The morbidity

rate associated with mycoplasma pneumonia is very low, even when the disease is not treated.

Aspiration (chemical) **pneumonia** is caused by acid vomitus aspirated into the lower respiratory tract, resulting in a chemical pneumonitis. It may follow anesthesia, alcoholic intoxication, or stroke that causes loss of the cough reflex. Chest radiography reveals edema produced by irritation of air passages (Fig. 3.32), appearing as densities radiating from one or both hila into the dependent segments. The treatment of aspiration pneumonia is strictly supportive and includes correction of hypoxia, control of secretions, and replacement of fluids. Further infection is treated by antimicrobial drugs based on laboratory results.

Viral (interstitial) **pneumonia** is caused by various viruses, most commonly influenza virus A and B. It is more common than bacterial pneumonia but less severe. This disease is spread by an infected person shedding the virus, which is transmitted to a nonimmune individual. Most cases of viral pneumonia are mild, and radiographic findings are often minimal. The diagnosis of this disease is based on clinical findings and serologic tests. Symptoms include a dry cough and fever. Complications include secondary bacterial infections, termed *superinfections*, which result from a lowered resistance brought on by the inflammatory response to the virus. Otherwise, treatment of viral pneumonia usually focuses on relief of symptoms because viral infections do not respond to antibiotic agents.

Bronchiectasis

Bronchiectasis is a permanent, abnormal dilation of one or more large bronchi as a result of destruction of the elastic and muscular components of the bronchial wall. The basic pathogenesis is either congenital or an acquired weakness, typically following inflammation of the bronchial walls, because of a viral or bacterial infection. In the early stage of the disease, the most common symptom is a chronic cough; however, some individuals may initially remain asymptomatic. As the bronchiectasis progresses, the cough becomes more productive because the weakened wall allows the bronchus to become dilated, forming a sac-like structure that harbors the pathogenic organism. As the infection grows, the bronchial wall is destroyed, resulting in an abscess. Nonreversible bronchiectasis results in saccular and varicose dilations and constrictions which are permanent alterations to the bronchial tree (Fig. 3.33). These individuals may also complain of pleuritic pain, demonstrate recurrent fevers, wheezing, and shortness of breath, or both during the physical examination.

Conventional chest radiography generally demonstrates increased bronchovascular markings and parallel lines outlining the dilated bronchi ("tram lines") because of peribronchial fibrosis and inflammation and intrabronchial secretions (Fig. 3.34). Occasionally, areas of honeycombing or cystic areas may be present. Bronchography is rarely performed in cases of

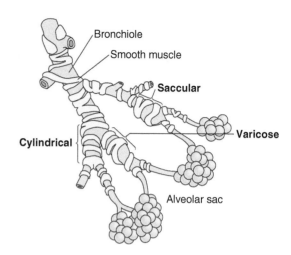

FIG. 3.33 Types of bronchiectasis.

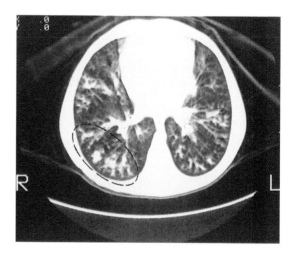

FIG. 3.34 Bronchiectatic changes are seen peripherally on this computed tomography scan of the lungs from the 9-year-old patient with cystic fibrosis.

bronchiectasis; it has been replaced by high-resolution CT (HRCT) of the chest, through which 1- to 2-mm slice images are obtained. HRCT, with or without contrast enhancement, is able to demonstrate bronchiectasis better than clinical findings and conventional radiography alone. It clearly shows dilated airways (those with a luminal diameter more than one and a half times that of the adjacent vessel in cross-section), extension of the bronchi as a result of the destruction of lung parenchyma, thickening of bronchial walls, and obstruction of airways either by a mucous plug or by air trapping (Fig. 3.35).

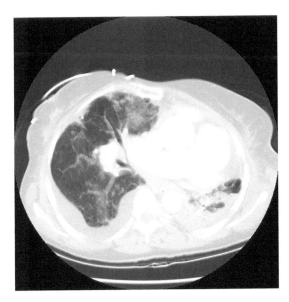

FIG. 3.35 High-resolution computed tomography scan demonstrating bilateral lung bronchiectasis with associated left lung pneumatoceles.

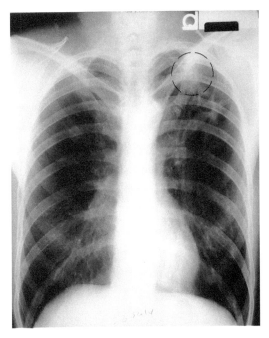

FIG. 3.36 Tuberculosis of left upper lobe in a 49-year-old man admitted with esophagitis and dull pain in the left subclavicular region.

Pulmonary Tuberculosis

Pulmonary tuberculosis is an infection caused by inhalation of *Mycobacterium tuberculosis*. Although *M. tuberculosis* generally affects the lungs, it may also affect other systems of the body such as the genitourinary system, the skeletal system, and the CNS. *M. tuberculosis* organisms are captured by macrophages within the alveoli but are not killed. This creates a cell-mediated immune response, which results in granulomatous lesions that infiltrate the tracheobronchial lymph nodes. These lesions eventually result in necrosis, fibrous scarring, and calcifications, which are visible on chest radiographs. It is more prevalent in persons born outside of the United States, individuals in correctional facilities and homeless shelters, and intravenous (IV) drug users. An estimated one third of the world's population is infected with TB. In the United States, a total of 9421 cases were reported in 2014 according to the CDC.

Early pulmonary TB is asymptomatic in 90% to 95% of cases and may be identified only with a skin test. Signs appear when the lesion or nodular scars are large enough to be seen on a chest radiograph. Lesions are most commonly seen in the apical region of the chest (Fig. 3.36); therefore, the apical lordotic projection of the chest is useful in the evaluation of TB.

The primary means for diagnosing TB requires identifying the organism from a sputum culture or by using a microbacterial nucleic acid amplification technique for laboratory confirmation. A positive response to an intradermal injection of purified protein derivative (the Mantoux test) is the primary means of diagnosing latent TB. Because reading the results of this test is not conclusive, a two-step testing procedure may be used if the first step is negative. The most common symptom is a morning cough producing minimal mucus. As the disease progresses, the cough becomes more productive, the patient may complain of dyspnea, and a spontaneous pneumothorax or pleural effusion may develop.

If the patient is in good health, and the bacterial load is fairly small, healing with scarring of the lung tissue is the most common result of infection. The presence of TB scars may be demonstrated radiographically in the apex of one or both lungs. These scars result from the body's immune system surrounding the bacilli with fibrous tissue, which invades and destroys the infectious agent. Fibrocaseous TB is usually the course of the disease if the patient demonstrates active signs of TB. Necrosis is a prominent feature of the disease because

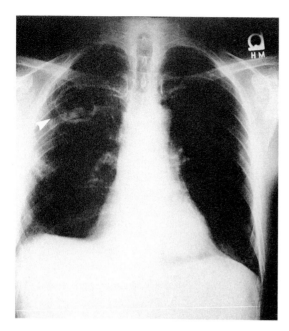

FIG. 3.37 Cavitation in the right lung resulting from expansion of tubercular lesion.

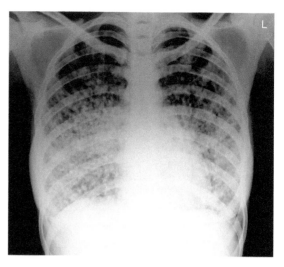

FIG. 3.38 Miliary tuberculosis (TB) resulting from hematogenous spread of TB, demonstrating small, distinct nodules throughout the lung fields.

its infiltration affects the lung parenchyma. This infiltration may expand and produce the formation of a cavity (cavitation) (Fig. 3.37). If these cavities spread to communicate with the bronchus, the bacteria are spread throughout the lung. In older adults, dormant TB may reactivate and remain undiagnosed for weeks or months. Infection spreads to the lobar or segmental bronchus, causing a persistent pneumonia resistant to antibiotic therapy. As a result, these individuals are especially susceptible to **miliary tuberculosis,** which occurs when large numbers of bacteria are picked up and carried via the bloodstream throughout the body. *Miliary* refers to its characteristic resemblance to millet seeds, which are small, white grains (Fig. 3.38). Initially, the disseminated miliary pattern may not be radiographically identifiable, but when disseminated TB is suspected, chest radiography should be repeated in a few days to better visualize the millet-sized tubercles.

In immunocompromised patients, the infection is much more aggressive. It overwhelms the immune system and progresses through the lungs at a rapid rate to cause acute tuberculous pneumonia. The body does not develop fibrous tissue to surround the bacteria, so the infection spreads quickly. Without medical treatment, acute TB pneumonia may result in death within a few

months. If the particular bacterial strain is resistant to drug therapy, the result is a 50% mortality rate within a median time of 60 days.

Patients with pulmonary TB are contagious and should be placed in isolation. The bacteria are spread through sputum and airborne droplets expelled while coughing. Modern treatment of TB consists primarily of various chemotherapeutic agents that are effective and usually curative if the full course is taken. TB must be treated with at least two anti-TB drugs, including both bactericidal and bacteriostatic drugs that act through different mechanisms. In extreme cases where the disease shows drug resistance, surgical resection of a persistent TB infection may be performed to eliminate the bacteria.

Chronic Obstructive Pulmonary Disease

Chronic obstructive pulmonary disease (COPD) refers to a group of disorders that cause chronic airway obstruction. The most common forms are chronic bronchitis and emphysema, which frequently coexist and may be associated with varying degrees of asthma and bronchiectasis—two other causes of airway obstruction.

Because it may be difficult to determine whether the pulmonary obstruction is caused by chronic obstructive bronchitis, emphysema, or a combination of the two diseases, the designation COPD is commonly used.

This disease is irreversible and results in limited airflow and, in the case of emphysema, decreased elastic recoil of the alveoli. Statistics show that the mortality rate of COPD has dramatically increased over the past 20 years, and it is ranked as the third most common cause of death in the United States. In addition, the number of individuals diagnosed with COPD in the United States continues to increase each year, currently there are 15 million Americans suffering with this disease. The predominant risk factor associated with COPD is cigarette smoking. Air pollution, airborne chemical fumes, and inhalation of hazardous dust such as silica may also increase the risk of COPD but are minimal compared with the effects of cigarette smoke.

Chronic obstructive bronchitis most often arises from long-term, heavy cigarette smoking or prolonged exposure to high levels of industrial air pollution. Cigarette smoke and industrial air pollutants irritate the mucous lining of the bronchial tree and increase the susceptibility to both bacterial and viral infections. Chronic exposure to these respiratory irritants leads to hyperplasia of the mucous glands, hypertrophy of the smooth muscle, and thickening of the bronchial wall.

Persistent cough and expectoration (expulsion of mucus or phlegm from the throat) are the primary symptoms of chronic bronchitis. The effects of the disease develop slowly and progressively over months and years, gradually resulting in bronchial obstruction from excess secretion of mucus. Eventually, the lungs remain in a chronically inflated state because more air is inhaled than is exhaled. Additional signs and symptoms of chronic bronchitis include wheezing, shortness of breath, and arterial hypoxemia leading to right-sided heart hypertrophy and failure (cor pulmonale). No dependable radiographic criteria exist for a definitive diagnosis of chronic bronchitis.

Chest radiography may demonstrate hyperinflation of the lungs. Elimination of the causative agent (e.g., cigarettes) is an important first step in treatment. Pulmonary rehabilitation, including breathing exercises and physical conditioning, helps manage the disease. Antibiotics may reduce the presence of infection; adrenergic and anticholinergic bronchodilators are used to reduce bronchospasm; and oxygen therapy may be prescribed for patients with severe hypoxemia.

Emphysema is a condition in which the lung's alveoli become distended, usually from loss of elasticity or interference with expiration. It is characterized by an

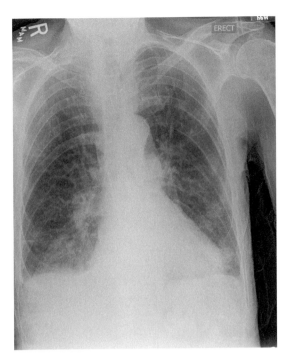

FIG. 3.39 Posteroanterior chest radiograph demonstrating hyperinflation and blunting of costophrenic angles caused by emphysema.

increase in the air spaces distal to the terminal bronchioles, with destruction of the alveolar walls.

The primary symptom of emphysema is dyspnea, which at first occurs only during exertion but eventually even at rest. In the early stages of emphysema, chest radiography may show normal results. However, as the disease progresses, hyperinflation results (Fig. 3.39), and the AP diameter of the chest increases because of increased air in the lungs. Emphysema appears radiographically as a depressed or flattened diaphragm, abnormally radiolucent lungs, and an increased retrosternal air space (barrel-shaped chest). Conventional chest radiography helps differentiate emphysema from other lung disorders such as TB or lung cancer, which have similar symptoms. Conventional chest radiography may demonstrate large bullae (>1 cm in diameter), prominent hilar markings, or blisters filled with air (Fig. 3.40), but smaller lesions are best demonstrated by CT examinations of the chest. HRCT using thin section cuts (1–2 mm) clearly demonstrate areas of hypovascularity and bullae associated with emphysema (Fig. 3.41).

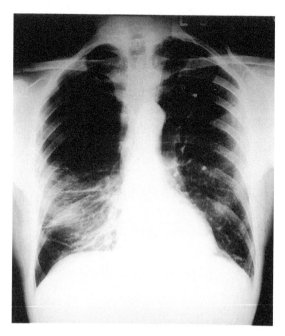

FIG. 3.40 Pulmonary emphysema with a giant emphysematous bleb occupying the upper half of the right lung.

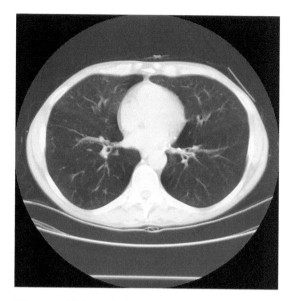

FIG. 3.41 High-resolution computed tomography scan of the chest demonstrating parenchymal changes associated with emphysema.

Treatment for emphysema is much like that for chronic obstructive bronchitis. The goals are to alleviate the symptoms, treat any reversible elements (e.g., infection), and prevent further progression of the disease, if possible.

Because these two forms of COPD represent chronic deterioration of the pulmonary system, the continued problems eventually lead to heart failure. The heart begins to wear out over time in its effort to increase blood flow to compensate for the decreased airflow caused by COPD. This may result in death from associated complications such as respiratory failure, pneumonia, cardiac arrhythmias, or pulmonary embolism. However, some individuals may live for many years with COPD and will eventually develop pulmonary edema and cor pulmonale. Both these conditions are discussed in Chapter 4.

Asthma is a chronic inflammation of the bronchial system resulting in airway obstruction and bronchial hyperresponsiveness. It may affect individuals at any age, most commonly before the age of 40 years. The incidence of asthma has increased over the past 20 years, and it is estimated that over 22 million individuals in the United States have this pathologic condition. Genetics play a major role in the development

of asthma. Additional risk factors include exposure to allergens, air pollution, cigarette smoke, and recurrent viral respiratory infections. The signs and symptoms of asthma include intermittent attacks of coughing, wheezing, dyspnea, and chest tightness caused by airflow obstruction. Radiography plays a limited role in the diagnosis of asthma. Diagnosis is made through the assessment of ABG tests and expiratory flow rates. Management of asthma most frequently includes the use of inhaled bronchodilators and oral corticosteroids and the administration of oxygen.

Pneumoconioses

Pneumoconioses result in pulmonary fibrosis from inhalation of foreign inorganic dust, most commonly from a particular work environment. The effects of an inhaled foreign material depend on its physical and chemical properties, the dose of the agent, and the site of deposition within the bronchial tree. The size of the dust particle inhaled is of particular importance. Most occupationally generated dusts and those occurring naturally are too large to cause pneumoconioses. Dusts greater than 10 μm are filtered out in the nasal passages or the mucous lining of the tracheobronchial tree; those smaller than 1 μm generally remain suspended in the air and are exhaled. Those most likely to be trapped are

1 μm to 5 μm. In addition to the size criterion, exposure to a substance capable of causing disease for a sufficient duration (dose) and the susceptibility of the host are factors required to cause pneumoconiosis. Fibrogenic inorganic dusts responsible for pneumoconiosis generally include silica, coal, asbestos, and beryllium.

Radiography assists in the detection and follow-up of this disease group. Lesions produced by the different pneumoconioses vary but may include nodules, cavitation, and pleural thickening. The three primary types of pneumoconioses are (1) silicosis, (2) anthracosis, and (3) asbestosis. Treatment is focused on preventing infection, relieving any respiratory symptoms, and maintaining adequate oxygenation.

Silicosis, the oldest known pneumoconiosis, results from inhaling silica (quartz) dust and is common among miners, grinders, and sand-blasters. It is the most widespread and most serious type of pneumoconiosis. This disease occurs following 10 to 30 years of exposure to silica dust. Phagocytes located within the bronchioles carry silica dust into the septa of the alveoli. In response to the foreign dust particles, the alveoli form large amounts of fibrous connective tissue, thus destroying normal lung tissue. This disease is clearly visible on conventional chest radiographs as multiple small, rounded, opaque nodules throughout the lungs, resulting from the creation of the fibrous tissue. With the exception of lung transplantation, no treatment exists for silicosis. Therefore prevention through the use of protective masks and adequate ventilation is the key to controlling this occupational disease.

Anthracosis (black lung disease) results from inhalation of coal dust (Fig. 3.42) over an extended period of about 20 years. As coal dust is deposited in the lungs, "coal macules" develop around the bronchioles and cause their dilation. This dilation does not affect the alveoli or the airflow; thus, impairment of the function of the lungs and the lung architecture is limited. Other than suppressing coal dust in the work environment to prevent anthracosis, no real treatment for anthracosis exists, and usually efforts to treat this condition are futile.

Asbestosis results from the inhalation of asbestos dust, which causes chronic injury to the lungs. Asbestos dust is found in building materials and insulation. Radiographically, diffuse, small irregular or linear opacities may be demonstrated in the lower lungs, and diaphragmatic pleural calcifications suggest asbestosis. Pleural changes in asbestosis are considered far

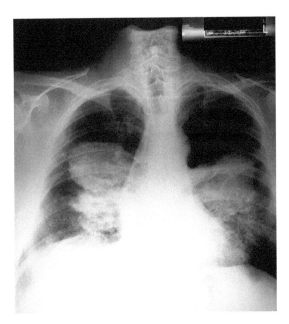

FIG. 3.42 Chest radiograph demonstrating large perihilar nodules. Thoracotomy revealed heavy anthracotic pigmentation, with the two largest nodules containing black fluid, consistent with anthracosis.

more striking than parenchymal changes. Pleural thickening may also be present. This disease may be prevented by effectively suppressing asbestos dust in the air of the work environment. Because of a heightened awareness of asbestosis, advances in industry, and the use of occupational face mask ventilators, the incidence of asbestosis has decreased, and further advances are likely to eliminate it in the United States. A cumulative, extended exposure to asbestos dust has been shown to increase the risk of mesothelioma, a rare malignant neoplasm of the pleura. This neoplasm develops at least 15 years after a high exposure to asbestos.

Fungal Diseases

Fungi are plants without chlorophyll and are widely found in nature. Many fungi found in nature are not usually pathogenic unless they enter a compromised host. Therefore most severe fungal infections are termed *opportunistic*. They are more likely to disseminate, causing severe illness in patients undergoing therapy with corticosteroids or immunosuppressants or in individuals with human immunodeficiency virus (HIV) infection, diabetes mellitus, bronchiectasis, emphysema, TB, lymphoma, leukemia, or serious burns.

Histoplasmosis is a systemic fungal infection caused by a dimorphic fungus, *Histoplasma capsulatum*, which thrives in the soil, especially soil that is fueled by bird or bat excreta. The infectious agent, which is particularly endemic to the Ohio, Missouri, and Mississippi River valleys, enters the body through the respiratory system. Most cases are classified as acute primary histoplasmosis and are so mild that they may go undiagnosed. Symptoms of acute primary histoplasmosis are nonspecific and include fever, cough, and general malaise. However, if the immune system is not effective at controlling and overcoming the fungal infection, it may spread from the lungs to other parts of the body. This condition is termed **progressive disseminated histoplasmosis.** This is considered an opportunistic infection in acquired immunodeficiency syndrome (AIDS), often leading to severe acute pneumonia. Disseminated histoplasmosis that leads to cavitary formations (chronic cavitary histoplasmosis) is more serious. The cavities resemble those in TB, often affecting the apical portion of the lungs. Dyspnea, cough, and fatigue may persist for months or even years. Diagnosis of histoplasmosis is made by histologic laboratory analysis. Chest radiography eventually may reveal small calcifications as a late manifestation of the disease, although these do not usually appear for 4 or 5 years (Fig. 3.43).

Less than 1% of those who acquire histoplasmosis require treatment because most forms of the disease (acute primary histoplasmosis) are self-limiting and may remain undiagnosed. If undiagnosed, however, advanced cases such as chronic cavitary histoplasmosis may result in death. Antifungal therapy is used to treat progressive disseminated histoplasmosis when first diagnosed, and patients with AIDS often receive intermittent doses of IV antifungal medications necessary for chronic suppression of the infectious agent.

Coccidioidomycosis is also a systemic fungal infection. It is caused by a dimorphic fungus, *Coccidioides immitis*, which thrives in semiarid soil, particularly the southwestern United States and northern Mexico. Infective spores in the soil become airborne by winds, digging, or other disruptions. For this reason, agricultural and construction workers are particularly at risk. As with histoplasmosis, most primary coccidioidomycosis infections are mild, usually self-limiting, and may

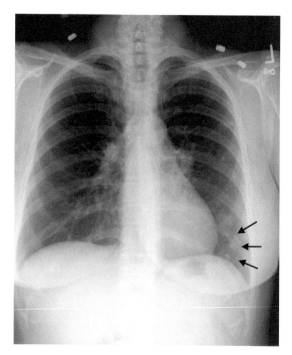

FIG. 3.43 Posteroanterior chest radiograph demonstrating old histoplasmosis with calcified nodes in left lower lobe.

go unrecognized. The most common radiographic finding of primary coccidioidomycosis, if present, is a small area of pulmonary consolidation. Lesions may comprise nodules of varying sizes that appear similar to malignant nodules and thus require biopsy or surgical excision. The typical treatment is bed rest because most occurrences are mild. However, in a few cases, progressive coccidioidomycosis may develop weeks or months after the primary infection, especially in immunosuppressed individuals. If disseminated coccidioidomycosis is not treated, it may lead to meningitis. The treatment for meningeal coccidioidomycosis must be continued for many months or years. Progressive coccidioidomycosis could be a deadly disease, as over 70% of individuals infected with HIV who develop this disease die of disseminated coccidioidomycosis within 1 month of initial diagnosis.

Lung Abscess

A lung abscess is a localized area of dead (necrotic) lung tissue surrounded by inflammatory debris. These abscesses may result from periodontal disease, pneumonia, neoplasms, or other organisms that invade the lungs. Lung abscess is more common in the right lung because of the vertical orientation of the right main bronchus. When the abscess reaches a bronchus, it drains into the bronchus forming a cavity (cavitation), which is visible on a chest radiograph. Clinical manifestations of a lung abscess include fever, cough, expectoration of pus, and foul sputum. Radiographically, an abscess generally appears as a lobar or segmental consolidation that becomes globular in shape as pus accumulates, or it may appear as a round, thick-walled capsule containing air and fluid. CT may be used to provide better anatomic information or to detect cavity formations. Empyemas consist of an accumulation of pus in the pleural cavity, usually caused by some primary lung infection. They may be caused by the invasion of a lung abscess that results in a bronchopleural fistula.

Treatment of an abscess and empyema centers on treatment of the primary condition causing it, including antibiotic therapy, chest physical therapy, postural drainage, and possible drainage of fluids via bronchoscopy. If the abscess is resistant to antibiotics, surgical resection of the abscess may be necessary, and in cases of multiple drug-resistant abscesses, the entire lobe may be surgically removed.

Pleurisy

Inflammation of the pleura is loosely termed *pleurisy*, a word often used to indicate inconsequential thoracic pain. True **pleurisy** is often indicative of a serious condition such as pneumonia, pulmonary embolism, TB, or malignant disease. Pain, varying in intensity, is usually distributed to one side or the other and along the intercostal nerve roots. Because the parietal layer of the pleura contains sensory receptors (the visceral layer does not), pain indicates that the parietal layer is involved in the inflammatory process.

Chest radiography does not generally demonstrate pleurisy, but it is helpful in confirming the presence of pleural fluid associated with the disease. Diagnosis and treatment of any underlying condition are important in relieving the symptoms of pleurisy.

Pleural Effusion

Pleural effusion results when excess fluid collects in the pleural cavity. It is a frequent manifestation of

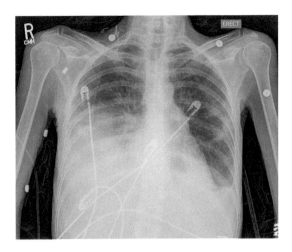

FIG. 3.44 Posteroanterior erect chest radiograph demonstrating bilateral pleural effusion with right lower lobe atelectasis.

serious thoracic disease, usually pulmonary or cardiac in origin. It should be regarded not as a disease entity, but rather as a sign of an important underlying condition. Pleural effusion may be caused by inflammation, as in pleurisy, a pulmonary embolism, or a neoplasm. These pleural effusions are termed **exudates.** Pleural effusions may also result from microvascular changes such as those associated with heart failure or ascites and are termed **transudates.** A pleural effusion containing blood is called a **hemothorax** and most frequently follows trauma to the thorax or thoracic surgery.

Conventional chest radiography is commonly used in the diagnosis of pleural effusion. The radiographic signs of pleural effusion include a blunting of the costophrenic angles (Fig. 3.44), which is often best demonstrated on an erect lateral chest radiograph. The blunting occurs as a part of the healing process, and the fibrous changes in the lung tissue may remain even after the pleural effusion has resolved. Lateral decubitus chest radiographs are also valuable (Fig. 3.45) because they can better demonstrate smaller amounts (<100 mL) of fluid in the pleural space compared with either erect PA radiographs or lateral chest radiographs. In severe cases, an entire lung may be opacified, and the mediastinum may be shifted to the contralateral side of the chest. Because a pleural effusion is indicative of an underlying medical problem, CT may be used to evaluate the lung parenchyma in search of a neoplasm, abscess, or pneumonia hidden by the effusion. Diagnostic sonography is also an excellent modality for locating or localizing pleural effusion (Fig. 3.46) and assisting the clinician in performing thoracocentesis.

Thoracocentesis or interventional techniques may be used to remove excess fluids for symptom alleviation and laboratory analysis, and to confirm the presence and type of fluid present in the pleural cavity (Fig. 3.47). In the case of a hemothorax, blood rarely clots within the pleural cavity, so a water-sealed chest tube is placed within the pleural cavity to drain blood, provided the bleeding has stopped.

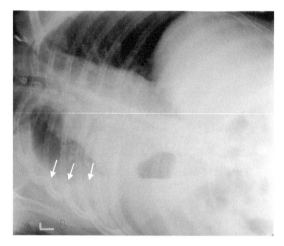

FIG. 3.45 Left lateral decubitus chest shows free pleural fluid layering out against the chest wall.

Sinusitis

The communication with the nasal cavities that subjects the paranasal sinuses to infection and inflammation is called **sinusitis**. Common causes of acute sinusitis include streptococcal, pneumococcal, *H. influenzae*, and staphylococcal bacteria. Sinusitis often follows acute viral infection of the respiratory tract, and the ethmoid sinuses tend to be the most commonly affected because of their proximity to the nose. Exposure to extremes in humidity or temperature, poor oral hygiene, the presence of a deviated septum, or all of these factors may exacerbate the condition. The symptoms of sinusitis include nasal discharge, headache, tenderness over the affected area, a toothache, and general malaise.

Radiography is important in the diagnosis of sinusitis. CT is the modality of choice because it clearly demonstrates the swollen mucous membrane and retained exudate caused by the infection. Although upright sinus radiographs do demonstrate the increased density and possible air–fluid levels (Fig. 3.48) from both mucosal swelling and fluid accumulation, CT provides better definition of the extent and degree of the sinusitis (Fig. 3.49). Chronic sinusitis may cause nasal polyps.

Treatment of sinusitis typically involves a saline nasal spray, antibiotic therapy, and an analgesic for pain relief. A deviated septum that contributes to sinusitis can be corrected surgically, if necessary.

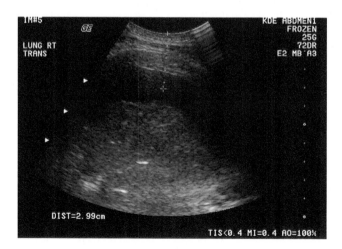

FIG. 3.46 Sonograms demonstrating pleural effusion, which help the clinician in preparation for performing a thoracocentesis.

Neoplastic Diseases

Bronchial Carcinoid Tumors

Bronchial carcinoid tumors (adenomas) are usually considered benign but are included in the World Health Organization's classification of "lung cancer" because they tend to invade local tissues, sometimes metastasize to regional lymph nodes, and are treated much like other malignant neoplasms. They are rare in occurrence, accounting for less than 1% of all lung tumors. Bronchial carcinoid tumors occur equally in both sexes, generally affecting adults in their mid-40s, and often have a prolonged course of disease. Although they are adenomas,

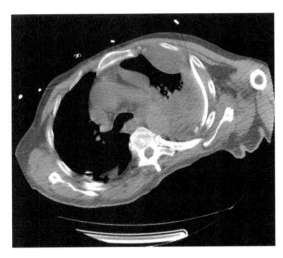

FIG. 3.47 Chest computed tomography scan for placement of a pigtail catheter into the pleural space to drain a large, loculated pleural effusion.

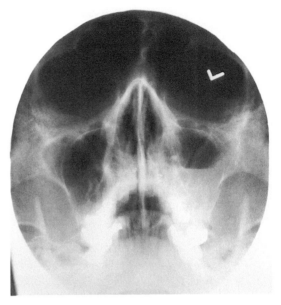

FIG. 3.48 Air–fluid level present in the left maxillary sinus reflects sinusitis secondary to an oral–antral fistula in this 26-year-old woman.

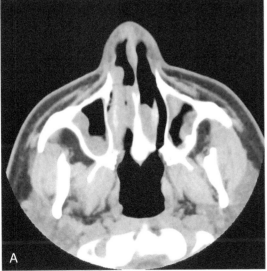
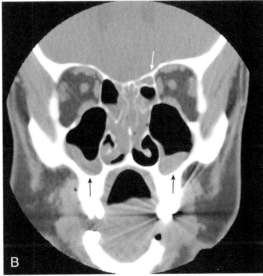

FIG. 3.49 A, Axial and B, coronal computed tomography scans of paranasal sinuses, demonstrating bilateral mucosal thickening of the maxillary sinuses and opacification of the nasal cavity.

they rarely produce the endocrine symptoms associated with most carcinoid tumors. Bronchial carcinoid tumors are slow growing and often asymptomatic. The radiographic appearance of this neoplasm shows opacity; bronchial narrowing, obstruction, or both; and possible collapse of the affected segment of the lung. Bronchial obstruction is the most common presentation, and recurrent pneumonia within the same area of the lung, in combination with pleural pain, is a common occurrence in affected individuals. If the disease is discovered before metastasis, surgical resection may be curative.

Bronchogenic Carcinoma

Bronchogenic carcinoma, the most common fatal primary malignancy in the United States, accounts for over 90% of all lung tumors and has a very low 5-year survival rate (20%). Interestingly incidence in lung cancer have been declining since 2001 which reflects the pattern of smoking prevalence. It accounts for more deaths in males and then in females and usually occurs in individuals between the ages of 45 and 70 years, especially among cigarette smokers. Lung cancers are divided into two major categories: (1) non–small cell lung cancer (NSCLC) and (2) small cell lung cancer (SCLC). The four main histologic types of bronchogenic cancer are (1) squamous cell carcinoma, (2) adenocarcinoma, (3) undifferentiated large cell carcinoma (NSCLC); and (4) undifferentiated small cell carcinoma (SCLC) (Fig. 3.50). These tumors arise from epithelial tissue in the major bronchi near the hilar area and metastasize via the lymph nodes, the bloodstream, or both. Adenocarcinomas are the most common type of bronchogenic cancers, accounting for almost 40% of the cases diagnosed in the United States. A decline in the incidence of squamous cell carcinoma has been noted over the past 20 years, with this tumor currently accounting for about 30% of all bronchogenic cancers. Undifferentiated large cell carcinomas and small cell carcinomas occur equally in approximately 10% to 15% of individuals diagnosed with bronchogenic cancer; however, small cell carcinoma has a much higher mortality rate, accounting for about one quarter of deaths from lung cancer in the United States.

In addition to a thorough patient history, chest radiography is essential for the diagnosis of bronchogenic carcinoma. The most common radiographic presentation of squamous cell carcinomas is airway obstruction caused by a unilateral hilar mass (Fig. 3.51); however,

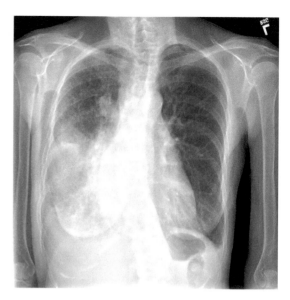

FIG. 3.50 Posteroanterior chest radiograph demonstrating advanced small cell lung carcinoma.

the lesion must be larger than 6 mm to be visible on a conventional radiograph. As the tumor grows, it may occlude the bronchus, producing atelectasis and pneumonitis. These secondary effects provide more opacity radiographically than does the actual tumor. Adenocarcinomas usually are relatively small and are found in the peripheral regions of the lung parenchyma. The radiographic presentation of this neoplasm consists of a solitary radiopaque lung nodule, sometimes called a **coin lesion.** Histologic confirmation is necessary to make a definitive diagnosis.

CT is essential in demonstrating nodules smaller than 6 mm, which are not visualized with conventional chest radiography. CT has the ability to show calcifications to help differentiate malignant lung tumors from benign and is useful in staging the disease by demonstrating the presence or absence of spread to the lymph nodes in the thoracic and upper abdominal areas. Malignant lesions are rarely calcified (Fig. 3.52), whereas benign lesions generally have a calcified center. Staging bronchogenic carcinoma is critical to the selection of treatment for the disease. CT or PET imaging can assist in determining metastases to the liver, brain, and adrenal glands (Fig. 3.53, A and B), so it is now common practice to include a portion of the upper abdomen during an oncologic CT examination of the chest and from the base of the skull through the midfemur during a PET scan. Advances in

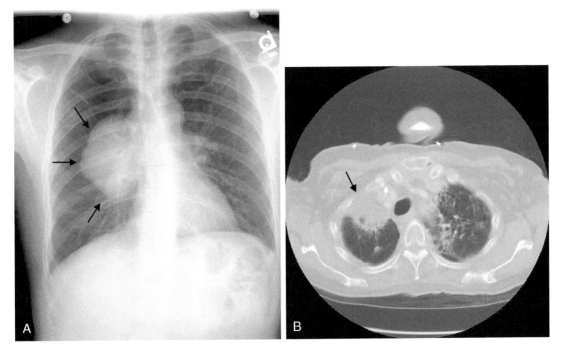

FIG. 3.51 A, Bronchogenic carcinoma in a posteroanterior projection, indicated by a large right hilar mass. B, Chest computed tomography scan demonstrating a large bronchogenic mass in the anteromedial aspect of the right lung with a cavitary lesion just above the level of the right main stem bronchus.

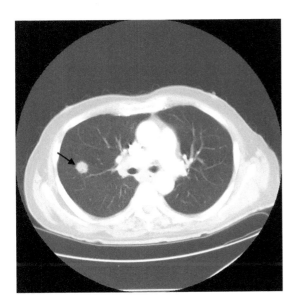

FIG. 3.52 Chest computed tomography scan of a bronchogenic lesion (*arrow*) in the upper lobe of the right lung.

technology have made it possible to perform virtual bronchoscopy to assess the location and extent of the carcinoma. Thoracic magnetic resonance imaging (MRI) is of limited value, but it is helpful in assessing tissue planes and the chest wall before surgery and in cases where apical tumors have invaded the vertebral column. Nuclear medicine bone scans may be used to screen for bone metastases, which are often confirmed with either conventional skeletal radiography or MRI.

The patient may undergo percutaneous lung biopsy, bronchoscopy, or brush biopsy. During a brush biopsy, a device with tiny brushes is introduced through a bronchoscope or bronchial catheter to procure cells and tissues under fluoroscopic guidance.

The prognosis is very poor for bronchogenic carcinoma, with a 5-year survival rate of only 12% to 14%. Fairly good results are associated with a lobectomy in individuals with peripheral nodular lesions; however, second primary lesions occur in 6% to 10% of survivors. Small cell tumors tend to be the most deadly because

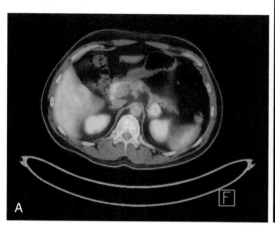

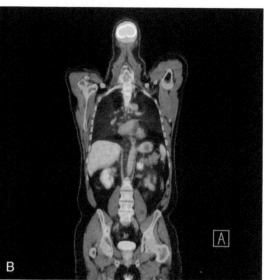

FIG. 3.53 A, Axial and B, coronal positron emission tomography and computed tomography demonstrating metastasis of bronchogenic carcinoma to the left adrenal gland.

the cancer almost always has metastasized before diagnosis. Cigarette smoking is, by far, the most important etiologic factor, accounting for over 90% of cases in men and over 80% of cases in women. Exposure to potentially carcinogenic substances from air pollution and occupational exposure are also etiologic factors.

This disease process may be treated with surgery, chemotherapy, external radiation therapy, brachytherapy, or any combination of these modalities, depending on the type, location, and stage of disease. Chemotherapy, radiation therapy, or a combination of both may be administered before surgical resection, and radiation therapy may also be used for palliative treatment to control the pain associated with skeletal metastasis, spinal cord compression, or brain metastasis (Fig. 3.54). Recent research has led to developments in targeted growth factor receptor therapy, gene therapy, antiangiogenic therapy, and immunotherapeutic treatments. As mentioned earlier, CT, MRI, SPECT, and PET scans are all vital in staging the carcinoma and determining the optimal treatment. In addition, CT of the chest and upper abdomen should be performed for all patients before surgical resection.

Metastases from Other Sites

Pulmonary metastases are much more common than primary lung neoplasms. Many malignancies progress to pulmonary metastases, which are detectable on chest

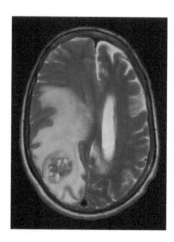

FIG. 3.54 Axial magnetic resonance imaging of the brain, demonstrating metastatic spread from a primary bronchogenic neoplasm.

radiographs. The most common primary sites for these tumors are the breast, the gastrointestinal tract, the female reproductive system, the prostate, skin (melanoma), and the kidneys.

Malignancy spreads to the lungs from a primary site via five different routes: (1) through the bloodstream in hematogenous metastases, (2) through the lymph system in lymphogenous metastases, (3) by direct extension in local invasion, (4) through the tracheobronchial system in

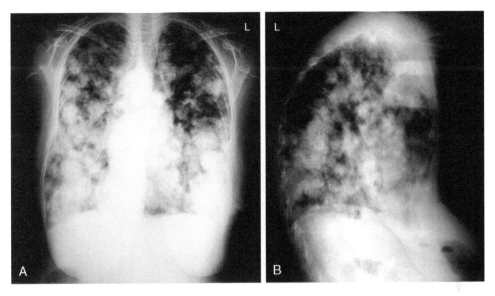

FIG. 3.55 A, Pulmonary metastases from uterine cancer demonstrate multiple lesions with the characteristic "cotton ball" appearance. B, Lateral projection of pulmonary metastases resulting from uterine cancer.

bronchogenic metastases, and, rarely, (5) by direct implantation from biopsies or other surgical procedures. Radiographically, these metastatic lesions appear as single or multiple rounded opacities throughout the lungs (Fig. 3.55, A and B). CT is more sensitive than conventional chest radiography in the detection of small metastatic lesions.

Pathology Summary the Respiratory System

Pathology	Imaging Modality of Choice
Cystic fibrosis	Chest radiography
Respiratory distress syndrome	Chest radiography
Pneumonias	Chest radiography
Bronchiectasis	Chest radiography, high-resolution chest CT
Tuberculosis	Chest radiography, chest CT
COPD	Chest radiography, high-resolution chest CT
Pneumoconioses	Chest radiography
Fungal disease	Chest radiography
Lung abscess	Chest radiography, chest CT
Pleurisy	None
Pleural effusion	Chest radiography, chest CT, sonography
Sinusitis	Sinus CT
Bronchial adenoma	Chest CT
Bronchogenic carcinoma staging	Chest CT, FDG-PET
Metastatic lung disease	Chest CT, FDG-PET, brain MRI

COPD, Chronic obstructive pulmonary disease; *CT,* computed tomography; *FDG-PET,* fluorodeoxyglucose–positron emission tomography; *MRI,* magnetic resonance imaging, *SPECT,* single photon emission computed tomography.

Review Questions

1. By use of what radiographic position can bony structures such as clavicles be removed from the apices of the lungs?
   a. Anteroposterior
   b. Lateral decubitus
   c. Lordotic
   d. 45-degree oblique

2. The "sail sign" in an infant is commonly associated with enlargement of the:
   a. Heart
   b. Pulmonary arteries
   c. Thymus
   d. Thyroid

3. Posterior mediastinal masses most commonly originate from_____tissue.
   a. Lymphatic
   b. Nervous
   c. Thymus
   d. Thyroid

4. An infant born after only 6 months of gestation could have:
   a. Cystic fibrosis
   b. Respiratory distress syndrome
   c. Mediastinal emphysema
   d. Pectus excavatum

5. Lack of respiratory function or lack of proper oxygen and carbon dioxide exchange best describes:
   a. Cardiac arrest
   b. Cardiac arrhythmia
   c. Respiratory failure
   d. Tachypnea

6. Which of the following is the most common type of bacterial pneumonia?
   a. Aspiration pneumonia
   b. Legionnaires' disease
   c. Pneumococcal pneumonia
   d. Streptococcal pneumonia

7. Loss of elasticity of the bronchial walls, as a result of bacterial infection, may result in:
   a. Bronchiectasis
   b. Bronchogenic carcinoma
   c. Pneumococcal pneumonia
   d. Tuberculosis

8. Pulmonary fibrosis resulting from occupationally inhaled dusts is characteristic of:
   a. Atelectasis
   b. Chronic bronchitis
   c. Pleural effusion
   d. Pneumoconiosis

9. An accumulation of pus in the pleural cavity is known as a(n):
   a. Coin lesion
   b. Empyema
   c. Pleural effusion
   d. Pleurisy

10. The most common etiologic factor in the development of bronchogenic carcinoma is:
    a. Automobile emissions
    b. Cigarette smoking
    c. Dust
    d. Iatrogenic treatment

11. Explain how technical exposure factors must be changed to compensate for the additive and subtractive pathologies of the chest. Give one example of each type of pathology.

12. Specify the reasons for obtaining chest radiographs taken in the erect position at a 72-inch source-to-image distance.

13. What specialized radiographic projection of the chest is used to demonstrate tuberculosis? Why is this projection of benefit?

14. Chronic obstructive pulmonary disease (COPD) includes both emphysema and chronic bronchitis. Compare and contrast these two pathologic conditions, and explain how both can be considered COPD.

15. Metastasis to the lungs from other primary tumors occurs via five routes. What are they?

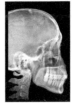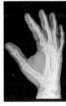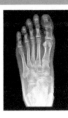

Cardiovascular System

http://evolve.elsevier.com/Kowalczyk/pathology/

LEARNING OBJECTIVES

On completion of Chapter 4, the reader should be able to do the following:

1. Describe the anatomic components of the cardiovascular system.
2. Explain the appearance of the various portions of the heart on conventional chest radiographs.
3. Describe each segment of the cardiac cycle.
4. Discuss the role of other imaging modalities in the diagnosis, treatment, and management of cardiovascular disorders.
5. Differentiate among the major congenital anomalies of the cardiovascular system.
6. Identify the pathogenesis of the diseases cited and the typical treatment(s) for each.
7. Describe, in general, the radiographic appearance of each of the given pathologies.

OUTLINE

Anatomy and Physiology
  Heart
  Cardiac Cycle
  Circulatory Vessels
Imaging Considerations
  Radiography
  Echocardiography
  Nuclear Cardiology
  Computed Tomography
  Magnetic Resonance Imaging
  Angiography

Congenital and Hereditary Diseases
  Patent Ductus Arteriosus
  Coarctation of the Aorta
  Septal Defects
  Transposition of the Great Vessels
  Tetralogy of Fallot
Valvular Disease
Congestive Heart Failure
  Left-Sided Failure
  Right-Sided Failure

Cor Pulmonale
Degenerative Diseases
  Atherosclerosis
  Coronary Artery Disease
  Myocardial Infarction
Aneurysms
Venous Thrombosis
Pulmonary Emboli

KEY TERMS

2-D echocardiography
Adventitia
Aneurysm
Arteries
Atherosclerosis
Atrial septal defects
Capillaries

Cardiomegaly
Coarctation of the aorta
Congestive heart failure
Cor pulmonale
Coronary artery disease
Diastole
Dissecting aneurysm

Doppler echocardiography
Ductus arteriosus
Embolization
Endocardium
Epicardium
Foramen ovale

87

Fusiform aneurysm

Gated cardiac blood
  pool scans

Heart

Infarct

Intima

Ischemia

Lumen

Media

M-mode
  echocardiography

Murmur

Myocardial perfusion
  scan

Myocardium

Patent ductus arteriosus

Percutaneous
  transluminal
  angioplasty

Permanent
  catheterization

Phlebitis

Pulmonary embolus

Rheumatic fever

Right and left atria

Right and left ventricles

Saccular aneurysm

Sinoatrial node

Stent

Systole

Tetralogy of Fallot

Thrombolysis

Thrombophlebitis

Thrombus

Transesophageal
  echocardiography

Transjugular
  intrahepatic
  portosystemic shunt

Transposition of the
  great vessels

Valvular stenosis

Veins

Venous thrombosis

Ventricular septal
  defects

Anatomy and Physiology

The cardiovascular system consists of the heart, arteries, capillaries, and veins and may be further divided into two subsystems of circulation: (1) The *pulmonary circulation* transports blood between the heart and lungs for exchange of blood gases, and (2) the *systemic circulation* transports blood between the heart and the rest of the body.

Heart

The **heart** acts as a pump to propel the blood throughout the body via the circulatory vessels. It lies in the anterior chest within the mediastinum and is generally readily visible on a chest radiograph. The interior of the heart is divided into two upper chambers, termed the **right and left atria,** and two lower chambers, termed the **right and left ventricles** (Fig. 4.1). Note that the heart lies in an oblique plane within the mediastinum; therefore, a conventional posteroanterior (PA) chest radiograph does not clearly demonstrate all chambers of the heart.

A frontal projection of the chest shows a cardiac silhouette, with two thirds of the heart lying to the left of midline; the right side is composed mainly of the right atrium, and the left side is composed mainly of the left ventricle. The right ventricle lays midline within the cardiac shadow and is located anterior to the right atrium and left ventricle. The left atrium is located midline and is the most posterior aspect of the heart (Fig. 4.2). Therefore it is necessary to obtain a lateral projection of

the chest to best demonstrate the right ventricle and the left atrium. In a lateral projection of the chest, the right ventricle constitutes the anterior portion of the cardiac silhouette, and the left atrium and the left ventricle constitute the posterior portion of the cardiac shadow (Fig. 4.3).

The heart contains three tissue layers. The innermost layer, termed the **endocardium,** is smooth. The valves located within and between the various chambers are also composed of endocardium. Although the valve tissue is relatively thin, in a normal heart, it is able to prevent the backflow and passage of blood when the valve is closed. The middle layer is muscular and is termed the **myocardium.** This is the thickest layer of heart tissue, and the cardiac muscle receives blood supply from the right and left coronary arteries, which arise directly from the aorta, just superior to the aortic valve. When the myocardium contracts (systole), blood is pumped out of the heart. The outermost layer is a protective covering termed the **epicardium.** The entire heart is enclosed within a pericardial sac, which contains a small amount of fluid to lubricate the heart as it contracts and relaxes, thus reducing friction between the heart and other mediastinal structures.

In the normal heart, the right atrium receives deoxygenated blood from the body via the superior and inferior venae cavae. The deoxygenated blood passes through the right atrioventricular or tricuspid valve into the right ventricle. The right ventricle contracts during systole, thus propelling blood to the lungs through the pulmonary

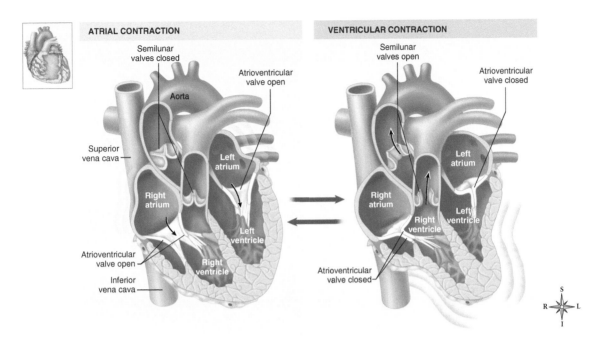

FIG. 4.1 Blood flow through the heart.

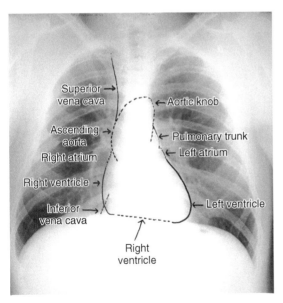

FIG. 4.2 Posteroanterior chest radiograph with heart chambers and great vessels outlined.

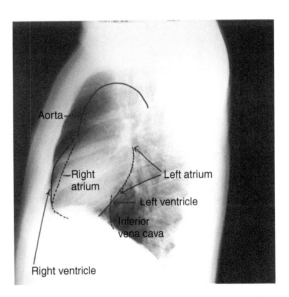

FIG. 4.3 Lateral chest radiograph with heart chambers and great vessels outlined.

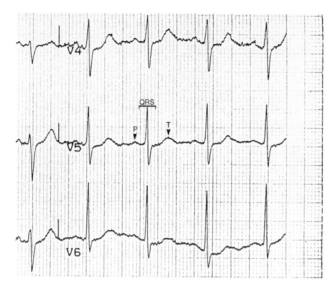

FIG. 4.4 Electrocardiogram demonstrating P wave, QRS wave, and T wave.

valve and pulmonary trunk, which bifurcates into the right and left main pulmonary arteries, respectively. Approximately 60% of deoxygenated blood enters the right lung, and approximately 40% enters the left lung.

The exchange of gases occurs at the capillary–alveolar level within the lungs, and the now-oxygenated blood is returned to the left atrium via the four pulmonary veins. Oxygenated blood flows from the left atrium to the left ventricle via the left atrioventricular, or mitral valve. The left ventricle is responsible for pumping oxygenated blood throughout the systemic circulatory system; therefore, the left ventricle has a thicker layer of myocardium and contracts with greater force than does the right ventricle. Oxygenated blood flows through the aortic valve into the aorta when the left ventricle contracts.

Cardiac Cycle

The contraction of the myocardium is termed **systole**, and the subsequent relaxation is termed **diastole**. The pacemaker of the heart is the **sinoatrial** (SA) **node**, which is located in the upper portion of the right atrium near the superior vena cava. An electrical current is transmitted through the myocardium, resulting in a heartbeat.

Electrocardiography graphically demonstrates this electrical activity. The elements of an electrocardiogram (ECG) include the P wave, PR interval, QRS complex, T wave, and QT duration (Fig. 4.4). The P

wave is the graphic display of the spread of the electrical impulse from the atria. The PR interval shows the amount of time required for the electrical impulse to travel from the SA node to the ventricular muscle fibers. The spread of the electrical impulse through the ventricles is displayed by the QRS complex, and the period in which the ventricles recover from the spent electrical impulse is graphically displayed by the T wave. The QT duration represents the total time from ventricular depolarization (QRS) to ventricular repolarization (T).

Circulatory Vessels

Arteries are blood vessels that carry blood away from the heart and are generally named for their location or the organ they supply (e.g., splenic artery). They are composed of three layers. The outermost layer is termed the **adventitia,** the middle layer is the **media,** and the innermost layer is the **intima.** The internal, tubular structure of the vessel is termed the **lumen.** **Veins** are blood vessels that carry blood to the heart. They are composed of the same three layers; however, venous walls are thinner than arterial walls, and veins contain valves at set intervals to help with blood return to the heart. **Capillaries** are microscopic vessels that connect arteries and veins (Fig. 4.5). They are responsible for the exchange of substances necessary for nutrient and waste transport.

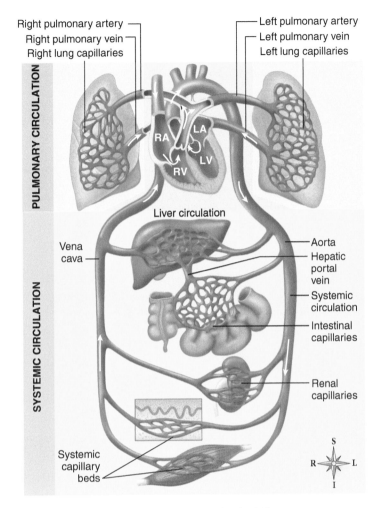

FIG. 4.5 General systemic circulation.

Imaging Considerations

Radiography

Several imaging modalities play an important role in the evaluation of the cardiovascular system and the management of cardiovascular disease. Chest radiography provides information about heart shape and size. Chest radiography is also excellent for demonstrating the great vessels and vascular changes within the lung fields. Radiographers do need to be aware that many factors may affect the cardiac image.

Factors that the radiographer can control include patient posture, degree of inspiration, correct positioning, geometric factors, and exposure technique selection. Whenever possible, chest radiographs should be taken with the patient in the erect position. If a patient is semirecumbent or recumbent, the heart appears to be enlarged because abdominal organs push the diaphragm and the heart superiorly into the thoracic cavity. It is important to identify cases in which the patient is not able to assume the erect position to aid the physician in diagnosis and interpretation.

Chest radiographs obtained without a good inspiration also distort heart shape and size (Figs. 4.6 and 4.7). Keep in mind that at least 10 posterior ribs should be visible within the lung fields on a chest radiograph taken with a good inspiration. The sternoclavicular

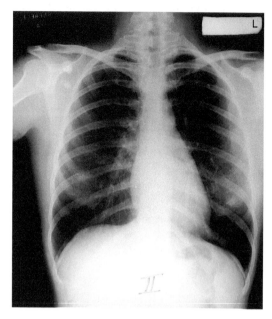

FIG. 4.6 Posteroanterior chest radiograph with adequate level of inspiration.

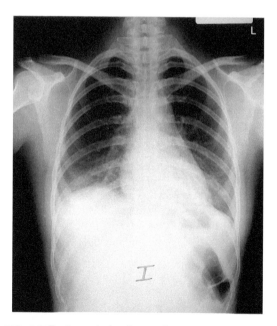

FIG. 4.7 Posteroanterior chest radiograph with expiration on the same patient as in Fig. 4.6; note the enlargement of the cardiac shadow on this radiograph.

joints should be an equal distance from the spine, and the scapulae should be rolled laterally out of the lung fields on a well-positioned PA chest radiograph. To position a patient for a lateral chest radiograph, the arms and shoulders should be placed above the patient's head to ensure that they are superior to the apices.

Geometric factors affecting heart shape and size include source-to-image receptor distance (SID) and object-to-image receptor distance (OID). Conventional chest radiographs are generally obtained using a 72-inch SID to decrease magnification of the heart to an approximate factor of 10%. Again, it is important to document variations in SID to aid in the proper diagnosis of heart disorders. Because the heart is fairly anterior in the mediastinum, it is preferable to obtain PA chest images, whenever possible. This places the heart closest to the image receptor, allowing for the smallest OID. Positioning the patient for a PA projection also helps decrease magnification of the cardiac silhouette. A third geometric factor that is frequently overlooked is the anode-heel effect. Radiographers can use this phenomenon to their advantage by placing the anode over the apical region and the cathode toward the base of the lungs, when possible, thus distributing the radiographic density more evenly throughout the chest radiograph.

Adequate penetration of the mediastinal structure is also critical in chest radiography and requires the use of a relatively high kilovoltage. A minimum of 100 kilovolts peak (kVp) should be used. Vascular markings within the chest help the physician assess ventricular function. The pulmonary vessels also provide information about pulmonary artery pressure. Dilation of these vessels often indicates problems with the right ventricle. Exposure times of one tenth of a second or less should be used, whenever possible, to decrease involuntary cardiac motion. It has been documented that heart motion may increase the size of the cardiac shadow. The heart may look larger if the radiograph is exposed during diastole.

In most institutions, chest radiography is the most commonly performed procedure, and radiographers all too often underestimate the importance of these basic radiographic principles. Well-positioned diagnostic chest radiographs are crucial in the diagnosis and treatment of cardiovascular disorders. In a normal adult, the transverse diameter of the cardiac shadow should be less than half the transverse diameter of the thorax on a PA erect chest radiograph. An enlarged heart is termed **cardiomegaly** (Fig. 4.8), which is indicative of many cardiovascular disorders and is a nonspecific finding.

Factors affecting cardiac shape and size that are not under the technologist's control include patient body habitus, bony thorax abnormalities, and pathologic conditions such as pneumothorax or pulmonary emphysema. Bone abnormalities of special concern include scoliosis and pectus excavatum. Individuals with pectus excavatum present a funnel-shaped depression of the sternum. The abnormal placement of the xiphoid causes displacement of the heart to the left and distortion of the cardiac shadow. Some pathologic conditions may require special tubes or lines to be inserted into the vessels or chest cavity. Vascular lines and tubes are discussed in Chapter 3 of this text.

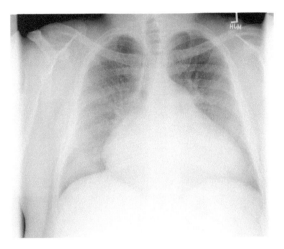

FIG. 4.8 Posteroanterior chest radiograph demonstrating cardiomegaly secondary to congestive heart failure.

Echocardiography

Echocardiography encompasses a group of noninvasive sonographic (ultrasound) procedures that can provide detailed information about heart anatomy, function, and vessel patency (Fig. 4.9). Sonographic imaging may be performed using M-mode, two-dimensional (2-D) imaging, spectral Doppler, color Doppler, or stress echocardiography.

M-mode echocardiography uses a stationary ultrasound beam to provide an examination of the atria, ventricles, heart valves, and aortic root, allowing evaluation of left ventricular function. The "M" refers to motion, as this technique allows for the recording of the rate of motion and the amplitude of moving objects. This technique has the advantage of being able to demonstrate subtle motion of the cardiac structures. M-mode cardiac sonography is also used to measure the thickness of the ventricular walls; however, it has largely been replaced

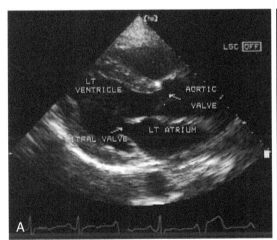
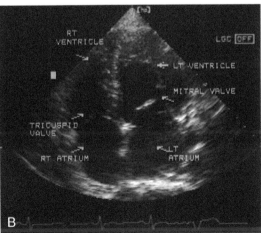

FIG. 4.9 A, Echocardiographic visualization of heart anatomy of a 47-year-old man as seen in a parasternal sagittal view. B, Coronal view of the same heart demonstrated by echocardiography.

by **2-D echocardiography.** Use of 2-D imaging allows for spatially correct, real-time imaging of the heart. It provides multiple tomographic projections of the heart and great vessels in a cinelike (dynamic imaging) presentation. In addition, it is an excellent modality for visualizing the ascending and descending thoracic aorta in cases of suspected aneurysm. Both M-mode and 2-D images are obtained by placing the transducer over the thorax at the sternal borders, at the cardiac apex, between the ribs, or at the suprasternal notch. Smaller transducers have been developed to allow for **transesophageal echocardiography** (TEE), in which the patient swallows a mobile, flexible probe containing the transducer. With TEE, the heart's structure can be readily visualized without interference from such structures as the skin, rib cage, and chest muscles. It is especially helpful in imaging the aortic arch and root.

Intravascular ultrasound (IVUS) is commonly performed following angioplasty with stent placement or during cardiac catheterization to provide for accurate measurement of the vessel lumen and to determine the plaque volume and type. In IVUS, smaller transducers are placed on intravascular catheters to assess vessel anatomy and blood flow. Stress echocardiography combines an exercise test with an echocardiogram to check the heart's contraction ability and its pumping efficiency. If exercise is not possible, a drug, dobutamine, may be used to increase cardiac output to assess how well the heart pumps during infusion.

Doppler sonography is an adjunct, noninvasive procedure used to study the peripheral vasculature. It has been a mainstay of vascular imaging since the 1970s and is used to determine the direction and velocity, as well as the presence or absence, of blood flow in both arteries and veins. The Doppler Effect is the principle that the sound coming toward you has a higher pitch than the sound going away from you. The return of pulsed ultrasound allows calculation of the shift in the direction of blood flow and creates a spectral display from which velocity is calculated (Fig. 4.10). The spectral signal is displayed on a strip chart or videotape. With Doppler sonography the flow of blood is not affected until any obstruction present is at least 60% complete. The percentage of stenosis present dictates the treatment of vascular disease, and usually this consists of surgery (e.g., endarterectomy). Such vascular

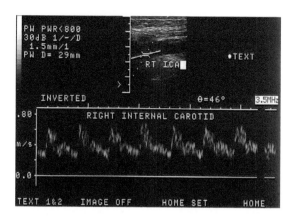

FIG. 4.10 Doppler effect with normal arterial flow in the internal carotid artery depicted above a graph of the arterial flow.

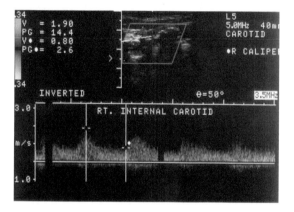

FIG. 4.11 Doppler sonogram of an abnormal internal carotid artery spectrum caused by heterogeneous calcified plaque. Note the difference in appearance of the graphic representation compared with Fig. 4.10.

imaging is said to be *duplex* in that it helps reveal physiologic characteristics, and the imaging component defines anatomy (e.g., plaque morphology). The most common conditions imaged by 2-D Doppler sonography are carotid stenosis (significantly reducing carotid angiography) (Figs. 4.11 and 4.12), lower extremity arterial stenosis, and deep venous thrombosis (Figs. 4.13 and 4.14), largely supplanting traditional venography. Blood flow may be encoded with color to differentiate blood flowing toward the transducer (red) from blood flowing away from the transducer (blue); this is termed *color Doppler echocardiography.*

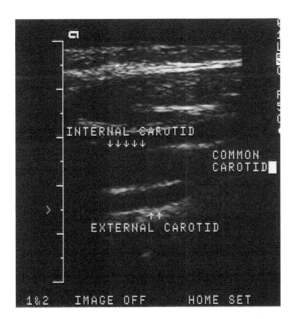

FIG. 4.12 Doppler sonogram of a normal carotid bifurcation from the common carotid into the internal and external carotid arteries.

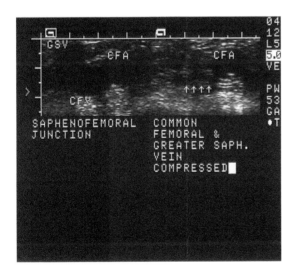

FIG. 4.13 Doppler sonographic portrayal of normal flow on the left of the image through the greater saphenous vein (*GSV*), common femoral vein (*CFV*), and common femoral artery (*CFA*). Compression on the right side of the image depicts normal closure of the common femoral vein and greater saphenous vein, as expected.

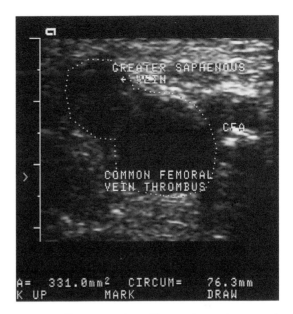

FIG. 4.14 Transverse view of the greater saphenous vein and common femoral vein indicating failure to close on compression because of the large venous thrombus contained within.

Nuclear Cardiology

Nuclear medicine procedures used in the assessment of cardiovascular disease include myocardial perfusion scans, gated cardiac blood pool scans, and positron emission tomography (PET). They are useful in assessing coronary artery disease (CAD), congenital heart disease, and cardiomyopathy.

A **myocardial perfusion scan** is the most widely used procedure in nuclear cardiology. It may be performed on patients with chest pain of an unknown origin, to evaluate coronary artery stenosis, and as a follow-up to bypass surgery, angioplasty, or thrombolysis. It is especially useful in detecting regions of myocardial ischemia and scarring (Figs. 4.15 and 4.16). In this study, a radionuclide, usually radioactive technetium sestamibi or thallium, is injected through a vein. It concentrates in the areas of the heart that have the best blood flow. Those areas lacking blood flow demonstrate filling defects, visualized by comparing images taken at rest and during stress. Stress may be induced by exercise on a treadmill or by the use of pharmaceuticals such as regadenoson. Myocardial perfusion scanning is performed

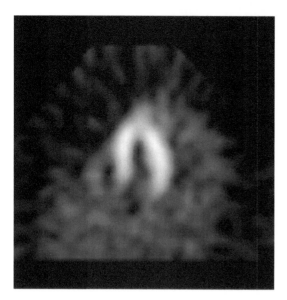

FIG. 4.15 Appearance of a normal heart on a nuclear medicine perfusion scan, with the isotope distribution equal throughout the myocardium at rest.

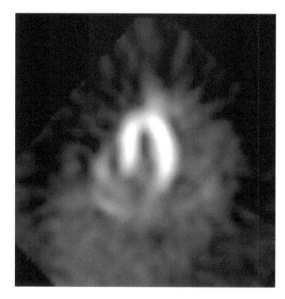

FIG. 4.16 The appearance of a normal heart on a nuclear medicine perfusion scan on the same patient as in Fig. 4.15 during exercise. Notice the increased activity in the myocardium

using single photon emission computed tomography (SPECT), allowing the camera to rotate around the patient to obtain tomographic images of the heart parallel to the short and long axes of the left ventricle. SPECT myocardial perfusion scans can detect significant CAD in 90% of patients presenting with CAD. PET may also be used for imaging myocardial perfusion employing a variety of positron perfusion and metabolic agents. A PET unit is more sensitive than conventional nuclear medicine cameras, and spatial resolution is superior to that of conventional cameras. It is highly accurate for detecting CAD that interferes with blood flow to the heart muscle and can identify injured but viable heart muscle. PET can also provide quantitative data about the distribution of the radionuclide within the body.

Gated cardiac blood pool scans, sometimes called *radionuclide ventriculograms* or *multiple gate acquisition scans (MUGA)*, are used to evaluate ventricular function and ventricular wall motion. These images are obtained with the patient at rest and during exercise. They are synchronized with the patient's heartbeat using electrocardiography to image the heart during specific phases of the cardiac cycle with the use of the radionuclide technetium-99. Images are obtained over a 5- to 10-minute period. The images are displayed in a cinelike format, allowing the wall motion of the beating heart to be evaluated. Ventricular function is assessed by calculating the ejection fraction, ejection and filling rates, and left ventricular volume.

Computed Tomography

Computed tomography (CT) is a noninvasive modality used to assess cardiac and vascular disease. Multidetector (or multislice) scanners provide the highest image quality, and electron beam CT (EBCT) may also be used to image the heart. Calcium scoring of the coronary arteries is performed without the use of a contrast agent. It was introduced in 1990, and a scoring algorithm was developed for evaluating the amount of calcium (hard plaques) present in the coronary arteries.

EBCT was introduced in the mid-1980s and is a technique used primarily to examine the heart, particularly as related to coronary artery calcifications. It uses a scanning focused x-ray beam to provide complete cardiac imaging in 50 ms—fast enough to "freeze" heart motion without the need for ECG gating. An electron gun produces an electron stream that is magnetically focused onto four tungsten targets. Each target emits two fan beams of x-rays, which are directed through the patient and registered on detectors arranged in a semicircle above the patient. The net result is that extremely thin slices are readily demonstrated, either as a cine loop or as single images. This allows for coronary calcium scoring, which may represent a predictor of atherosclerosis and current heart disease. A low calcium score implies a low risk for obstructive coronary disease. EBCT should not be relied on for a final diagnosis of CAD, as it is limited in its ability to detect noncalcified (soft) plaques. EBCT is not of value in patients with a history of a previous heart attack, angioplasty, or bypass surgery.

Multidetector volumetric CT units with specialized cardiac software are most commonly used to perform calcium scoring and have better reproducibility compared with EBCT examinations. The software enables ECG gating and fast, multiple-section scans to obtain images without interference from the normal heart motion. Images are generally captured during the R wave to acquire the image during the diastolic phase of the heart. The gating may occur prospectively or retrospectively. Images with a slice thickness of 2.5 mm are obtained, generally at 2.5-mm intervals. Images can also be obtained at much smaller thicknesses such as 0.6 mm and then reconstructed at a larger thickness, but at the cost of increased patient dose. As with EBCT, multidetector CT calcium scoring uses software to analyze the histogram information obtained during the scans and computes image and region scores.

ECG-gated CT is also used to perform noninvasive angiography (CT angiography [CTA]) allowing for the evaluation of the right and left coronary arteries, the circumflex artery, and the anterior descending artery. Currently, by using CTA, it is possible to identify a stenotic cardiac vessel in almost 70% of cases because of CTA's ability to image soft atherosclerotic plaque. Postprocessing software can reproduce three-dimensional (3-D) images of the heart to assess the coronary arteries, heart chambers, coronary stents, and coronary anomalies and to assess bypass grafts. Contrast-enhanced CT images may also be reviewed in a cine loop to allow for the evaluation of heart motion and assessment of cardiac function and perfusion.

Contrast-enhanced CTA is approved by the U.S. Food and Drug Administration (FDA). It is noninvasive (requiring only a peripheral intravenous [IV] line for contrast media administration) and is more cost-effective than conventional angiography. In combination with 3-D reconstruction, it is used to image vascular structures for organ donors, to diagnose pulmonary embolisms, to evaluate vascular stenosis and peripheral vascular disease, and to image abdominal aortic aneurysms (Fig. 4.17). CTA helps the surgeon determine the necessary stent type and size in the presurgical planning of abdominal aortic aneurysms and in the evaluation after surgery to assess the stent's effectiveness.

Magnetic Resonance Imaging

Magnetic resonance imaging (MRI) is also a common imaging modality used to evaluate many cardiac, mediastinal, and great vessel anomalies (Fig. 4.18). It may be used to evaluate myocardial wall thickness and chamber volumes and is especially helpful in diagnosing right ventricular dysplasia. MRI is highly effective in the evaluation of viable *versus* nonviable myocardium. Most protocols involve obtaining imaging sequences and putting them into motion using a cine loop to evaluate how well the valves of the heart are functioning. Like nuclear cardiology, contrast-enhanced MRI can demonstrate myocardial perfusion and blood flow velocities within the heart can be measured. The advantage of MRI is the production of images with high spatial resolution and, thus, higher quality images. As with many other imaging modalities, information may be ECG gated to acquire the images during specific portions of the cardiac cycle. MRI is a valuable tool for imaging the anatomy, function, and disease of the heart and is fast becoming a "one-stop shop" for noninvasive cardiac imaging.

MRI is also used to evaluate aortic aneurysms, dissections, and aortic stenosis, especially in patients who are unable to have contrast-enhanced CT scans because of renal failure. Contrast-enhanced magnetic resonance angiography (MRA) is widely used to evaluate the vasculature from the aorta to the brain (Fig. 4.19). This technology takes only about 1 minute to acquire data and is considered noninvasive. The larger coronary arteries may also be assessed with MRA.

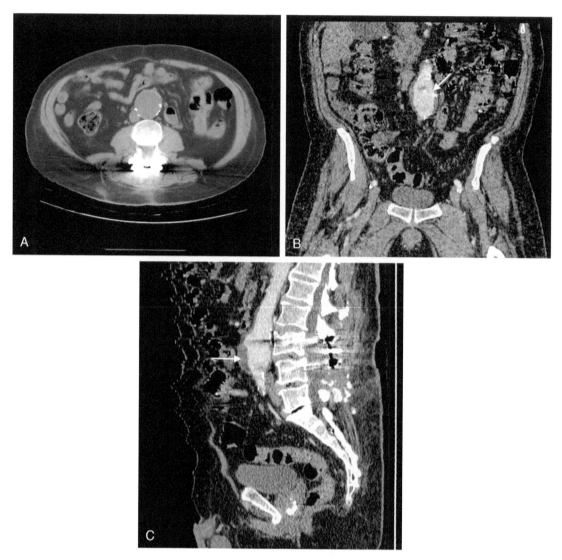

FIG. 4.17 Computed tomography angiogram demonstrating an abdominal aortic aneurysm in three planes: A, axial. B, coronal. C, sagittal.

Angiography

Angiography is a procedure commonly performed to evaluate cardiovascular disease. It may be performed for diagnostic purposes or for therapeutic reasons. As discussed earlier, traditional diagnostic angiography is being challenged by less invasive procedures such as MRA and CTA. Cardiac catheterization is an invasive procedure specific to the heart and the great vessels. It is performed in patients with CAD, conduction disturbances, or congenital heart disease and provides information about heart and vessel anatomy. Intracardiac and arterial pressures are measured as the catheter passes through the various areas of the heart. This provides information about the function of the cardiac valves. Angiocardiography is performed by injecting the contrast material

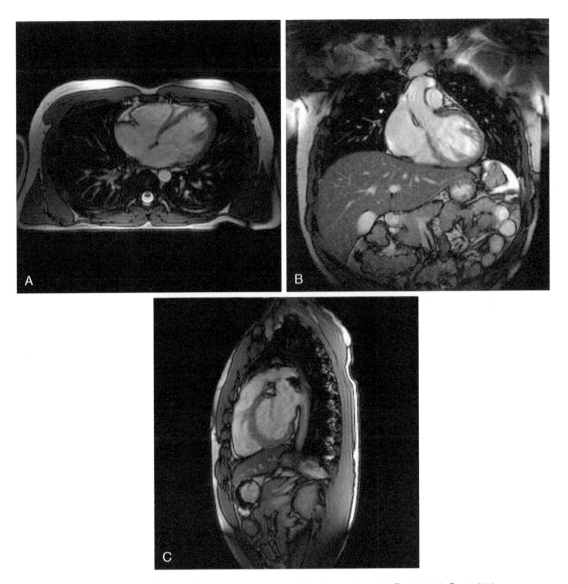

FIG. 4.18 Normal magnetic resonance image of the heart. A, axial. B, coronal. C, sagittal.

into the left ventricle of the heart and/or coronary arteries and obtaining cine images of the heart and the great vessels in motion.

Therapeutic angiography continues to steadily increase through expanded use of interventional procedures. Percutaneous transluminal coronary angioplasty (PTCA) is a therapeutic procedure commonly performed to open stenotic coronary vessels and to place a stent in a narrowed vessel to maintain its patency. Thrombolysis is a procedure in which a high-intensity anticoagulant such as streptokinase is dripped over a period of hours directly onto a clot to dissolve it (Fig. 4.20). With embolization, devices such as coils are used to clot off vessels (Fig. 4.21). Common examples of the use of embolization include clotting of vessels feeding brain tumors, arteriovenous

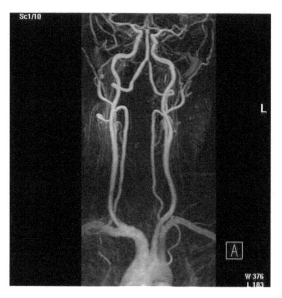

FIG. 4.19 Contrast-enhanced three-dimensional magnetic resonance angiography image of the aortic arch, carotid and vertebral arteries, and circle of Willis.

malformations, or other abnormalities of the brain to prevent excessive bleeding during open cranial surgery. In a **transjugular intrahepatic portosystemic shunt** (TIPS) procedure, a catheter is used to connect the jugular vein to the portal vein to reduce the flow of blood through a diseased liver (Fig. 4.22). Arterial stents are devices placed in arteries (Fig. 4.23), typically the iliac, aorta, renal, or coronary arteries, to open occluded vessels. Insertion of a stent is often preceded by **percutaneous transluminal angioplasty** (PTA) with a balloon catheter to open up the vessel's occlusion before stent placement (Fig. 4.24). In **permanent catheterization,** a catheter is placed in the subclavian or jugular vein and tunneled under the skin to allow for improved dialysis access. This is similar to a central venous line with a port for easy access. Inferior vena cava (IVC) filters are basket-like devices placed in the inferior vena cava to catch clots before they enter the heart (Fig. 4.25). Besides typical contrast media, some of these procedures use carbon

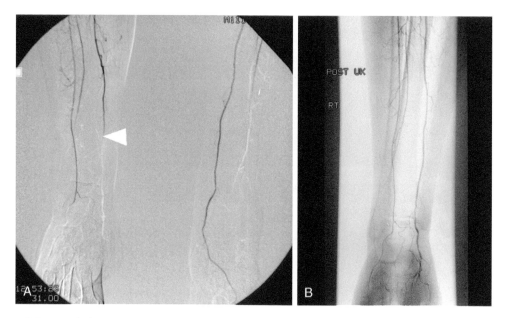

FIG. 4.20 A, An apparent embolus in the right popliteal artery prevents blood flow to the foot in this 91-year-old woman. B, In this thrombolysis procedure, urokinase is sprayed onto the embolus and allowed to drip over a 30-minute period. Patency is restored.

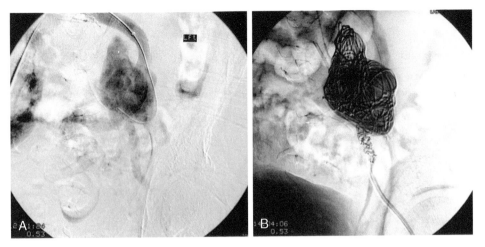

FIG. 4.21 A, A large aneurysm is seen angiographically in the left common iliac artery of this 74-year-old man. B, Embolization of this large aneurysm was accomplished by progressive insertion of a variety of coils and guidewire fragments.

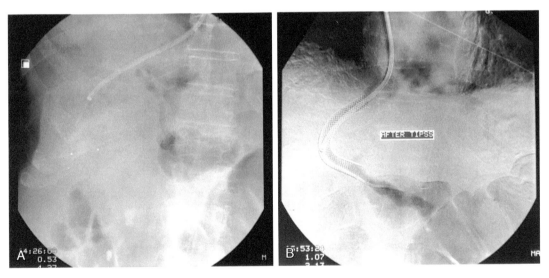

FIG. 4.22 A, A specialized catheter is used to create an opening through a cirrhotic liver of a 69-year-old man for the beginning of a transjugular intrahepatic portosystemic stent procedure. B, After dilation of the pathway, using standard angioplasty technique, a shunt is installed to connect the right hepatic vein to the right portal vein, restoring blood flow.

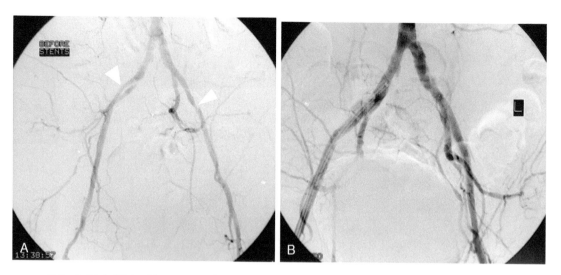

FIG. 4.23 A, Bilateral lower extremity arteriogram reveals stenosis of both external iliac arteries. B, After balloon angioplasty, stent placement in each external iliac artery results in restored flow of blood.

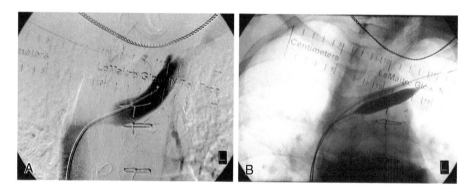

FIG. 4.24 A, Catheterization and angiography of the left brachiocephalic vein of this 56-year-old man reveal significant narrowing. B, Balloon angioplasty and a stent are used to open up the stenotic left brachiocephalic vein. Excellent blood flow was restored in subsequent images.

dioxide (CO_2) as the contrast agent in patients who do not tolerate normal agents (Fig. 4.26). The use of CO_2 is helpful in assessing patients who are in renal failure, but should not be utilized as an arterial contrast agent in sites above the diaphragm because of the increased risk for gas embolism of the spinal, coronary, and cerebral arteries. The role of interventional angiography will continue to grow and reduce costs and complications associated with certain surgical procedures it replaces.

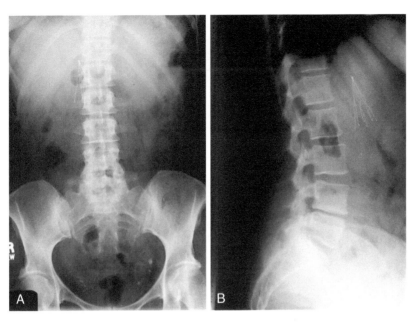

FIG. 4.25 A, Greenfield filter placement in the inferior vena cava, as seen on an anteroposterior abdominal radiograph. B, Greenfield filter placement in the inferior vena cava, as seen on a lateral abdominal radiograph.

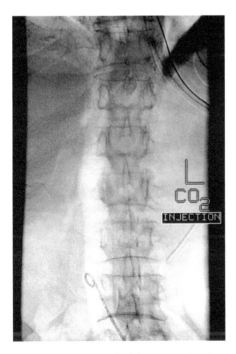

FIG. 4.26 Use of carbon dioxide as a contrast medium demonstrated in inferior vena cavogram (appearing white along the right of the spine) on a frail 75-year-old man.

Congenital and Hereditary Diseases

Because fetal circulation and blood–gas exchange occur within the placenta, certain characteristics are present in the fetal circulatory system that should normally disappear at birth. These characteristics include an opening in the septum between the atria, termed the **foramen ovale,** which allows the blood to bypass the pulmonary circulatory system, and a small vessel termed the *ductus arteriosus,* which connects the pulmonary artery and the descending aorta. If these anatomic structures persist, a variety of congenital anomalies may develop in the newborn. The incidence of congenital cardiovascular anomalies is approximately 1 per 120 live births.

Etiology of congenital heart disease includes inherited genetic disorders, chromosomal aberrations (such as Down syndrome), and environmental factors (such as drugs, alcohol, infection, radiation, and maternal disease). In addition, individuals with congenital anomalies of the heart are at an increased risk for developing endocardial infections. Immediate diagnosis to determine the type and severity of the anomaly and treatment of the cardiac anomaly are vital to survival. The outcome of the disease depends on the pressure differences created between the right and left sides of the heart, abnormal ventricular load, and defects that obstruct blood flow.

Radiography and diagnostic medical sonography play a critical role in the diagnosis and treatment of congenital anomalies, along with the diagnosis of heart murmurs by physical examination, and abnormal heart rates and ventricular hypertrophy demonstrated by ECG. A **murmur** is an abnormal heart sound resulting from disturbed or turbulent flow, often through malformed valves. Although echocardiography is generally used to diagnose congenital heart disease, MRI and CT have become valuable tools for the continued evaluation of congenital heart diseases as affected patients are living longer. Three-dimensional reconstructions allow for visualization of defects as well as any repair of the defect.

Patent Ductus Arteriosus

The **ductus arteriosus** is a temporary vessel that is used during in utero life. It shunts blood from the pulmonary artery into the systemic circulation because the pulmonary circulation is not needed during this time. If it does not close at birth, **patent ductus arteriosus** results (Figs. 4.27 and 4.28). This condition is more common in premature infants, occurring in approximately 80% of infants born before 28 weeks of gestation, especially in those with respiratory distress syndrome.

Because the left ventricle contracts with more force compared with the right ventricle, arterial blood within the aorta is shunted into the pulmonary trunk via the open ductus arteriosus instead of out into the systemic circulation. This increases the volume of blood propelled into the lungs, thus increasing pulmonary vascular congestion and the volume of blood returning to the left atrium. Infants with this condition generally have a heart murmur and display cyanotic features resulting from the shunting. Echocardiography is the imaging

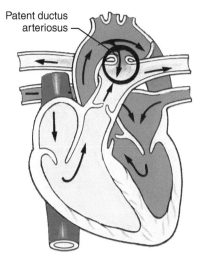

Patent ductus arteriosus

FIG. 4.27 Patent ductus arteriosus.

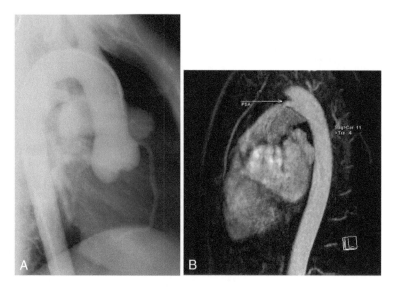

FIG. 4.28 A, Aortogram demonstrating patent ductus arteriosus. Note the filling of the pulmonary vessels as well as the aorta. B, Magnetic resonance imaging demonstrating patent ductus arteriosus.

method of choice for evaluating the severity of this anomaly and usually demonstrates a left atrial diameter larger than the aortic root. Color Doppler technology demonstrates the reverse pulmonary artery flow during diastole and shows the full length of the ductus arteriosus. Chest radiography demonstrates cardiomegaly with prominence of the left side of the heart and ascending aorta and increased pulmonary vascular congestion. In premature infants, treatment includes fluid restriction and diuresis, the use of drugs, or surgical intervention. Surgery is used as a last resort in premature infants and generally is not performed until the child is 1 to 2 years of age. In full-term infants, surgical ligation is necessary in cases of heart failure. In full-term infants without distress, elective surgery is generally performed between the ages of 6 months and 3 years to decrease the risk of the infant developing infective endarteritis.

Coarctation of the Aorta

Although the ductus arteriosus may close normally at birth, a narrowing of the aorta may occur at the junction site. This anomaly is termed **coarctation of the aorta** (Fig. 4.29); it is the cause of 7% to 8% of all congenital cardiac anomalies and is more common in boys. It occurs anatomically inferiorly to the vessels responsible for circulation to the head, neck, and upper extremities, so circulation to these anatomic regions is not affected. However, blood flow to the abdomen and lower extremities is compromised, and the femoral pulse is very weak in most individuals with this anomaly. This anomaly may lead to heart failure. Radiographically, two bulges of the aorta are demonstrated in the aortic arch region, one superior to and one inferior to the stenosis. *Rib notching*, another radiographic indication of coarctation of the aorta, refers to well-defined bone erosions along the lower rib margins as a result of the enlargement of anastomotic vessels. Coarctation of the aorta may be successfully treated surgically by removing the narrowed region of the aorta and reattaching the normal aorta superiorly and inferiorly to the coarctation.

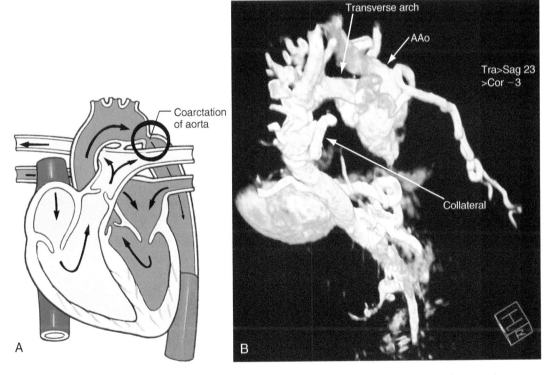

FIG. 4.29 A, Coarctation of the aorta. B, Computed tomography volume three-dimensional rendering of coarctation of the aorta.

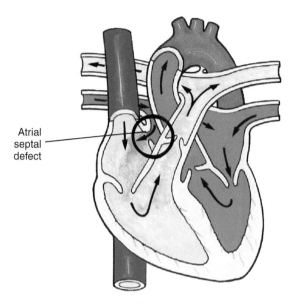

FIG. 4.30 Atrial septal defect.

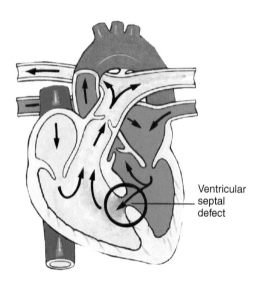

FIG. 4.31 Ventricular septal defect.

Septal Defects

A defect in either the ventricular septum or the atrial septum allows the blood to be shunted between the two chambers (Figs. 4.30 and 4.31), mixing pulmonary and systemic blood. Blood is generally shunted from the left chamber to the right chamber because of increased pressure on the left side of the heart. This shunting of the blood results in an enlargement of the right side of the heart and increased pulmonary vascularity as the lungs overload with blood.

If the foramen ovale does not close at birth, an opening remains between the right and left atria. **Atrial septal defects** are the most common congenital heart defect, responsible for about 10% of all cases of congenital heart disease. Such defects occur twice as frequently in girls as in boys and are generally detected clinically by an audible heart murmur at the upper left sternal border around the age of 1 year as well as by atrial dysrhythmias on ECG evaluation. Doppler and 2-D echocardiography may also be performed to confirm the diagnosis. Radiographically, the right atrium and ventricle are enlarged, resulting in cardiomegaly. Evidence of increased pulmonary blood flow within the lung fields is also present. In most cases, these close on their own and do not require surgical intervention. However, if surgical intervention is necessary, a preoperative cardiac catheterization may be performed to evaluate the size of the defect, left ventricular function, and the vessel anatomy.

Ventricular septal defects involve defects between the two ventricles and are more serious because the pressure difference is greater between the ventricles than between the atria. Clinically, patients with these defects also have an audible heart murmur; however, it is heard a little lower on the left sternal border and at a younger age than the murmur associated with an atrial defect. In significant cases of ventricular septal defect, the murmur may be audible in infants as young as 2 to 3 weeks old. In these cases, intervention is necessary, as signs of heart failure may develop between 6 and 8 weeks of age. In addition, these infants are at an increased risk for developing severe viral or bacterial pneumonia and infective endocarditis. Again, color flow **Doppler echocardiography** is the imaging method of choice. Radiographically, the left atrium and ventricle are enlarged, resulting in cardiomegaly (Fig. 4.32). Increased pulmonary flow is also evident in the lung fields. Surgical intervention depends on the size of the defect and the risk of developing bacterial endocarditis at the site of the defect.

Transposition of the Great Vessels

Transposition of the great vessels is an anomaly in which the aorta arises from the right ventricle instead of the left ventricle, and the pulmonary trunk arises from the left ventricle instead of the right ventricle (Figs. 4.33 and 4.34). This serious congenital defect does not allow the pulmonary and systemic subsystems to communicate and comprises over 5% of all cardiac anomalies. Deoxygenated blood returns to the right atrium, travels through the right ventricle, and

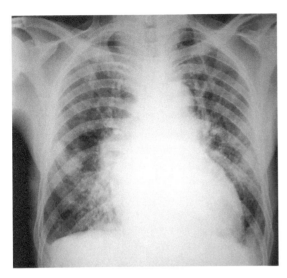

FIG. 4.32 Chest radiograph depicting ventricular septal defect. Note the enlargement of the right heart border.

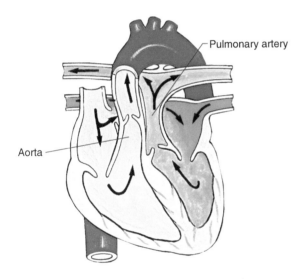

Pulmonary artery

Aorta

FIG. 4.33 Transposition of great vessels.

is pumped through the aorta back into the systemic subsystem without becoming oxygenated. Oxygenated blood returns to the left atrium, travels through the left ventricle, and is pumped through the pulmonary trunk back to the lungs for gas exchange to occur. Conventional chest radiography demonstrates a narrow mediastinum because the vessels are superimposed and the main pulmonary trunk is not in the usual location. Pulmonary congestion is also visible in the lung fields. Obviously, this anomaly is incompatible with life.

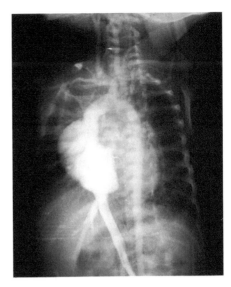

FIG. 4.34 Angiogram demonstrating transposition of great vessels. Note the "closed" system of the right side of the heart. Blood is returned via the venae cavae and redistributed via the aorta, thus bypassing the lungs.

Because immediate recognition and treatment of this defect are imperative, echocardiography is performed to confirm the diagnosis. Emergency cardiac catheterization and balloon septostomy must be performed to enlarge the opening between the atria to increase mixing of venous and arterial blood and to decompress the left atrium. Surgical correction of this anomaly is indicated within the first 10 days of life.

Tetralogy of Fallot

Tetralogy of Fallot is a combination of four defects: (1) pulmonary stenosis, (2) ventricular septal defect, (3) overriding aorta, and (4) hypertrophy of the right ventricle (Fig. 4.35). Narrowing of the pulmonary valve prevents passage of a sufficient volume of blood from the right ventricle to the lungs and results in the most common cause of cyanosis in infants with cardiovascular anomalies. Normally, the aorta should arise from the left ventricle, but in patients with tetralogy of Fallot, the aorta arises from a ventricular septal defect. In other words, it overrides the right ventricle, which, in turn, results in hypertrophy of the right ventricle. Enlargement of the right ventricle is demonstrated radiographically as a boot-shaped cardiac shadow caused by displacement of the heart apex (Fig. 4.36). Corrective surgery is usually performed after the age of 1 year.

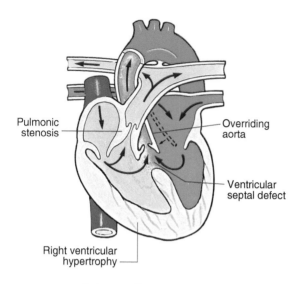

Pulmonic stenosis

Overriding aorta

Ventricular septal defect

Right ventricular hypertrophy

FIG. 4.35 Tetralogy of Fallot.

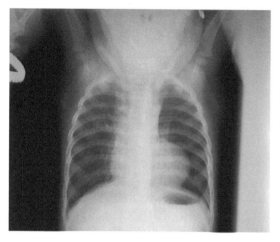

FIG. 4.36 Chest radiograph on an infant with tetralogy of Fallot. Note the "boot-shaped" cardiac shadow.

Valvular Disease

Abnormalities of the heart's valves often cause cardiac symptoms such as dyspnea, fatigue, syncope, or chest pain and signs such as murmurs. In addition, lesions of the valves often result in abnormal pulses detectable through palpation. Clinicians are often able to diagnose most valve abnormalities by assimilating historical and physical findings. Noninvasive techniques add to the precision of diagnosis, and invasive studies are reserved for surgical candidates.

The most common cause of chronic valve disease of the heart is **rheumatic fever.** This condition most frequently affects the bicuspid (mitral) and aortic valves and is more common in women than in men. Because of advances in pharmaceuticals, technology, and medical care, the incidence of rheumatic heart disease is on the decline. Rheumatic fever produces inflammatory changes within the connective tissues of the body, thus affecting the valves within the heart. It may result in stenosis, insufficiency, or incompetency. Individuals with rheumatic heart disease have a distinct heart murmur audible during physical examination.

Valvular stenosis (Fig. 4.37) is caused by a scarring of valve cusps that eventually adhere to one another. The results of valvular stenosis become apparent in adult life because it generally takes years for the scarring to affect valve function. Mitral valve stenosis inhibits blood flow from the left atrium into the left ventricle. It slows the blood flow through the lungs and the right side of the heart, resulting in an enlargement of the right side of the heart and the left atrium. Insufficiency and incompetency occur when the valves do not close properly and allow blood to reflux during systole. This complication often follows endocarditis or is seen in the case of mitral valve prolapse. Mitral valve prolapse, a genetic disease caused by an autosomal dominant inheritance, occurs in about 6% of the population and is generally diagnosed by clinical examination. Echocardiography, which is usually performed to confirm the diagnosis, has an accuracy rate of approximately 95%. Patients with mitral valve prolapse are at an increased risk for developing endocarditis, so prophylactic treatment is necessary.

Damaged valves are often replaced surgically, especially in patients experiencing symptoms of heart failure. Patients with a reduced ejection fraction diagnosed by either nuclear medicine studies or echocardiography are also candidates for surgery. These patients must receive prophylactic medication to prevent endocarditis both preoperatively and postoperatively. Cardiac catheterization is performed before surgery to assess valve function and to detect CAD. After surgery, patients are generally placed on a regimen of medications to help maintain proper cardiac function.

Radiographically, manifestations of mitral stenosis may be subtle. More progressed cases may show the heart silhouette as enlarged, with a straightening of the left cardiac border and a prominent main pulmonary

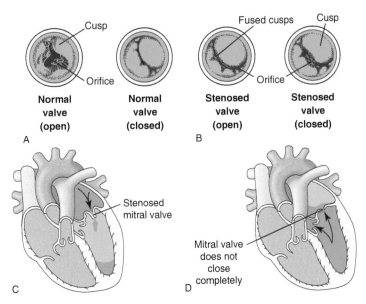

Valvular stenosis and regurgitation. A, Normal position of the valve leaflets, or cusps, when the valve is open and closed. B, Open position of a stenosed valve (*left*) and open position of a closed regurgitant valve (*right*). C, Hemodynamic effect of mitral stenosis. The stenosed valve is unable to open sufficiently during left atrial systole, inhibiting left ventricular filling. D, Hemodynamic effect of mitral regurgitation. The mitral valve does not close completely during left ventricular systole, permitting blood to reenter the left atrium.

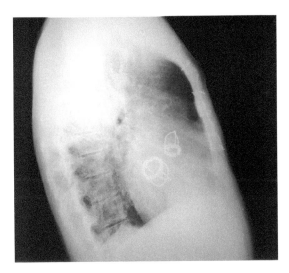

Lateral chest radiograph demonstrating two prosthetic valve replacements clearly visible within the heart.

artery. The diseased valves may contain small calcifications visible during echocardiographic or CT evaluation. Mitral valve insufficiency appears radiographically as an enlargement of the left atrium and ventricle with right upper lobe pulmonary congestion. Color Doppler echocardiography provides quantification or grading of the severity of regurgitation; however, TEE provides the most information in terms of mitral valve function. In cases of aortic valvular disease, both conventional chest radiography and echocardiography may demonstrate calcification of the cusps of the valve and hypertrophy of the septum. Left ventricular enlargement is generally present only when the left ventricular myocardium is damaged. In cases of tricuspid damage, the right side of the heart is affected, and chest radiography will reveal enlargement of the superior vena cava, right atrium, and right ventricle. The right ventricular enlargement is best demonstrated on the lateral projection radiograph of the chest. Doppler and 2-D echocardiography confirm the diagnosis by demonstrating increased dimensions in the right side of the heart. After valve replacement, the prosthetic devices are clearly visible on conventional chest radiographs (Fig. 4.38).

Congestive Heart Failure

Congestive heart failure (CHF) occurs when the heart is unable to propel blood at a sufficient rate and volume. This results in congestion of the circulatory subsystems and does not allow a sufficient supply of blood to reach the tissues of the body. CHF is most commonly caused by hypertension but may result from other disease processes that overburden the heart, such as valvular disease. CHF may affect either side of the heart, but both sides are commonly affected together. It may develop gradually or have a quick onset in combination with pulmonary edema. Regardless of the side affected initially, prolonged strain on the heart eventually affects the entire organ. Signs and symptoms may vary with the extent and location of the disease. The treatment of CHF is usually medical but depends on the cause and severity of the disease and may include surgical intervention, especially in cases of valvular disease.

Left-Sided Failure

When the left ventricle of the heart cannot pump an amount of blood equal to the venous return in the right ventricle, the pulmonary circulatory subsystem becomes overloaded. The fluid that accumulates in the capillaries of the lungs leaks into the interstitial tissue within the lungs. This results in rales and pulmonary edema, which may be a life-threatening condition. Radiographically, the heart is enlarged, and the hilar region of the lungs is congested with increased vascular markings (Fig. 4.39). During the physical examination, individuals with left-sided heart failure are found to have an increased heart rate because the heart tries to compensate for the deficiency. Individuals commonly complain of difficulty breathing or shortness of breath during exertion and respiratory distress severe enough to awaken them during the night. As the disease progresses, sleeping in a recumbent position becomes impossible. The most common cause of left-sided failure is hypertension, but other causes include aortic and mitral valvular disease and CAD.

Right-Sided Failure

Right ventricular failure is not as common as left-sided failure and occurs when the right ventricle cannot pump as much blood as it receives from the right

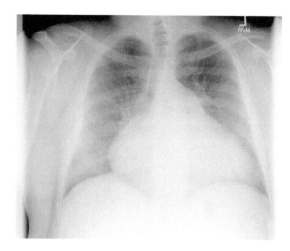

FIG. 4.39 Chest radiograph demonstrating cardiomegaly resulting from congestive heart failure.

atrium. This causes the venous blood flow to slow down, producing engorgement of the superior and inferior venae cavae and edema of the lower extremities. A common complaint from individuals with right-sided failure is swelling of the ankles. Radiographically, the right atrium and the right ventricle appear enlarged. Common causes of true right-sided failure are pulmonary valve stenosis, emphysema, and pulmonary hypertension secondary to pulmonary emboli.

Cor Pulmonale

Cor pulmonale results from a lung disorder producing hypertension in the pulmonary artery and an enlargement of the right ventricle of the heart. It may be acute, in the case of a pulmonary embolism, or chronic, as a result of chronic obstructive pulmonary disease (COPD). This disease results from alveolar hypoxia, and common symptoms include dyspnea and syncope during exertion. Patients may also experience chest pain. Conventional chest radiography reveals enlargement of the right ventricle and a proximal pulmonary artery. Echocardiography and nuclear medicine examinations are performed to demonstrate and evaluate right ventricular function. Right-sided heart catheterization may be performed to confirm the diagnosis. Patients with cor pulmonale are at an increased risk for venous thrombosis and may be placed on long-term anticoagulants.

Degenerative Diseases

Atherosclerosis

Atherosclerosis is a degenerative condition that affects the major arteries of the body, often termed *hardening of the arteries*. It is the most prevalent disease in humans and occurs in epidemic proportions in the United States. It tends to affect men at an earlier age compared with women. Atherosclerosis may occur in any artery (Fig. 4.40), but it has a predilection for the aorta, coronary arteries, and cerebral arteries (Fig. 4.41). Risk factors associated with this disorder that cannot be controlled include increased age and a strong family history of atherosclerosis. Risk factors that can be altered include decreased serum low-density lipoprotein (LDL), which is known as the "bad" cholesterol. High levels of LDL can lead to plaque buildup in the arteries. Increased levels of high-density lipoprotein (HDL), the "good" cholesterol can reduce the risk of heart disease and stroke. Other risk factors that can be controlled are hypertension, cigarette smoking, obesity, and a sedentary lifestyle. In addition, some other disease processes such as diabetes mellitus predispose individuals to atherosclerotic disease.

Atheroma formations (fibrofatty plaques) are composed of intracellular and extracellular lipids, muscle, and connective tissue. They begin as fatty streaks and progress to fibrous plaque, which collects within the vessel and reduces its ability to expand during systole (Fig. 4.42). The cause of the development of these formations within the vessel is currently being debated, but two hypotheses, the chronic endothelial injury theory and the lipid theory, are most prominent. The chronic endothelial injury theory suggests that the disease process first affects the intima, or inner layer, of the artery as a result of injury, resulting in an accumulation of platelets, monocytes, and T-cell lymphocytes at the site of injury. These cells cause a migration of the smooth muscle tissue from the media, forming a fibrous plaque. The lipid theory suggests that an increase in LDL within blood plasma causes lipid accumulation in smooth muscle cells. The LDL becomes oxidized and this modification affects the monocytes, creating fat-laden macrophages and foam cells. As these cells enlarge and project into the vessel lumen, platelets aggregate to the site. Oxidized LDL has been found to be toxic to endothelial cells and may be responsible for their dysfunction. The reality may be a combination of the

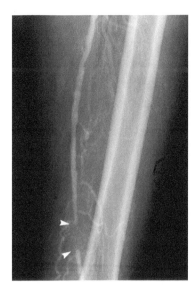

FIG. 4.40 Arteriogram from a 47-year-old man demonstrates atherosclerosis occluding the femoral artery.

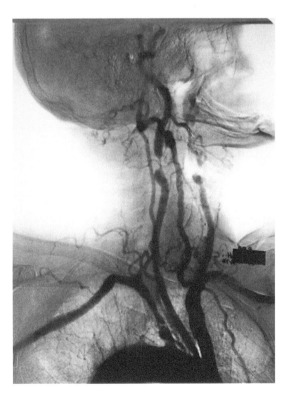

FIG. 4.41 Digital subtraction arteriogram demonstrating atherosclerotic disease of the carotid artery. Note that the carotid artery is almost completely occluded.

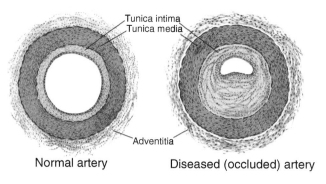

Tunica intima
Tunica media
Adventitia

Normal artery

Diseased (occluded) artery

FIG. 4.42 Development of arteriosclerosis.

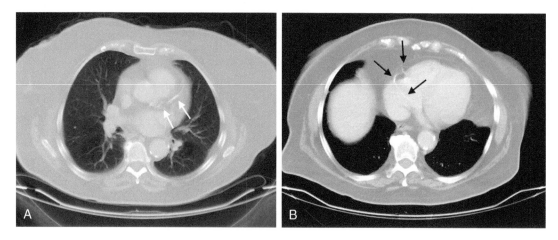

FIG. 4.43 A & B Computed tomography of chest demonstrating extensive coronary artery calcification. The patient's major complaint was shortness of breath. A, Calcifications within the superior arteries of the heart (*arrows*) and the descending aorta. B, Calcifications in the inferior arteries of the heart (*arrows*) and the descending aorta.

two theories because the oxidized LDL may injure the endothelium, attracting the monocytes and macrophages as described in the endothelial injury hypothesis. As the disease slowly progresses, the vessel becomes stenotic, and the atheroma may calcify (Fig. 4.43), hemorrhage, ulcerate, or include a superimposed thrombosis. These arterial changes often occur silently, and symptoms may not manifest until atheroma formation occludes more than two-thirds of the vessel. In some cases, this slow narrowing allows enough time for the formation of collateral vessels to maintain blood supply distal to the stenotic site. If normal blood supply is decreased or stopped completely, ischemia occurs. Unfortunately, the most common signs and symptoms associated with atherosclerotic disease result from ischemia of a vital organ such as the

heart or the brain, or a weakening of a vital artery resulting in an aneurysm. Atherosclerotic disease is the most common cause of coronary heart disease (CHD) and cerebrovascular accidents (CVAs).

Cardiovascular angiography is often used in the diagnosis and treatment of atherosclerosis through the use of PTA. CTA is becoming more popular for imaging atherosclerosis and provides results rapidly (Fig. 4.44). Doppler sonography also plays a major role in the diagnosis of atherosclerosis (Fig. 4.45). MRI (Fig. 4.46) and echocardiography are both noninvasive modalities that may also visualize blood flow without the use of contrast agents.

Some researchers believe that a simple blood test, C-reactive protein (CRP), may be helpful in determining who is at risk for developing atherosclerosis.

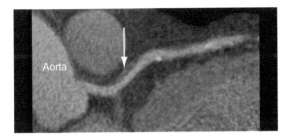

FIG. 4.44 Multislice computed tomography angiogram image demonstrating soft plaque (*arrow*) in the left anterior descending artery.

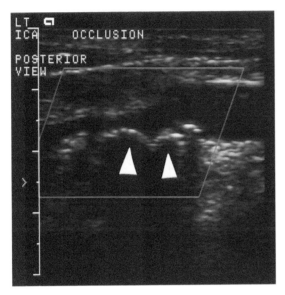

FIG. 4.45 Atherosclerosis as seen in Doppler sonography of the internal carotid artery in a 75-year-old man. *Arrows* point to the "hilly" plaque deposit on the lower surface of the artery; the lack of echo signal beneath them indicates calcium contained within the plaque.

CRP is a marker of inflammation and it is now believed that inflammation plays a major role in the formation of atherosclerosis. This particular blood test (specifically the high sensitivity test, hs-CRP) is sometimes ordered in conjunction with a lipid profile (cholesterol, triglycerides, LDL, HDL). An increased level of CRP may point to an increased future risk of heart attack, stroke, and peripheral arterial disease (PAD). It is important to note that an increased CRP may also indicate inflammation associated with another disease process, such as infection or an autoimmune disease.

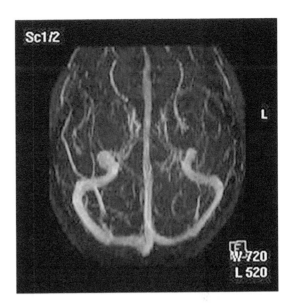

FIG. 4.46 Two-dimensional time flight magnetic resonance imaging of normal venous blood flow of the brain within the sagittal and transverse sinuses.

Coronary Artery Disease

CAD results from the deposition of atheromas in the arteries supplying blood to the heart muscle. As plaques accumulate in the coronary arteries, blood supply to the heart muscle is decreased, resulting in **ischemia,** a local and temporary impairment of circulation caused by obstruction of circulation, and myocardial damage as an **infarct,** which is an area of ischemic necrosis (Fig. 4.47). Major complications of CAD include angina pectoris (chest pain), myocardial infarction (MI), and subsequent myocardial necrosis, if the patient survives the heart attack. CAD is responsible for over 30% of all deaths annually in the United States and is the single most frequent cause of death in both men and women. Most cases, during autopsy, demonstrate significant widespread atherosclerotic disease of the coronary arteries.

As noted earlier, the exact cause of plaque formation is unknown. However, risk factors for CAD are well known and include tobacco use, diets high in fats and calories and low in phytochemicals and fiber, and poor physical fitness. Recent research has demonstrated the possibility that a common variant of the platelet fibrinogen receptor may also be a strong predictor of CAD.

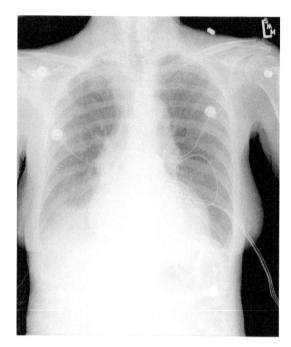

FIG. 4.47 Posteroanterior chest radiograph on a patient with known coronary artery disease. The radiograph demonstrates cardiomegaly with left ventricular configuration and mild dilation of the thoracic aorta.

Medical treatments of CAD may include antianginal drugs to improve circulation and decrease the amount of oxygen consumed by the myocardium. Other cases may be treated surgically with coronary artery bypass grafting (CABG), which involves bypassing the obstruction with a segment of the saphenous vein. A portion of the saphenous vein is removed from the patient's leg, and one end is attached to the aorta superior to the level of the coronary arteries. The distal end of the graft is attached to the coronary artery, distal to the site of the occlusion.

Nuclear medicine studies such as myocardial perfusion scans and gated examinations are important noninvasive methods of determining the presence and extent of CAD; these studies also assist in the clinical management of patients after an MI. In addition, echocardiography may be used to provide needed clinical information in the diagnosis, treatment, and management of CAD. It is also helpful in demonstrating abnormalities in the left ventricular wall motion when the diagnosis of MI is uncertain. Highly advanced MRI and CT are noninvasive, efficient methods of diagnosing CAD. MRI is often considered a "one-stop shop" for imaging of the heart. Although it is not widely used to image the coronary

vessels, MRI provides high quality images of the function and structure of the heart without the use of radiation. CT is a highly effective method for imaging the coronary arteries. With contrast injection, CT can produce high quality images of plaque build-up in the vessels.

Myocardial Infarction

MI is most commonly caused by an acute thrombus of the coronary arteries and primarily affects the left ventricle of the heart. The ability of the heart to continue pumping blood depends on the extent of muscle damage. Clinical signs and symptoms of MI include a sudden onset of severe, crushing chest pain that may radiate down the left arm or up into the neck. It may be accompanied by profuse sweating, shortness of breath, nausea, or vomiting. In milder cases, it may be dismissed as indigestion. It is important to note that although the signs and symptoms are similar in men and women, women often experience atypical chest discomfort. Immediate medical attention is critical to the survival of individuals experiencing an MI. Approximately 20% to 25% of these patients die before reaching the hospital, primarily from ventricular fibrillation. Early medical intervention significantly increases survival. Survival rates are approximately 85% in those having the first attack and receiving medical attention within the first 30 minutes after the attack. The prognosis of CAD is variable, depending largely on the location of the occlusion, the extent of damage to the heart muscle, and the amount of collateral circulation available.

Cardiac angiography plays a major role in the diagnosis of stenotic or occluded heart vessels (Figs. 4.48 and 4.49). PTCA with stent placement is routinely performed to open stenotic vessels and is quite effective. Thrombolytic therapy may also be used, and it is most effective if administered within hours of the onset of an MI. If therapy is started within 3 hours, the chances of long-term survival are approximately 80%. The most common thrombolytic agents include streptokinase, anistreplase, alteplase, and reteplase.

Acute coronary syndrome (ACS) may be diagnosed by performing cardiac biomarker tests. A biomarker is a characteristic that can be measured and evaluated as an indicator of a normal biologic process or a pathogenic process. Common cardiac biomarkers include troponin I or T, creatine kinase (CK), and CK–muscle-type or brain-type (CK-MB). Troponins are proteins found in skeletal and heart muscles. Troponin I and T are specific to cardiac muscle and are normally present in very small quantities. When heart muscle is damaged, troponins I

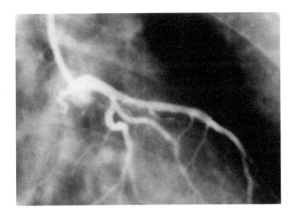

FIG. 4.48 Coronary angiography demonstrating a normal left anterior descending artery as shown in this right anterior oblique projection.

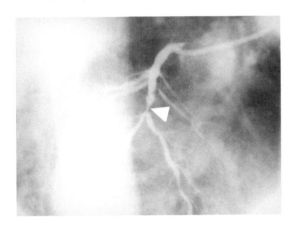

FIG. 4.49 A major stenosis is seen in this coronary arteriogram in a left anterior oblique projection, just as the left coronary artery bifurcates into the left anterior descending artery to the right and a major diagonal branch to the left.

and T are released into the circulation. Thus an elevated level of troponin indicates that an individual has suffered a heart attack. CK is an enzyme found in the heart, brain, skeletal muscle, and other tissues. Enzymes are proteins that help cells perform their normal functions. CK-MB is found mostly in the heart and its levels are elevated when muscle or heart cells are injured. These tests are completed with a simple blood draw from a vein.

Aneurysms

A localized "ballooning" or outpouching of a vessel wall is called an **aneurysm.** It results when the vessel wall has been weakened by atherosclerotic disease, trauma,

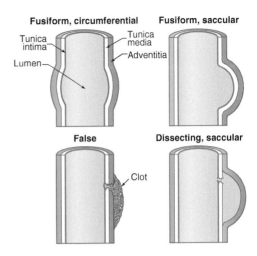

FIG. 4.50 Types of aneurysms.

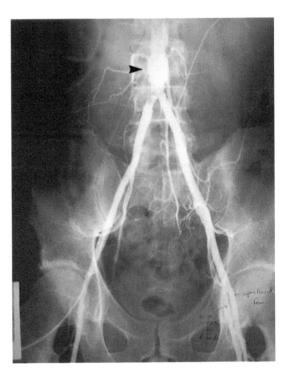

FIG. 4.51 Abdominal aortogram from a 53-year-old man demonstrating a saccular abdominal aneurysm and bilateral areas of stenosis at the bifurcation of the aorta into the common iliac arteries.

infection, or congenital defects. Aneurysms are usually classified as saccular, fusiform, or dissecting (Fig. 4.50). A **saccular aneurysm** is a localized bulge involving one side of the arterial wall (Fig. 4.51). It usually occurs in a cerebral artery. If this bulging includes the entire

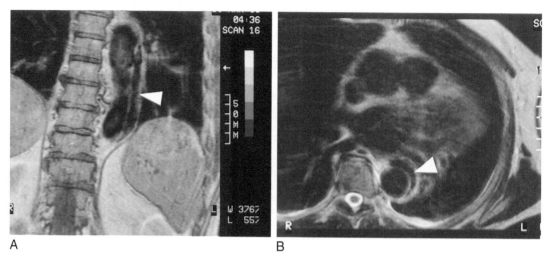

A   B

FIG. 4.52 A, A dissecting aneurysm in a 79-year-old man seen in a coronal magnetic resonance imaging (MRI) scan, with clear depiction of the extraluminal flow. B, A dissecting aneurysm in a 79-year-old man, seen as extraluminal flow in this transverse MRI scan, which represents a view looking down into the aorta.

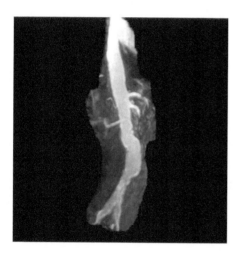

FIG. 4.53 Three-dimensional reconstruction of a magnetic resonance angiogram demonstrating an abdominal aortic aneurysm below the level of the renal arteries.

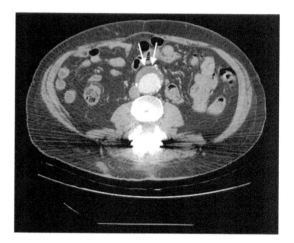

FIG. 4.54 Contrast-enhanced axial computed tomography image showing an infrarenal abdominal aortic aneurysm approximately 4 cm in diameter.

circumference of the vessel wall, it is termed a **fusiform aneurysm.** This type is often found in the distal abdominal aorta. A **dissecting aneurysm** results when the intima tears and allows blood to flow within the vessel wall, thus forming an intramural hematoma (Fig. 4.52). Symptoms of a dissecting aneurysm often mimic those of a heart attack.

Although an aneurysm may occur anywhere in the aorta, the majority (75%) occur in the abdominal

aorta, with 90% of those occurring below the level of the renal arteries. Abdominal aortic aneurysms (AAAs) may cause pain, or the patient may remain symptom-free. Conventional abdominal images are of little value; however, a cross-table lateral abdomen radiograph may show enlargement of the aorta with calcification of the vessel wall. Diagnostic medical sonography, MRI, and CT are fairly noninvasive and are of value in determining the size and extent of the aneurysm (Figs. 4.53 and 4.54). Aortography is an invasive procedure that

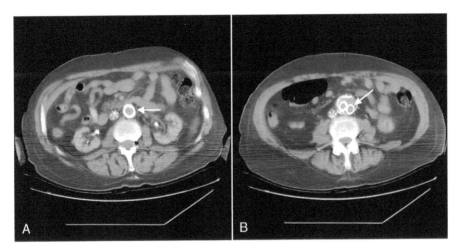

FIG. 4.55 Computed tomographic examination of a patient after graft placement for abdominal aortic aneurysm. Images A and B show the graft at different levels within the aorta.

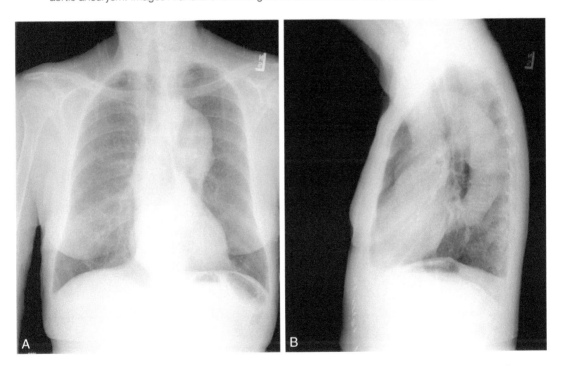

FIG. 4.56 A, Posteroanterior chest radiograph demonstrating a widened mediastinum as a result of a thoracic aortic aneurysm. B, Lateral projection of the chest on the same patient as in A.

also helps delineate the aneurysm, especially in cases in which the aneurysm extends above the renal arteries. Surgical repair is necessary for AAAs larger than 6 cm in diameter. The aneurysm is removed, and the section of the vessel is replaced with a synthetic graft (Fig. 4.55), possibly extending to the iliac arteries. In the case of an endograft, the aneurysm is not removed. This device is

introduced into the aneurysm through an incision made in the femoral artery. The endograft stays within the aneurysm to prevent rupture.

Thoracic aortic aneurysms most commonly result from congenital anomalies or blunt chest trauma. These are visible on conventional chest radiographs (Fig. 4.56); however, CT, MRI, and transesophageal ultrasonography are most helpful in assessing the size and extent of the aneurysm. As in the case of AAAs, thoracic aortic aneurysms are surgically repaired if they are 6 cm or larger in diameter. Aneurysms may also occur in the extremities, most commonly in the popliteal artery. These often are bilateral and occur in conjunction with an abdominal aortic aneurysm. Popliteal aneurysms are generally confirmed by ultrasonic evaluation or CT. Arteriography may also be performed.

Venous Thrombosis

The formation of blood clots within a vein is called **venous thrombosis.** These clots commonly form in the veins of the lower extremities (Fig. 4.57) and result from a slowing of the blood return to the heart. The contraction of leg muscles assists with venous blood return; therefore, postoperative or bedfast patients are especially prone to this disorder. **Phlebitis,** an inflammation of the vein, is often associated with venous thrombosis. The medical term used to specify the combination of these disorders is **thrombophlebitis.** The thrombus formation generally begins in the valves of the deep calf veins, where thromboplastin traps red blood cells to create the blood clot. Patients may be placed on anticoagulant drugs or they may receive thrombolytic therapy.

Sonography is performed to determine the location and the extent of this disease, primarily in the lower extremities, and venography may be of use in confirming the diagnosis. One major complication associated with deep vein thrombosis (DVT) is the development of a pulmonary embolism. Filters may be placed in the patient's inferior vena cava to prevent these clots from reaching the kidneys and the chest. These filters may be inserted under fluoroscopic control and are clearly visible on plain radiographs of the abdomen (Fig. 4.58).

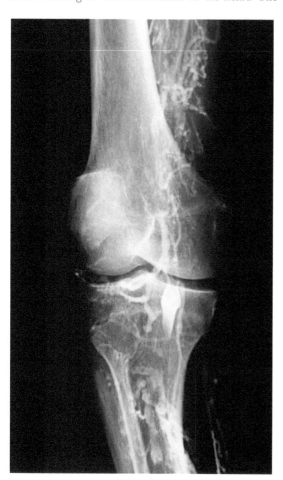

FIG. 4.57 Venogram of the left lower extremity demonstrating deep vein thrombosis.

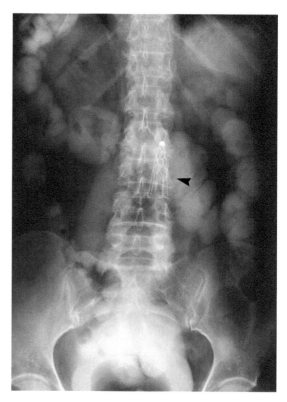

FIG. 4.58 Abdominal radiograph from an older woman demonstrating the proper placement of a vena caval filter.

Pulmonary Emboli

A **pulmonary embolus** (PE), or thromboembolism, occurs when a blood clot forms or becomes lodged in a pulmonary artery. Most commonly, this arises from a **thrombus** that originates in a lower extremity, migrates to the lungs, and becomes lodged there, resulting in an obstruction of blood supply to the lungs. Pulmonary emboli are also caused by fat emboli resulting from skeletal fractures or from amniotic fluid emboli. The resulting decrease in blood supply to the lungs may lead to acute respiratory distress and heart failure or cardiogenic shock, depending on the extent of the obstruction and the individual's cardiovascular status before the embolism. Pathophysiologically, the pulmonary embolus changes the pulmonary hemodynamics and the gas exchange capabilities of the lungs. Prolonged periods of inactivity or bed rest increase the risk for pulmonary embolism. Symptoms generally occur abruptly and include a sudden onset of coughing, acute shortness of breath, and chest pain.

Pulmonary angiography and nuclear perfusion and ventilation lung scans (VQ scan) are commonly used in the diagnosis of a PE; however, multidetector CT has been demonstrated to be the most time-saving and cost-effective imaging modality for diagnosis of pulmonary emboli (Fig. 4.59). The prognosis is dependent on the size and location of the PE as well as the patient's prior cardiovascular status. Thrombolytic agents such as streptokinase, urokinase, or tissue plasminogen activator (tPA) and placement of inferior vena cava filters may be used in the treatment of a PE. In some cases, a pulmonary embolectomy may be required. Anticoagulant therapy with agents such as heparin or warfarin is always indicated after the initial episode because it decreases the probability and intensity of recurrent pulmonary emboli. Approximately 50% of patients who survive the initial PE experience a recurrent episode.

Thrombolytic therapy (with streptokinase or urokinase) is used in life-threatening situations and is administered in the cardiovascular or interventional area of the radiology department. In less severe cases, patients may be treated with anticoagulation medications.

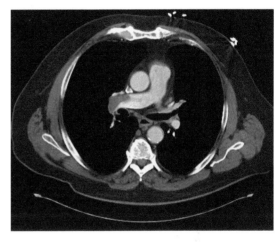

FIG. 4.59 Computed tomographic angiogram demonstrating a large pulmonary embolism in the right pulmonary artery.

Pathology Summary Cardiovascular System

Pathology	Imaging Modalities of Choice
Patent ductus arteriosus	Echocardiography, MRI
Coarctation of the aorta	Echocardiography, chest radiography, MRI
Septal defects	Echocardiography, MRI heart, chest radiography, CT heart, cardiac catheterization
Transposition of great vessels	Echocardiography, cardiac catheterization, MRI
Tetralogy of Fallot	Echocardiography, chest radiography, MRI
Valvular disease	Echocardiography, cardiac catheterization, chest radiography
Congestive heart failure	Chest radiography
Cor pulmonale	Echocardiography, nuclear medicine cardiac studies, chest radiography
Atherosclerosis	Sonography and angiography

Continued

Pathology Summary Cardiovascular System—cont'd

Pathology	Imaging Modalities of Choice
Coronary artery disease	Echocardiography, nuclear medicine cardiac studies, CT, CTA
Myocardial infarction	Cardiac catheterization, nuclear medicine, SPECT, MRI rest and stress, echocardiography rest and stress, CTA coronary arteries
Aneurysm	Sonography, MRI, CT
Aortic dissection	Chest radiography, CTA chest and abdomen, trans-esophageal sonography, MRA chest and abdomen, sonography
Venous thrombosis	
Pulmonary embolism	CTA chest, chest radiograph, nuclear medicine, V/Q lung scan, angiography

CT, Computed tomography; *CTA*, computed tomographic angiography; *MRI*, magnetic resonance imaging; *SPECT-MRI*, single photon emission computed tomography-MRI.

Review Questions

1. The heart chamber located most anteriorly and forming the anterior border of the cardiac shadow on a lateral chest radiograph is the:
   a. Left atrium
   b. Left ventricle
   c. Right atrium
   d. Right ventricle

2. The bicuspid valve is also known as the:
   a. Left atrioventricular valve
   b. Right atrioventricular valve
   c. Aortic valve
   d. Pulmonary valve

3. Contraction of the myocardium is termed:
   a. Diastole
   b. Systole
   c. Peristole
   d. Myostole

4. How many posterior ribs should be visible on a good inspiration PA chest radiograph?
   a. 12
   b. 10
   c. 8
   d. 6

5. In a fetus, the ductus arteriosus connects the:
   a. Aorta and the superior vena cava
   b. Aorta and pulmonary trunk
   c. Right and left atria
   d. Right and left ventricles

6. Which of the following defects are included in tetralogy of Fallot?
   a. Pulmonary stenosis
   b. Ventricular septal defect
   c. Hypertrophy of right ventricle
   d. a and c
   e. a, b, and c

7. A condition in which the left ventricle cannot pump an amount of blood equal to the venous return of the right ventricle is:
   a. Coronary artery disease
   b. Left-sided congestive heart failure
   c. Right-sided congestive heart failure
   d. Patent ductus arteriosus

8. Risk factors associated with atherosclerosis include:
   a. Low blood sugar levels
   b. Hypertension
   c. Cigarette smoking
      a. a and b
      b. a and c
      c. b and c
      d. a, b, and c

9. A decrease in tissue blood supply is termed:
   a. Atheroma
   b. Infarction
   c. Ischemia
   d. Necrosis
10. The single most frequent cause of deaths in the United States is:
    a. Congestive heart failure
    b. Coronary artery disease
    c. Transposition of the great vessels
    d. Valvular disease
11. Clinical signs of a myocardial infarction include:
    a. Shortness of breath
    b. Crushing chest pain
    c. Neck pain
       a. a and b
       b. a and c
       c. b and c
       d. a, b, and c
12. Which type of vessel is used as the graft material for coronary artery bypass grafts?
    a. Arteries
    b. Capillaries
    c. Veins
13. Aortic aneurysms most commonly occur in the:
    a. Abdominal aorta above the level of the renal arteries
    b. Abdominal aorta below the level of the renal arteries
    c. Thoracic aorta

14. Imaging procedures that may be used to demonstrate an abdominal aneurysm include:
    a. Angiography
    b. CT
    c. Sonography
       a. a and b
       b. a and c
       c. b and c
       d. a, b, and c
15. Venous thrombosis most often affects the:
    a. Deep veins of the upper extremities
    b. Deep veins of the lower extremities
    c. Superficial veins of the upper extremities
    d. Superficial veins of the lower extremities
16. What common imaging procedures provide functional information regarding the heart?
17. Which type of aneurysm results when the intima tears and allows blood to flow within the vessel wall?
18. An older adult has shortness of breath during exertion and overall respiratory distress. The chest radiograph reveals an enlarged heart and a congested hilar region, with some pulmonary edema. What is the likely cause?
19. Identify at least two common sites where atherosclerosis occurs.
20. What is the cause of ischemia in coronary artery disease?

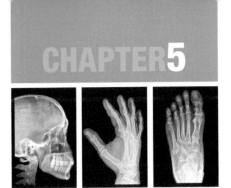

Abdomen and Gastrointestinal System

http://evolve.elsevier.com/Kowalczyk/pathology/

LEARNING OBJECTIVES

On completion of Chapter 5, the reader should be able to:

1. Describe the anatomic components of the abdomen and the gastrointestinal system and how they are visualized radiographically.
2. Compare and contrast the various imaging modalities used in the evaluation of the abdomen and gastrointestinal system.
3. Identify the tubes and catheters related to the gastrointestinal system by type, and explain their use.
4. Characterize a given condition as congenital, inflammatory, neurogenic, or neoplastic.
5. Identify the pathogenesis of the gastrointestinal diseases cited and typical treatments for them.
6. Describe, in general, the radiographic appearance of each of the given pathologies.
7. Understand which imaging modalities foster the diagnosis of the cited abdominal and gastrointestinal pathologies.

OUTLINE

KEY TERMS

Achalasia

Adenocarcinomas

Adynamic ileus

Anal agenesis

Appendicitis

Atresia

Carbohydrate
  intolerance

Colostomy

Crohn's disease

Diverticulitis

Diverticulum

Dysphagia

Endoscopy

Esophageal varices

Gallstone ileus

Gastroenteritis

Gastroesophageal reflux
  disease

Gluten-sensitive
  enteropathy

Granulomatous colitis

Hernia

Hiatal hernia

Hirschsprung disease

Hypertrophic pyloric
  stenosis

Ileostomy

Imperforate anus

Intussusception

Leiomyomas

Malrotation

Mechanical bowel
  obstruction

Paralytic ileus

Peptic ulcer

Reflux esophagitis

Regional enteritis

Situs inversus

Ulcerative colitis

Volvulus

Anatomy and Physiology

Abdomen

The abdomen is composed of the abdominal and pelvic cavities and is often divided into nine anatomic regions: right hypochondriac, epigastric, left hypochondriac, right lateral, umbilical, left lateral, right inguinal, hypogastric, and left inguinal (Fig. 5.1). It may also be described in terms of quadrants: right-upper (RUQ), right-lower (RLQ), left-upper (LUQ), and left-lower (LLQ) (Fig. 5.2). The abdominal cavity contains organs of the digestive system (stomach and intestines), the hepatobiliary system (liver, gallbladder, and pancreas), the urinary system (kidneys and proximal ureters), and the circulatory system (spleen). The pelvic cavity contains the distal ureters, bladder, portions of the intestines, and the reproductive organs.

The abdominal cavity is lined by a serous membrane known as the peritoneum (Fig. 5.3, A). The serous lining that covers the abdominal organs is called the visceral peritoneum. The serous lining that covers the abdominal and pelvic walls and extends to the abdominal organs is called the parietal peritoneum.

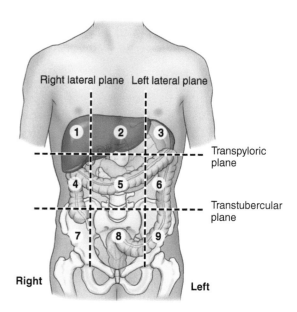

FIG. 5.1 The nine regions of the abdomen. (1) Rt. Hypochondriac, (2) Epigastric, (3) Lt. Hypochondriac, (4) Rt. Lateral (lumbar), (5) Umbilical, (6) Lt. Lateral (lumbar), (7) Rt. Inguinal (iliac), (8) Pubic (hypogastric), (9) Lt. Inguinal (iliac).

The mesentery is a double fold of parietal peritoneum projecting from the posterior abdominal wall and attaching to the intestines (see Fig. 5.3, B). The mesentery offers support and allows for nerves, blood vessels, and lymph vessels to travel to the abdominal organs. The mesentery of the small intestine is simply called the mesentery. The mesentery of the large intestine is called the mesocolon. It is classified by the portion of the colon to which it attaches, for example the transverse mesocolon attaches to the transverse colon, whereas the sigmoid mesocolon attaches to the sigmoid colon.

The greater omentum is a double fold of peritoneum that attaches to the greater curvature of the stomach, the proximal duodenum and the transverse colon. It hangs loosely over the intestines. The lesser omentum is a fold of peritoneum that attaches the lesser curvature of the stomach and the proximal duodenum to the liver (Fig. 5.4).

The abdominal organs are often classified as intraperitoneal, retroperitoneal or intraperitoneal. Intraperitoneal organs include the following: stomach, first portion of the duodenum, jejunum, ileum, cecum, appendix, transverse colon, sigmoid colon, proximal one-third of the rectum, liver, spleen, and tail of the pancreas. Retroperitoneal organs include: the remainder of the duodenum, the ascending colon, the descending colon, the middle one-third of the rectum, the pancreas (except for the tail), the kidneys, the proximal ureters, and the adrenal glands. Intraperitoneal structures include the distal one-third of the rectum, distal ureters, urinary bladder and female reproductive organs.

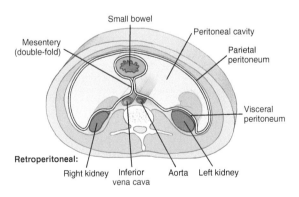

FIG. 5.2 The four quadrants of the abdomen.

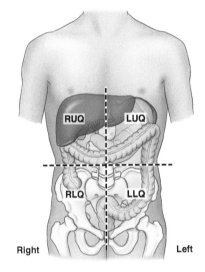

FIG. 5.3 A cross-sectional drawing of the abdomen demonstrating the mesentery, peritoneum, and retroperitoneal areas.

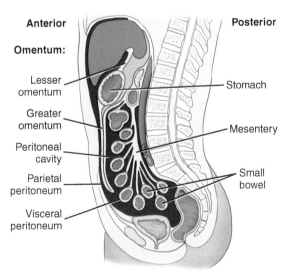

FIG. 5.4 A cross-sectional drawing of the abdominal cavity demonstrates the omentum.

Gastrointestinal System

A major portion of the gastrointestinal (GI) system is the alimentary tract, which serves to digest and absorb food. Extending from the mouth to the anus, the alimentary tract consists of the mouth, pharynx, esophagus, stomach, small bowel and large bowel.

The esophagus is the first part of the GI system. It is approximately 10 to 12 inches long and extends from the pharynx to the stomach (Fig. 5.5). The upper esophagus is midline, but it courses to the left to pass behind the aortic arch, which results in a normal indentation upon the proximal esophagus (Fig. 5.6). A second normal indentation occurs at the level of the left main stem bronchus (Fig. 5.6). As it passes downward, the esophagus follows the curvature of the thoracic spine and thoracic descending aorta. The distal one-third of the esophagus is indented by the left atrium of the heart (Fig. 5.6).

The stomach is located within the LUQ of the abdomen. The stomach is typically classified into the following portions: cardia, fundus, body, antrum and pylorus. The medial side of the stomach is the lesser curvature and the lateral side of the stomach is the greater curvature. The cardiac orifice is at the level of the tenth or eleventh thoracic vertebra and the pyloric canal is just to the right of the first or second lumbar vertebra (Fig. 5.7). Peristalsis churns the gastric content (chyme) and propels it toward the pylorus. Gastric emptying of liquids is accounted for by the peristalsis initiated in the fundus of the stomach, whereas gastric emptying of solids requires to-and-fro action of the antrum and pylorus. In the presence of masses, inflammation or diabetes, the peristaltic activity may be diminished. When the stomach is filled with barium, the entire gastric lumen should have a generally smooth contour. The rugae are folds that appear on barium studies as smooth longitudinal ridges predominately within the fundus and body of the stomach. The antrum often lacks rugal folds.

The small bowel is segmented into the duodenum, jejunum, and ileum. It arises from the stomach at the duodenal bulb and courses to the ileocecal valve (Fig. 5.8), over a length of nearly 21 feet. The duodenal C-loop moves posteriorly from the gastric antrum to its ending at the ligament of Treitz. The jejunum begins here and coils in the LUQ before terminating at the ileum in the RUQ. The ileum then courses through the lower abdomen and pelvis to terminate at the ileocecal junction in the RLQ. The mucosal folds of the small intestine are called valvulae conniventes. When filled with barium, the segments of the small bowel are normally distinguishable by the appearance of the mucosal folds. The duodenal mucosa has the appearance of transverse ridges. The jejunal mucosa

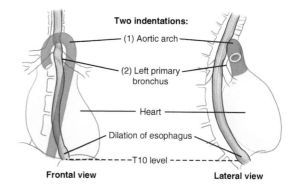

FIG. 5.5 The esophagus in the mediastinum.

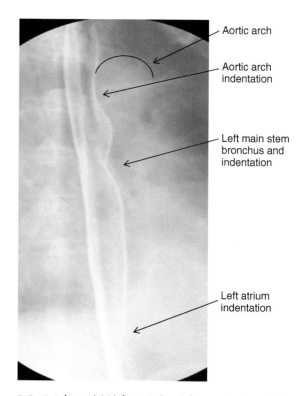

FIG. 5.6 An upright left posterior oblique projection of the esophagus during a double-contrast esophagram. Note the normal indentations upon the esophageal lumen.

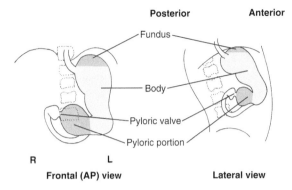

Fundus

Body

Pyloric valve

Pyloric portion

R   L

Frontal (AP) view   **Lateral view**

FIG. 5.7 The stomach depicted in its average orientation when empty.

has a greater number of folds (four to seven per inch) and thus appears delicate and feathery. Ileal folds are less in number than in the jejunum (two to four per inch) and have a transverse appearance like those of the duodenum, although not as large. The last section of the ileum is referred to as the terminal ileum and it inserts into the large bowel at the ileocecal valve.

The large bowel extends from the terminal ileum to the anus for a length of about 6 feet (Fig. 5.9). Its distinct regions are the cecum, ascending colon, hepatic flexure, transverse colon, splenic flexure, descending colon, sigmoid, rectum, and anus. The cecum is usually located in the RLQ and lies against the anterior abdominal wall. The cecum has orifices for the appendix and the

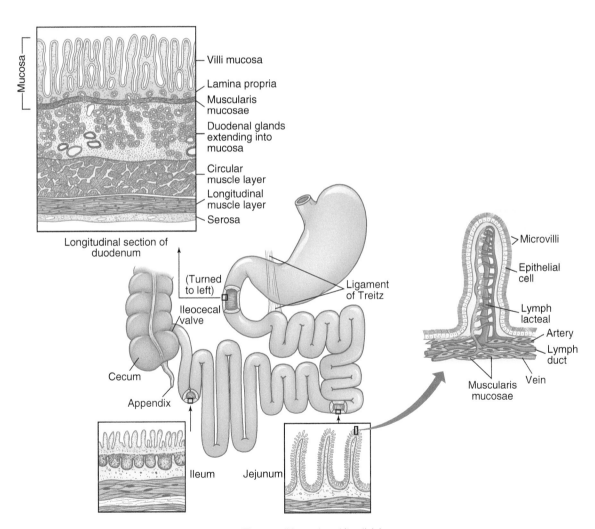

Mucosa

Villi mucosa

Lamina propria

Muscularis mucosae

Duodenal glands extending into mucosa

Circular muscle layer

Longitudinal muscle layer

Serosa

Longitudinal section of duodenum

(Turned to left)

Ileocecal valve

Ligament of Treitz

Cecum

Appendix

Ileum   Jejunum

Microvilli

Epithelial cell

Lymph lacteal

Artery

Lymph duct

Muscularis mucosae   Vein

FIG. 5.8 The small bowel and its divisions.

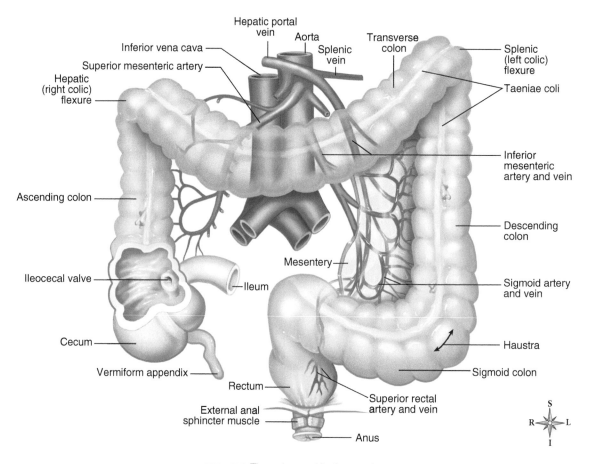

FIG. 5.9 The colon and its four parts.

ileocecal valve. The ascending colon is retroperitoneal and becomes more posterior as it ascends to lie adjacent to the inferior surface of the liver. The hepatic flexure, transverse colon, and splenic flexure are all intraperitoneal. The descending colon is retroperitoneal, moving posteriorly as it descends. The sigmoid colon lies in the pelvis and is quite mobile. Structures located anterior to it include the bladder and, in women, the uterus. Posterior structures include the iliac arteries and sacral nerves. The rectum courses intraperitoneal, beginning at the third sacral segment and following the sacrococcygeal curve to the anus. The mucosal folds of the colon are termed haustra and they have a sacculated appearance. The valves of Houston are prominent transverse folds in the rectum that support fecal matter. The anus forms the distal one to two inches of the large bowel and contains no peritoneal covering.

Imaging Considerations

Radiography

Abdomen

Abdominal radiography is often performed for survey purposes, without contrast agents. The usual starting point is a supine radiograph taken to include the kidneys, ureters, and bladder (KUB). Although the frequency of abnormal findings on a conventional abdominal radiograph can be fairly low and nonspecific, the KUB is of most value for patients complaining of severe abdominal tenderness to rule out bowel obstructions and perforations. In addition, abdominal radiographs are invaluable in assessing the placement of various tubes and catheters, as discussed later in this chapter.

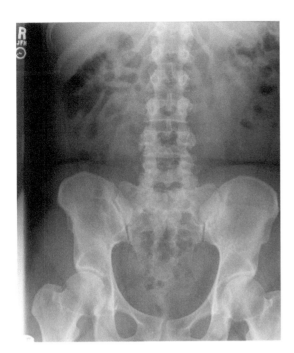

FIG. 5.10 Radiographic appearance of a normal abdomen, demonstrating kidney shadows, liver shadow, psoas muscles, and transverse processes of the lumbar spine.

Anteroposterior (AP) projections of the abdomen are generally taken in the supine position. An AP radiograph allows for examination of the air distribution within the bowels, the size of the viscera, vascular and other types of calcifications, body or soft tissue trauma, and also serves as a preliminary radiograph for other procedures.

During inspection of the abdominal radiograph, the technologist should verify that the technique chosen is correct or diagnostic, motion is nonexistent, and the anatomy under consideration has been properly visualized. Normal peristalsis often results in motion of the final radiographic image. As with other body areas, evaluation of the abdomen should be done systematically. This should include inspection of the renal outlines, ureters, psoas muscles, spleen, liver, gallbladder, and peritoneal fat stripes.

In a normal abdomen (Fig. 5.10) of an unprepared patient, varying amounts of gas and fecal material are always present. The liver, kidney, spleen, and psoas muscle shadows are variably outlined because of the lucent layer of fat surrounding them. Properitoneal fat stripes are visible as radiolucencies extending laterally from the costal margins down to the iliac crests. The

aorta and pancreas are not normally seen unless they are calcified, as might be expected in an older patient in the case of the aorta or in a patient with chronic calcific pancreatitis. The inferior margin of the liver should lie at or above the level of the right twelfth rib. The left kidney is usually slightly higher than the right kidney because of the presence of the liver superior to it. The top of the left kidney generally lies at the vertebral level of T11-T12, whereas the top of the right kidney is approximately 1 cm lower in position. In terms of renal size, the kidneys are generally the length of three vertebrae in children over 1 year of age. By adulthood, the kidneys reach the length of approximately two and a half vertebrae.

Few, if any, air–fluid levels are present in the normal patient who is radiographed in the erect position. Limited fluid levels in the small bowel and large bowel, however, may be considered normal. Fluid levels are abnormal when they are seen in dilated bowel loops or when they are numerous. The intestinal gas pattern may be confusing to the diagnostician. In infants and children, gas may be scattered throughout the bowel, but in adults, gas is normally seen only in the stomach and colon. Small bowel gas in an adult, therefore, may indicate a pathologic process. In some patients, gas may be recognizable only on erect radiographs because of the presence of intraluminal fluid. Free air should not be visible in the peritoneal cavity and is indicative of a bowel perforation or other pathologic entities that introduce air into the peritoneum. Erect abdominal radiographs must include the diaphragm to assess for free air, and in instances in which the patient is unable to stand, a left lateral decubitus abdomen should be obtained (Fig. 5.11).

Gastrointestinal System

Some contents of the abdomen can be seen without contrast media, as explained earlier. However, most of the GI tract cannot be examined directly with conventional radiographs. The internal surfaces of the GI tract can be directly visualized through endoscopy that employs lighted optical instruments. Endoscopy allows abnormal areas to be visualized, biopsied, and examined histologically. An upper endoscopy is the test that assesses the esophagus, stomach, and duodenum. A video capsule endoscopy can be performed to evaluate the small intestine. A lower endoscopy or colonoscopy examines the colon and sometimes the terminal

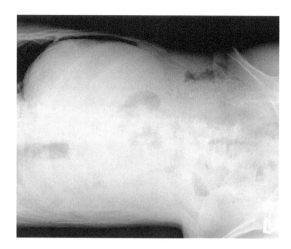

FIG. 5.11 A left lateral decubitus abdomen demonstrating free air over the dome of the liver.

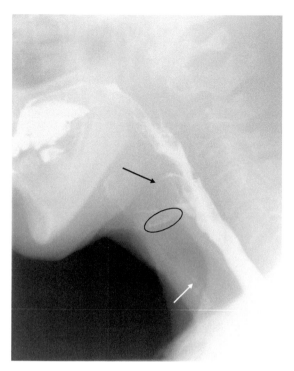

FIG. 5.12 Lateral spot image of the oropharynx and neck captured during a modified barium swallow examination shows laryngeal penetration (*black arrow*) and aspiration (*white arrow*) of liquid barium during the examination. Penetration is the term used for material entering the laryngeal vestibule. Aspiration is the term used for material that migrates below the level of the vocal cords (*black circle*) and into the trachea.

ileum. Computed tomographic (CT) colonography, also known as a virtual colonoscopy, is another means of colonic visualization and has become more common with improvements in technology allowing for more detailed studies. Virtual endoscopic studies are less invasive than conventional endoscopic procedures and provide greater patient comfort.

Radiographic investigation of the GI system is commonly a combination of fluoroscopy and radiography. Fluoroscopy provides dynamic information, whereas radiography provides a permanent static record of the examination. Fluoroscopic examination of the GI system requires positive and negative contrast agents for visualization. Barium sulfate is generally used as the positive contrast agent, but is contraindicated in cases of GI tract perforation. If a perforation is suspected, a water-soluble contrast agent should be used. Although infrequently used alone, a negative contrast agent (e.g., air or carbon dioxide) may be used to distend the GI tract for better visualization of the mucosal lining. A combination of both positive and negative contrast agents is commonly used so that the thicker barium sulfate adheres to the mucosa while the carbon dioxide expands the lumen, thus allowing optimal visualization of small variances in the walls of the GI organs. A study performed with both positive and negative contrasts is known as double contrast, whereas a study performed using only one contrast agent is known as single contrast. Some studies of the upper

GI tract may be referred to as biphasic because double and single contrast methods are used during the same examination.

Oropharynx

The modified barium swallow (MBS) is a fluoroscopic examination that focuses on the oropharyngeal swallow. Images are generally limited to the mouth, pharynx and neck. The examination is performed in conjunction with a Speech and Language Pathologist (SLP). The MBS test assesses swallowing safety so that an SLP can make appropriate diet and therapy recommendations for the patient. A primary goal of MBS studies is to determine whether and why a patient is aspirating liquids or foods (Fig. 5.12). Reasons for oropharyngeal swallowing impairment include: stroke, neuromuscular disease, brain injury, cervical spine injury, head and neck cancer, prolonged mechanical ventilation, debilitation, elderly status, respiratory issues, cognitive impairment and some medications. Patients may present with dysphagia (difficulty swallowing), odynophagia (painful swallowing), globus sensation, choking, coughing, pneumonia, weight loss, malnutrition and/or altered vocal quality.

Esophagus

An esophagram or barium swallow study may be performed to demonstrate anomalies and abnormalities of the esophagus. Transport of the food or liquid bolus through swallowing is the sole function of the esophagus and is accomplished by gravity and peristalsis. Most esophagrams are biphasic with a double contrast (thick barium sulfate and carbon dioxide) portion for mucosal assessment and a single contrast (thin barium sulfate) portion used to obtain functional information. For postoperative or perforation evaluations, a single contrast esophagram using water soluble contrast would be performed. Barium-coated solids and/or barium sulfate tablets may also be administered during esophagrams for enhanced functional imaging or in cases of possible luminal narrowing called strictures.

The chief complaint from most patients undergoing a traditional esophagram is **dysphagia**, or difficulty swallowing. The causes for dysphagia are numerous and are discussed later in this chapter. Esophagram indications may also include gastroesophageal reflux disease (GERD), odynophagia, atypical chest pain with a negative cardiac workup, esophageal cancer, fistula, diverticulum, hiatal hernia, pneumomediastinum (free air in the mediastinum), and postoperative evaluation.

During fluoroscopy, the clinician is able to visualize mechanical problems presented while the patient is swallowing the barium sulfate mixture. When assessing for motor disorders such as achalasia or cricopharyngeal spasm the barium swallow may be recorded for dynamic viewing. For patients with motor disorders, care needs to be taken to avoid aspiration of the barium sulfate into the bronchus, which could lead to aspiration pneumonia.

Stomach

One common radiologic procedure of the GI tract is an upper GI (UGI) series. The UGI includes fluoroscopic

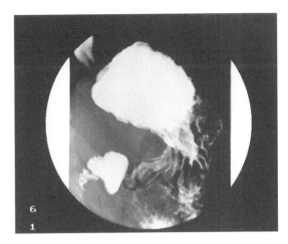

FIG. 5.13 Normal stomach as seen on this radiograph of an 18-year-old man.

evaluation of the esophagus, stomach, and duodenum. The clinician evaluates the contour, position, rugae appearance, and the peristaltic changes occurring as the stomach fills and empties. Indications for UGI examination include: hiatal hernia, abdominal pain, dyspepsia, nausea, vomiting, anemia, GI tract bleeding, and postoperative evaluation.

If the clinician wishes to diminish peristalsis, glucagon may be given to relax the stomach musculature. In many instances, the UGI is performed as a biphasic examination using a gas-producing substance (carbon dioxide crystals) with thick barium sulfate for double-contrast imaging followed by thin barium sulfate for single contrast imaging. The purpose is to expand the stomach and promote coating of the gastric mucosa. The duodenal bulb and C-loop are studied as barium sulfate progresses into the small bowel. Compression may be used for better visualization of specific anatomic areas of the stomach and duodenum.

A series of images are obtained during or after fluoroscopy, with the projections differing from one institution to another. Typical patient positions include recumbent posteroanterior (PA) projection to demonstrate the entire stomach and duodenal bulb, right anterior oblique (RAO) to highlight the pyloric canal and duodenal bulb (Fig. 5.13), right lateral to show the duodenal bulb, duodenal loop and retrogastric space, and left posterior oblique (LPO) to demonstrate the gastric fundus. Proper positioning relates significantly to the patient's body habitus. Generally, the more hypersthenic a patient is, the higher and more transverse the stomach tends to lie. For other body habitus types (i.e., sthenic, hyposthenic, and asthenic), the stomach is more J-shaped, lying lower and closer to the spine.

Small Bowel

In some instances, the barium sulfate mixture may be followed as it progresses through the small intestines. This fluoroscopic test is typically called a small bowel follow through (SBFT). A SBFT may directly follow the UGI examination or be performed independently when small bowel pathology is of primary concern. Radiographs are exposed at set intervals to determine GI tract motility and to demonstrate abnormalities within the small bowel. Once the contrast agent reaches the ileocecal valve, the small bowel study is complete, typically within 2 to 3 hours (Fig. 5.14). Indications for a SBFT include: abdominal pain, nausea, vomiting, diarrhea, anemia, GI tract bleeding, staging of inflammatory bowel disease, malabsorption, unexplained weight loss, and postoperative evaluation.

The small intestines may also be studied radiographically by means of enteroclysis, a small-bowel enema. This is accomplished by advancing an intestinal tube through the patient's mouth or nose to the end of the duodenum at the ligament of Treitz. Contrast agents, both positive and negative (barium sulfate and methylcellulose, respectively), are directly injected into the small bowel with tube advancement as needed.

Abdominal radiography may often depict abnormalities in patients with known inflammatory bowel disease (IBD). Because negative findings will rarely preclude the need for further imaging studies, radiography typically is reserved for evaluating the presence of obstruction, perforation, or toxic colon distention associated with advanced disease. Although small bowel barium studies were, at one point, the primary method for diagnosing suspected IBD cases, the introduction of video capsule endoscopy is playing an increasingly larger role in making the initial diagnosis.

Large Bowel

The lower GI tract is examined by administering barium or water soluble contrast as an enema through the rectum. This examination demonstrates abnormalities of the large bowel such as intraluminal neoplasms.

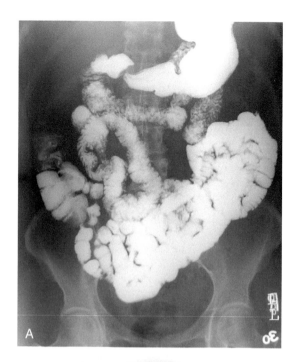

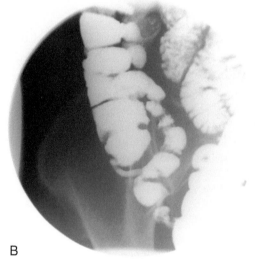

FIG. 5.14 **A,** Small-bowel radiograph demonstrating barium filled terminal ileum. **B,** Spot image demonstrating ileocecal junction.

Indications for contrast enemas include: incomplete or poorly prepped colonoscopy, colorectal cancer screening, anemia, GI tract bleeding, abdominal pain, diarrhea, constipation, fistula, inflammatory bowel disease, and pre- and postoperative evaluation.

The barium enema is performed in a single-contrast fashion with only barium or as a double-contrast study using barium sulfate in combination with a negative contrast agent (e.g., air). The negative contrast agent distends the lumen, allowing for improved visualization of the mucosal lining (Fig. 5.15), especially for detection of small polyps and intraluminal tumors. In cases of suspected perforation or during postoperative evaluation, water soluble contrast is substituted for barium sulfate. In either case, the clinician typically obtains a series of images during fluoroscopy, with the patient in various positions to highlight certain areas of the colon (e.g., flexures). The radiographer may also expose a series of radiographs of the contrast-enhanced large bowel per the clinician's instructions (Fig. 5.16). After evacuation of the barium sulfate mixture, the radiographer will obtain a "post evacuation" radiograph to visualize colon contraction and to demonstrate the mucosa.

Ostomies

If a patient has had a surgical enterostomy procedure, the contrast medium may be administered through the opening in the abdominal wall to the specific area of the GI system. A **colostomy** is a procedure in which a stoma is surgically created on the abdominal wall to allow drainage of large bowel contents into a closed pouch hung outside the body. Those in the sigmoid and descending colon are most frequently placed because of rectal or sigmoid cancer. Those placed in the transverse or ascending colon are often for indications that allow the colostomy to be placed for temporary purposes, for the diversion of colonic content flow of (e.g., sigmoid diverticulitis, rectovaginal fistula, colon obstruction).

A colostomy variation includes the wet or double barrel colostomy. This is a diversion of the large bowel and the urinary tract used to expel both fecal contents and urine into one external pouch. The wet colostomy is usually an irreversible procedure in patients who require bladder and colon removal generally as treatment for pelvic cancers.

An **ileostomy** is a similar opening that is placed from the ileum to divert bowel contents from entering the colon. As with colostomies, patient problems with ileostomies include proper skin protection and odor control. Proper fit of the appliance for drainage is essential to prevent problems caused by excoriating digestive enzymes. Other enterostomies (i.e., jejunostomies and

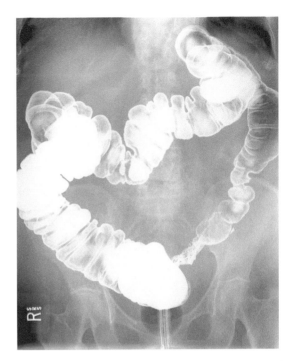

FIG. 5.15 Normal air-contrast enema as demonstrated on this anteroposterior projection.

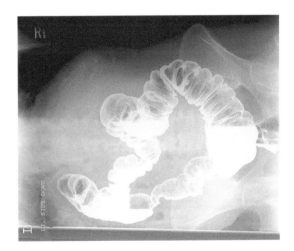

FIG. 5.16 Normal air contrast barium enema as demonstrated on this left lateral decubitus posteroanterior projection.

duodenostomies) are more rarely used, and only under very specific circumstances because of the loss of electrolytes that occurs before their absorption through the small bowel. Affected patients often require total parenteral nutrition (TPN) to maintain life.

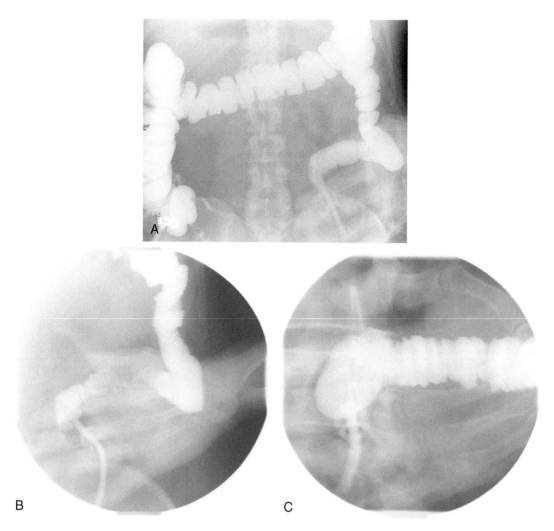

FIG. 5.17 **A**, Barium enema via a colostomy demonstrating enema tip within the ostomy. **B** and **C**, Spot images demonstrating administration of barium sulfate via the ostomy.

If a patient has had a surgical enterostomy procedure, the contrast agent may be administered through the opening in the abdominal wall to the specific area of the GI system (Fig. 5.17). Special enema tips are manufactured to administer contrast agents directly into an ostomy opening. Varying sizes of Foley catheters are also useful for ostomy contrast administration. Fluoroscopic contrast studies of the bowel via ostomies are generally single contrast and may be performed with barium sulfate or water soluble contrast depending on the indication for the study. Special

care needs to be taken when imaging the patient with a stoma because this area can be particularly sensitive. Adhesive removal wipes should be kept on hand for removing ostomy bags. Also, patients should be notified to bring extra ostomy supplies with them to their examination.

Computed Tomography

Computed Tomography (CT) is an important modality in abdominal survey and in the examination of the GI system. Because CT can visualize small differences in tissue density, it clearly demonstrates abdominal organs, which are normally not apparent on conventional abdominal radiographs without the use of contrast, resulting in good visualization of structures in the upper abdomen close to the diaphragm.

During CT examination, the liver, spleen, pancreas, and kidneys appear as homogeneous soft tissue densities, making any alteration in the density resulting from pathologic conditions readily visible, even without contrast media. Abscesses and solid and cystic masses all have a respective range of densities between that of water and normal soft tissue densities. CT is also quite useful in the evaluation of retroperitoneal pathologies such as lymph node enlargement resulting from neoplastic disease or infection. In combination with conventional abdominal radiography, CT of the abdomen is recommended when a bowel obstruction is suspected. Finally, it has become the accepted modality for tracking the progress of GI malignancies and also plays a role in the diagnosis of inflammatory conditions (e.g., abscess). CT of the colon is commonly performed to evaluate neoplastic disease, diverticulitis, and appendicitis. It has the capability of locating the exact site of neoplasms and allowing the clinician to measure the size of the tumor and the presence of infiltration into surrounding tissues. It is also useful in planning radiation therapy protocols. An increase in the availability of CT dose reduction techniques results in a decrease of associated radiation exposure levels.

Routine CT examination of the abdomen requires good opacification of the bowel and vascular structures because poorly opacified bowel loops may be mistaken for abdominal masses. Patients must be given an oral contrast agent approximately 45 minutes to 1 hour before abdominal CT scanning. This time allows the contrast agent to reach the distal ileum before examination. Contrast agents may also be administered rectally, depending on the anatomic structures to be imaged.

Multidetector CT (MDCT) units, in combination with oral contrast and gaseous distention of the colon, have the capability to perform a noninvasive endoscopic procedure called *virtual colonoscopy* (or CT colonography). This technique produces two-dimensional (2-D) and three-dimensional (3-D) images of the colon, thus enabling the radiologist and endoscopist to view anatomic landmarks and structures that

may not be seen with conventional colonoscopy. This, in turn, can reduce risk and discomfort to the patient. This application is a benefit to those who may not be able to or choose not to have a traditional colonoscopy procedure, which remains the gold standard for colorectal screening. Additionally, virtual colonoscopy has a high sensitivity for detection of polyps greater than 10 mm as well as lesions that may be missed with fecal blood tests, barium enemas, and sigmoidoscopy. However, it is important to note that residual stool may cause problems with accuracy of image reconstruction, potentially simulating pathology such as polyps or masses.

CT enterography is also an increasingly used technique, in which optimal visualization of the small bowel mucosa is attained through the use of MDCT scanners. For these examinations, patients are given large volumes (approximately 1350 mL) of 0.1% barium sulfate before imaging. CT enterography is an excellent diagnostic tool for patients with inflammatory bowel diseases and has largely replaced the SBFT in that patient population. Additionally, for certain indications such as obscure GI bleeding, small bowel tumors, and chronic ischemia, a biphasic contrast-enhanced study may be performed. Because of the ability to acquire both intraluminal and extraluminal information of the entire GI tract in a noninvasive manner, techniques such as CT enterography and CT colonography are quickly supplanting the standard small bowel series and barium enema examinations.

Magnetic Resonance Imaging

The role of magnetic resonance imaging (MRI) in the abdomen has expanded as a result of faster sequences and shorter scan times. Evaluation of the GI tract is still limited by bowel motion; however, a hypomotility medication, such as glucagon can be administered to slow bowel peristalsis. MRI is useful in demonstrating the presence of retroperitoneal masses impinging on the GI system. Breath-hold imaging using MRI allows the technologist to visualize abdominal organs in a matter of seconds (Fig. 5.18). A few different imaging sequences are used to differentiate between normal tissue and pathology. The most common of the imaging sequences are T1-weighted images for optimal visualization of anatomic structures and T2-weighted images for optimal visualization of diseased tissues. Three-dimensional contrast-enhanced magnetic resonance

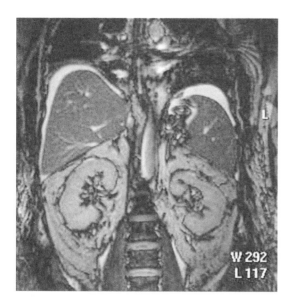

FIG. 5.18 A T2-weighted coronal breath-hold magnetic resonance image of the abdomen.

angiography (MRA) is also used for the imaging of the arterial vessels of the abdomen.

For imaging of the small bowel, magnetic resonance enterography (MRE) is gradually being incorporated into routine clinical practice, as published literature highlighting the benefits of its use is becoming more prevalent. Because of its ability to display both intraluminal and extraluminal information, similar to that of CT, MRE is often the preferred imaging modality for pediatric populations and pregnant women, in whom radiation exposure is of high concern. MRE has the ability to demonstrate areas of active bowel inflammation, and complications including bowel obstruction, fistulas, and abscesses. Furthermore, MRE sequences have the ability to depict bowel motility, which is a potential advantage when attempting to distinguish between fixed and transient segments of luminal narrowing. Subsequently, sequences can be repeated to capture various vascular phases, reassess abnormal bowel segments, or improve image quality without increasing the radiation risk to the patient. The examination is performed by having the patient ingest 1 L to 2 L of a 0.1% barium suspension containing sorbitol, before MRE of the abdomen. Use of this agent produces high signal intensity in the bowel lumen on T2-weighted images and low signal intensity in the lumen on T1-weighted images. The "dark lumen" appearance that results

with the administration of the contrast is critical for the detection of mural enhancement on postcontrast T1-weighted images, which rarely can be achieved through use of water alone.

Sonography

Sonography is occasionally useful in imaging the GI system, although successful examination is highly dependent on the skill of the operator. When water is used as a contrast agent, it can be highly successful in imaging gastric emptying, gastroesophageal reflux disease (GERD), and duodenal abnormalities. More commonly, however, it is used to image the retroperitoneum because of the flexibility of angling the transducer to image that region. Structures posterior to the bowel, such as the aorta, kidneys, lymph nodes, and adrenal glands can be imaged with ultrasound to assess for various abnormalities. Most commonly used in the evaluation of appendicitis, graded compression ultrasonography is a technique performed using a 5 MHz or 7 MHz linear transducer to firmly compress the anterior abdominal wall, displacing normal bowel loops in an effort to locate a potentially inflamed appendix.

Nuclear Medicine Procedures

Nuclear medicine also has applications for abdominal and GI tract imaging. GI bleed scans, which are quick, noninvasive procedures useful in demonstrating GI bleeding, direct angiographers to the site of bleeding if therapeutic intervention is to be performed. This is accomplished by using either technetium-99m (Tc-99m) to label red blood cells (RBCs) or Tc-99m–labeled colloid to identify the origin of the bleed. Tc-99m is a short-lived (half-life of about 6 hours) nuclear isomer that emits β-rays, enabling its use as a contrast agent. Active bleeding sites are identified through evaluation of focal areas of the tracers that conform to the bowel anatomy, increase with time, and move with peristalsis. This study is typically performed in patients with significant hemorrhage and an unprepared bowel, in whom endoscopic evaluation is not optimal.

Gastric emptying scans are nuclear medicine tests used to assess the rate food exits the stomach into the duodenum. The examination is performed by having the patient consume either a solid or liquid radiolabeled meal followed by observation with a gamma

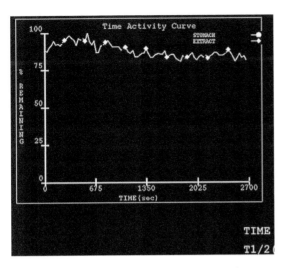

FIG. 5.19 A nuclear medicine gastric emptying scan demonstrates a marked delay in emptying of the stomach.

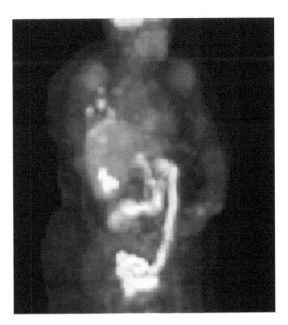

FIG. 5.20 A positron emission tomography (PET) scan for staging of colon cancer demonstrates new hypermetabolic activity of metastatic disease in the liver and right hemithorax.

camera as it passes out of the stomach. Typically, a high level of radioactivity maintained within the stomach after an extended period would indicate poor gastric emptying (Fig. 5.19). In addition, the test may also be used to monitor the response of promotility drug treatments such as that of metoclopramide or erythromycin. One drawback of the test is that it cannot differentiate between physical obstruction and gastroparesis; that is, further diagnostic studies will often need to be ordered if the patient exhibits a delay in gastric emptying.

Urea breath tests are performed on patients with gastric ulcers to identify the presence of *Helicobacter pylori (H-pylori)*. Infection with this bacterial species is a common cause of gastric ulcers and can be treated quite effectively with antibiotic therapy. The procedure begins by having the patient drink radioactive urea. If the bacteria are present in the stomach, they will break down the urea, and the patient will release radioactive carbon dioxide. This is captured in the breath test.

Meckel scans can be utilized in identifying ectopic gastric mucosa, as in a Meckel's diverticulum. This is accomplished through injection of Tc-99m pertechnetate, which is taken up by mucus-secreting cells of the gastric mucosa. Focal uptake outside of the stomach and in the small bowel would be positive for the pathologic condition.

Positron emission tomography (PET) may be used to evaluate and stage GI cancers (Fig. 5.20). PET has been proven to demonstrate approximately 20% of esophageal cancerous lesions (Fig. 5.21) undetected by CT.

Endoscopic Procedures

As noted earlier, **endoscopy** is the use of tubular fiber optic devices to look inside the GI tract and other hollow organs or cavities of the body. As its sophistication and specificity have increased, it is assuming a greater role in diagnosis and therapy of the GI tract. Upper endoscopy provides direct visualization of the mucosal surface of the esophagus, stomach, duodenum (including the ampulla of Vater), and even the proximal jejunum. Colonoscopy allows retrograde visualization of the colon as far as the terminal ileum. Sigmoidoscopy is an abbreviated version of the colonoscopy used to visualize the rectum, sigmoid, and possible descending colon.

The small bowel is still largely out of reach through traditional endoscopy; however, the advent of video capsule endoscopy, which involves the ingestion of a small camera pill, has resulted in its increased use in the diagnosis of small bowel tumors. The capsule encases

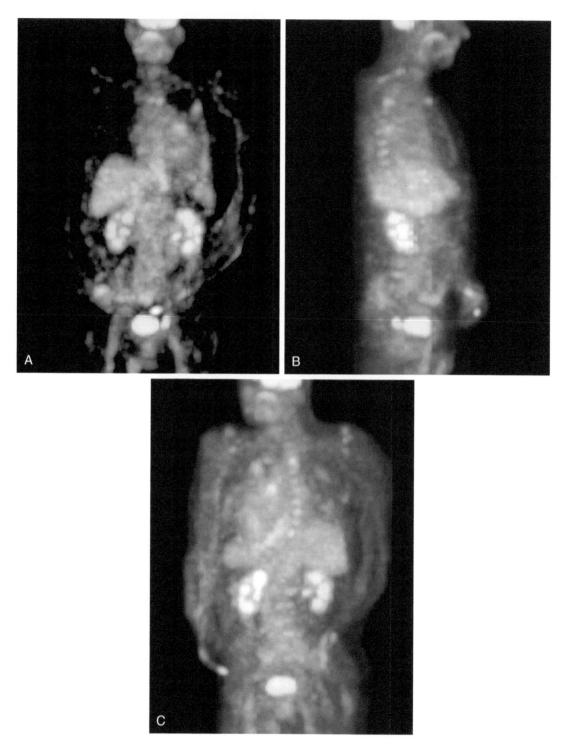

FIG. 5.21 A positron emission tomography (PET) scan (**A**, frontal; **B**, lateral; **C**, oblique) of a patient with known esophageal cancer ordered for staging of the disease. Hypermetabolic focal activity is demonstrated at the level of the gastroesophageal junction designating the primary tumor and in the upper thoracic spine, right lobe of the liver, and left lung suggesting metastatic disease.

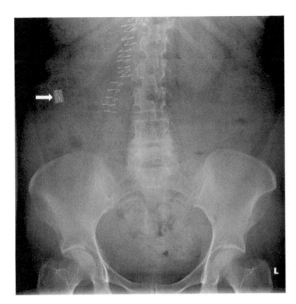

FIG. 5.22 Kidneys, ureters, and bladder radiograph providing visualization of a patency capsule (*white arrow*) retained within the region of the ascending colon.

a digital camera that transmits images to a recording device worn on a belt. The capsule has a gastric transit time of approximately 1 hour and small-bowel transit time of 3 to 4 hours. This technology is indicated in diagnosis of obscure GI bleeding, which is often caused by a lesion. This technology, however, has several drawbacks such as inability to identify the precise location of pathology, inability to biopsy or treat located pathology, and lack of reimbursement by insurance companies. The contraindications to performing capsule endoscopy are a bowel obstruction and strictures. Patients may be asked to swallow a patency capsule before the actual camera capsule to screen for possible transit obstructions. The patency capsule is radiopaque and can be located using a conventional supine abdominal radiograph if the capsule does not pass (Fig. 5.22). The patency capsule will dissolve whereas the actual camera capsule will not and may require surgical intervention if it becomes lodged in the GI tract. Photographic views of the interior of the small intestine provide readily diagnosable information (Figs. 5.23 and 5.24).

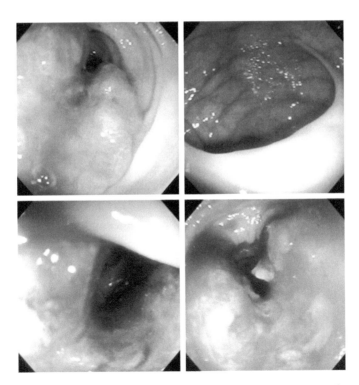

FIG. 5.23 Endoscopic image of a sigmoid colon mass in a 72-year-old woman; the mass is seen bulging into the lumen of the colon.

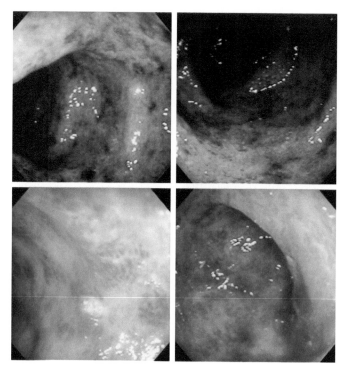

FIG. 5.24 Endoscopic image of diffuse colitis with a bacterial cause in this 40-year-old man, indicated by the splotchiness of the bowel mucosa.

In addition to the diagnostic value of endoscopy, the therapeutic applications are numerous. They include polyp removal, stricture dilation, injection and thermal methods to stop hemorrhaging, sclerosing and banding of esophageal varices, lesion biopsy, sealing of tracheoesophageal fistulae, foreign body removal, upper GI tract stent insertion, and laser tumor removal (both generally for palliative purposes). In addition, endoscopically placed enteric wall stents have been used to open lesions in nonoperative malignancies of the colon. There is even an endoscopically performed version of antireflux surgery called a transoral incisionless fundoplication (TIF).

Abdominal Tubes and Catheters

As with the chest, a variety of tubes and catheters can be placed within particular portions of the abdomen and GI tract. The technologist must be familiar with each type of tube and exercise great caution in attempting to move patients with abdominal tubes in place. The technologist should also ask the patient's nurse or consult the patient's medical record before altering the patient's

position. In addition, some abdominal tubes and catheters allow entry into body systems that are normally sterile and require special care to avoid infection.

Gastric tubes may be placed for a variety of diagnostic and therapeutic purposes. They may be indicated for aspiration of gastric contents to help control nausea and vomiting, for decompression and removal of gastric contents because of bowel dysfunction or surgery, and for nutritional support tube feedings (gastric gavage) or medication administration. Gastric tubes placed through the mouth are termed orogastric (OG) tubes. More commonly, gastric tubes are placed via the nose and are called nasogastric (NG) tubes. The Salem Sump tube is the most commonly used NG tube for adults. It is a double lumen tube with multiple openings at its distal end that also has a radiopaque strip down the length of the tube with a small lucent section near the distal tip to detect proper placement on a radiograph (Fig. 5.25). The tube may also be placed as an OG tube. The Levin tube is another type of NG tube. It is a fairly small, single-lumen tube with a plain tip, and it may be visualized radiographically. Proper placement is

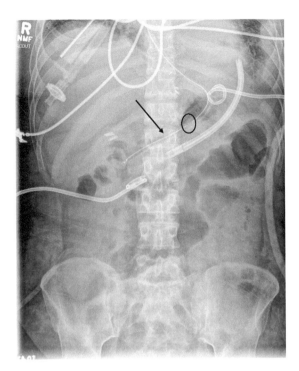

FIG. 5.25 Supine abdominal radiograph showing a naso-gastric (NG) tube (*black arrow*) with the tip in the region of the pylorus of the stomach. The small lucent section (*black circle*) is located in the region of the gastric body.

commonly assessed through aspiration of gastric juices and listening over the stomach via a stethoscope as air is injected through the tube. If an NG tube is placed for feeding, the patient's head must remain elevated to prevent the tube from becoming displaced, leading to aspiration of the gastric contents. If an emergent condition exists that requires large amounts of gastric contents to be aspirated quickly (gastric lavage), the Ewald tube or the Edlich tube may be used. These tubes are placed through the mouth, are wider than the Levin tube, and contain several openings that allow quicker aspiration. The Levacuator tube may also be used for the evacuation of gastric contents. This is a wide, double-lumen tube placed through the patient's mouth. The larger lumen is used for gastric lavage, and the smaller lumen allows instillation of an irrigant.

An enteral tube is a small-caliber tube used to deliver a liquid diet directly to the duodenum or jejunum. Postpyloric feeding tube placement lessens the risk of gastroesophageal reflux and aspiration of reflux from tube feeding. It is generally inserted via the nose with

the mouth being a less common insertion route. Enteral tubes commonly have weighted ends to maintain proper placement. The Dobhoff tube is a common radiopaque enteral tube (Fig. 5.26). Other common types of prolonged enteral tubes include the Corpak tube and the Entriflex tube.

Nasoenteric decompression tubes are used to remove gas and fluids in the prevention and treatment of abdominal distention. At one end, these tubes have a balloon or rubber bag filled with air, mercury, or water to stimulate peristalsis and facilitate passage through the pylorus into the intestinal tract. The Miller-Abbott tube is a common type of double-lumen decompression tube. It is passed through the nose, pharynx, and esophagus with the balloon uninflated. Once the end of the tube reaches the stomach, the balloon is inflated and the tube is pulled back until it stops at the cardiac sphincter. The patient is then placed on his or her right side in the semierect position, and the air is withdrawn from the balloon and replaced with mercury. Progress of the tube is assessed by taking abdominal radiographs at regular intervals. The Harris and Cantor tubes are other types of decompression tubes. Unlike the Miller-Abbott tube, however, the Cantor tube (Fig. 5.27) and the Harris tube contain a single lumen.

The Levin tube or the Foley catheter may also be surgically placed directly into any portion of the GI system. A gastrostomy tube (G-tube), as the name indicates, is a tube placed through the wall of the stomach, whereas a duodenostomy or a jejunostomy tube (J-tube) is specific to that portion of the small intestine. A percutaneous endoscopic gastrostomy (PEG) tube is frequently placed endoscopically. These tubes provide a direct route for administering liquid nutrition.

Congenital and Hereditary Anomalies

Esophageal Atresia

Atresia is a congenital absence or closure of a normal body orifice or tubular organ. Esophageal atresia is a rare congenital anomaly in which the esophagus fails to develop past some point, resulting in discontinuation of the esophagus (Fig. 5.28). This anomaly is caused by a defect in cell differentiation of the trachea and esophagus during the fourth to sixth week of embryonic development. The symptoms of esophageal atresia are

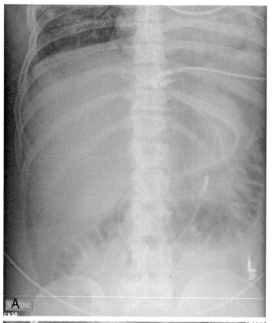

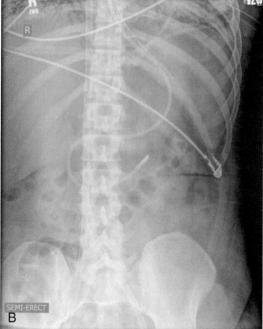

FIG. 5.26 **A,** Supine abdominal radiograph demonstrating Dobhoff tube reaching to the fourth segment of the duodenum (ligament of Treitz). **B,** Semierect abdominal radiograph demonstrating Dobhoff tube placement in the same patient.

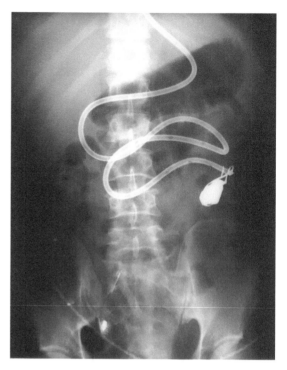

FIG. 5.27 Radiographic appearance of the Cantor tube in this 50-year-old man with a mechanical bowel obstruction. Approximately 4 hours after placement, it has advanced into the second portion of the duodenum.

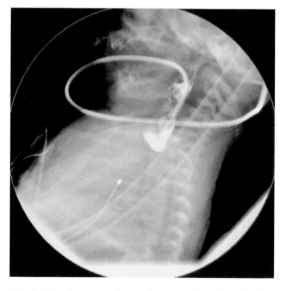

FIG. 5.28 Lateral neck image following injection of barium sulfate demonstrating esophageal atresia.

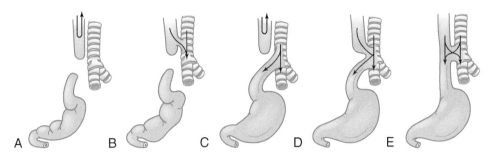

FIG. 5.29 Five types of esophageal atresia and tracheoesophageal fistulae.

visible soon after birth and include excessive salivation, choking, gagging, dyspnea, and cyanosis. Diagnosis of this congenital anomaly may be established by inability to pass an NG tube into the stomach. If a radiopaque NG tube is used, the terminal end of the pouch may be demonstrated radiographically with a chest radiograph without the use of a contrast agent. Immediate surgery is required to alleviate the problem, and preoperative care must be taken to prevent aspiration pneumonia. The infant may not receive oral feedings and continuous suction is necessary to prevent aspiration. Under most circumstances, this increased risk of aspiration contraindicates the use of a contrast agent to visualize the extent of the atresia.

Usually a tracheoesophageal (TE) fistula is coexistent with atresia (Fig. 5.29). This consists of an atresia at the level of the fourth thoracic vertebra with a fistula—an abnormal tube-like passage from one structure to another—to the trachea (Fig. 5.30). In addition, a gastrostomy tube may be placed in the infant's stomach to prevent reflux of gastric secretions into the trachea through the fistula. Such a condition is incompatible with life for more than 2 to 3 days, but the prognosis is good if the infant is handled appropriately before surgery to prevent aspiration.

Bowel Atresia

Ileal atresia, a congenital discontinuation of the ileum, is the most frequent type of bowel atresia, followed by duodenal atresia. This anomaly manifests a few days after birth. The most common signs and symptoms of ileal atresia are abdominal distention and the inability of the infant to pass stool. Eventually, the infant regurgitates feedings. Treatment consists of surgery to resect the atretic portion of the bowel and reconnect the bowel proximal and distal to the discontinuation. In

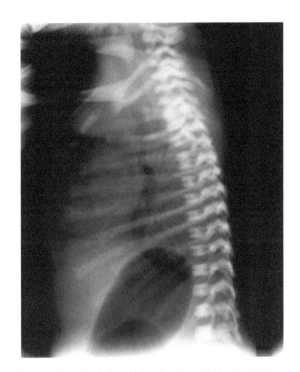

FIG. 5.30 Lateral view of the chest on a 1-day-old premature infant demonstrates distention of the distal esophagus with air and discontinuity with the trachea. Marked gastric distention is also present. Appearance is consistent with esophageal atresia and a tracheoesophageal fistula.

some cases, the proximal ileum may be grossly dilated, necessitating a double-barrel ileostomy. Once the lumen of the proximal ileum returns to a more normal size, the ileostomy is reversed, and bowel anastomosis can be performed.

Duodenal atresia is a congenital anomaly in which the lumen of the duodenum does not exist, resulting in

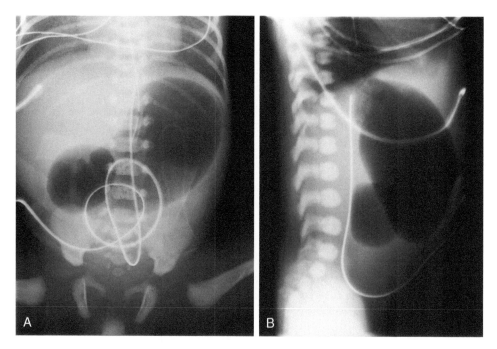

FIG. 5.31 **A**, Marked distention of the stomach and duodenal bulb with bowel gas distal to the duodenum. Visualization of the classic "double bubble sign" indicates duodenal atresia. **B**, The "double bubble sign" in a lateral projection of the same 1-day-old infant.

complete obstruction of the GI tract at the duodenum. In some cases, the atresia may be identified before the birth of the infant with the use of sonography. Sonographic evaluation of the fetus should demonstrate a normal stomach with amniotic fluid coursing through it. Atresia is suggested during sonography if a dilated stomach is noted without other fluid collections noted in the fetal abdomen. Although rare (one in approximately 20,000 births), it is evident soon after birth when vomiting begins and the epigastrium becomes distended. A radiographic indication of duodenal atresia is the "double bubble sign." Gaseous distention of the stomach creates one bubble, and gas in the proximal duodenum creates a second bubble (Fig. 5.31). As with esophageal atresia, oral feedings should be withheld in infants with duodenal atresia. Nasogastric decompression of the stomach is indicated to prevent vomiting and possible aspiration of gastric contents. Treatment consists of surgery to open the duodenum for connection to the pylorus. During surgery, it is common to examine the other areas of the small bowel and the large bowel for other sites of atresia and malrotation, which often accompany duodenal atresia.

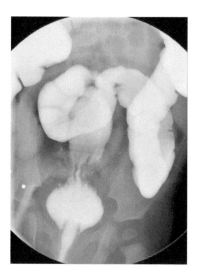

FIG. 5.32 Spot image demonstrating imperforate anus in a pediatric patient.

Colonic atresia is a congenital failure of development of the distal rectum and anus, which may occur to a variable extent (Fig. 5.32). A frequent complication is fistula formation to the genitourinary system (Fig. 5.33),

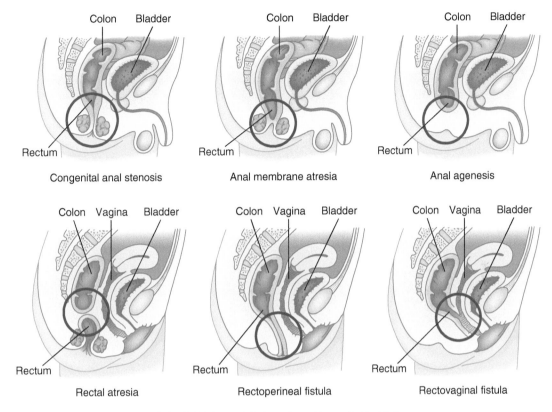

Congenital anal stenosis

Anal membrane atresia

Anal agenesis

Rectal atresia

Rectoperineal fistula

Rectovaginal fistula

FIG. 5.33 Anorectal stenosis and imperforate anus.

which often can be repaired surgically. Prognosis is excellent after surgical intervention for all three types of bowel atresia.

Imperforate anus or **anal agenesis** is a congenital disorder in which the anal opening to the exterior body is absent. A fistula may be present between the colon and the perineum or the urethra in boys or between the colon and the vagina in girls. This condition can be demonstrated radiographically with a cross-table lateral rectum projection with the patient lying prone or by performing a fistulogram. It is corrected surgically shortly after birth and may require a temporary colostomy.

Hypertrophic Pyloric Stenosis

Hypertrophic pyloric stenosis (HPS) is a congenital anomaly of the stomach in which the pyloric canal leading out of the stomach is greatly narrowed because of hypertrophy and hyperplasia of the pyloric sphincter (Fig. 5.34). It is the most common indication for surgery

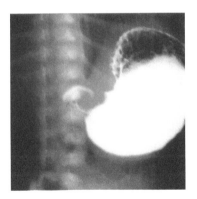

FIG. 5.34 A thin column of barium flowing from the stomach into the pylorus in this 1-month-old boy with projectile vomiting indicates hypertrophic pyloric stenosis.

in infants. Its exact cause is unknown, but it seems to be genetically related. Current literature suggests that infants born to mothers with a history of pyloric stenosis, or instances of increased gastrin secretion by the mother within the third trimester of pregnancy, may increase the probability of HPS occurring in the infant. Researchers believe the muscle mass is stimulated by the transforming growth factor-alpha (TGF-α) and the nerves within the muscular layer are not functioning properly. HPS occurs more frequently in Caucasians than in African Americans or Asians, four times more often in male children (1 in 200), and most often in first-born male children. HPS is typically suggested by projectile bile-free emesis in a previously healthy infant around 2 to 6 weeks of age. Affected infants often become dehydrated and fail to gain weight. It is most commonly confused with pylorospasm, which, in contrast, is an incomplete obstruction to fluid flow into the duodenal bulb resulting from spasmodic changes in pyloric muscle tone.

When the classic "olive" sign of hypertrophied pyloric muscle is palpated, the diagnosis of HPS can be made clinically, and the patient can be sent to surgery without the need for imaging examinations. Accurate measurements of pyloric muscle thickening are useful in surgical planning, even when the diagnosis is clinically evident. When no "olive" is palpated, imaging by radiography, sonography, fluoroscopic UGI series, or a combination of these modalities can be performed for initial diagnosis.

Abdominal radiography may show gastric distention with HPS. On occasion, a mass impression of the thickened pyloric muscle on an air-filled gastric antrum may be noted; however, initial radiography is usually limited to determining a strategy for further workup.

Sonography has become the standard and highly accurate method for diagnosing HPS without the need for radiation exposure. It allows for imaging of the pyloric muscle and channel, and the constant imaging of an elongated, thick-walled pylorus is indicative of HPS. Prolonged sonographic observation of the passage of gastric contents may be tedious but helps avoid surgery in cases simulating HPS. Measurements of pyloric channel length, pyloric diameter, and muscle thickness are often used for diagnosis. Abnormal muscle wall thicknesses can range from 4.8 ± 0.6 mm in HPS patients, compared with 1.8 ± 0.4 mm in normal persons.

An upper GI study demonstrates delayed gastric emptying accompanied by the mass impression of the hypertrophied pyloric muscle on the barium-filled antrum ("shoulder sign"), the filling of the proximal pylorus ("beak sign"), or the entire elongated pylorus ("string sign") as barium trickles through the narrowed pyloric canal. However, because of delayed gastric emptying in cases of HPS, the demonstration of the beak and string signs may be difficult to detect, requiring considerable fluoroscopic time and an increased radiation risk to the patient.

Scintigraphy, a nuclear medicine test, is seldom indicated but may provide useful information about gastric emptying if other tests fail to reveal a delay. Furthermore, delayed images in standard positions allow scintigraphy to assess gastric transit without additional radiation exposure. Delayed gastric emptying has been defined as more than 50% retained labeled liquid within the stomach after 120 minutes in children younger than 2 years of age.

A surgical pyloromyotomy procedure is used to incise the hypertrophied muscle fibers and thus increase the opening of the pyloric channel. Affected infants generally are able to begin normal feedings within a few days after the surgical procedure. Pylorospasm is said to be the most common cause of gastric outlet obstruction in pediatrics and, unlike HPS, it is treated conservatively.

Malrotation

Aberrations in the normal process of intestinal rotation in utero may result in the anomalous position of the small bowel and the large bowel, with abnormal fixations predisposing the patient to internal herniation and volvulus. **Malrotation** exists when the intestines are not in their normal position (Fig. 5.35), which occurs in an equal male-to-female ratio. Varying degrees of malrotation of the intestinal tract exist, ranging from failure of fixation of the cecum in the RLQ to complete transposition of the bowel, a condition in which the small bowel is on the right and the colon is on the left. Complete reversal of all abdominal organs, although rare, is known as **situs inversus**.

When malrotation is suspected in an infant with bilious vomiting, a UGI series should be the examination of choice and is considered the gold standard. During the examination, the focus is on following the initial column of oral contrast media through the upper GI system. Evaluation involves the search for any deviation in the normal route of the duodenum from right to left of midline, as well as its turn upward to the duodenojejunal flexure at the ligament of Treitz, which is generally at the same height as the duodenal bulb

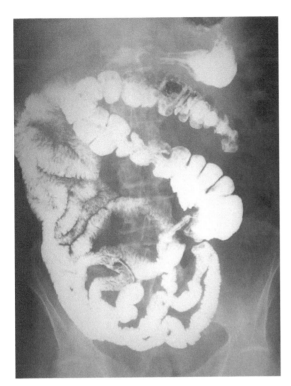

FIG. 5.35 Malrotation of the bowel indicated by the position of the small bowel on the right side of the abdomen and the colon on the left. Note how the terminal ileum enters the cecum from the right.

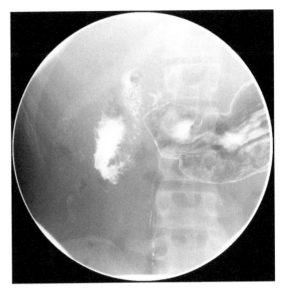

FIG. 5.36 Double-contrast upper gastrointestinal tract image (UGI) showing a malrotation of the duodenal c-loop that does not cross to the left of midline as it should, but instead remains in the right upper quadrant (RUQ) with the fourth portion of the duodenum overlapping the duodenal bulb. A sparse amount of barium can be seen in jejunal loops located in the RUQ as a result of the malrotation.

(Fig. 5.36). Additionally, a UGI study may demonstrate a high greater curvature, a greater curvature crossing the esophagus, a downward-pointing pylorus, two air–fluid levels, or a lowering of the gastric fundus, all of which are suggestive of gastric torsion, commonly associated with malrotation of the bowel. A barium enema examination may also be useful in evaluating the location of the cecum, which is normally located in the RLQ of the abdomen. Such errors of intestinal fixation are often asymptomatic, but they may lead to bowel volvulus or incarceration of bowel in an internal hernia.

Sonography is useful as a complementary tool to confirm the diagnosis of malrotation, with demonstration of the position of the third part of the duodenum between the aorta and the superior mesenteric artery (SMA) in the transverse and sagittal planes. However, it is important to note that the obscuration of the entire course of the normal fluid-filled duodenum by overlying gas may limit the usefulness of sonography in the acute setting.

In some instances of malrotation, the patient may have clinical signs of bowel obstruction, as discussed later in this chapter. Another complication is that a volvulus or bowel incarceration resulting from a malrotation can compromise the blood supply to the involved bowel leading to ischemia (inadequate blood supply) and subsequent infarction (tissue death or necrosis). Surgery is the treatment for correction of a volvulus or bowel incarceration, with resection of the involved bowel to remove the intestinal infarction.

Hirschsprung Disease (Congenital Aganglionic Megacolon)

Hirschsprung disease or congenital aganglionic megacolon refers to the absence of neurons (Meissner and Auerbach autonomic plexus) in the distal large bowel wall, typically in the sigmoid colon. Occurring in approximately 1 in 5000 births, this defect is a familial

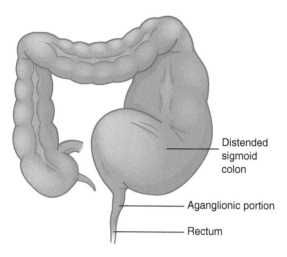

FIG. 5.37 Congenital aganglionic megacolon.

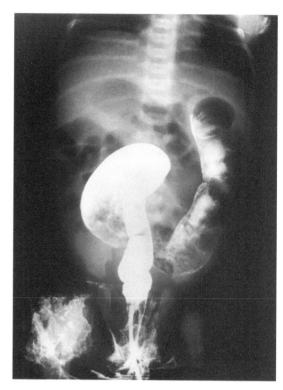

FIG. 5.38 Barium enema on a 6-day-old infant demonstrates a normal rectosigmoid leading to a distended large bowel consistent with Hirschsprung disease.

disease, primarily affecting males. Although the exact cause of Hirschsprung disease is unknown, a link to inheritance of the "rearranged during transfection" (RET) proto-oncogene localized to chromosome 10 has been established. A malformation of the parasympathetic nervous system results in the absence of neurons in the bowel wall preventing the normal relaxation of the aganglionic colon and subsequently impairing normal colon peristalsis. This anomaly results in a functional obstruction with gross dilation of the colon to the point of the aganglionic segment that is narrow and constricted (Fig. 5.37).

This generally becomes apparent shortly after birth, when the affected infant passes little meconium and the abdomen becomes distended. As the patient ages, the continued effects include severe constipation and recurrent fecal impactions. It is important to diagnose this disease early because it can progress to toxic megacolon if left untreated. Toxic megacolon develops from bacterial overgrowth leading to fluid and electrolyte imbalances that could result in death.

Barium enemas demonstrate a transition from the narrow, distal rectum to a dilated proximal colon (Fig. 5.38). However, it should be noted that barium enema examination is strictly contraindicated in patients with known or suspected toxic megacolon. Initial treatment in an infant may consist of a temporary colostomy until surgical resection is possible later. In some cases, multiple surgeries may be performed during infancy to correct the anomaly.

Meckel's Diverticulum

Meckel's diverticulum is a congenital diverticulum of the distal ileum. This sac-like anomaly is located within 6 feet of the ileocecal valve and is a remnant of a duct, called the vitelline or omphalomesenteric duct, connecting the small bowel to the umbilicus in the fetus. A Meckel's diverticulum may be asymptomatic in some cases. Children with a Meckel's diverticulum often develop an ulcer in the adjacent bowel, and a common sign is repeated episodes of bleeding from the ulcerated site resulting in hematochezia (blood in the stool). Symptoms in adolescents and adults include cramping, vomiting, and bowel obstruction. The symptoms mimic those of appendicitis except for the location of the pain.

Diagnosis of a Meckel's diverticulum is difficult, as it is likely not be visible on radiographic or fluoroscopic studies of the small bowel. Abdominal radiographs may show signs of obstruction or free air if those complications are present. However, nuclear medicine Meckel scans are useful in diagnosing this anomaly by identifying ectopic gastric mucosa, which is present in over half of all cases. This is accomplished through injection of Tc-99m pertechnetate, which is taken up by the mucus-secreting cells of the gastric mucosa. If hematochezia is present, a nuclear medicine GI bleed scan or vascular interventional arteriogram may also lead to diagnosis. Enterography, CT enterography, MR enterography and video capsule endoscopy have also been used for diagnosis. Treatment of a symptomatic Meckel's diverticulum involves surgical resection of the diverticulum.

Gluten-Sensitive Enteropathy

Gluten-sensitive enteropathy, formally known as celiac sprue or celiac disease, is an autoimmune hereditary disorder involving increased sensitivity to the gliadin fraction of gluten, an agent found in wheat, barley, and rye products such as bread, which interferes with normal digestion and absorption of food through the small bowel. The gliadin acts as an antigen and combines with antibodies within the intestinal mucosa, which promotes the aggregation of K lymphocytes. These lymphocytes cause mucosal damage in combination with an increase in crypt cells within the mucosa. With such a condition, the bowel dilates, mucosal folds atrophy, and peristalsis slows or stops. Common symptoms include diarrhea, flatulence, weight loss, abdominal distention, and abdominal pain. In addition, patients often present with nutritional deficiencies specific to the primary disease and the area of the GI system affected by the disorder.

Radiographic changes during SBFT examination generally seen with gluten-sensitive enteropathy are segmentation of the barium column, flocculation (resembling tufts of cotton), and edematous mucosal changes (Fig. 5.39). The mucosal changes cause the jejunum to have a dilated appearance with folds that resemble that of the ileum instead of the normal delicate and feathery folds of normal jejunum. Laboratory tests demonstrate low albumin, calcium, potassium, and sodium levels in combination with elevated alkaline phosphatase and prothrombin time. Diagnosis is confirmed by biopsy of the small bowel. Treatment of gluten-sensitive enteropathy consists of avoidance of substances containing gluten. Vitamin therapy is also used to ensure adequate amounts of nutrients that are not available because of malabsorption in the small bowel.

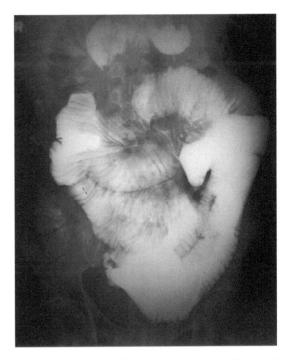

FIG. 5.39 Gluten-sensitive enteropathy in a 15-year-old patient with a history of diarrhea, indicated on this small bowel study by dilated bowel loops, thickened folds, a grayish appearance of the barium (because of excess fluid in the bowel), and a delayed transit time.

Carbohydrate Intolerance

Carbohydrate intolerance is the inability to digest certain carbohydrates, including lactose, because of an acquired lactase deficiency. This disorder affects approximately 60% of the nonwhite population and 20% to 30% of the Caucasian population. In this condition, the small bowel lacks enough of the enzyme lactase, which is used to break down lactose into simple sugars that can be absorbed. The result is that lactose stays in the bowel and acts as an osmotic agent, causing fluid to weep from the wall into the lumen of the colon, creating cramping and diarrhea. The diarrhea also leads to other nutritional deficiencies because the nutrients are purged before they can be absorbed through the intestinal mucosa. Lactose mixed with barium shows the barium moving quickly through the bowel and becoming diluted in the distal ileum and colon (Fig. 5.40). Patients affected by this condition avoid symptoms by abstaining from consumption of dairy products.

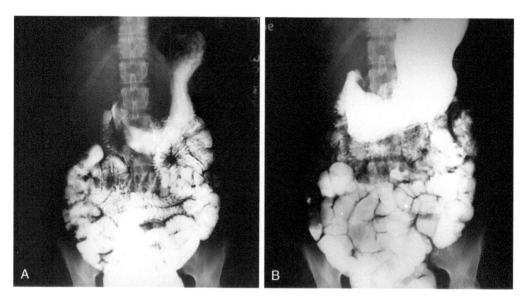

FIG. 5.40 **A,** Abdominal distention, pain, and diarrhea led to this small bowel examination, diagnosed as normal for this 35-year-old patient. **B,** Mixing of lactose with barium on a repeat study led to mild bowel dilation, rapid transit time, and dilution of barium in the distal small bowel, indicative of lactase insufficiency.

Inflammatory Diseases

Esophageal Strictures

A stricture is an abnormal narrowing. Strictures may be benign or malignant. Esophageal strictures occur in varying degrees, with the symptoms displayed differing according to the amount of obstruction produced. Strictures may be secondary to the ingestion of caustic materials such as strong acids or alkalines (Fig. 5.41) or from any factor that inflames the mucosa and creates scarring (Fig. 5.42 A & B). Common types of caustics include household cleansers and detergents containing sulfuric acid and sodium hydroxide. These caustic agents burn the esophagus and cause edema, swelling, and possibly perforation. Endoscopy is usually performed to assess the damage to the esophagus, and the esophageal lesions are treated with corticosteroid therapy. Strictures can also be a result of a tumor or scarring after radiation therapy treatment. Narrowing of a segment of the esophagus related to external compression by other adjacent structures is also a form of an esophageal stricture.

Strictures can be differentiated radiographically from normal peristalsis by their fixed or unchanging

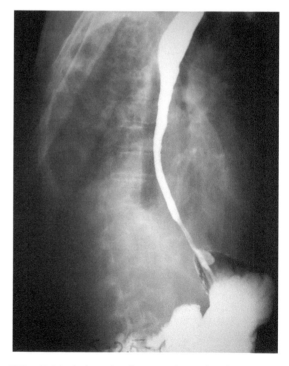

FIG. 5.41 A longstanding esophageal stricture in a 78-year-old man caused by accidental ingestion of a caustic agent at age 3 years.

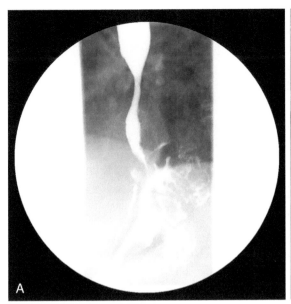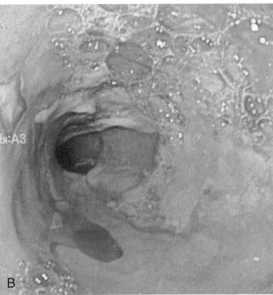

FIG. 5.42 **A,** Esophagram image demonstrating a long segment stricture of the distal esophagus related to reflux esophagitis. Note that the stricture is continuous from the GE junction upward and that the proximal margin is smoothly tapered without abrupt margins. The mucosal lining of the narrowed segment does not have smooth margins but instead has a ragged appearance with several areas of small projections. This appearance is seen with a reflux stricture that has active inflammation and mucosal erosions. **B,** Image taken during an upper endoscopy on the same patient demonstrating narrowing of the esophageal lumen that has red and inflamed mucosa.

appearance; peristalsis is transitory. The mucosa of a benign stricture appears normal with a smooth contour and smoothly tapered proximal and distal margins; the contour of a malignant stricture typically appears ragged and often has acute or "shouldered" proximal and distal margins. Esophageal strictures require repeated dilation with special mercury-filled tubes of varying diameters to maintain proper patency. Common tubes for this purpose include the Hurst dilator, the Maloney dilator and pneumatic balloon dilators that are passed over a guidewire. Esophageal stents can be placed for palliative treatment of esophageal stricture symptoms. Malignant strictures generally require surgical resection to remove the neoplastic portion. Benign strictures may also require surgical intervention if they are not responsive to dilation efforts.

Gastroesophageal Reflux Disease

Gastroesophageal reflux disease (GERD) results from an incompetent cardiac sphincter, which allows the backward flow of gastric acid and contents into the esophagus. **Reflux esophagitis** is the primary cause

of esophageal inflammation; however, reflux is not necessarily always abnormal. Heartburn, or symptomatic reflux, has been experienced by most people at one time or another. Furthermore, regurgitation, or gastroesophageal reflux, is common in the first 3 months of life and resolves with time. It usually has no definitive pathologic cause and is unrelated to a functional defect. It is only when the normal event leads to chronic symptoms and complications such as esophagitis, a stricture, or an esophageal ulcer that it becomes of concern.

Many tests are used to confirm the diagnosis of gastroesophageal reflux. These tests include esophageal manometry to determine the pressure in the upper and lower esophageal sphincters, pH monitoring of the esophagus, acid perfusion (Bernstein) testing, upper endoscopy, and fluoroscopic evaluation in the form of an esophagram or UGI procedure. Of the previously mentioned diagnostic examinations, the pH monitoring is considered the current gold standard. Fluoroscopy studies are performed to assess the structure and function of the esophagus. Depending on clinical circumstances, the degree of reflux based on the number of events over a given period of time, the height of the refluxing column, the quality of the esophageal mucosa, and evidence of aspiration into the lungs are assessed and reported. It is important to note that reflux may often not be evident on a barium swallow. The associated sensitivity and specificity of esophagram and UGI examinations range from 31% to 86%. The brief duration of observation for reflux often results in false-negative results, whereas the frequent occurrence of nonpathologic reflux may result in false-positive results. Thus the esophagram or UGI series is not considered a useful test to reliably determine the presence or absence of GERD but more so to identify pathology such as ulcers and strictures caused by chronic irritation that may be associated with a predetermined diagnosis of GERD.

Reflux scintigraphy with Tc-99m–labeled sulfur colloid mixed with food has shown comparable sensitivity and specificity to that of barium studies in the diagnosis of GERD. Furthermore, nuclear medicine scintigraphy can be used over a prolonged time without increasing radiation exposure and at a lesser radiation dose than the UGI series. A 1-hour scintigraphic study formatted in 60-second frames provides a quantitative representation of postprandial GERD, particularly if gastric emptying is not rapid. The use of this study is typically limited to patients in whom other modalities have already identified an anatomic cause.

Sonographic diagnosis of reflux is made by noting water, which has been previously placed into the stomach, refluxing into the distal esophagus after tube removal. Because sonography typically demonstrates more episodes of reflux in comparison to a UGI series, some clinicians consider it too sensitive, and thus less specific, in diagnosing GERD. Sonography provides functional and morphologic information and therefore may be useful for identifying patients who should be referred for pH monitoring. Current literature suggests that color Doppler ultrasonography may be used in place of the more invasive pH-probe testing procedure.

GERD treatment may be conservative, medical, or surgical. Conservative treatment involves lifestyle and dietary changes such as elevating the head of the individual's bed and the patient avoiding drinks such as coffee or alcohol that stimulate acid secretion or foods such as chocolate that decrease sphincter competence. Smoking must be avoided because it also lowers sphincter competence. GERD is also treated with

medication therapy. Antacids aim to neutralize gastric acids producing temporary symptom relief but they do not heal existing inflammation. Histamine 2 receptor blockers (H_2 blockers) decrease acid production short term. Proton pump inhibitors (PPIs) hinder acid production by cells in the stomach and provide healing time for mucosal inflammation caused by reflux. Prokinetic agents can enhance motility reducing stasis of gastric acids and contents. Surgery as a treatment is the last option for those whose symptoms have failed to respond to medical therapy. It is performed using laparoscopic or endoscopic techniques aimed at strengthening or reconstructing the lower esophageal sphincter.

Peptic Ulcer

Normally, the GI system is protected by a mucosal barrier and epithelial cells that remove excess hydrogen ions. Mucosal blood flow also helps to remove excess acid, thus maintaining a normal pH balance. A **peptic ulcer** is an erosion of the mucous membrane of the lower end of the esophagus, stomach, or duodenum (Fig. 5.43). The most likely sites of a peptic ulcer are in the duodenal bulb and on the lesser curvature of the stomach. Duodenal ulcers are found in adults of all ages and are almost always benign. Gastric ulcers may affect individuals at any age but primarily those over 40 years of age.

Current studies suggest that peptic ulcers result from disruption of the normal mucosal defense and repair mechanisms. Nonsteroidal antiinflammatory drugs (NSAIDs) and the bacterium H. pylori alter the mucosa, making it more susceptible to the effects of acid normally residing in the GI tract. H. pylori is a gram-negative, spiral-shaped bacillus, which was identified in 1983. Researchers believe the H. pylori increases gastrin production, making the mucosa more susceptible to acid damage. NSAIDs inflame the mucosa because they are able to diffuse through the mucosa into the epithelium and damage the epithelial cells.

The main symptom of a gastric ulcer is pain, usually above the epigastrium and radiating to all parts of the abdomen. Food ingestion or antacids provide temporary relief, but the pain usually returns when the stomach is empty. In some patients, food may actually increase pain as it stimulates peristalsis, which irritates the ulcer. Symptoms of a duodenal ulcer are more consistent, and pain generally begins midmorning. The pain subsides with food ingestion but returns 2 to 3 hours later.

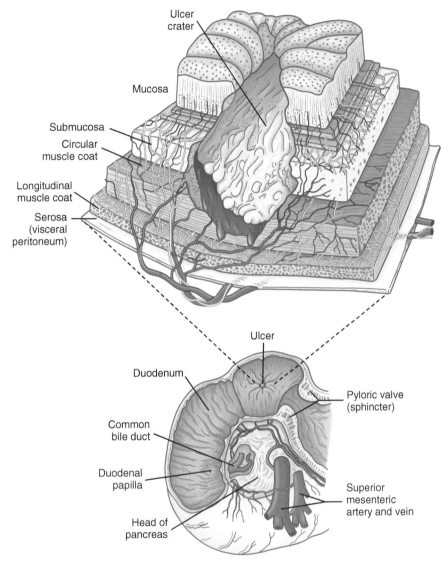

Ulcer crater

Mucosa

Submucosa

Circular muscle coat

Longitudinal muscle coat

Serosa (visceral peritoneum)

Ulcer

Duodenum

Pyloric valve (sphincter)

Common bile duct

Duodenal papilla

Superior mesenteric artery and vein

Head of pancreas

FIG. 5.43 Common location of duodenal ulcer.

Diagnosis is made primarily via upper endoscopy. However, double-contrast radiographic UGI studies may be performed. Intermittent healing in the midst of continuing inflammation leads to considerable scarring at the base of the ulcer. Gastric ulcers generally display as radiating, spike-like wheels of mucosal folds that run to the edge of the ulcer crater (Fig. 5.44). Seen en face, the edge of this ulcer appears round and regular (Fig. 5.45).

Ulcers are commonly treated with multidrug therapy in combination with a PPI. The drug regimen currently used is a combination of antibiotics and acid-blocking drugs. The most common drugs used to eradicate *H. pylori* include omeprazole or lansoprazole, clarithromycin, amoxicillin or metronidazole, and bismuth citrate or a PPI. Surgery is rarely performed and primarily is required only for complications of ulcers, such as obstruction, bleeding or perforation.

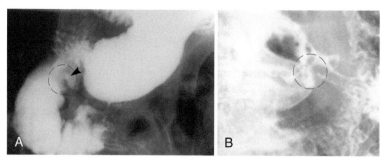

FIG. 5.44 **A**, Prone right anterior oblique projection of the duodenal bulb demonstrates a dense collection of barium in an ulcer crater, suggesting that it is on the anterior duodenal wall. **B**, Persistent collection of barium in the middle portion of the duodenal bulb indicating a superficial ulcer crater, with radiating folds extending from the ulceration. An incisura (fold) along the lower bulb margin points to the ulcer.

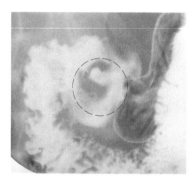

FIG. 5.45 A duodenal ulcer in a 25-year-old man, evidenced by a radiolucent ulcer crater resulting from the surrounding edema.

Complications may include pneumoperitoneum or peritonitis if the ulcer perforates into the abdomen. Perforations are generally confirmed by CT evaluation or conventional erect abdominal radiography. Ulceration into an artery, which is the most common complication associated with ulcers, may produce life-threatening hemorrhage. Finally, the edema, spasm, and scarring produced by ulceration may result in gastric outlet or bowel obstruction.

Gastroenteritis

A number of inflammatory disorders of the stomach and intestine fall into the general grouping of **gastroenteritis**, inflammation of the mucosal lining of the stomach and small bowel (Fig. 5.46). Erosive gastritis appears to be a precursor to gastric ulcer formation and results from a compromised mucosal barrier within the stomach. Causes of erosive gastritis include ingestion of aspirin and other NSAIDs, alcohol, and steroids; physical stress or trauma; and viral or fungal infections. Acute gastric erosions heal rapidly once the cause is eliminated. Gastric erosions may be identified on double-contrast examinations of the stomach. Complete erosion appears as slit-like collections of barium surrounded by radiolucent halos of swollen, elevated mucosa. In some cases, scalloped or nodular antral folds may also be visualized. Antral gastritis appears to result from alcohol, smoking, and *H. pylori* infection. Radiographically, it is demonstrated by decreased distensibility of the antrum in combination with thickened mucosal folds within the antrum, which tend to be oriented on its longitudinal axis and result in a narrowed antrum.

Ingestion of foods contaminated with *Salmonella* and other types of bacteria—most commonly, poultry, meat, dairy products, and eggs—may also result in gastroenteritis. Because of the methods used in the mass production of eggs, a dramatic increase in *Salmonella* infections occurred in the 1980s. Diarrhea results from mild mucosal ulcerations within the small bowel and the ability of the *Salmonella* bacteria to produce a secretory factor. This is a threat to the normal electrolytic balance of the body, with the diarrhea lasting 3 to 4 days. A good patient history often points out the offending agent, and treatment consists of proper fluid management and relief of nausea and vomiting.

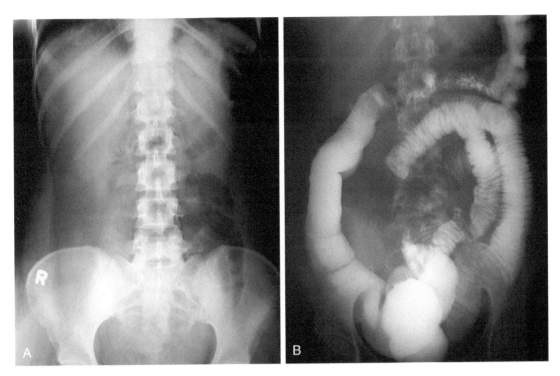

FIG. 5.46 **A,** Air-filled, dilated small bowel loops seen on this abdominal radiograph are suggestive of an obstruction in this 30-year-old patient with abdominal pain, nausea, and vomiting. **B,** Barium readily refluxes from a barium enema into the distal ileum, demonstrating dilation without obstruction. The dilation was secondary to inflammation caused by gastroenteritis.

Regional Enteritis (Crohn's Disease)

Regional enteritis, also known as Crohn's disease (CD) or granulomatous colitis, is a chronic IBD of unknown cause that is increasing in prevalence. Research indicates that affected individuals have a genetic predisposition for CD, with 10% to 20% of affected individuals having a positive family history. The discovery of the *NOD2/CARD15* gene on chromosome 16 has been indicated as a determinant in susceptibility to CD. Individuals with the disease are primarily affected by an unregulated intestinal immune response to various agents such as food or environmental factors, which results in crypt cell inflammation and abscesses, leading to the development of small ulcers. CD eventually affects all layers of the bowel wall. The bowel wall thickens in response to the inflammation and may form fistulas to adjacent loops of bowel, skin, or other abdominal viscera. CD typically occurs in the distal ileum but may be seen anywhere throughout

the GI tract, from the mouth to the anus. The small bowel alone is affected in about a third of patients, the colon alone in 20% to 30% of patients, and combined involvement of the colon and the small bowel is seen in 40% to 50% of patients.

This disease has a bimodal distribution, with initial diagnosis being made in young adults of both sexes between the ages of 14 and 24 years, and in older adults in their 50s and 60s, with presenting symptoms suggestive of appendicitis or acute bowel obstruction. Subsequent fibrotic scarring may give rise to mechanical obstruction of the bowel. The combination of mucosal edema and crisscrossing fine ulcerations gives the bowel a "cobblestone" appearance on barium studies (Fig. 5.47). The string sign (Fig. 5.48) is demonstrated when the terminal ileum is so diseased and stenotic that the barium mixture can only trickle through a small opening that looks like a string. Regional enteritis is a chronic disease characterized by periods of exacerbation

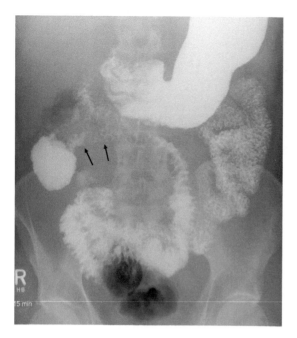

FIG. 5.47 Anteroposterior abdominal radiography obtained 15 minutes into a small bowel follow through examination demonstrates a "cobblestone" pattern (*black arrows*) to the mucosa of a segment of the ileum in a patient with Crohn's disease. Note that the lumen lacks the normal transverse appearing folds, which here are replaced with a rounded "cobblestone" appearing surface.

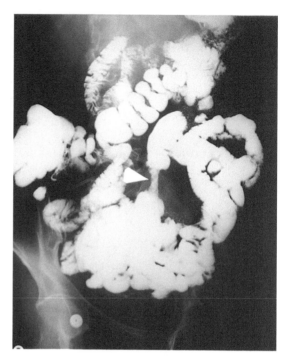

FIG. 5.48 The string sign, demonstrating a diseased, stenotic terminal ileum.

interspersed with periods of inactivity. Presentation of the disease in two or more areas with normal intervening bowel between is identified as "skip areas" (Fig. 5.49), thus the designation "regional" enteritis. In addition, these patients tend to have an increased chance of developing carcinoma of the bowel with a very poor prognosis. CD is classified as early stage, intermediate stage, or advanced stage. The progression of the disease may be demonstrated radiographically by performing a SBFT, enteroclysis, or a double-contrast barium enema.

The initial diagnosis of CD is based on a combination of clinical, laboratory, histologic, and imaging findings, with no single diagnostic test serving as the gold standard for reaching a diagnosis. Imaging is commonly used to distinguish CD from other conditions causing colitis through demonstration of small bowel involvement. Furthermore, imaging is also utilized to accurately assess the subtype of disease, location, and severity to determine the appropriate treatment protocol. Radiology studies, traditionally, have played a

smaller role in long-term surveillance of patients with known CD, but recent developments in imaging techniques using CT and MRI hold promise for predicting disease activity and monitoring therapy.

Although abdominal radiography may often depict abnormalities in CD patients, it has a low predictive value of only 62%, making this modality a poor screening test for patients presenting with initial symptoms. Because negative findings will rarely preclude the need for further imaging studies, radiography is typically reserved for evaluating the presence of obstruction, perforation, or toxic colon distention associated with advanced disease. Although small bowel barium studies were at one point the primary method for diagnosing CD, the introduction of capsule endoscopy is playing an increasingly larger role in making the initial diagnosis. However, a 5% incidence of capsule retention proximal to unsuspected bowel strictures often necessitates surgery for capsule removal, so initial testing with a patency capsule is used. Abdominal radiography may be used to locate a patency capsule if it does not pass within a certain time period. Imaging studies such as the SBFT can also serve as a screening tool

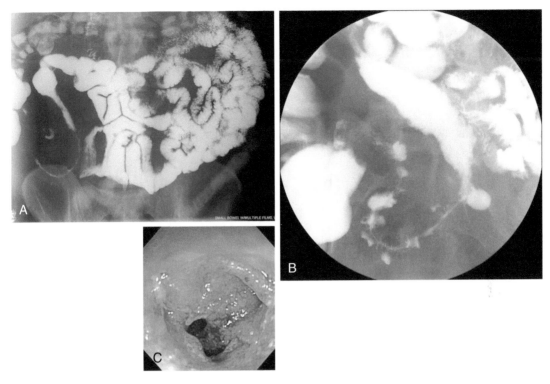

FIG. 5.49 **A**, Small bowel study demonstrating "skip areas" of normal bowel between segments of diseased bowel in a patient with regional enteritis (Crohn's disease). **B**, Spot image demonstrating Crohn's disease linear ulcerations. **C**, Endoscopic images of Crohn's disease linear ulcerations.

before capsule endoscopy examinations however, this has become less prevalent with the institution of the patency capsule. When evaluating the colon for possible CD involvement, endoscopy is the preferred initial examination of the colon and is superior to barium enema in detecting early changes. The barium enema is typically reserved for patients with unsuccessful colonoscopies or those with contraindications such as anticoagulation therapy.

CT has traditionally been thought to only be useful in assessing extraenteric complications of CD such as fistulas or abscesses; however, the advent of CT enterography has shown promise for its use in the initial diagnosis of suspected CD. Through the use of a neutral enteric contrast to dilate the bowel loops, as well as intravenous (IV) contrast timed specifically to best display bowel wall enhancement, active disease can be identified by bowel wall thickening along with mural hyperenhancement. Furthermore, utilization of cross-sectional CT imaging provides better visualization of pelvic small bowel loops that can often be

obscured by overlapping bowel during radiographic barium studies.

CT colonography (CTC) techniques are not usually indicated for the detection of CD because IV contrast is not typically administered and the blind administration of room air or carbon dioxide for colonic distention may be a contraindication in a severely inflamed colon (toxic megacolon). Furthermore, colonic cleansing, which is required for CTC, is not usually required for detecting inflammation by the CT enterography technique.

Similarly to CT, contrast-enhanced MRI, utilizing fast imaging and MRE techniques, has the ability to optimize bowel distention and accurately display bowel wall changes in patients with early-stage CD. Additionally, specific characteristics related to bowel changes, including bowel wall thickening, mural hyperenhancement, and high T2 mural signal, can be visualized without the radiation concerns that are associated with CT. This is a definite benefit when considering pediatric populations, pregnant women, and patients receiving serial imaging.

Transabdominal sonography is capable of demonstrating the presence of CD through findings of bowel wall thickening greater than or equal to 4 mm to 5 mm, visualization of the "target" sign when seen in cross-section, and reduced or absent peristalsis in the affected loops. One potential drawback of this imaging approach is the high dependency on user ability, with sensitivity in diagnosing CD increasing from 75% to 87% as experience is gained by the machine operator.

Although nuclear medicine currently has little effect in the evaluation of patients with suspected CD, an increased interest in the role of Tc-99m white blood cell (WBC) imaging has been gaining ground as a possible superior imaging modality compared with contrast-based radiographic imaging. Tc-99m WBC scans seem to be ideally suited for obtaining a precise temporal snapshot of inflammatory distribution and intensity within the GI tract, in just a single examination. In instances in which patients present with inconspicuous signs suggestive of CD, as well as relatively normal laboratory results, a negative Tcm-99m WBC study may eliminate the need for further endoscopic investigation. In situations where patients already have a histologically confirmed diagnosis of CD, technetium hexamethyl propylene amine oxime (HMPAO)–labeled WBCs, with single proton emission computed tomography (SPECT) imaging, can be utilized to monitor chronic CD and assess disease activity. HMPAO-labeled leukoscintigraphy has several advantages over barium studies, including simultaneous examination of both the large bowel and the small bowel in a single patient encounter, lower radiation exposure, and higher patient acceptance.

Treatment of regional enteritis includes drug therapy to decrease inflammation, relieve diarrhea, and treat the infection. Bowel resection to remove the involved section of the intestine is necessary approximately 70% of the time, particularly if perforation or hemorrhage is present. Recurrence of the disease in other areas of the bowel, however, is common. The disease is rarely cured, but rarely fatal.

Appendicitis

Appendicitis is an inflammation of the vermiform appendix resulting from an obstruction caused usually by a fecalith (Fig. 5.50) or more rarely by a neoplasm. It is the most common abdominal surgical emergency in the United States. Appendicitis is most frequent in

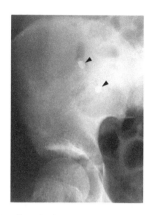

FIG. 5.50 Fecalith within the appendix, a common cause of appendicitis.

the late teens and 20s and has a fairly equal distribution between the sexes. Complications, usually resulting from gangrenous or perforated appendicitis, occur in approximately 3% to 5% of all cases. Delayed diagnosis and treatment of appendicitis account for much of the morbidity and mortality associated with this disease.

The obstruction leads to inflammation and distention and affects the blood supply to this portion of the bowel. Venous blood return is decreased, which, in turn, results in deoxygenation of the tissue. All of these factors leave the appendix susceptible to infection from bacteria such as *Escherichia coli*, which are normally found in the intestinal tract. Poor blood supply may also lead to gangrene, perforation, and possible rupture. Once the vermiform appendix ruptures, the infection spreads to the peritoneum, leading to general peritonitis that could result in death.

The signs and symptoms of appendicitis include initial pain in the epigastrium that moves to the RLQ and becomes persistent. Nausea and vomiting may occur as a reflex symptom because the vagus nerve supplies both the stomach and the appendix. Individuals also have a low-grade fever, sudden onset of constipation, and an elevated WBC count. The elevation of WBCs helps distinguish appendicitis from other colicky abdominal disorders.

Many patients presenting with acute appendicitis may not require imaging, because the clinical presentation is often sufficient enough for a reliable diagnosis to indicate the need for surgical treatment. Conventional radiography is relatively limited in its value of

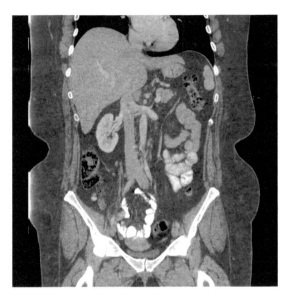

FIG. 5.51 Computed tomography of the abdomen and pelvis indicating appendicitis.

diagnosing acute appendicitis. Furthermore, fluoroscopic examinations such as SBFT or barium enema are more often useful as a follow-up to negative cross-sectional imaging studies, to evaluate for other causes of RLQ pain, including small bowel obstruction, infectious ileitis, and IBD.

Currently, CT is the most accurate imaging modality for evaluating patients who do not have a clear clinical diagnosis of acute appendicitis (Fig. 5.51). The use of CT in demonstrating appendicitis has a sensitivity of 91% and specificity of 90%, with increased confidence in identifying the appendix when thinner slices and multiplanar reformatting of collected data is utilized. Both IV and rectal contrast enhancement, if utilized in adult patients, increase the accuracy of a CT assessment of RLQ pain.

Sonography may be utilized as an alternative to CT. Sonographic imaging has a sensitivity of 78% and specificity of 83% when used for diagnosing suspected appendicitis. Although CT has an overall higher accuracy, when a sonographic examination is conducted by an experienced sonographer, it is almost as effective as a CT procedure but without the risks of ionizing radiation. Thus sonographic evaluation is preferred in children and pregnant women, especially when any questionable results are followed up by either CT or MRI (when available).

Because of slower acquisition time, higher cost, and relatively decreased availability in comparison with CT and sonography, MRI is yet to be utilized routinely for emergent diagnosis of this pathologic condition. Although nuclear medicine imaging with WBC scans can provide some useful information, its level of sensitivity and specificity is significantly inferior to that of CT, sonography, and MRI.

Surgical removal of the appendix is the most common treatment, and in cases of early surgical intervention, the mortality is low. However, complications such as abscess formation, perforation, or peritonitis place the individual at a greater risk and significantly increase the recovery period.

Ulcerative Colitis

Ulcerative colitis (UC) is an inflammatory bowel disease of the colonic mucosa. Its cause is unknown, but it is thought to be an autoimmune disease. It is four times more common in Caucasians, especially in Jewish persons of eastern European (Ashkenazi) descent, than in nonwhites. A familial tendency to develop this disease is believed to exist, with evidence of UC occurring in identical twins supporting the genetic theory of causation. Typically, it affects 15- to 25-year-olds, who develop excessive diarrhea with blood, pus, and mucus in the stool. The disease generally starts in the rectum and spreads to the sigmoid, sometimes involving the entire colon. Unlike CD, UC affects the colon in a continuous manner without skip areas. Its clinical course is highly variable in severity and prognosis.

Inflammation of the mucosa and submucosa (reticulin fibers beneath the mucosal epithelium) causes abscesses to form in the crypt cells, separating them from their blood supply and leading to epithelial necrosis and mucosal ulceration. Gradually, the mucosa is replaced by fibrous tissue whose crevices give a rough, cobblestone appearance to the involved colon (Fig. 5.52 A & B).

Signs and symptoms include intermittent spells of bloody diarrhea and abdominal cramping. Colon strictures are a rare complication of UC. Another complication of UC is toxic colitis or megacolon, an acute dilation of the colon from colonic paralytic ileus (Fig. 5.53). The dilated bowel is particularly susceptible to rupture; a barium enema is absolutely contraindicated if perforation is a concern. People with UC have a greatly increased incidence of colon cancer, especially if the entire colon is affected for over 10 years.

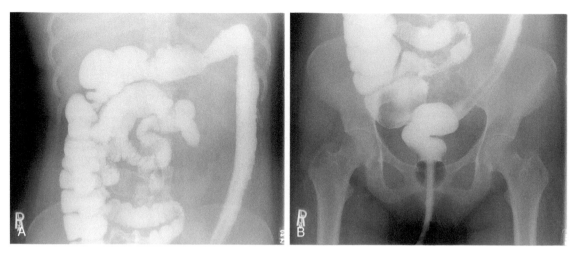

FIG. 5.52 Anteroposterior barium enema radiographs demonstrating ulcerative colitis in the left colon. **A,** Superior aspects of the large intestine. **B,** Lower aspects of the large intestine. The loss of haustral markings throughout the left side of the colon is what is responsible for the "lead pipe" sign.

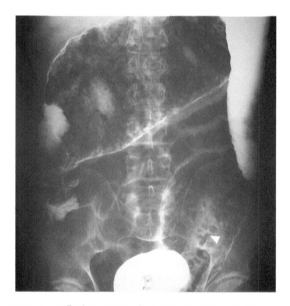

FIG. 5.53 Barium enema in a 61-year-old man demonstrates toxic megacolon secondary to ulcerative colitis. Pseudopolyps are seen in the descending colon.

Sigmoidoscopy and colonoscopy are the usual means of diagnosing UC because 90% to 95% of the cases involve the distal colon or rectum. Barium enemas are sometimes used to support the clinical diagnosis and to assess the progression of the disease and its complications. When filled with barium, the normally smooth colon outline becomes irregular because of the ulceration present.

Pseudopolyps are islands of unaffected mucosa that become visible when surrounded by affected mucosa. Another radiographic indication of UC is an easily recognized loss of colon haustration and mucosal edema, which may be referred to as the "lead pipe" sign.

Certain characteristics of UC distinguish it from regional enteritis (CD) (Fig. 5.54). UC is a disease of the mucosa of the colon, whereas regional enteritis affects all layers of the bowel wall. Also, UC typically begins at the anus and ascends, often resulting in megacolon and bowel perforations, and frequently progressing to cancer; by contrast, regional enteritis usually begins in the terminal ileum and cecum and descends through the bowel, often with skip areas. It rarely produces megacolon or bowel perforations.

Treatment of UC is initially medical in nature and often involves dietary restrictions. Steroid therapy is used to treat UC, and it may be administered either orally or rectally. Development of an obstruction or neoplasm may necessitate surgical intervention. This involves removal of the colon from cecum to sigmoid or rectum with establishment of an ileostomy or ileorectal or ileoanal anastomosis. Many patients who undergo a total proctocolectomy for UC treatment will have surgical creation of an ileal pouch. The most common types of ileal pouches are the J-pouch and the S-pouch, both named after the letter they resemble. The W-pouch is another version. Those three pouch reconstructions employ an ileal pouch-anal anastomosis (IPAA). Barium or water soluble enemas are frequently used to evaluate

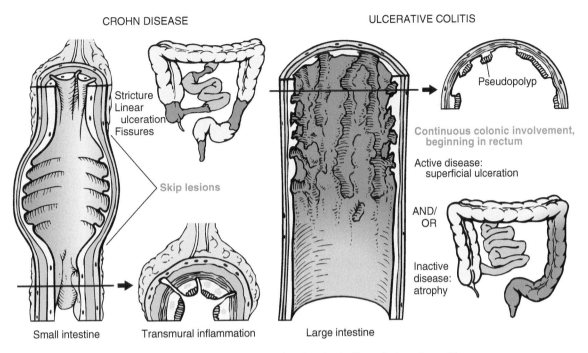

CROHN DISEASE

Stricture
Linear
ulceration
Fissures

Skip lesions

Small intestine   Transmural inflammation

ULCERATIVE COLITIS

Pseudopolyp

Continuous colonic involvement,
beginning in rectum

Active disease:
superficial ulceration

AND/
OR

Inactive
disease:
atrophy

Large intestine

FIG. 5.54 Distribution patterns of regional enteritis and ulcerative colitis.

the postoperative status of these pouches for surgical leaks, strictures, or recurrent disease.

Esophageal Varices

Varicose veins are abnormally lengthened, dilated, and superficial veins; those in the esophagus are referred to as **esophageal varices**. They occur in the esophagus as a result of portal venous hypertension. Conditions that cause resistance to the normal blood flow through the liver (such as cirrhosis) cause a bypass of the normal venous drainage mechanism. Instead, blood is directed through the esophageal and gastric collateral veins. The increase in blood flow through these channels results in venous dilation and formation of varices.

Esophageal varices are best demonstrated during barium studies in a recumbent position because gravity causes poor visualization in the erect position. A thin barium mixture shows the varices as smooth worm-like and serpiginous (wavy margins) filling defects within the column of barium on the radiograph (Fig. 5.55). Use of thick barium may be counterproductive because it can obscure the varices. Esophageal varices may also occasionally be visualized as a retrocardiac posterior mediastinal mass on a conventional chest radiograph obtained with the patient in the recumbent position. Sonography

does not provide adequate visualization of esophageal varices but it is an excellent and safe screening tool for portal hypertension. CT and MRI studies also allows for the visualization of esophageal varices and other effects of portal hypertension. Upper endoscopy is a common diagnostic method for esophageal varices.

Patients with esophageal varices are subject to rupture and hemorrhage, which may be massive and often fatal. Patients with hemorrhaging varices may present with hematemesis, melena, or hematochezia. Statistics show that ruptured varices have accounted for approximately one third of all deaths from cirrhosis. An erect image taken for this situation should be done with great caution because the patient's blood loss may be significant. The resultant reduced blood pressure along with the elevation may cause the patient to faint.

Treatment for esophageal varices may consist of endoscopic sclerotherapy, banding ligation, or infusion of vasopressin, a natural hormone useful in stopping hemorrhage. Compression of the varices through balloon tamponading may be occasionally used. Shunts such as transjugular intrahepatic portosystemic shunts (TIPSS), applied via interventional radiology or during surgery, may be used to help redirect liver blood flow, thus reducing portal hypertension and easing venous pressure in the esophageal and gastric collateral circulation. Sonography

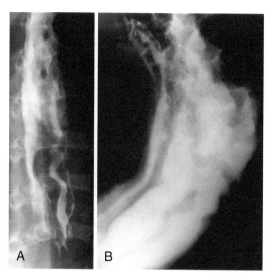

FIG. 5.55 **A**, Long, serpentine filling defects in the esophagus of a 41-year-old with chronic alcoholism, indicative of esophageal varices. **B**, Similar filling defects seen in the cardia of the stomach of the same patient, indicative of gastric varices.

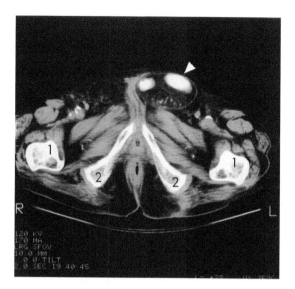

FIG. 5.56 Moderate left inguinal hernia (*arrow*) on this computed tomography image of a 96-year-old man. Also well-defined are (*1*) the femurs, showing the lesser trochanters projecting posteriorly, and (*2*) the ischial tuberosities.

has been helpful in affected patients over time to access the direction of flow with TIPSS. Occasionally the shunt may become blocked and not function correctly, which may be a clinical concern. Doppler interrogation with ultrasound may give quantitative analysis about the direction and magnitude of the flow of blood within the shunt.

Degenerative Diseases

Herniation

A **hernia** is a protrusion of a loop of bowel through a small opening, usually in the abdominal wall. Popularly referred to as a *rupture*, it occurs because of an anatomic weakness. As the bowel loop herniates, it pushes the peritoneum ahead of it. An inguinal hernia, which is common in men, occurs when a bowel loop protrudes through a weakness in the inguinal ring (Fig. 5.56) or inner groin and may descend downward into the scrotum (Fig. 5.57 A & B). Femoral (outer groin) and umbilical (belly button) herniations (Fig. 5.58) occur in both sexes. A ventral hernia occurs when bowel projects through a defect in the abdominal wall muscles. Bowel protruding through a location of a surgical incision is called an incisional hernia. A parastomal hernia is a

specific type of incisional surgery that results in bulging of bowel at the site of an ostomy.

If a herniated loop of bowel can be pushed back into the abdominal cavity, it is said to be *reducible*. If it becomes stuck and cannot be reduced, it is called an *incarcerated hernia*. As described previously, this can result in a bowel obstruction (Fig. 5.59). If the constriction through which the bowel loop has passed is tight enough to cut off blood supply to the bowel, it is called a *strangulated hernia*. Prompt surgical intervention is required in this case to avoid necrosis of that portion of the bowel. Bowel that has already become necrotic can generally be surgically resected.

Hiatal Hernia

A **hiatal hernia** is a weakness of the esophageal hiatus that permits some portions of the stomach to herniate into the thoracic cavity. Hiatal hernias occur in about half of the population over age 50 years. In its early stages, a hiatal hernia is reducible. Chronic herniation may be associated with GERD.

A direct, or sliding, hiatal hernia occurs when a portion of the stomach and gastroesophageal junction are both situated above the diaphragm (Fig. 5.60). This type of hernia constitutes the outstanding majority (about 99%) of all hiatal hernias. A Schatzki ring is often visible with this condition (Fig. 5.61) and consists of a mucosal

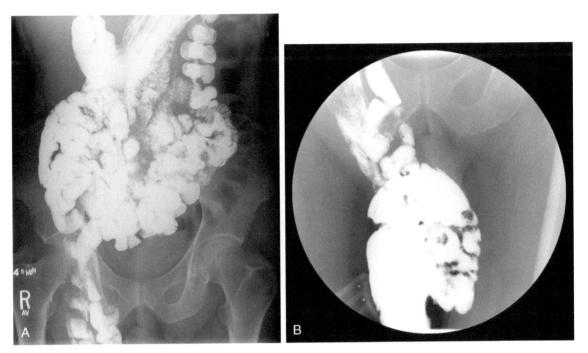

FIG. 5.57 **A,** Abdominal radiograph obtained during a small bowel follow through (SBFT) examination showing an inguinal hernia containing the ileum and proximal colon. **B,** A spot image taken during the same SBFT examination revealing descent of the bowel into the scrotum.

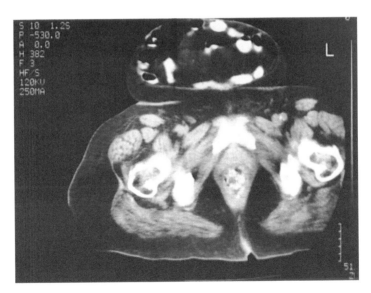

FIG. 5.58 Computed tomography demonstration of a large anterior abdominal hernia containing multiple loops of small bowel and possibly some large bowel without evidence of obstruction in this 70-year-old man.

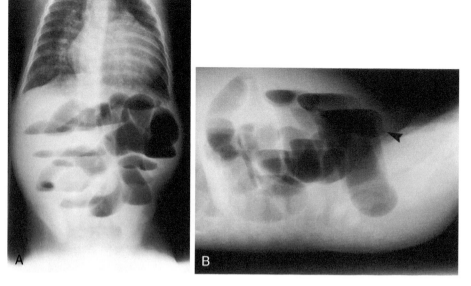

FIG. 5.59 **A**, Upright abdominal view of a 3-month-old indicates multiple dilated loops of bowel with air and fluid levels present, suggesting a mechanical bowel obstruction. **B**, A prone cross-table lateral view shows the small bowel forming a beak-like projection at the point of obstruction at the internal inguinal ring in this incarcerated hernia.

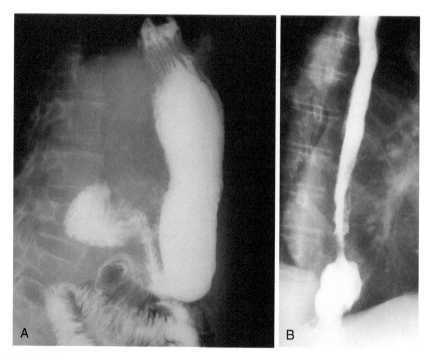

FIG. 5.60 **A**, Demonstration of contrast material above the hemidiaphragm on an upper gastrointestinal series of this 51-year-old woman. **B**, The esophagus narrows to the stomach, which is seen to empty passively, above the hemidiaphragm in this sliding hiatal hernia.

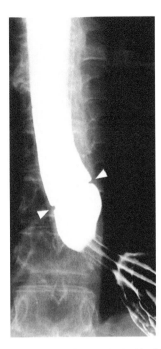

FIG. 5.61 Schatzki ring demonstrated in the case of a sliding hiatal hernia.

ring that protrudes into the lumen. Such a ring has traditionally been thought to be congenital but may be related to gastric reflux. It is, however, generally of no clinical significance unless it produces narrowing sufficient to cause dysphagia, usually less than 13 mm in diameter.

A far less common type of hiatal hernia is the rolling, or paraesophageal, hiatal hernia. This occurs when a portion of the stomach or adjacent viscera herniates above the diaphragm but the gastroesophageal junction remains below the diaphragm (Fig. 5.62). If all of the stomach slides above the diaphragm, an intrathoracic stomach (Fig. 5.63) results. Unlike the sliding hiatal hernia, a paraesophageal hernia is potentially life-threatening because of the risk of volvulus, incarceration, or strangulation of the hernia.

Most hiatal hernias are asymptomatic, but some are accompanied by reflux. Most patients experiencing reflux complain of a full feeling in the chest, particularly after meals. Some reflux of gastric contents leads to complaints of heartburn. An esophagram or UGI examination may pinpoint the herniation and provide classification of the type of hernia as well as measure the extent of the hernia. Treatment of hiatal herniation

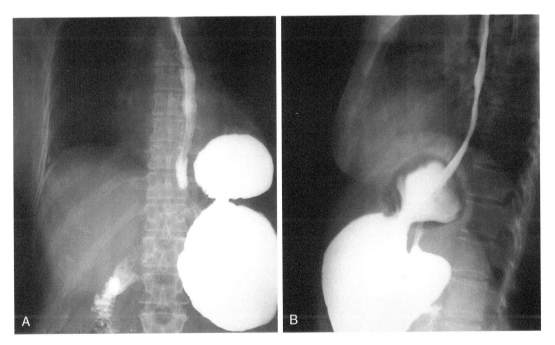

FIG. 5.62 **A**, Paraesophageal hiatal hernia, demonstrating narrowing in the fundus. **B**, Lateral view of the same patient demonstrates the cardioesophageal junction in its normal place below the hemidiaphragm. The fundus is highlighted by radiolucency of the lung.

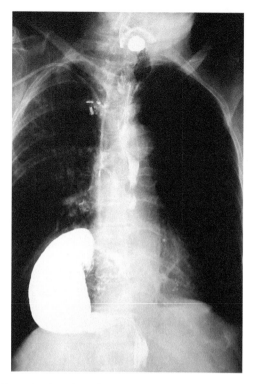

FIG. 5.63 Intrathoracic stomach indicated by the presence of the entire stomach above the diaphragm, also with malrotation of the stomach.

is generally conservative to minimize discomfort. Paraesophageal hernias generally require surgical treatment.

Gastric Volvulus

A gastric volvulus is an abnormal rotation of the stomach with greater than 180 degrees of rotation. A gastric volvulus may be organoaxial, mesenteroaxial, or a combination of the two. Organoaxial volvulus occurs when the stomach rotates around the long axis formed between the esophagogastric junction and the pylorus as the antrum rotates anterior and superior and the fundus rotates posterior and inferior. The greater curvature will lie more superior and the lesser curvature inferior. It is the more common type in adults and often occurs as a result of trauma or a paraesophageal hernia where a diaphragmatic defect is present. The mesenteroaxial gastric volvulus results when the antrum rotates around the short axis that bisects the greater and lesser curvatures so that the posterior surface of the stomach now lies anteriorly and the antrum is displaced superior to

the esophagogastric junction. This type is more common to the pediatric population but can occur in adults. A diaphragmatic defect is usually absent. A combined volvulus is usually a result of a chronic volvulus that begins either as organoaxial or mesenteroaxial.

A gastric volvulus may present as a gas distended stomach in the chest or upper abdomen on an upright chest radiograph. Radiographs may also demonstrate pneumoperitoneum if perforation has occurred. An UGI is helpful with diagnosis as the gastric contour can be evaluated and assessed for a gastric outlet obstruction. MDCT examination is also a valuable diagnostic tool as the stomach and vessels can be seen.

Symptoms of a gastric volvulus include severe epigastric pain, retching without vomiting, and an inability to advance a nasogastric tube. Patients with a chronic nonobstructive volvulus may be asymptomatic, but patients with symptoms require prompt surgical treatment to correct the rotation. There is a high risk of gastric ischemia that can lead to necrosis, perforation, and peritonitis.

Bowel Obstructions

Both the small and large bowel of the normal person are nearly always active in peristalsis. Many lesions of various types (e.g., inflammatory, degenerative) can interfere with this action and cause an obstruction of either the small bowel or the large bowel (Table 5.1). The resultant obstruction can be either a **mechanical bowel obstruction**, as occurs from a blockage of the bowel lumen, or a **paralytic ileus**, which results from a failure of peristalsis causing a functional bowel obstruction. Gradations of each exist, and both may be present at the same time. Initial diagnosis of a small bowel obstruction with conventional abdominal radiography may be difficult because of the frequency of vomiting and the use of nasogastric decompression. However, an acute abdominal series (AAS) is the recommended first radiologic evaluation in cases of suspected bowel obstruction.

General signs and symptoms of a bowel obstruction include vomiting, abdominal distention, and abdominal pain. Patients may also fail to pass flatus or stool. Sequential radiographs over 12 to 24 hours help to determine the diagnosis and to locate the level of the obstruction in individuals with mechanical obstructions. Most commonly, gas confined to the small bowel with multiple air and fluid levels visible on an erect abdominal radiograph indicates a mechanical obstruction, whereas gas

TABLE 5.1

Large and Small Bowel Obstruction

Cause	Pathophysiology
Small bowel obstruction	Adhesive secondary to previous abdominal surgeries: 50%–70% Hernia: inguinal, ventral, or femoral: 20%–25% Tumors: may be associated with intussusception: 10% Mesenteric ischemia: 3%–5%
Large bowel obstruction	Colon/rectal cancer: 90% Volvulus: 4%–5% Diverticular disease: 3% Other causes (inflammatory bowel disease, adhesions, hernia)

Table 39.2 *Common causes of intestinal obstruction protusion of the intestine through a weakness in the abdominal in McCance.* From McCance KL, Huether SE: Pathophysiology: the biologic basis for disease in adults and children, ed 5, St. Louis, 2006, Mosby.
From Feldman, M, Friedman LS, Brandt LJ: *Sleisenger & Fordtran's gastrointestinal liver disease,* ed 7, Philadelphia, 2003, Saunders;

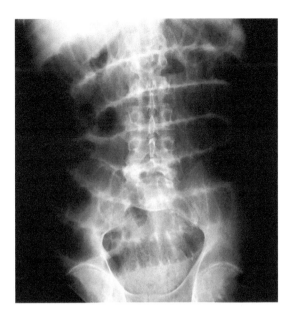

FIG. 5.64 Abdominal radiograph demonstrating a mechanical bowel obstruction. Numerous loops of dilated bowel are seen within the midabdomen. The patient had an acute onset of abdominal pain, nausea, and vomiting.

distributed throughout both the large and small bowel is indicative of paralytic ileus. The small bowel tends to be more distended in cases of mechanical obstruction. Physical signs are also helpful in distinguishing the type of obstruction present. Bowel sounds, the normal sounds of a bowel in motion as heard during auscultation, are absent with an ileus; they are present with a mechanical obstruction and are often hyperactive and high-pitched. Emesis containing bile may also indicate a mechanical obstruction.

Mechanical Bowel Obstruction

A mechanical bowel obstruction (Fig. 5.64) is one in which the lumen of the bowel becomes occluded, as might occur for a variety of reasons such as hernias, tumors, volvulus, intussusceptions, or postoperative adhesions (Fig. 5.65). A simple mechanical obstruction does not involve the blood supply to the bowel, whereas a strangulating obstruction may lead to bowel infarction. Nearly half of all strangulating mechanical bowel obstructions are caused by an incarcerated (i.e., trapped) hernia, a condition discussed earlier in this chapter as a degenerative disease. Entrapment of a hernia, usually involving the small bowel, causes impairment of blood flow and swelling of the affected tissues. The resultant edema affects arterial blood flow to the bowel and may lead to ischemic necrosis, perforation, and peritonitis. Prompt surgical intervention and reduction are required to relieve an incarcerated hernia.

A bowel **volvulus** is a twisting of a bowel loop about its mesenteric base, usually at either the sigmoid or the ileocecal junction (Fig. 5.66). This most commonly occurs in older adults and is identifiable on a conventional abdominal radiograph as a collection of air conforming to the shape of the affected, dilated bowel. MDCT provides visualization of not only distended bowel, but of the effect of the twisting on the mesentery, which presents as the "whirl sign." Some twists resolve spontaneously; however, bowel that is twisted more than 360 degrees requires surgical intervention. Surgical untwisting and resection are necessary to prevent necrosis and perforation of the bowel caused by a lack of blood supply.

An **intussusception** occurs when a segment of bowel, constricted by peristalsis, telescopes into a distal segment and is driven further into the distal bowel by peristalsis. Recall that the bowel is connected to the mesentery, so as the bowel telescopes into itself, the mesentery (with its rich blood supply) is also involved. Radiographically, the area of intussusception may appear as a "coiled

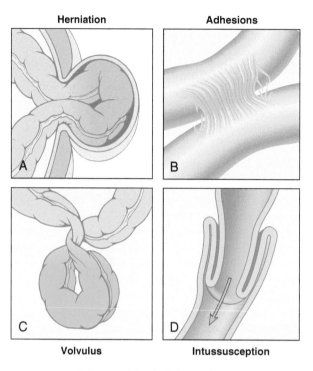

Herniation | Adhesions

A | B

Volvulus | Intussusception

C | D

FIG. 5.65 Intestinal obstructions.

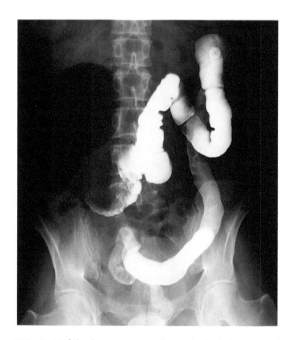

FIG. 5.66 A barium enema radiograph depicting a cecal volvulus. Note how the column of barium stops at the level of the volvulus.

spring." During sonography and CT studies, the intussusception appears as a "target sign" as bowel within bowel appears as concentric rings. Intussusception is responsible for approximately 5% of all mechanical obstructions and most frequently affects the ileocecal valve (Fig. 5.67). It is more common in children and infants than in adults. In children and infants, an intussusception can often be reduced by an air only enema, sparing a surgical intervention. Its presence in an adult generally signifies an accompanying intraluminal mass and is generally reduced surgically so that the physician can search for the cause of the intussusception and correct the condition. Although, intussusceptions in adults can often be transient and can be a common incidental finding on abdominal CT. A SBFT could be performed to determine whether an intussusception is transient in nature.

Gallstone ileus is another cause for a mechanical bowel obstruction. In this condition, a gallstone may erode from the gallbladder and create a fistula to the small bowel. This leads to an obstruction, usually when the gallstone reaches the ileocecal valve. Radiographic signs of this include air and fluid levels or air in the biliary tree (pneumobilia) (Fig. 5.68). The gallstone itself may also

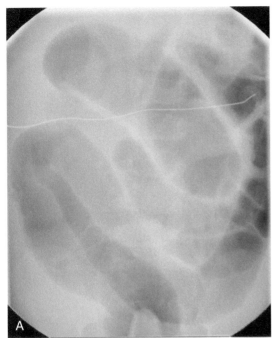

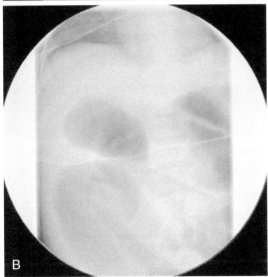

FIG. 5.67 **A**, Pediatric barium enema demonstrating in-tussusception before resolution and **B**, after resolution (*B*).

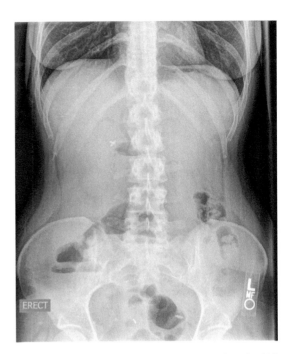

FIG. 5.68 Abdominal radiograph demonstrating air within the biliary ductal system.

be visible, often in the terminal ileum, where it causes the obstruction. Small bowel obstructions may also result from pathologic conditions such as Crohn's disease and appendicitis previously discussed in this chapter.

Diagnosis of mechanical bowel obstruction is initially based on clinical signs and symptoms including abdominal distention, abdominal cramps, and vomiting, sometimes progressing to bloody stools. The quality of regurgitated material may provide clues as to the possible location of obstruction, with bilious vomit indicating a proximal location and yellow colostrum or vomitus with meconium (in pediatric patients) being more indicative of a distal obstruction. Conventional supine and erect abdominal radiographs often confirm the diagnosis with air and fluid levels clearly visible in the erect position. Additionally, abdominal radiographs that are positive for bowel obstruction often direct the subsequent imaging workup. CT is a more advanced diagnostic method for diagnosing mechanical obstructions than a fluoroscopic study. CT provides visualization of the bowel loops despite overlap, which is a problem on SBFT examination, so that a transition zone and cause of obstruction can be better demonstrated. CT is also better tolerated by patients with an obstruction because of shorter examination time and improved intake of CT oral contrast agents. When fluoroscopic studies are to be performed, findings of proximal obstruction indicate an UGI or SBFT examination and distal or colonic obstruction can be clarified with a contrast enema. Additional examinations are more comprehensive in nature than conventional radiographs, providing important information related to the specific location of a transition point in which the lumen changes from being patent to being obstructed. Whether water-soluble or barium contrast agents are best for diagnosing small bowel obstructions (SBOs) is still being debated. Water soluble contrast agents are less than ideal as there is the potential for intravascular uptake, thus depleting the overall intraluminal volume. Water soluble contrast agents result in a fluid shift into the intestinal lumen, which dilutes the contrast column making fluoroscopic visualization and diagnosis difficult. A problem with barium is that it has the potential to convert a partial obstruction to a complete bowel obstruction as fluid is absorbed from the barium agent.

The use of CT to distinguish between high-grade SBO and ileus has been reported to have a diagnostic accuracy of 90%. Furthermore, no oral contrast administration is necessary, with the fluid in the bowel providing adequate contrast. A more efficient diagnosis can be reached by negating the need for a contrast agent when ruling out high-grade SBO while minimizing the potential related complications such as vomiting or aspiration. The use of CT enterography to detect the presence of lumen obliterating bowel abnormalities such as CD or neoplasms is another growing trend in SBO imaging. In comparison, MRI has shown promise for being used more frequently in the diagnosis of suspected low-grade SBO. Generally, mechanical obstructions require surgical intervention.

Paralytic Ileus

Paralytic ileus or **adynamic ileus** is a failure of normal peristalsis that may result from a variety of factors. The most common causes are surgery, especially those requiring manipulation of the bowel (postoperative ileus), and intraperitoneal or retroperitoneal infection. It may also be associated with bowel ischemia, certain drugs, electrolyte imbalance, pancreatitis, or it may occur simply as a reaction to any stressful illness. Paralytic ileus generally lasts no longer than 3 days with proper medical treatment.

Signs and symptoms of paralytic ileus include distention of the abdomen, abdominal cramping, and vomiting. The absence of peristalsis causes the lumen of both the small and large intestines to fill with gas and fluid, with the resultant dilation extending to the rectum (Fig. 5.69). Radiographically, gas is visible in the colon. Treatment for paralytic ileus generally consists of nasogastric suction and medical stimulation of the bowel to restore peristalsis. In some cases, colonoscopic or rectal tube decompression may be required.

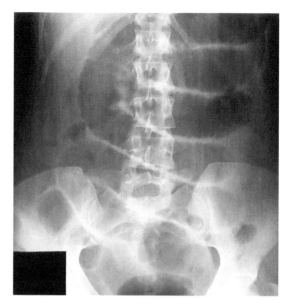

FIG. 5.69 Abdominal radiograph on a postoperative patient demonstrating paralytic ileus. Note the dilated bowel loops extending through the large intestine.

Neurogenic Diseases

Achalasia

Achalasia is a neuromuscular abnormality of the esophagus that results in failure of the lower esophageal sphincter (LES) of the distal esophagus to relax, leading to dysphagia. The LES is thus hypertonic. It occurs equally in men and women and most commonly affects individuals between the ages of 20 and 40 years. Clinically, these patients present with a slowly progressive dysphagia when swallowing both solids and liquids. Patients may also experience regurgitation, chest pain, and moderate weight loss.

Diagnosis of achalasia, generally involves esophageal manometry and an esophagram. Radiographically, the condition manifests as a dilated esophagus with little or no peristalsis. Normal esophageal peristalsis presents as a complete stripping motion that propels the bolus into the stomach. With achalasia, the normal stripping motion is absent and the walls of the dilated esophageal lumen may demonstrate a nonpropulsive and undulating or wave-like motion. The distal esophagus is smooth tapered resulting in a very narrow appearing LES, often described as having a "beaked," "bird-beak," or "rat tail" appearance (Fig. 5.70). Not only is the LES narrow

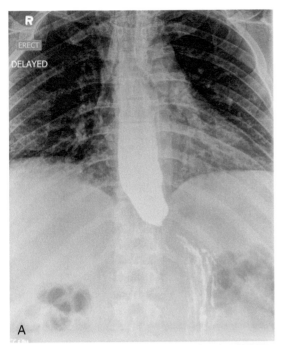

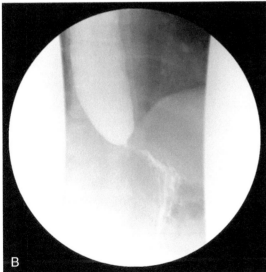

FIG. 5.70 **A**, Erect esophageal image demonstrating achalasia at the level of the gastroesophageal junction. The distal esophagus terminates into a beaked appearance. **B**, Spot image of achalasia at the gastroesophageal junction.

esophagus or even on a chest radiograph. Because the esophageal contents act as a water seal, the normal gastric gas bubble may be absent.

Initial treatment of achalasia is to reduce the pressure and obstruction at the cardiac sphincter. Esophageal dilation is effective in approximately 85% of patients affected by achalasia. Medications such as nitrates and calcium channel blockers may be used to reduce the sphincter pressure and reduce the frequency of repeated dilations. Botulinum toxin may also be injected into the sphincter to create chemical denervation, but this is generally effective for only 1 year. Patients not responding to dilation and medication protocols may require surgical myotomy (cutting of the sphincter muscle fibers). The Heller myotomy is a widely used laparoscopic surgical treatment for achalasia. It is often performed in combination with a Dor fundoplication, which is a partial wrap of the gastric fundus aimed at preventing GE reflux after the myotomy opens the LES. Another surgical procedure gaining popularity for achalasia treatment is the per-oral endoscopic myotomy or POEM procedure. The POEM procedure is performed endoscopically so there are no external incisions.

Diverticular Diseases

Esophageal Diverticula

A **diverticulum** is a pouch or sac of variable size that occurs normally or is created by herniation of a mucous membrane through a defect in its muscular coat. Esophageal diverticula occur when mucosal outpouchings penetrate through the muscular layer of the esophagus. The two primary types of esophageal diverticula are pulsion and traction.

A pulsion diverticulum involves only the mucosa and results from a motility disorder of the esophagus that allows the mucosa to herniate outward. A pulsion diverticulum may also form in an area of increased luminal pressure proximal to a stricture interfering with bolus transit. This type of diverticulum appears radiographically as a rounded projection with a narrow neck and occurs more frequently in the upper and lower thirds of the esophagus. A Zenker's diverticulum is a pulsion type found at the pharyngoesophageal junction at the cervical end of the esophagus on the posterior aspect just above the cricopharyngeal muscle (Fig. 5.71). A Killian-Jamieson diverticulum

but it is functionally impaired with intermittent and brief periods of relaxation and opening. Because the distal esophagus opens only intermittently, when the pressure is high enough, food residue may be seen in the distal

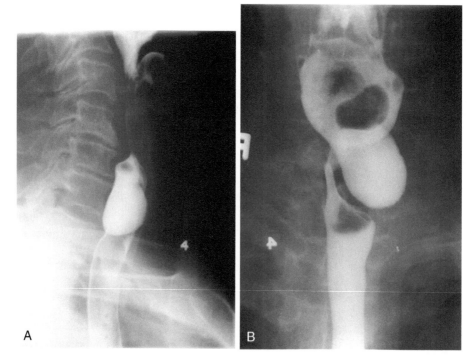

FIG. 5.71 **A,** Large Zenker diverticulum in the esophagus of a 67-year-old man with complaints of difficulty swallowing over the past 6 months. **B,** Zenker diverticulum in the same patient on a magnified view.

is similar to that of a Zenker's diverticulum except that it originates on the lateral aspect of the esophagus (Fig. 5.72). An epiphrenic diverticulum is another pulsion type, but it is found in the distal esophagus just above the hemidiaphragm (Fig. 5.73).

A traction diverticulum involves all layers of the esophagus and results from adjacent scar tissue that pulls the esophagus toward the area of involvement (Fig. 5.74 A & B). Such a diverticulum occurs more frequently in the middle third of the esophagus, often near the carina and appears radiographically as a triangular projection whose apex points toward the external source.

Usually, diverticula are asymptomatic until they reach a relatively large size, at which time complications may occur. For example, food and secretions may collect in the diverticulum and cause a mechanical obstruction of the esophagus. Diverticula of the cervical esophageal segment that are large enough to pocket food and secretions often result in halitosis. Such contents may also be aspirated by a recumbent patient, resulting in aspiration pneumonia. Failure to

control the effects of diverticula through diet modifications may result in the need for surgical removal, depending on the amount of food retention in the diverticulum or extent of aspiration.

Small Bowel Diverticula

Although less common, diverticula can also develop in any portion of the small bowel. Duodenal diverticula are approximately five times more common than diverticula of the jejunum or ileum. With the exception of the previously discussed Meckel diverticulum, small bowel diverticula are predominately asymptomatic. Complications are rare but include diverticulitis, bacterial overgrowth, hemorrhage, perforation, obstruction, and inversion of the diverticulum leading to intussusception. A periampullary duodenal diverticulum may interfere with the common bile duct or pancreatic duct leading to cholangitis or pancreatitis.

As most small bowel diverticula are asymptomatic, treatment is usually not indicated. In cases of complications, treatment depends on the complication.

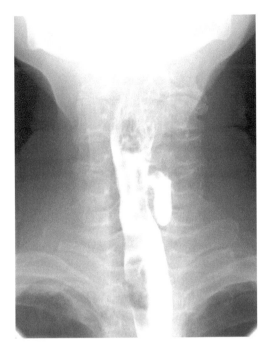

FIG. 5.72 A projection of the cervical esophageal lumen during an esophagram examination demonstrating a Killian-Jamieson diverticulum. These are best demonstrated by increasing the frame/second to visualize the barium column within the pharynx and cervical esophagus as the patient swallows.

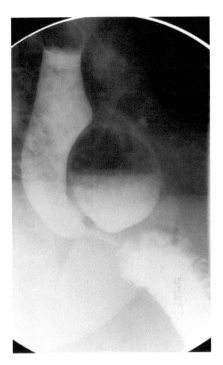

FIG. 5.73 A patient with achalasia who has also developed an epiphrenic diverticulum, shown as a large collection of barium connected and adjacent to the lower esophagus. Note the mottled appearance to the barium resulting from food debris collecting in the diverticulum and esophagus.

Conservative treatments such as dietary changes, bulking agents, and antibiotic therapy may be employed. Surgery may be warranted for complications of hemorrhage, obstruction, or perforation. A diverticulectomy is most common, however, surgical intervention varies with the severity of the complication.

Colonic Diverticula

Diverticulosis, the presence of diverticula without inflammation, is seen in all parts of the colon, most frequently in the sigmoid colon, and particularly among adults over the age of 40 years (Fig. 5.75). Diverticula are associated with hypertrophy of the muscular layer of the bowel. They occur most often where the terminal branches of the mesenteric vessels pierce the bowel wall and are present in 35% to 50% of patients over age 50 years. Factors contributing to the development of diverticula include a pressure gradient between the lumen and the serosa of the bowel and areas of weakness within the bowel

wall. The most common site for diverticula (95%) is the sigmoid colon, the narrowest portion of the colon, which generates the highest intrasegmental (between haustra) pressure.

Inflammation of a diverticulum, termed **diverticulitis**, occurs in approximately 10% to 20% of patients with known diverticulosis, especially in older adults. The inflammation is exacerbated by feces lodging in the diverticulum. Signs and symptoms include lower left quadrant pain and tenderness, fever, and an increased WBC count. Because of these symptoms, sigmoid diverticulitis has been termed *left-sided appendicitis*. This condition may lead to bowel obstruction, perforation, and fistula formation. In some instances, no imaging may be required to make a diagnosis of acute diverticulitis, especially in patients with a history of attacks of diverticulitis who present with symptoms of recurrent disease. The growing trend is toward greater use of radiologic examinations to confirm the diagnosis, to evaluate

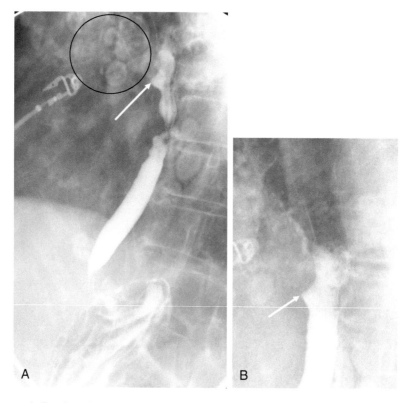

FIG. 5.74 A, Traction diverticulum (*white arrow*) indicated by the triangular-shaped outpouching of the esophagus seen in an esophagram. Multiple rounded opacities (*black circle*) resulting from calcified granulomas in the lungs, indicating prior inflammation that has tethered to the esophagus and formed a traction diverticulum. **B,** Magnified view of the same patient with a more distended barium column demonstrating persistence of the traction diverticulum.

the extent of disease, and to detect possible associated complications that may affect the selection of the most appropriate treatment protocol. Complications associated with acute diverticulitis include the presence of abscesses, fistulas, obstructions, and perforations. Abdominal radiography is of limited value unless complications of pneumoperitoneum or obstruction are suspected. Furthermore, nuclear medicine has no role in evaluating patients presenting with LLQ pain, and MRI is primarily only utilized in pediatric patients with recurrent episodes of diverticulitis to reduce radiation exposure.

Traditionally, a barium enema examination was the primary imaging test performed when evaluating for colonic diverticulitis. Reported diagnostic sensitivity for this imaging examination ranges between 59% and 90%. Radiographic signs of diverticulitis on

barium enema are limited, as diverticulitis is mainly an extramucosal process. A barium enema will only show the secondary effects of an inflamed colon and not the extraluminal abnormalities of abscesses and pericolonic inflammation that may be present. For this reason, the barium enema examination has largely been replaced by CT as the initial imaging examination and has been reserved for patients with equivocal CT findings or poor candidates for endoscopic evaluation because of their colonic narrowing. Patients with acute diverticulitis are at a high risk for perforation so if an enema must be performed, water soluble contrast should be considered. Barium is not contraindicated in cases of diverticulosis.

CT has a much higher sensitivity for diagnosing colonic diverticulitis with a range of 79% to 99% (Fig. 5.76). Additionally, its ability to detect extraluminal

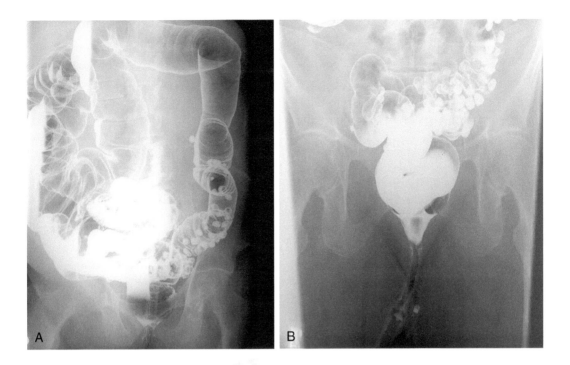

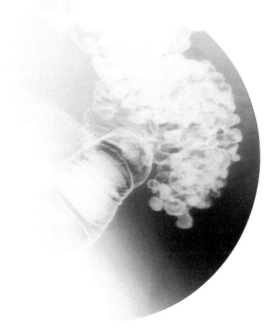

FIG. 5.75 An air-contrast barium enema demonstrating diverticulosis in various projections. **A**, Right lateral decubitus projection. **B**, Posteroanterior axial sigmoid projection. **C**, Digital spot image.

pathology enables potential diagnosis of other disease processes that may mimic the signs and symptoms of LLQ pain. In cases of suspected perforated colon as a result of cancer, in which clinical and radiographic findings mimic diverticulitis, the presentation of pericolonic lymphadenopathy adjacent to a segment of thickened colon wall indicates a diagnosis of diverticulitis over that of colon cancer.

As an alternative technique, transabdominal sonography with graded compression is reported to have a sensitivity of 77% to 98% and a specificity of 80% to 99% in diagnosing diverticulitis. However, sonographic imaging of the sigmoid portion of the colon, a relatively posterior structure, is highly dependent on body habitus in comparison with CT or MRI. The use of transvaginal sonography is often utilized in women of childbearing age to rule out conditions such as ectopic pregnancy or pelvic inflammatory disease that may mimic the signs and symptoms of diverticulitis.

Treatment of diverticulitis centers on reduction of inflammation and infection. Mild cases are treated with antibiotic therapy. Complications such as peritonitis may result if perforation of a diverticulum occurs, and these, of course, must be treated. Abscesses may often be treated via sonography-guided or CT-guided percutaneous drainage. Surgical resection of the bowel

may be used to remove the diseased portion in more severe cases.

Neoplastic Diseases

Tumors of the Esophagus

Although benign and malignant tumors could occur anywhere in the esophagus, tumors of the lower third are the most common. Benign tumors are almost always **leiomyomas**, which are smooth muscle tumors, although these have an incidence of less than 10% that of malignant tumors of the esophagus. Many are discovered during radiographic examination for complaints not related to esophageal problems. These benign lesions present as intramural filling defects in the barium-outlined esophageal wall (Fig. 5.77). The exact location of a leiomyoma, which appears as a homogeneous soft tissue mass, may be determined on CT. Treatment of a leiomyoma consists of surgical removal

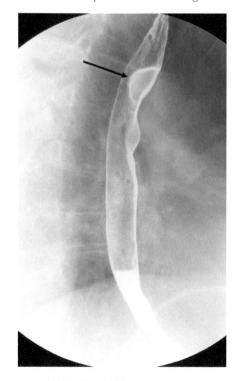

FIG. 5.77 Well-defined filling defect in the proximal esophagus indicative of a benign esophageal leiomyoma. Note the smooth mucosal surface and obtuse margins with the adjacent esophageal lumen suggesting that this is a benign tumor.

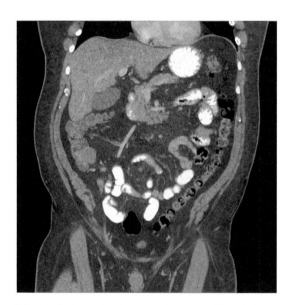

FIG. 5.76 Computed tomography scan of the abdomen demonstrating diverticulitis.

through a thoracic or abdominal incision that avoids esophageal resection.

Cancers of the esophagus constitute approximately 7% of cancers of the GI system but carry a poor prognosis, with an overall 5-year survival rate of less than 10%. Squamous cell carcinomas most commonly arise in the body of the esophagus; those at the gastroesophageal junction are typically **adenocarcinomas**. These two types of esophageal cancers have different clinical and radiographic features. Diagnosis is made by endoscopic biopsy of the lesion. Regardless of the type of esophageal cancer, however, CT of the neck, chest, and abdomen is helpful to stage the spread of the disease by demonstrating tumor size, lymph node involvement, and metastases. PET CT is often used for staging of esophageal cancers. Endoscopic ultrasonography (EUS), although highly accurate in detecting disease, is less available in many medical institutions.

Chronic irritation of the esophagus is thought to be a predisposing factor to squamous cell carcinomas, with such irritation caused by particular agents, including reflux, alcohol, and smoking, and disorders such as achalasia and esophageal diverticula. The chronic presence of irritation to the esophageal mucosa leads to Barrett (dysplastic) epithelium, with mutation of the *TP53* gene being an early event in the development of Barrett adenocarcinoma. The primary symptom of esophageal cancer is dysphagia. However, dysphagia may not become significant until the tumor has narrowed the lumen to 50% to 75% of its normal circumference, allowing metastatic spread to the adjacent lymph nodes and mediastinal structures before diagnosis. Surgery is used as a treatment, with the goal to excise the tumor and regional metastasis. Chemotherapy, radiation therapy, or both may be used as an adjunct to surgical intervention. The rapid spread of esophageal cancer, however, requires the goal to be palliation in many cases. The radiographic appearance of a malignant squamous cell tumor may include mucosal destruction, ulceration, narrowing, and a sharp demarcation between normal tissue and the malignant tumor.

As mentioned earlier, adenocarcinomas usually occur in the lower esophagus around the gastroesophageal junction. Many believe these begin as primary gastric carcinomas that invade the lower esophagus. Others believe that a direct link exists between a disorder termed *Barrett esophagus* and the development of adenocarcinoma of the esophagus. Barrett esophagus involves progressive columnar metaplasia of the distal esophagus as a result of chronic gastroesophageal reflux. More than 90% of adenocarcinomas of the esophagus have been found to arise from the mucosa. Similar to squamous carcinomas, adenocarcinomas spread via the lymph nodes; however, unlike squamous carcinomas, they also spread below the diaphragm. Metastasis to mediastinal structures and hematogenous spread to the liver, lung, and bone occur readily (Fig. 5.78). Radiographically, early adenocarcinomas appear as plaque-like lesions or as sessile polyps (Fig. 5.79), and advanced tumors appear as infiltrating lesions with irregular narrowing of the lumen and abrupt, asymmetric borders.

Tumors of the Stomach

Benign tumors account for fewer than 10% of all stomach tumors. Those that are clinically significant are quite rare. Most stomach tumors are malignant, and the outstanding preponderance (about 95%) of these are adenocarcinomas. Alterations in the tumor-suppressor *p53* gene, as well as cell cycle regulators, cell adhesion molecules, and DNA repair genes, all contribute in part to the development of gastric adenocarcinomas. The incidence of gastric cancer varies strikingly by geographic area, race, diet, heredity, and sex. For example, the rate is nearly five times greater in Japan than in the

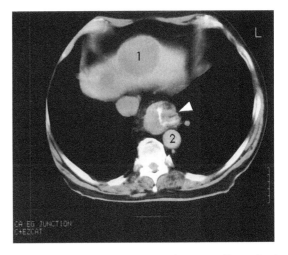

FIG. 5.78 A computed tomography scan with contrast demonstrates an increased thickening of the esophageal wall and distortion of the lumen (*arrow*), compatible with a gastroesophageal junction malignancy. Also seen are (*1*) a large metastatic lesion in the superior portion of the liver and (*2*) the aorta.

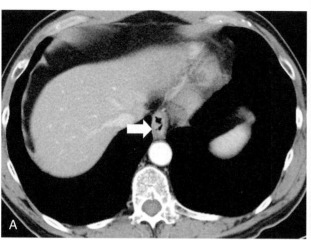

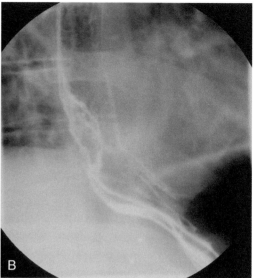

FIG. 5.79 **A**, Adenocarcinoma of the esophagus as seen on a CT scan with contrast showing thickening of the distal esophageal wall with an irregular shaped projection into the lumen. **B**, A double-contrast esophagram image on the same patient demonstrating the irregular and unsmooth mucosa of the tumor projecting into the esophageal lumen.

United States. The survival rate associated with gastric carcinoma depends on the stage of the disease. If the neoplasm is limited to the stomach mucosa, the 5-year survival rate is as high as 71%; however, advanced stages carry a poor prognosis, with overall 5-year survival rates less than 4%.

Current research indicates that the presence of *H. pylori* results in a threefold to sixfold increase in the risk of gastric adenocarcinoma. Most gastric carcinomas develop in the pyloric and antrum regions, particularly along the lesser curvature, although they may occur anywhere (Fig. 5.80). Gastric carcinomas may also be polypoid with a plaque-like, lobulated appearance. Most gastric carcinomas are diagnosed at an advanced stage because early stomach cancers do not have specific symptoms. They invade other structures by a variety of routes. These tumors metastasize fairly readily outside the stomach to involve the omentum, liver, pancreas, and colon. Liver involvement creates the possibility of discharge into the bloodstream and dispersal throughout the body. Because of the abundance of lymphatics in the stomach, approximately 75% to 85% of these patients also demonstrate metastases via the lymphatic system.

Patients who complain of persistent GI pain should have a thorough workup. The most appropriate primary diagnostic procedure is an upper endoscopy with

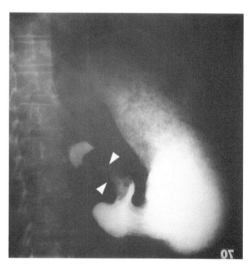

FIG. 5.80 Adenocarcinoma of the stomach in a 66-year-old woman, resulting in gastric outlet obstruction. Note the area of narrowing and the abrupt transition between normal stomach and the acutely narrowed area.

biopsy. Endoscopy is often followed by a fluoroscopic UGI series. Symptoms of gastric tumors are often vague but include bleeding, vomiting, loss of appetite, weight loss, and early satiety. Tumors are radiographically indicated by a relative rigidity of peristalsis and filling defects on compression. Filling defects manifest as areas of total or relative radiolucency within the barium column. Polypoid tumors are clearly visible during CT examination. By identifying lymphatic involvement and extragastric spread of the cancer, CT is also useful in the staging of gastric cancers.

Surgical removal of gastric cancer has been the only successful treatment; a subtotal gastrectomy is the usual procedure. Resection of the stomach to attach to the jejunum via a gastrojejunostomy usually accompanies this procedure. If a total gastrectomy is warranted, the jejunum is attached to the esophagus forming an esophagojejunostomy. Radiation therapy and chemotherapy treatments for stomach carcinoma have been less effective.

Small Bowel Neoplasms

Small bowel tumors represent fewer than 5% of all benign and malignant GI neoplasms; however, this may be an underestimate because of limitations in current imaging modalities for the small bowel. The incidence of malignancy for this small amount is about 50%. The low overall incidence is surprising, considering that the small bowel constitutes 75% of the entire GI tract, with an enormous mucosal surface. Also, it is in constant contact with enteric carcinogenic substances. Reasons for this low incidence of tumors are not entirely known or understood. Most small bowel cancers occur in the duodenum and proximal jejunum.

One predisposing factor for small bowel neoplasms seems to be the degree of polyposis in other areas of the GI tract, a condition frequently determined by heredity. Another predisposing factor is Kaposi sarcoma, most common in patients with acquired immunodeficiency syndrome (AIDS). Up to 60% of these patients have GI involvement, with the tumors arising anywhere in the stomach, small bowel, or distal colon. In addition, patients who have Crohn's disease also have an increased risk for developing adenocarcinoma of the small bowel. Intermittent abdominal pain, sometimes described as cramps, is the most common symptom. Endoscopy with biopsy is the most common means of identifying small bowel neoplasms, but small bowel barium studies may assist in the diagnosis. Surgical resection is the primary means of treating small bowel neoplasms, both benign and malignant.

Colonic Polyps

Colonic polyps are small masses of tissue arising from the bowel wall to project inward into the lumen (Fig. 5.81). An adenomatous polyp is a tumor of benign neoplastic epithelium that may undergo dysplastic changes to become malignant. It consists of a saccular projection into the bowel lumen and is either sessile, that is, attached directly to the bowel wall with a wide base, or pedunculated, that is, attached by a narrow stalk (Fig. 5.82). Polyps are more frequently noted in the left colon, and particularly in the rectosigmoid areas. Other types of polyps are inflammatory, hyperplastic, and juvenile.

Although most polyps are asymptomatic, all should be removed, especially adenomatous polyps, which pose a greater risk of malignancy (Fig. 5.83). Those over 2 cm in size have a malignancy rate of over 50%. Most never reach this size, however. The complications of polyps include ulceration from chronic irritation or bowel obstruction from inflammation. Most cancers of the colon and rectum arise from previously benign polyps. Patients with polyps may have rectal bleeding, constipation, diarrhea, or flatulence, but most are asymptomatic. Radiographically a double-contrast barium enema is the examination of choice, with the polyps manifesting as rounded filling defects or contour defects in the barium shadow. CT colonography is gaining popularity as availability and reimbursement improve. Although pedunculated polyps are easily recognized and often considered benign, size is a better indicator of malignancy *versus* benignancy, as noted. At times, it is difficult to discriminate between fecal matter and a polyp. In general, fecal matter is mobile, whereas a polyp stays fixed to the stalk. Sigmoidoscopy and colonoscopy are the gold standard for diagnosis and are critical in the evaluation and removal of polyps. Patients with polyps

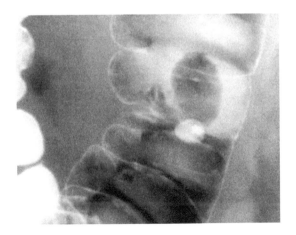

FIG. 5.81 Filling defect in the transverse colon near the splenic flexure indicates a polyp projecting into the lumen. A barium-filled diverticulum is seen immediately above it in this patient, who had blood in his stools.

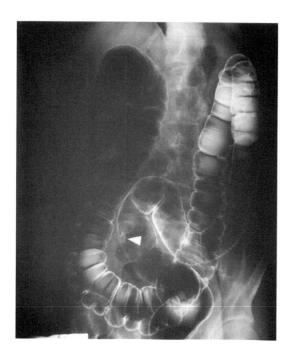

Pedunculated polyp seen attached to the wall of the sigmoid colon by a long stalk on an air-contrast barium enema.

are monitored closely after discovery and are often treated with aspirin and cyclooxygenase 2 (COX-2) inhibitors to prevent new polyp formation.

Colon Cancer

Colorectal cancers are the third most common tumors in the United States and the most common GI cancer. Additionally, carcinoma of the colon is the third most common cause of mortality from cancer. The incidence of colon cancer rises significantly after age 40 years and doubles with each decade, reaching a peak at about age 75 years. In the United States adults have a 1 in 20 chance of developing colorectal cancer in their lifetime and a 1 in 40 chance of dying from this disease. Predisposing factors include a family history of familial polyposis and UC. Colon cancer tends to cluster in families, with the risk of the disease in people with one affected first-degree relative being two to three times higher than in the general population. The *APC* gene, which is responsible for the colon cancer subset of adenomatous polyposis, has been mapped to chromosome 5, and mutations of the gene are found in at least 85% of all colon tumors. Hereditary nonpolyposis colorectal cancer, which accounts for as many as 5% of all colorectal

Adenomatous polyp

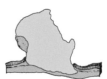

Focal atypia (cancer in situ)   Focal cancer (malignant adenoma)

Focal cancer invading stalk with some "benign" polyp still in body   Invasive cancer containing piece of polyp

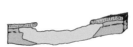

Polypoid invasive cancer without polyp remnant   Ulcerated invasive cancer without polyp remnant

Adenomatous polyp transformation.

cancer cases, has also been tied to mutations to as many as six different genes. Furthermore, allelic deletion on chromosomes 5, 17, and 18 is believed to be responsible for promoting the transition from normal to malignant colonic mucosa. Environmental factors also seem to correlate with colorectal cancer; countries with a higher intake of sugar and animal fats (e.g., the United States) have a higher incidence, when compared with countries (e.g., Western Asia, Central America, and Africa) that have a higher fiber intake.

Recent guidelines have divided colorectal cancer risk levels into three categories. The first category is of those with an average risk, including patients 50 years of age or older. The second category is of moderate risk, and includes those with a first-degree relative with a history of adenoma or carcinoma, or a personal history of similar pathology. Finally, the third category is of those with high risk, and includes hereditary syndromes such as hereditary nonpolyposis colorectal cancer (HNPCC) and familial polyposis, or patients with a personal history of UC or CD.

Adenocarcinoma is the most common type of colorectal cancer and is derived from the glandular epithelium of the colon. It begins as a benign adenoma that undergoes a slow malignant transformation. Although the transformation may take up to 7 years to complete, all polypoid lesions larger than 1 cm should be removed from the colon. Adenocarcinoma is characterized by infiltration of the colon wall, as opposed to being a bulky, intraluminal mass.

Although the incidence of proximal colon cancers is increasing, nearly 50% still occur below the mid-descending colon. Most of these (70%) occur in the rectosigmoid area and are detectable by flexible sigmoidoscopy. Right colon lesions differ considerably from left colon lesions in terms of symptoms produced. Lesions in the right colon may produce no early symptoms, often becoming quite large, ulcerating, and even bleeding without other significant symptoms. They also tend to penetrate and extend into surrounding tissues without causing obstruction. Patients often present initially with anemia and blood in their stools. Left colon lesions, in contrast, present more often with obstruction and bleeding, largely because of a smaller lumen and an annular (ring-like) growth pattern.

Detection of colorectal cancer, when localized, is associated with a 5-year survival rate of approximately 80%. The evaluation of colon cancer includes fecal blood testing, sigmoidoscopy, colonoscopy, barium enema, CT, CT colonography (CTC), transrectal ultrasonography (TRUS), and PET imaging. The use of clinical fecal occult blood testing (FOBT) has demonstrated a 15% to 33% reduction in mortality rates. Additionally, use of screening sigmoidoscopy examinations may decrease colorectal cancer mortality rates by two-thirds for cancers within reach of the scope. When proximal GI lesions are suspected, a colonoscopy may be ordered. Colonoscopy is currently considered to be the most sensitive and specific test for detecting colorectal polyps and cancers because of its ability to obtain abnormal tissue for biopsy and histologic identification of dysplasia. The primary benefits unique to the use of endoscopic imaging are the ability to directly visualize the luminal mucosal lining and availability of biopsy upon identification of abnormal tissue. CTC may be useful to screen for colorectal cancer when a fibrostenotic stricture in the colon prevents traditional colonoscopy techniques from evaluating proximally to the diseased colon.

Double-contrast barium enema (DCBE) has been noted to produce more accurate diagnoses compared with the limited single-contrast study because of the enhanced display of subtle mucosal abnormalities otherwise masked by a dense barium column. Although appropriate for colorectal cancer screening, DCBE is typically utilized when colonoscopy is unsuccessful or CTC is unavailable. One benefit of DCBE over diagnostic colonoscopy is the dramatic reduction in the number of bowel perforations, 1 out of 25,000 *versus* 1 out of 2000, respectively. The radiographic appearance of adenocarcinoma has led to its designation as the "napkin-ring" carcinoma or the "apple-core" lesion, as the edges of the lesion tend to overhang and form acute angles with the bowel wall (Fig. 5.84). Although it may be difficult to distinguish between carcinoma and an inflammatory lesion (e.g., regional enteritis or UC), a carcinoma generally has a more clear-cut transition between the malignant mucosa and the normal mucosa. In addition, the length of bowel involved is usually shorter with carcinoma than with an inflammatory lesion.

Compared with CT, MRI is quickly gaining ground as an equal and even superior method for detecting rectal neoplasms and associated liver metastases. Prior imaging with MRI required the use of endorectal coils to attain optimal cancer staging information, which was limited to the length of the endorectal coil length. However, with the move to higher strength 3.0 T magnets, most colon cancer imaging can now be performed with only the phased array coils, although such a technique may still have limited use in patients who are obese. Additionally, MRI has the ability to depict the layers of the rectal wall and assess the depth of neoplastic bowel wall penetration, and with an accuracy of 86% in predicting the circumferential margin of cancer involvement, surgeons can more reliably reduce the area of resected tissue. Diffusion-weighted imaging (DWI) techniques have shown to be more sensitive and specific compared with standard contrast-enhanced MRI with gadolinium and are believed to be superior for tumor detection and characterization when monitoring tumor response to treatment. The use of the magnetic resonance colonography (MRC) technique has the benefit over CTC of not involving ionizing radiation. However, the spatial resolution of MRC is currently less than that of CTC, decreasing its overall accuracy. In recent MRC research studies, evidence has shown that "dark lumen" imaging (utilizing water as a negative contrast) has proven to be more effective in identifying colorectal cancer compared with "bright lumen" imaging (utilizing gadolinium as a positive contrast agent).

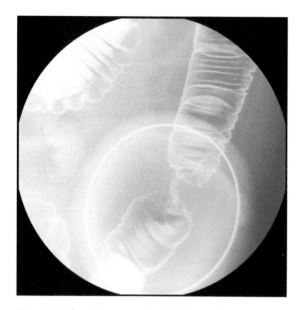

FIG. 5.84 Spot image captured during a double contrast barium enema delineating an "apple core" lesion of the descending colon consistent with adenocarcinoma. Note the characteristic appearance of abrupt change from normal to abnormal colon with the shelf-like appearance of overhanging edges caused by the mass and creating the apple core contour.

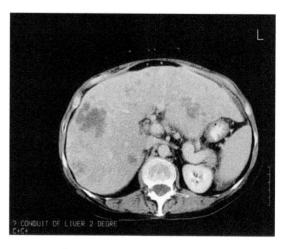

FIG. 5.85 Computed tomography demonstration of extensive metastatic disease from the colon to both lobes of the liver, ranging from punctate to up to 5 cm in this 50-year-old woman.

TRUS is currently the standard imaging procedure for staging superficial rectal carcinomas. Similar to MRI, TRUS helps distinguish between the layers within the rectal wall and has displayed an accuracy of up to 97% in detecting the depth of tumor penetration and perirectal spread. In its ability to detect local lymph node involvement, again, TRUS is comparable with MRI with an overall accuracy of 62% to 83%. It should be noted that studies comparing the use of frontal ultrasound probe types and radial ultrasound probe types found the frontal probe to have a higher overall accuracy in staging rectal cancer. Additionally, techniques utilizing sonographic imaging of the colon dilated with water have been established; however, experience with this technique is extremely limited, and the procedure is currently not recommended for colorectal cancer screening.

It is important to note that imaging modalities, including CTC, barium enema, and MRI are usually not appropriate for colorectal cancer screening in high-risk patients with hereditary nonpolyposis colorectal cancer and IBD. These patients are almost always examined by using colonoscopy.

PET alone or combined with CT has been shown to alter treatment protocols in almost a third of patients with advanced primary rectal cancer. PET with CT is particularly accurate in identifying hepatic and peritoneal metastases compared with CT alone. In fact, a relatively new concept of PET with CTC has been reported to be significantly more accurate in GI cancer staging compared with CTC alone. PET has a potential role in restaging colorectal cancer after chemoradiotherapy by measuring the pre- and posttreatment standard uptake volume (SUV). Limitations of PET include decreased sensitivity in detecting small colonic lesions 5 mm to 10 mm in diameter and decreased 18F-fluorodeoxyglucose (FDG) uptake by mucinous tumors.

Without treatment, cancer spreads by invasion of local tissue via the lymphatics to the mesenteric nodes and on to the liver (Fig. 5.85) and lungs. Fortunately the lesion does not metastasize early, leading to a good prognosis. The primary means of treatment are surgical excision of the primary tumor and its margins and resection of the bowel, if possible. A colostomy may be required, depending on the site of the tumor. Radiation therapy or chemotherapy is generally given before and after surgery for rectal cancers, especially in those with lymph nodes positive for metastasis. For inoperable tumors, radiation therapy is given to reduce the tumor size and its resultant complications (e.g., obstruction), and also to provide pain relief. Chemotherapy is given when the cancer has metastasized.

Pathologic Summary of the Gastrointestinal System

Pathology	Imaging Modality of Choice
Esophageal atresia	Radiography
Bowel atresia	Radiography in infant, sonography in fetus
Hypertrophic pyloric stenosis	Sonography abdomen, radiography, UGI
Malrotation	CT abdomen and pelvis with contrast, SBFT and BaE, sonography
Hirschsprung disease	BaE
Meckel diverticulum	Nuclear medicine Meckel scan
Gluten-sensitive enteropathy	UGI, SBFT, BaE
Carbohydrate intolerance	UGI barium mixed with lactose
Esophageal strictures	Esophagram and endoscopy
GERD	Endoscopy, esophagram, UGI, nuclear medicine reflux scintigraphy, abdominal sonography
Peptic ulcer	Endoscopy, double-contrast UGI, nuclear medicine urea breath test
Regional enteritis (Crohn's disease)	CT enterography (abdomen and pelvis with contrast), MRI enterography (abdomen and pelvis with contrast), routine CT abdomen and pelvis with contrast, SBFT and double-contrast BaE
Appendicitis	CT abdomen and pelvis with contrast, RUQ abdominal sonography, abdomen radiography
Ulcerative colitis	Sigmoidoscopy and colonoscopy
Esophageal varices	Esophagram,
Bowel obstruction	CT abdomen and pelvis with contrast, MRI abdomen and pelvis with contrast, supine and erect abdominal radiography
Achalasia	Esophagram
Diverticular disease	CT abdomen and pelvis with contrast, MRI abdomen and pelvis with or without contrast, double-contrast Ba studies, TRUS, transabdominal graded compression sonography
Polyps	Colonoscopy and double-contrast BaE
Neoplastic disease of the GI system	CT colonography, colonoscopy, double-contrast BaE, CT

Ba, Barium; *BaE*, barium enema; *CT*, computed tomography; *GERD*, gastroesophageal reflux disease; *GI*, gastrointestinal; *MRI*, magnetic resonance imaging; *TRUS*, transabdominal graded compression sonography; *UGI*, upper gastrointestinal study; *SBFT*, small bowel follow through.

1. Esophageal atresia is classified as a(n)_____ condition of the gastrointestinal (GI) system.
   a. Congenital
   b. Degenerative
   c. Inflammatory
   d. Neurologic

2. An outpouching of the bowel wall caused by a weakening in its muscular layer is a(n):
   a. Atresia
   b. Carcinoma
   c. Diverticulum
   d. Polyp

3. The radiographic string sign is associated with:
   a. Achalasia
   b. Adenocarcinoma
   c. Regional enteritis
   d. Ulcerative colitis

4. Celiac disease is a type of:
   a. Atresia
   b. Herniation
   c. Malabsorption syndrome
   d. Ulcerative colitis

5. The appearance of a Schatzki ring is associated with a(n)_____hernia.
   a. Inguinal
   b. Rolling
   c. Sliding
   d. Umbilical

6. A congenital, neurogenic disease of the GI system characterized by an absence of neurons in the bowel wall is:
   a. Achalasia
   b. Diverticulosis
   c. Hirschsprung disease
   d. Toxic megacolon

7. The fewest GI tumors, both benign and malignant, occur in the:
   a. Colon
   b. Esophagus
   c. Large bowel
   d. Small bowel

8. Which of the following statements are true of colon cancer?
   1. The majority of adenocarcinomas of the colon occur in the rectosigmoid area.
   2. The appearance of the "apple core" lesion is indicative of colon cancer.
   3. Adenomatous polyps may develop into adenocarcinoma of the colon.
   a. 1 and 2
   b. 1 and 3
   c. 2 and 3
   d. 1, 2, and 3

9. A twisting of bowel about its mesenteric base best refers to a(n):
   a. Ascites
   b. Intussusception
   c. Incarcerated hernia
   d. Volvulus

10. The condition in which a gallstone erodes from the gallbladder and creates a fistula to the small bowel is:
    a. Gallstone ileus
    b. Intussusception
    c. Incarcerated hernia
    d. Volvulus

11. Describe the differences, both clinical and radiographic, between a mechanical bowel obstruction and paralytic ileus.

12. Explain the connection between colonic polyps and the development of colorectal cancer.

13. Describe the role of computed tomography (CT) in the staging of various GI cancers.

14. Explain the physiologic alteration that causes esophageal varices, and describe the radiographic appearance of this disorder.

15. Compare and contrast the various gastric tubes in terms of their uses and radiographic appearance.

CHAPTER 6

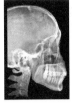
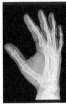
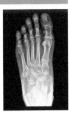

Hepatobiliary System

http://evolve.elsevier.com/Kowalczyk/pathology/

Anatomy and Physiology

The hepatobiliary system is composed of the liver, gallbladder, and biliary tree (Fig. 6.1). The pancreas is closely related and shares a portion of the biliary ductal system, hence its inclusion in this chapter.

Liver

The liver is the second largest organ in the body and is sheltered by the ribs in the right upper quadrant (RUQ) of the abdomen. It is kept in position by peritoneal ligaments and intraabdominal pressure from the muscles of the abdominal wall. The liver is typically divided into the right lobe and a smaller left lobe. The two are separated by the falciform ligament. The functions of the liver are multiple: metabolism of substances delivered via its portal circulation; synthesis of substances, including those concerned with blood clotting; storage of vitamin B, and other materials; and detoxification and excretion of various substances.

The liver has a dual supply of blood, coming from the hepatic artery and the portal vein. The hepatic artery usually originates from the celiac axis and it delivers oxygenated blood to the liver. The portal vein is formed by the union of the superior mesenteric and splenic veins. It is located within the liver and serves to return venous blood from the abdominal viscera to the inferior vena cava (IVC). Any interference with blood flow, which may occur with liver disease, results in consequences elsewhere in the abdominal viscera and spleen.

Biliary Tree

The biliary tree is a system of ducts that act to drain bile produced by the liver into the duodenum (Fig. 6.2). Bile from the liver's two main lobes is drained by small intrahepatic branches that join to form the right and left hepatic ducts. These unite to form the common hepatic duct, which is joined usually in its midportion by the cystic duct from the gallbladder. Together, the cystic duct and the common hepatic duct form the common bile duct.

The common bile duct descends posterior to the descending duodenum (second portion) to enter at its posteromedial aspect. Before its entrance into the duodenum, the common bile duct may be joined by the pancreatic duct from the head of the pancreas (Fig. 6.3). The short part of the common bile duct, after joining the pancreatic duct, is known as the *hepatopancreatic ampulla* or, more commonly, the *ampulla of Vater*.

The flow of both bile and pancreatic juice into the duodenum is regulated by the hepatopancreatic sphincter, more commonly known as the *sphincter of Oddi* (Fig. 6.2). The release of bile into the duodenum is triggered by cholecystokinin, a hormone released by the presence of fatty foods within the stomach. The purpose of bile is to emulsify fats so that they may be absorbed by the GI tract.

Gallbladder

The gallbladder, a digestive organ, is a pear-shaped sac located on the undersurface on the right lobe of the liver. Normally, the walls are quite thin, but they often thicken in the presence of inflammation. The sole function of the gallbladder is to store and concentrate bile that has been produced in the liver. The gallbladder receives bile from the liver via the hepatic duct and empties bile into the duodenum to aid in the digestion and absorption of fats.

Pancreas

The pancreas is an elongated, flat organ that obliquely crosses the left side of the abdomen behind the stomach; it is a powerful digestive organ. Its functions are both exocrine and endocrine. Exocrine function is concerned with production of the three digestive enzymes trypsin, amylase, and lipase. Trypsin assists in the digestion of proteins. Amylase helps to break down large molecules of starch into smaller molecules of maltose, which eventually are broken down into glucose and stored in the liver. Lipase assists in breaking down lipids into fatty acids and glycerol. These are discharged through the pancreatic duct into the duodenum. The endocrine portion of the pancreas consists of multiple clusters of specialized cells, which are termed the *islets of Langerhans*. The specialized cells are classified as α-cells (alpha) and β-cells (beta). The function of β-cells is to produce insulin, and α-cells produce glucagon, both of which are discharged directly into the blood from the pancreas. Insulin and glucagon regulate carbohydrate metabolism. Insulin's role includes making and storing glucose in the liver and muscle tissue throughout the body while enabling the body to burn the stored glucose. When the blood flowing from the pancreas to the liver through the portal vein is hyperglycemic, insulin is released into the bloodstream via the portal vein. Glucagon acts in a similar manner, but it functions to increase the glucose level in blood. If the blood released into the portal vein is hypoglycemic, glucagon stimulates the liver to break down glycogen into glucose, thus increasing the glucose level in the bloodstream.

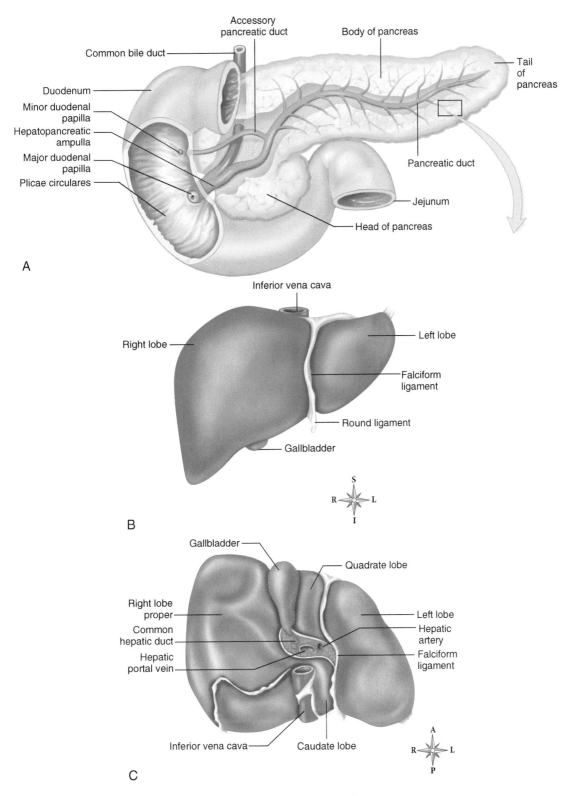

FIG. 6.1 The hepatobiliary system and the pancreas.

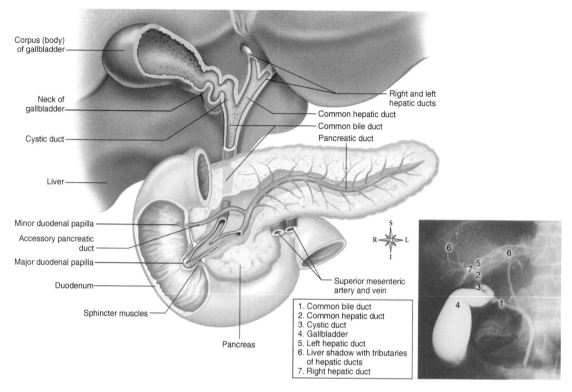

Corpus (body) of gallbladder

Neck of gallbladder

Cystic duct

Liver

Minor duodenal papilla

Accessory pancreatic duct

Major duodenal papilla

Duodenum

Sphincter muscles

Pancreas

Right and left hepatic ducts

Common hepatic duct

Common bile duct

Pancreatic duct

Superior mesenteric artery and vein

1. Common bile duct
2. Common hepatic duct
3. Cystic duct
4. Gallbladder
5. Left hepatic duct
6. Liver shadow with tributaries of hepatic ducts
7. Right hepatic duct

FIG. 6.2 The biliary system.

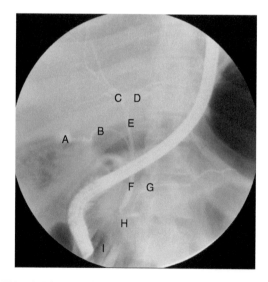

FIG. 6.3 Image of a normal appearing biliary tree and pancreatic duct as visualized during an ERCP examination with retrograde contrast injection of the ducts. The anatomy is labeled as follows: A. gallbladder, B. cystic duct C. right hepatic ducts, D. left hepatic ducts, E. common hepatic duct, F. common bile duct, G. pancreatic duct, H. hepatopancreatic ampulla, and I. duodenum.

Imaging Considerations

Radiography

A conventional abdominal radiograph may contain information about the hepatobiliary system through the demonstration of faint calcifications that might otherwise be obscured by contrast media. A plain radiograph of the gallbladder may demonstrate radiopaque gallstones composed of a mixture of cholesterol, bile pigment (bilirubin), and calcium salts or milk of calcium, which is a semiliquid sludge composed of calcium carbonate mixed with bile in the gallbladder (Fig. 6.4). The hazy radiopacity results from a settling of bile as a result of an obstruction at the neck of the gallbladder, or it may develop in patients who have been fasting or have been on hyperalimentation. Only about 10% to 30% of gallstones are radiopaque and able to be visualized on an abdominal radiograph. Thus abdominal radiography is often used to exclude other causes of abdominal pain.

Gas may occasionally be seen in the wall or lumen of the gallbladder because of the presence of

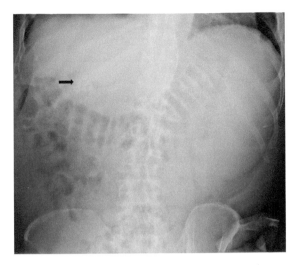

FIG. 6.4 Abdominal radiograph demonstrating multiple gallstones (*black arrow*) that are radiopaque in their composition.

gas-forming organisms in the gallbladder walls. This is more often seen in patients with poorly controlled diabetes because of poor blood supply to the organ. Gas visualized in the biliary tree, termed pneumobilia, may occur as a result of a spontaneous fistula, as might be seen in gallstone ileus, a postoperative biliary anastomosis or a sphincterotomy procedure (Fig. 6.5).

Contrast Studies

Percutaneous Transhepatic Cholangiography

Percutaneous transhepatic cholangiography (PTC) is a method of visualizing the biliary tree using a puncture through the wall of the abdomen to insert a needle directly into the biliary tree. With the use of a flexible, 22-gauge, skinny needle (Chiba), this procedure is safe and fairly easy to perform. The subsequent injection of iodinated contrast medium (Fig. 6.6) is useful in distinguishing **medical jaundice**, caused by hepatocellular dysfunction, from **surgical jaundice**, which results from biliary obstruction. Also, the examination is useful for detecting the presence of calculi or a tumor in the distal common bile duct. It has a high success rate in imaging the biliary ductal system, is less expensive than an endoscopic retrograde cholangiopancreatogram, and has a low complication rate of approximately 3.5%. PTC also may be immediately followed by a therapeutic procedure such as biliary drainage, stone removal or crushing via contact lithotripsy or laser fragmentation,

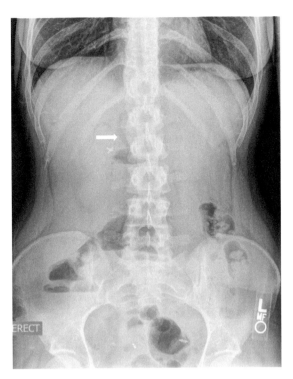

FIG. 6.5 Abdominal radiograph with visualization of pneumobilia shown as a gas filled biliary tree with the white arrow pointing toward the common bile duct segment. Cholecystectomy clips are also seen in the right upper quadrant.

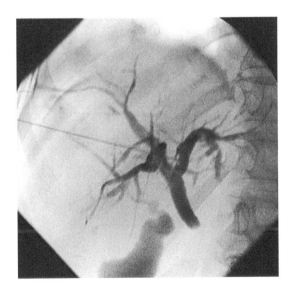

FIG. 6.6 Demonstration of the biliary system via a percutaneous transhepatic cholangiogram.

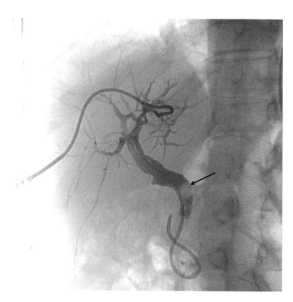

FIG. 6.7 Percutaneous transhepatic cholangiogram examination with placement of a biliary tube known as an internal-external biliary drainage catheter, which is used to bypass an obstruction within the biliary tree. In this case the cause of the obstruction is a large gallstone (*black arrow*) within the distal common bile duct.

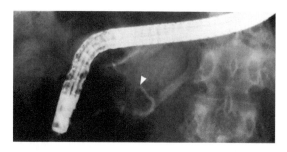

FIG. 6.8 An endoscopic retrograde cholangiopancreatogram showing abrupt termination of the pancreatic duct about 4 cm from its opening.

stent placement, or biopsy (Fig. 6.7). This procedure is preferred in the evaluation of proximal obstructions involving the hepatic duct bifurcation, which is difficult to image with the retrograde approach via an endoscopic retrograde cholangiopancreatogram (see next section).

Endoscopic Retrograde Cholangiopancreatogram

The endoscopic retrograde cholangiopancreatogram (ERCP), an imaging procedure performed by a gastroenterologist, is a means of visualizing the biliary system

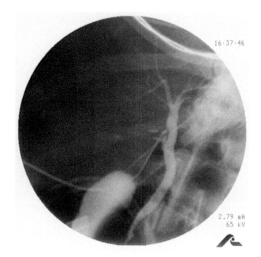

FIG. 6.9 A digital image of an operative cholangiogram taken during surgery.

and main pancreatic duct. A fiberoptic endoscope is passed through the mouth and gastrointestinal (GI) tract to the duodenal C-loop to visualize the hepatopancreatic ampulla (ampulla of Vater). A thin catheter is then directed into the orifice of the common bile duct and/or pancreatic duct, followed by a retrograde injection of contrast medium (Fig. 6.8). In many cases, the ERCP is preferred over the PTC and is often preceded with a sonographic examination or computed tomography (CT) investigation of the pancreas. Although an ERCP is more expensive than PTC, it is often used to visualize nondilated ducts, distal obstructions, bleeding disorders, and the pancreas. The complication rate (2%–3%) is similar to that of PTC. The ERCP also offers the ability to perform therapeutic procedures such as sphincterotomy, stone extractions, stent placement, and biliary dilatation. Cytology and biopsy may also be performed.

Operative Cholangiography

Operative cholangiography is performed during surgery at the time of a cholecystectomy to detect biliary calculi and the need for common bile duct exploration (Fig. 6.9). A needle is placed directly into the cystic duct or common bile duct by the surgeon, and a small volume (6 mL) of iodinated contrast material is injected, followed by radiography. A second injection of 5 mL is made, followed by radiography a second time. A more modern imaging method for operative cholangiography is to use intraoperative fluoroscopy produced by a portable fluoroscopic C-arm unit to obtain real-time visualization during the

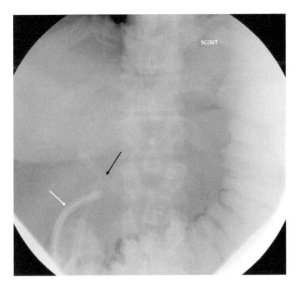

FIG. 6.10 Fluoroscopic scout image of a T-tube (*black arrow*). A surgical drain (*white arrow*) is also present in the field of view.

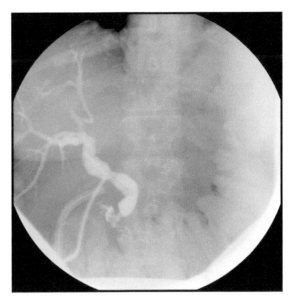

FIG. 6.11 T-tube cholangiogram image with contrast filling the biliary tree and flowing into the duodenum indicating patency of the sphincter of Oddi.

injection of contrast. The resulting images are reviewed for possible areas of concern before the surgery is completed. It is imperative that no air bubbles be injected into the ductal system with the contrast agent during this procedure because they can mimic stones.

T-Tube Cholangiography

T-tube cholangiography is used after a cholecystectomy to demonstrate patency of the common bile duct and to check for residual calculi. With a T-shaped tube already inserted surgically into the common bile duct, iodinated contrast medium is injected to verify removal of all calculi and to evaluate for any other abnormalities of the biliary tree (Fig. 6.10). The contrast should flow retrograde, filling the right and left hepatic ducts and smaller branches, and it should also flow antegrade into the common bile duct and eventually the duodenum (Fig. 6.11).

The radiologist must take care not to inject air bubbles because they may give the radiographic appearance of radiolucent calculi. A technologist preparing the contrast should make certain that all air bubbles are purged from the syringe and that any extension tubing is flushed with contrast before being connected to the T-tube. A tip for avoiding air bubbles is to employ a three-way stopcock with one end attached to the T-tube, the second end attached to an empty syringe, and the third end attached to the contrast syringe (with or without extension tubing). The three-way stopcock system allows for contrast

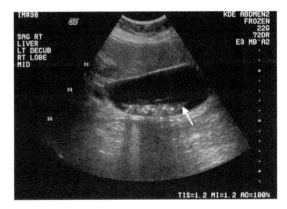

FIG. 6.12 A sagittal sonographic view of the gallbladder demonstrating stones.

from one direction and bile from the other to be aspirated individually into the empty syringe to aspirate small air bubbles that would occur when connecting the tubes. This injection set-up can be utilized when injecting any type of biliary tube or drain.

Diagnostic Medical Sonography

Real-time diagnostic medical sonography is now the modality of choice for evaluating the gallbladder (Fig. 6.12) and biliary tree. This procedure is noninvasive, performed without exposure to ionizing radiation, and the gallbladder can be imaged in almost all fasting patients regardless of the body habitus or clinical condition of the patient. When sonography is performed by a skilled sonographer, it has been proven to be almost 100% accurate in detecting gallstones with the capability of detecting stones as small as 2 mm in size. Gallstones are demonstrated as echogenic areas, meaning white or bright, within the echo-free gallbladder that is dark or black because it is filled with liquid bile. A gallstone results in shadowing, which

means that below the bright echogenic stone there will be a dark shadow caused by a lack of sound wave penetration through the stone (Fig. 6.13). Thickening of the gallbladder wall is easily identified. Sonography is also an excellent tool for determining the presence of common bile duct obstruction, evaluation of the intrahepatic biliary ductal system, and identification of abscesses.

The liver may be evaluated by sonography because of its ideal location in the RUQ and broad contact with the abdominal wall. Hepatic lesions of 1 cm or greater are easily identified, with cystic lesions appearing echo-free (dark) and solid masses appearing echogenic (bright), making sonography an excellent guidance method for aspiration and biopsy of liver lesions.

Doppler sonography enhances the diagnostic capabilities of sonography to allow for clear analysis of the circulatory dynamics, including portal blood flow and hepatic artery thrombosis following liver transplantation. Doppler sonography can also differentiate between vessels and biliary ducts based on flow characteristics.

Computed Tomography

The role of CT in the hepatobiliary system is similar to its role in the GI tract. It is the accepted modality for following malignancies and assessing masses, particularly of the gallbladder, liver, and pancreas. It is also helpful in evaluating complications of cholecystitis such as perforations and abscess formations. Although a high percentage of gallstones are visible with CT, it is not a screening tool for uncomplicated cholelithiasis, as sonography is the preferred modality (Fig. 6.14).

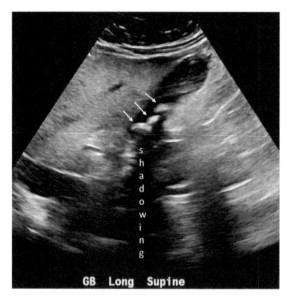

FIG. 6.13 Sonogram image depicting multiple stones within the gallbladder. Note the dark area of shadowing below the stones.

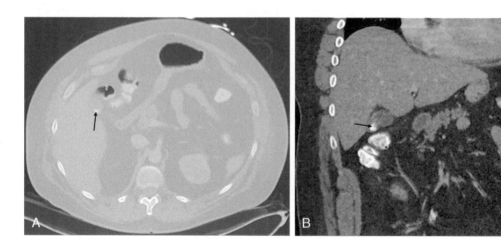

FIG. 6.14 Cholelithiasis as seen on axial computed tomography (CT) image A and coronal CT image B.

The use of spiral or helical CT ensures that the entire liver is imaged in one breath hold, eliminating respiratory artifacts and in many cases demonstrating the liver parenchyma and associated structures better than sonography. In addition to the excellent contrast resolution offered by CT, the use of large-bolus intravenous (IV) iodinated contrast media injections during dynamic CT examination has also improved evaluations of the hepatobiliary ductal system and blood flow via three-phase imaging of the liver to capture the arterial and portal venous blood flow (Fig. 6.15). If a biliary obstruction is not visible during a sonographic examination, CT is generally used to identify the location and extent of the obstruction because it is not limited by patient size or the presence of bowel gas. Lacerations of the liver and resultant abdominal bleeding are readily detected by CT (Fig. 6.16), as are metastatic lesions within the liver. CT also demonstrates good visualization of pancreatic tumors

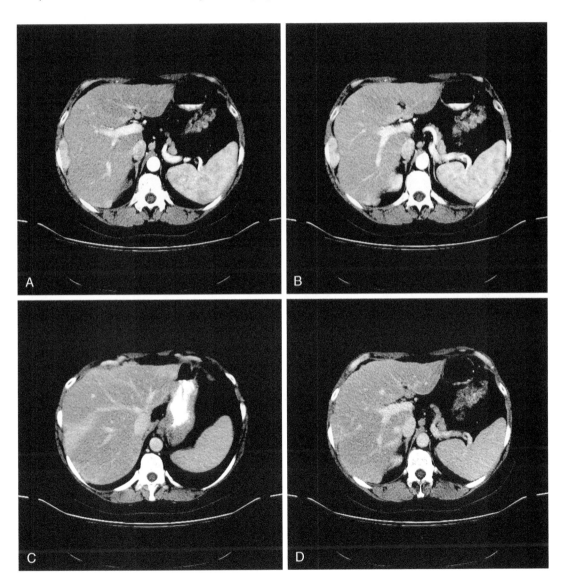

FIG. 6.15 A and B, Three-phase computed tomography (CT) of the liver following a bolus injection of intravenous contrast, demonstrating the arterial circulation. C and D, Three-phase CT of the liver, delayed images demonstrating the portal venous flow.

and pseudocysts. In addition, CT-guided biopsy procedures for the liver (Fig. 6.17), pancreas, and kidney allow for analysis and drainage and offer significant advantages over more invasive conventional surgical biopsy and drainage techniques.

Nuclear Medicine Procedures

Single photon emission computed tomography (SPECT) examinations permit excellent detection of hepatobiliary lesions, especially those located deep within the liver parenchyma. SPECT provides a noninvasive method of evaluating hepatic function and

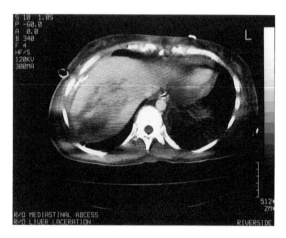

FIG. 6.16 Computed tomography of a 39-year-old woman after a car accident reveals large lacerations of the liver.

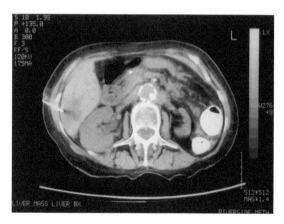

FIG. 6.17 Computed tomography of needle biopsy in an 87-year-old woman clearly demonstrates the needle in the liver.

hepatic and splenic perfusion. Because nuclear medicine imaging provides information regarding physiologic function, combining SPECT and CT can often provide information about both anatomic changes and physiologic function, thus enhancing the ability to diagnose pathologies earlier than using any one modality alone. Labeling of white blood cells (WBCs) with radioactive indium is useful in locating sites of infection for treatment.

Cholescintigraphy performed in nuclear medicine is very useful to confirm cholecystitis and for distinguishing acute from chronic cholecystitis (Fig. 6.18). Radioactive technetium is cleared from blood plasma into bile, demonstrating the physiologic function of the liver, excretion into the biliary ductal system, and visualization of the gallbladder about 1 hour after injection. Delayed visualization or nonvisualization of the gallbladder indicates pathology. In addition, it is a noninvasive method of evaluating biliary drainage, hepatobiliary leaks following trauma or surgery, and segmental obstruction.

Magnetic Resonance Imaging

The role of magnetic resonance imaging (MRI) of the hepatobiliary system has improved greatly as a result of shorter scan times, which allows for the acquisition of several images of the abdomen in a single breath. MRI is often used in conjunction with CT to evaluate pathologies and anomalies of the peritoneum, especially the liver and pancreas. MRI

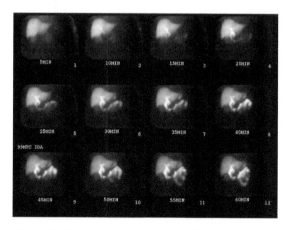

FIG. 6.18 Nuclear medicine hepatobiliary scan demonstrates ready ejection of the radionuclide from the gallbladder through sequential images into the duodenum.

may also be used to identify retroperitoneal bleeds following trauma (Fig. 6.19). Contrast-enhanced three-dimensional dynamic scans of the liver imaged at timed intervals help to differentiate certain tumors from hemangiomas.

Magnetic resonance cholangiopancreatography (MRCP) is an imaging procedure that uses magnetic resonance to visualize the gallbladder and biliary system.

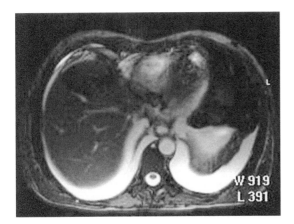

FIG. 6.19 T2-weighted true fast imaging with steady state precession (TrueFISP) axial magnetic resonance image of the abdomen demonstrating a retroperitoneal hemorrhage.

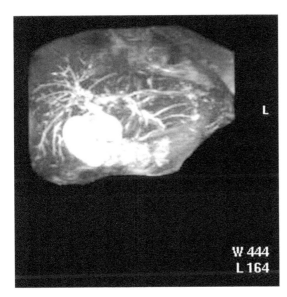

FIG. 6.20 Magnetic resonance imaging is capable of imaging the biliary system without the use of contrast agents.

MRCP is noninvasive and does not require the use of a contrast agent (Fig. 6.20). A heavily T2-weighted sequence is used to suppress the tissues around the biliary system, allowing the gallbladder and bile ducts to appear bright and enabling visualization of stones or other obstructions. MRCP usually accompanies other imaging sequences of the liver and takes about 15 seconds to acquire an image.

The American College of Radiology (ACR) provides highly researched guidelines for determining which of the diagnostic imaging studies is best suited for specific clinical conditions. The guidelines, called the ACR Appropriateness Criteria, are available online to assist referring physicians, radiologists, and others in making suitable imaging decisions for diagnosis and treatment. For patients who present with RUQ pain that may be attributed to the biliary system, sonography of the abdomen is the highest rated imaging examination. CT of the abdomen (with and without contrast), cholescintigraphy, and MRI of the abdomen (with or without contrast) are also recommended and may be appropriate for obtaining the diagnosis. Additionally, if the patient is suspected of having inflammation of the gallbladder (cholecystitis), a percutaneous cholecystostomy with placement of a cholecystostomy tube for drainage may be appropriate for patients in the intensive care unit, who are likely considered nonsurgical candidates (Fig. 6.21).

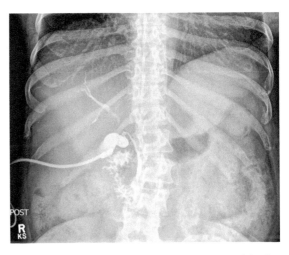

FIG. 6.21 Radiograph obtained after contrast injection of a cholecystostomy tube placed within the gallbladder for bile drainage in a patient who is not a candidate for surgery.

Inflammatory Diseases

Alcohol-Induced Liver Disease

Alcohol is a known toxin, which, when metabolized by the liver, causes cellular damage. Alcohol abuse has long been associated with liver disease. Approximately two million Americans have alcohol-induced liver disease, ranging from alcoholic fatty liver to alcoholic cirrhosis of the liver. Alcohol cannot be stored in the human body, and therefore, the liver must convert it, through oxidation, to alcohol dehydrogenase, acetaldehyde, and acetate, all of which reduce cellular function. This leads to interference with carbohydrate and lipid metabolism. Oxidation also results in reduced gluconeogenesis and increased fatty acid synthesis associated with alcohol metabolism. Chronic alcohol abuse often leads to **fatty liver**, followed by hepatitis, cirrhosis, hepatocellular carcinoma, or all of these diseases. Fatty liver is the most frequent early response to alcohol abuse. Changes in liver function result in a buildup of lipids such as triglycerides, which are deposited in the liver cells. This condition is usually asymptomatic; however, patients may have **hepatomegaly**. Fatty infiltration may be demonstrated by using CT or sonography, but CT is currently the examination of choice. CT demonstrates the fatty deposits as hypodense areas throughout the liver (Fig. 6.22). Inflammation often follows fatty changes within the liver, leading to **alcoholic hepatitis**. At this stage, many patients present with jaundice. This inflammation is diffuse throughout the liver cells and culminates in liver necrosis. This disease may be fatal, progressing quickly to liver failure; or if the individual survives the hepatitis, the condition progresses to alcoholic cirrhosis of the liver, which is an end-stage disease.

Fatty Liver Disease

Factors other than alcohol abuse may also lead to fatty infiltrates within the liver. Obese individuals with type 2 diabetes mellitus, metabolic syndrome, hyperlipidemia, or all of these diseases are at an increased risk of developing nonalcoholic fatty liver disease (NAFLD). This pathology develops as lipids accumulate within the hepatocytes forming free radicals. At some point, the liver cannot rid itself of the excessive triglycerides. This results in an excess of fatty acids within the liver, which leads to fatty infiltration of the liver, termed **steatosis**, and fatty liver disease. In the early stages, NAFLD is often asymptomatic and diagnosis requires biopsy of liver tissue. Although the disease progresses slowly, it may advance to cirrhosis of the liver if left untreated. Management includes implementation of weight loss and exercise programs as treatment for insulin resistance and associated metabolic disturbances.

Cirrhosis

Cirrhosis is a chronic liver condition in which the liver parenchyma and architecture are destroyed, fibrous tissue is laid down, and regenerative nodules are formed. In its early stages, it is usually asymptomatic, as it may take months or even years before damage becomes apparent. Cirrhosis affects the entire liver and is considered an end-stage condition resulting from liver damage caused by chronic alcohol abuse, drugs, autoimmune disorders, metabolic and genetic diseases, chronic hepatitis, cardiac problems, and chronic biliary tract obstruction. In 2014 the CDC ranked chronic liver disease and cirrhosis as the twelfth leading cause of death in the United States and the 2014 mortality statistics by race indicate chronic liver disease and cirrhosis is the fourth leading cause of death among Native Americans and the sixth leading cause among those of Hispanic origin.

The scarring and formation of regenerative nodules associated with cirrhosis result in serious complications. The functional impairments caused by cirrhosis are impaired liver function caused by hepatocyte damage, generally resulting in jaundice, and portal hypertension. Because of interference of portal blood flow through the liver, portal hypertension may lead to development of collateral venous connections to the

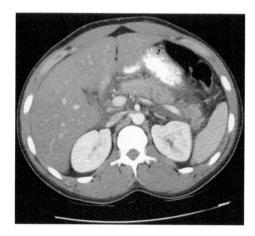

FIG. 6.22 Computed tomography shows fatty liver infiltration.

venae cavae (Fig. 6.23). Most commonly, such connections involve the esophageal veins, which dilate to become esophageal varices, as described in the preceding chapter. These are best evaluated with endoscopy, but may be seen with an esophagram or by CT examination. Also, the patient with cirrhosis has a tendency to bleed because the liver is unable to make the necessary clotting factors found in plasma or as a result of an esophageal variceal rupture. Such hemorrhaging may be, in fact, the first indication of portal hypertension.

Ascites, the accumulation of fluid within the peritoneal cavity (Fig. 6.24), is also seen as a result of portal hypertension and the leakage of excessive fluids from the portal capillaries. Much of this excess fluid is composed of hepatic lymph weeping from the liver surface. It is associated with approximately 50% of deaths from cirrhosis. Ascites may also result from chronic hepatitis, congestive heart failure, renal failure, and certain cancers. Abdominal sonography is commonly used in the detection or confirmation of ascites. Diagnostic and therapeutic paracentesis may be conducted with sonographic guidance to locate a site that will allow fluid to be removed and to avoid damage to the floating bowel loops. A diagnostic paracentesis involves removal of 50 mL to 100 mL of peritoneal fluid for analysis. Therapeutic paracentesis involves draining larger amounts of peritoneal fluid, or even the placement of an intraperitoneal drainage catheter for continued drainage. Patients with ascites generally complain of nonspecific abdominal pain and dyspnea. Medical treatment of ascites includes bed rest, dietary restrictions of sodium, use of diuretics to avoid excess fluid accumulation, and treatment of the underlying cause.

It is important for the radiographer to be aware of the clinical diagnosis of ascites because the fluid accumulation makes it difficult to adequately penetrate the abdomen. An increase in exposure factors is necessary to obtain a diagnostic-quality radiograph. Radiographically, large amounts of ascitic fluid give the abdomen a dense, gray, ground-glass appearance (Fig. 6.25). When the patient is in the supine position, fluid accumulates in the pelvis and ascends to either side of the bladder to give it a dog-eared appearance.

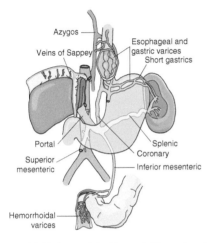

FIG. 6.23 Varices related to portal hypertension.

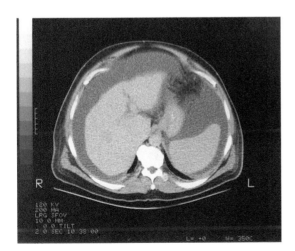

FIG. 6.24 Cirrhosis of the liver as indicated on this computed tomography scan showing a shrunken liver with significant ascites around it within the abdomen.

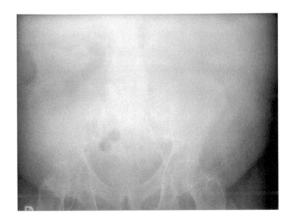

FIG. 6.25 Supine abdominal radiograph of the lower abdomen and pelvis demonstrating the gray and hazy appearance caused by abdominal ascites.

Gradually, the margins of the liver, spleen, kidneys, and psoas muscles become indistinct as the volume of fluid increases. Loops of bowel filled with gas float centrally, and a lateral decubitus radiograph demonstrates the fluid descending and the gas-filled loops of bowel floating on top.

Conventional radiographic signs of cirrhosis are few and not specific. Morphologic changes in the liver from cirrhosis may cause displacement of other abdominal organs such as the stomach, duodenum, colon, gallbladder, and kidney. CT is the primary modality for evaluating complications arising from cirrhosis. Fatty infiltration of the liver is well visualized by CT. The most characteristic finding of cirrhosis is an increase in the ratio of the caudate lobe and the right lobe. This occurs with cirrhosis because of atrophy of the right lobe and medial segment of the left lobe and hypertrophy of the caudate lobe and the lateral segment of the left lobe. Because of its dual arterial blood supply, the caudate lobe of the liver is usually spared in cases of cirrhosis. Studies show that individuals with cirrhosis have an increased risk of developing hepatic carcinoma, so CT is also of value when assessing for the presence of complications as a result of cirrhosis, such as ascites and hepatocellular carcinoma.

Diagnostic medical sonography is helpful in identifying liver cirrhosis and enlargement of the liver and spleen. Doppler is used to detect portal hypertension and evaluate portosystemic collateral circulation. It is used to measure the vessel size of the portal vein, which ranges from 0.64 cm to 1 cm in a normal adult. A portal vein larger than 1.3 cm in diameter is indicative of portal hypertension. In addition, the portal vein should distend with deep inspiration, but in patients with portal hypertension the vein lacks distensibility. Doppler integration of the portal vein allows for tracing of the blood flow within the vessel. Normal portal vein flow is toward the liver; however, with portal hypertension, the flow is shunted away from the liver because of the diseased liver's inability to accept the flow of blood. As a result, the splenic vein tries to handle this resistance by diverting the flow toward the spleen. In many cases, affected persons develop splenic varices from the increased flow from the portal vein. Sonographic evaluation of venous structures such as the superior mesenteric and splenic veins adds additional information for the clinician. However, final diagnosis of cirrhosis is generally accomplished by biopsy of liver tissue, often performed under sonographic guidance.

Treatment of cirrhosis depends on the extent of liver damage and the involvement of other organs (e.g., the esophagus and stomach). The primary goal of treatment is to eliminate the underlying causes of the disease and to treat its complications. Surgical treatment of portal hypertension may be achieved by diverting blood from the portocollateral system into the lower-pressure systemic circulation. This is accomplished by placing a shunt, eliminating the chance of variceal bleeding. A distal splenorenal shunt, in which the splenic vein is divided, with the distal portion anastomosed to the left renal vein, is most commonly used. If the patient is not a candidate for this type of shunt, a total shunt, either portocaval or mesocaval, must be placed. A palliative procedure, the transjugular intrahepatic portosystemic shunt (TIPSS), may also be used to divert the pressure of portal hypertension. The TIPSS procedure is commonly performed in the cardiovascular interventional area of a radiology department. A catheter is placed in the right internal jugular vein and pushed through the right atrium into the IVC. The needle end of the catheter is inserted into the closest portal vein in the liver, commonly the right portal vein. Through use of angioplasty, the tract is enlarged such that a shunt can be placed to reroute the flow of portal blood through the liver and into the IVC. Sonography is invaluable for assessing the long-term effect of this shunt. Typically, Doppler tracings are taken at the portal end, the midshunt, and the hepatic vein end of the shunt to ensure that flow through it allows the flow of blood to proceed through the liver to the IVC. However, all of these shunts have a tendency to thrombose, requiring patency to be assessed by angiography, CT, or sonography. The prognosis for patients with associated complications of cirrhosis such as ascites is poor, but advances in liver transplantation have changed the long-term outcome for many patients.

Lesions in the liver that have been identified by sonography, MRI, or CT are highly recommended to be further evaluated with MRI of the abdomen, with and without contrast, to conclusively differentiate between benign and malignant lesions. If the patient is unable to tolerate MRI contrast, CT of the abdomen is the next modality recommended to delineate the liver lesion in question.

If abdominal ascites is suspected in a patient with acute abdominal pain, the use of helical CT is highly recommended to document the presence of free fluid in the abdomen, as it is sensitive and very cost-effective in evaluating the patient with acute abdominal pain.

Viral Hepatitis

Hepatitis is a relatively common liver condition, with an estimated 70,000 cases reported annually in the United States. At least six types of viral agents that cause acute inflammation of the liver have been identified (Table 6.1). This inflammation interferes with the liver's ability to excrete bilirubin, the orange or yellowish pigment in bile. Clinical evidence of the disease includes nausea, vomiting, discomfort, and tenderness over the liver area, and laboratory results indicate a disturbance in liver function. Additional signs and symptoms include fatigue, anorexia, photophobia, and general malaise. Jaundice may also develop within 1 or

2 weeks because of the disturbance of bilirubin excretion. If the liver inflammation lasts 6 months or more, the condition is classified as chronic.

Hepatitis A virus (HAV) is a single-stranded ribonucleic acid (RNA) picornavirus. It is excreted in the GI tract in fecal matter and is spread by contact with an infected individual, normally through ingestion of contaminated food such as raw shellfish or through contaminated water. It is the most common form of hepatitis and is highly contagious. The incubation period of the disease is relatively short (15–50 days), and its course is usually mild. HAV infection does not lead to chronic hepatitis or cirrhosis of the liver.

Hepatitis B virus (HBV) is transmitted parenterally through infected serum or blood products. Its incubation period is much longer (50–160 days), and its effects are more severe than those of HAV. The etiologic makeup of

TABLE 6.1
Characteristics of Viral Hepatitis

Characteristic	Hepatitis A	Hepatitis B	Hepatitis D	Hepatitis C	Hepatitis E	Hepatitis G
Size of virus	27 nm DNA virus	47 nm DNA virus	36 nm RNA virus, defective with HbsAg coat	30–60 nm RNA virus	32 nm RNA virus	30–60 nm RNA virus
Incubation period	30 days	60–180 days	30–180 days	35–60 days	15–60 days	Unknown
Route of transmission	Fecal–oral, parenteral, sexual	Parenteral, sexual	Parenteral, fecal–oral, sexual	Parenteral	Fecal–oral	Parenteral, sexual
Onset	Acute with fever	Insidious	Insidious	Insidious	Acute	Unknown
Carrier state	Negative	Positive	Positive	Positive	Negative	Positive
Severity	Mild	Severe; may be prolonged or chronic	Severe	Mild to severe	Severe in pregnant women	Unknown
Chronic hepatitis	No	Yes	Yes	Yes	No	Unknown
Age-group affected	Children and young adults	Any	Any	Any	Children and young adults	Any
Prophylaxis	Hygiene, immune serum globulin HAV vaccine	Hygiene, HBV vaccine	Hygiene, HBV vaccine	Hygiene, screening blood, interferon-alpha	Hygiene, safe water	

DNA, Deoxyribonucleic acid; *HAV,* hepatitis A virus; *HbsAg,* hepatitis B surface antigen; *HBV,* hepatitis B virus; *RNA,* ribonucleic acid.
From McCance KL, Huether SE, Brashers VL, & Rote NS, *Pathophysiology: The biologic basis for disease in adults and children,* 6 ed, Mosby Elsevier, St. Louis, MO.

HBV is very complex, consisting of a viral core of deoxyribonucleic acid (DNA), which replicates within the cells of the liver. The viral core is covered with a surface coat. HBV may result in an asymptomatic carrier state, acute hepatitis, chronic hepatitis, cirrhosis, and hepatocellular carcinoma. Three distinct antigen–antibody systems have been shown to have a link to HBV. These include hepatitis B surface antigen (HBsAg), which appears in the incubation stage and is the first indication of HBV infection; hepatitis B core antigen (HBcAg), which is found in liver tissue but not in serum; and hepatitis B extracellular antigen (HbeAg), which reflects active viral replication. Most health care workers are now required to receive HBV vaccination. Vaccination has dramatically reduced the incidence of infection, and the vaccines are safe with very few side effects.

Hepatitis C virus (HCV) is caused by a parenterally transmitted RNA virus. Type C accounts for 80% of the cases of hepatitis that develop after blood transfusions. A routine test for anti-HCV antibody has been developed, so transmission via transfused blood has been significantly decreased. HCV may cause either acute or chronic hepatitis, with 10% to 20% of affected patients eventually developing cirrhosis of the liver.

Hepatitis D virus (HDV) is caused by an RNA virus and occurs only concurrently with acute or chronic HBV. It cannot occur alone. Hepatitis E virus (HEV) is also an RNA viral agent. It is most commonly responsible for outbreaks of waterborne epidemic acute hepatitis in developing countries. Although the infection may be severe, it does not progress to a chronic state. Hepatitis G virus (HGV), which has been recently isolated, may also be transmitted via blood products and may cause chronic hepatitis.

The diagnosis of viral hepatitis is usually made through laboratory testing because the disease is carried in the bloodstream during the acute phase. Evidence of hepatitis may be seen on radiographs of the abdomen that demonstrate *hepatomegaly* (enlargement of the liver), although this is a nonspecific finding. Cellular necrosis may be confirmed through nuclear medicine scanning of the liver, CT, or liver biopsy. Sonography is also useful in distinguishing the characteristics of the liver.

HAV is usually mild; the majority of patients recover without complications. Treatment generally consists of bed rest and medication for nausea and vomiting. In a healthy individual, the liver regenerates after hepatitis damage, and complete recovery is gained. Patients with type B, type C, type D, and type G generally go on to develop chronic hepatitis. In some, the disease may progress to liver failure.

Percutaneous liver biopsy is the gold standard for determining the type of disease that may be present in the liver. This is a recommended diagnostic step when the liver appears irregular on sonography, CT, or MRI. A pathologist examines the liver specimen and makes the final diagnosis regarding the type of disease that is present in the sample provided.

Cholelithiasis

Cholelithiasis (gallstones) is fairly common, with at least 20% of all persons in the United States developing them by the age of 65 years. Women are more likely than men to have them. Their occurrence is also more common in people with diabetes mellitus, those who are obese, older adults, and individuals who eat primarily a diet high in saturated fat, sugar, and sodium and low in fiber and nutrient density (Western diet). Heredity plays a role in the development of gallstones. Although most commonly found in the gallbladder, gallstones can be located anywhere in the biliary tree. The presence of stones within the common bile duct is termed choledocholithiasis (Fig. 6.26). Symptoms associated with cholelithiasis may be vague, including bloating, nausea, and

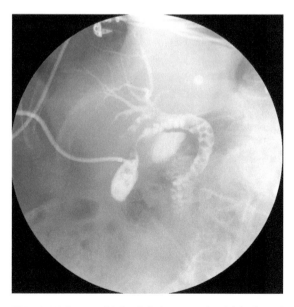

FIG. 6.26 Image obtained during a contrast injection of a cholecystostomy tube showing a patent cystic duct and the presence of many filling defects within the common bile duct, which is consistent with choledocholithiasis.

pain in the right upper quadrant. Sludge may develop within the gallbladder and may be identified sonographically. Sometimes sludge develops in patients who have been fasting or who have been treated with hyperalimentation and is a normal variant from underusage of the bile in the gallbladder; in other cases, sludge may be a precursor to the development of gallstones.

The characteristics of gallstones, also known as choleliths, are quite varied. They may occur as a single stone or as multiple stones. About 80% of all stones are composed of a mixture of cholesterol, bile pigment (bilirubin), and calcium salts. The remaining 20% are composed of pure cholesterol or a calcium–bilirubin mixture. Most stones are radiolucent because only approximately 10% of all stones contain enough calcium to be radiopaque. Those that are radiopaque may be difficult to distinguish from renal stones, but oblique radiographs help separate the two structures (kidney and gallbladder) from each other, demonstrating the gallbladder anterior to the kidney (Fig. 6.27). As noted before, sonography readily demonstrates cholelithiasis (Fig. 6.28). The best image is obtained when the gallbladder is distended and filled with bile, so patients should fast 8 hours before sonographic examination.

The three major sonographic criteria for gallstones include an echogenic focus, acoustic shadowing below the stone, and gravitational dependence. Gallstones may be the size of a pinhead to that of a large marble. The small stones tend to travel into the biliary tree and may result in obstruction. Obstruction of the bile duct causes pain and jaundice and may result in cholangitis, which is an infection of the biliary ductal system.

It is highly recommended that patients who do not have fever, have normal WBC counts, and have gallstones as demonstrated by sonograms undergo cholescintigraphy, CT of the abdomen (with or without contrast), and MRI of the abdomen (with or without contrast) to ensure that other forms of biliary disease are not present.

Surgical removal of the gallbladder (cholecystectomy) is usually the treatment of choice, with more than 500,000 such procedures performed annually in the United States. Since its introduction in 1988, laparoscopic cholecystectomy has replaced many traditional open cholecystectomies. This technique allows a less traumatic entry, excision, and removal of the gallbladder, resulting in shortened hospitalization and reduced costs. Radiographers are commonly called to the operating environment to image injections of contrast medium into the exposed biliary duct to determine whether all stones have been removed. If additional stones are suspected but not visualized, a T-tube may be inserted to allow for later postoperative study, as noted earlier. The T-tube will also provide a means for draining bile if the residual stones are compromising flow of bile from the CBD into the duodenum.

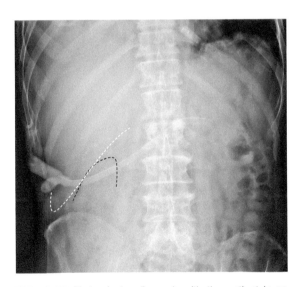

FIG. 6.27 Abdominal radiograph with the patient in an oblique position separating the liver border (*white dash line*) from the upper renal margin (*black dash line*), allowing for the small calcifications to be projected anterior to the kidney, and thereby confirming that they are gallstones and not kidney stones.

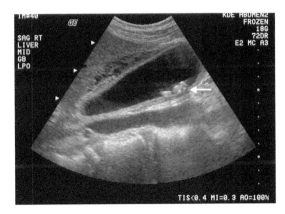

FIG. 6.28 A sagittal sonographic image of a dilated gallbladder containing stones.

Cholecystitis

Cholecystitis is an acute inflammation of the gallbladder. It is characterized clinically by a sudden onset of pain, fever, nausea, and vomiting. It is common in individuals with chronically symptomatic cholelithiasis. Its diagnosis is clinically suspected and supported through a sonographic examination or radionuclide cholescintigraphy. A radiopharmaceutical composed of technetium-99m (^{99m}Tc) in combination with diisopropyl iminodiacetic acid (DISIDA) allows for the visualization of the biliary ductal system and results in a highly sensitive examination with consistently reliable results. Nonvisualization of the gallbladder is a good indicator of acute cholecystitis. Repeated attacks of acute cholecystitis cause damage to the gallbladder, thickening of the walls (Fig. 6.29), and decreased function.

Complications of untreated gallbladder disease include infarction and a possible gangrenous state, prompting rupture of the walls. Perforation of the gallbladder occurs in approximately 5% to 15% of all patients with acute cholecystitis and can be diagnosed in several ways. Cholescintigraphy provides the best images of perforation; however, stones may be visible outside of the gallbladder on conventional abdominal radiographs, CT images, or sonographic images. Sonography and CT often also demonstrate a nonspecific pericholecystic fluid collection. If a rupture does occur, bile peritonitis may result and require immediate treatment.

Occasionally, a stone may erode through the wall of the gallbladder in cases of chronic cholecystitis and create a fistula to the bowel, most frequently the duodenum. If the stone becomes impacted in the small bowel and causes an obstruction, the condition is referred to as **gallstone ileus**. Gallstone ileus is characterized by air in the biliary ductal system, termed pneumobilia, which is clearly visible on a conventional abdominal radiograph. A radiopaque gallstone may also be visible within the bowel surrounded by intestinal gas. Surgical removal of the stone is necessary to relieve the obstruction. Treatment of chronic cholecystitis also includes laparoscopic removal of the inflamed gallbladder.

Pancreatitis

Inflammation of the pancreatic tissue is known as **pancreatitis**. It is one of the most complex and clinically challenging disorders of the abdomen and is classified as acute or chronic, according to clinical, morphologic, and histologic criteria. Acute pancreatitis resolves without impairing the histologic makeup of the pancreas and most often results from biliary tract disease. However, chronic pancreatitis does impair the histologic makeup of the pancreas, resulting in irreversible changes in pancreatic function. Its causes include excessive and chronic alcohol consumption, obstruction of the hepatopancreatic ampulla by a gallstone or tumor, and even the injection of contrast media during ERCP. Once activated by any of these causes, trypsin, the pancreatic enzyme that is normally excreted through the ducts into the duodenum, begins to autodigest the organ itself. This has serious consequences and carries a high mortality rate. Hemorrhagic pancreatitis is a complication of pancreatitis and consists of erosion into local tissues and blood vessels, with subsequent hemorrhaging into the retroperitoneal space. A **pseudocyst** is a fluid collection caused by pancreatitis. It is readily visualized by sonographic or CT examination (Fig. 6.30).

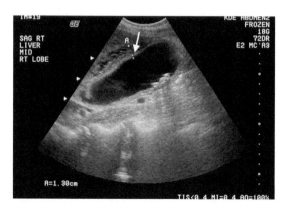

FIG. 6.29 Sonogram demonstrating a thickened wall of the gallbladder, often indicative of cholecystitis.

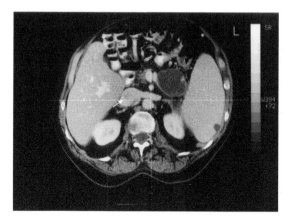

FIG. 6.30 Pancreatitis with demonstration of a 5-cm pseudocyst in the head as seen on computed tomography.

Symptoms of pancreatitis vary from mild abdominal pain, nausea, and vomiting to severe pain and shock. Radiographic indications of pancreatitis are subtle and previously centered on displacement of the duodenal C-loop or the stomach by the diseased pancreas or calcified stones within the pancreatic or biliary ducts. However, CT has made a major contribution to the diagnosis and staging of acute pancreatitis. It adequately demonstrates not only the pancreas itself but also the retroperitoneum, the ligaments, the mesenteries, and the omenta. The infected pancreas is usually enlarged, with a shaggy and irregular contour. In advanced cases, fluid collections are demonstrated within the pancreas and within the retroperitoneum. ERCP is of value in determining the reasons for acute recurrent pancreatitis, chronic pancreatitis, or the complications associated with pancreatitis. Because pancreatic disease is often asymptomatic in the early stages, sonography is good for assessing the texture and size of the organ. The pancreas is routinely imaged as part of the RUQ sonogram. In most sonographic examinations, the head and body of the pancreas can be measured and compared with normal values for the age of the patient. Pancreatitis is suggested on a sonogram by the decreased echo texture and an associated enlargement in the size of the organ (Fig. 6.31). In addition, recent advances in MRI allow for noninvasive, contrast-free imaging of the biliary tree. Laboratory testing is the most common way to diagnose pancreatitis, through evaluation of serum and occasionally urine amylase levels.

Sonography and CT of the abdomen with contrast are equally recommended by the ACR for diagnosis of acute pancreatitis. MRI of the abdomen (with and without contrast) is appropriate if the aforementioned imaging modalities are not available.

Management of patients with pancreatitis consists of a pain-relieving drug in mild cases and maintaining proper fluid levels to prevent shock, a frequent occurrence in acute pancreatitis. Proper dietary restrictions (e.g., abstinence from alcohol) are also important. The role of surgery in chronic pancreatitis remains controversial with regard to the effectiveness of results. The prognosis is excellent in patients with mild pancreatic inflammation and edema. However, a swollen pancreas, with extravasation of fluid within the retroperitoneum or pancreatic necrosis as demonstrated by CT, results in a more severe prognosis. Although most CT examinations are performed with the use of IV contrast agents, research has shown that use of contrast agents during the onset of acute pancreatitis may cause necrosis in areas with poor blood supply. Pancreatic necrosis increases mortality and the incidence of infection, so patients should be well hydrated before a contrast-enhanced CT examination is performed. Chronic pancreatitis also increases the risk for pancreatic cancer, so most patients are continuously monitored for malignancy.

Jaundice

Jaundice, a yellowish discoloration of the skin and whites of the eyes, is not a disease itself but rather a sign of disease. The accumulation of excess bile pigments (i.e., bilirubin) in the body tissues "stains" the skin and eyes this yellowish color. Normally, bile and its pigments are secreted into the bowel and eliminated. Bilirubin is a type of bile pigment that is produced when hemoglobin breaks down. Normal serum bilirubin levels are equal to or less than 1 mg per 100 mL but must exceed 3 mg per 100 mL to be visible to the observer.

Medical (nonobstructive) jaundice occurs because of hemolytic disease, in which too many red blood cells (RBCs) are destroyed or because of liver damage from cirrhosis or hepatitis. Its most common appearance is transient in the first few days after birth, when more bile pigments are released than can be handled. A liver that is damaged from disease simply cannot excrete the bilirubin in a normal fashion, and it enters the bloodstream.

Surgical (obstructive) jaundice occurs when the biliary system is obstructed and prevents bile from entering the duodenum. A common cause of this obstruction is blockage of the common bile duct caused

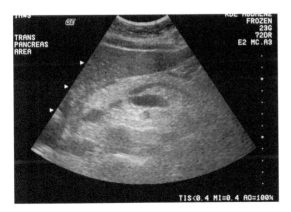

FIG. 6.31 Transverse sonographic image of the pancreas.

by stones or masses. The longer the obstruction persists, the more likely it is that complications (e.g., liver injury, infection, bleeding) will arise.

The jaundiced patient often undergoes a sonographic examination of the liver, biliary tree, and pancreas to determine whether the jaundice is obstructive (Fig. 6.32) or nonobstructive. The common bile duct is readily identified; generally, a normal size implies nonobstructive jaundice, and a dilated common bile duct suggests an obstruction. A normal size CBD is typically less than 6 mm in diameter, but the diameter is found to increase normally with advanced age and post cholecystectomy status. A variety of other methods may be used to diagnose the cause of jaundice, including ERCP, MRCP, and CT. A sonographic or CT-directed needle biopsy may be used if an intrahepatic cause of hepatitis is suspected. Treatment of jaundice centers on the diagnosis and treatment of its underlying cause. In the case of obstructive jaundice, surgical excision of the obstructing body may be necessary. Endoscopic removal of common duct stones is frequently done, and endoscopy also offers the opportunity to stent or bypass a tumor.

Neoplastic Diseases

Hepatocellular Adenoma

Hepatocellular adenoma is a benign tumor of the liver. Most tumors are asymptomatic, but the incidence of this disease has increased over the past few years.

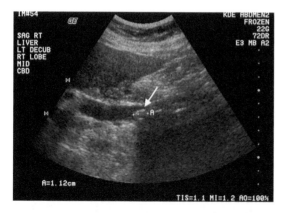

FIG. 6.32 A sagittal sonographic image demonstrating a stone (*arrow*) lodged in the distal portion of the common bile duct close to the ampulla of Vater (*A*) resulting in dilation and obstruction of the common bile duct.

Hepatocellular adenomas occur most often in women using oral contraceptives, which play a role in the development of these benign lesions. In terms of imaging, both CT and sonography are useful in demonstrating hepatic lesions.

Hemangioma

A **hemangioma** is the most common tumor of the liver. It is a benign neoplasm composed of newly formed blood vessels, and these neoplasms may form in other places within the body. For instance, a port-wine stain on the face (a superficial purplish red birthmark) is an example of a hemangioma elsewhere in the body. Hemangiomas are generally well-circumscribed, solitary tumors. They may range in size from microscopic to 20 cm. They are more common in women than in men, especially in postmenopausal women.

Normally, the texture of the liver is homogeneous during sonographic evaluation, but an area of increased echogenicity may occasionally be demonstrated. When this appears as a solitary, round lesion, the diagnosis is usually a hemangioma. These lesions generally do not become malignant; however, sonography may be used to assess the lesion if it is suspected that it has changed in size or character. In most cases, a hemangioma is insignificant, but it may manifest symptoms such as RUQ pain as a result of tissue displacement or bleeding. Diagnosis may be complicated when it occurs with a known malignancy because its characteristics may be difficult to distinguish from metastasis. Nuclear medicine scans using labeled RBCs that are attracted to the highly vascular tumor are virtually diagnostic in assessing the presence of a hemangioma. These scans demonstrate the tumor as a defect in the early phases and display prolonged and persistent uptake on delayed scans. A CT of the liver following an injection of IV contrast medium demonstrates the hemangioma with peripheral enhancement. MRI demonstrates marked hyperintensity on T2-weighted images, which corresponds with fibrosis within the tumor. After an IV injection of a gadolinium contrast agent, peripheral enhancement of the hemangioma occurs in early scans, followed by filling in of the tumor (Fig. 6.33), similar to the appearance seen during an enhanced CT examination.

A study completed on focal nodules in the liver and comparing the use of sonography, CT, and MRI found that MRI had a diagnostic advantage. MRI appears to have a higher sensitivity and specificity, especially when MRI contrast is administered, and provides physiologic information regarding the mass.

Hepatocellular Carcinoma (Hepatoma)

Hepatocellular carcinoma, a primary neoplasm of the liver, accounts for approximately 3% of all cancers in the United States. An association between cirrhosis and hepatocellular carcinoma exists, with chronic hepatitis B or hepatitis C and alcoholism associated with each. Thus the incidence of this neoplasm is on the rise because of an increase in chronic hepatitis B and hepatitis C infections in the United States. Most primary hepatomas originate in the liver parenchyma, creating a large central mass with smaller satellite nodules. Although vascular invasion is common, death occurs from liver failure, often without extension of the cancer outside the liver.

Hepatocellular carcinoma is suspected in patients with cirrhosis who experience an unexpected deterioration and in patients with increased jaundice, abdominal pain, weight loss, a RUQ mass, ascites, or a rapid increase in liver size. Plain abdominal radiographs may demonstrate hepatomegaly. Sonography and CT are often used to reveal the extent of the tumor (Fig. 6.34). Arteriography may demonstrate the increased vascularity associated with a carcinoma. A definitive diagnosis requires a liver biopsy, generally under sonographic guidance.

Surgical resection of the hepatocellular carcinoma represents the only possibility for cure. Hepatomas that are diffuse or have multiple nodules generally preclude surgery. The general lack of radiosensitivity of these tumors makes radiotherapy ineffective. Patients treated with chemotherapy demonstrate tumor shrinkage and an addition of a few months to their lives. The disease, however, is generally fatal except in those who have had successful resection of a single liver mass.

The ACR highly recommends resection of the tumor and possible liver transplantation as the best treatment for patients with hepatocellular carcinoma. Transarterial embolization may also be an appropriate treatment for lesions that are solid and are at least 5 cm in size. Selective radiation therapy treatments that are directed internally are also possible, depending on the extent of the disease and whether it has invaded the portal vein.

Metastatic Liver Disease

Metastatic liver lesions are much more common than primary carcinoma because of the liver's role in filtering blood. The liver is a common site for metastasis from other primary sites such as the colon, pancreas, stomach, lung, and breast (Fig. 6.35). Primary cancers located in the abdomen, especially those drained by the portal venous system, often metastasize to the liver (Fig. 6.36). Sonography is most commonly used to screen patients for **metastatic liver disease**; however, CT and MRI also produce an accurate diagnosis. Again, liver biopsy, often under sonographic guidance, provides the definitive diagnosis.

The recommended treatment for metastatic liver disease is to use a combination of intramuscular injection of long-acting octreotide (a somatostatin analog) and transarterial embolization, especially if the medication

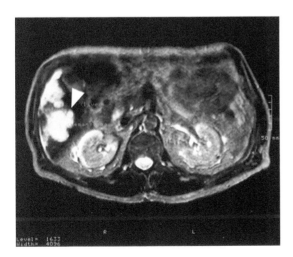

FIG. 6.33 An axial magnetic resonance imaging slice through the liver reveals a hemangioma.

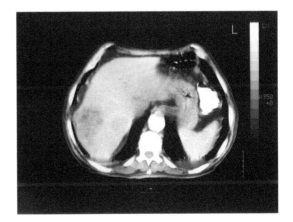

FIG. 6.34 Large, heterogeneous lesion in the liver consistent with hepatoma.

fails to decrease the tumor size. Selective radiation therapy treatments that are directed internally may also be used if the patient continues to be symptomatic and medication fails to provide some relief.

Carcinoma of the Gallbladder

Carcinoma of the gallbladder occurs infrequently, but most neoplasms within the gallbladder are malignant. Most primary carcinomas of the gallbladder, approximately 85%, are adenocarcinomas, with the remaining 15% being anaplastic or squamous cell cancers. Carcinoma of the gallbladder is more common in women and

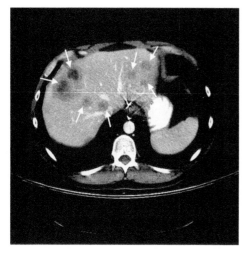

FIG. 6.35 Computed tomography scan of the liver demonstrating metastatic spread from bronchogenic carcinoma (*arrows*).

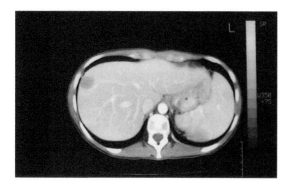

FIG. 6.36 Computed tomography scan after duodenal cancer resection in a 21-year-old woman demonstrates local recurrence and metastases to the liver on its lateral border in this slice.

older adults, with gallstones present in about 75% of all cases. The symptoms are nonspecific, including RUQ pain, jaundice, and weight loss. Another risk factor associated with the development of gallbladder carcinoma is a "porcelain" gallbladder, which results from chronic cholecystitis (Fig. 6.37). Approximately 22% of patients with porcelain gallbladders develop carcinoma.

The best methods for imaging gallbladder carcinoma include CT and sonography. Radiographically, the appearance of the carcinoma may vary. It may appear as a mass replacing the gallbladder or as a polypoid mass within the gallbladder, or the appearance may be as subtle as focal thickening of the gallbladder wall. Clinically and radiographically, this cancer may be difficult to differentiate from cholecystitis with pericholecystic fluid accumulation or an abscess. Unfortunately, the prognosis with gallbladder carcinoma is often poor because metastases to the liver usually occur before the primary disease is diagnosed (Fig. 6.38). It may spread via direct invasion of the liver, via intraductal tumor extension, or via the lymphatic system to regional lymph nodes. Approximately 88% of patients die within 1 year of diagnosis, and the 5-year survival rate following diagnosis is only 4%.

Cholangiocarcinoma

A cholangiocarcinoma is a malignancy of the bile ducts. Greater than 90% of cholangiocarcinomas are ductal

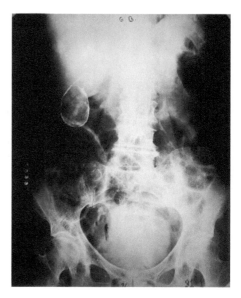

FIG. 6.37 A "porcelain" gallbladder in a 70-year-old man with a history of recurrent indigestion.

adenocarcinomas and the rest are squamous cell tumors. The etiology is unknown but increased risk is reported in those with chronic cholangitis, chronic parasitic infections, ulcerative colitis, and chronic cholecystitis. Incidence is higher in Native American and Asian populations with the range of 60 to 70 years of age being most affected. Cholangiocarcinomas invade the walls of the biliary ducts and can extend into the liver, porta hepatis, and regional lymph nodes. The prognosis is poor as most are unresectable or associated with metastatic disease and life expectancy from diagnosis is typically around 6 months.

Sonography and CT are generally the initial imaging studies for patients with suspected cholangiocarcinoma. Those will be followed by cholangiography to better visualize the bile ducts either in the form of a MRCP, an ERCP, or a PTC. Cholangiography images will often reveal an irregular and nonsmooth contour of normally smooth biliary ducts as a result of infiltration of the tissue of the ducts (Fig. 6.39).

Carcinoma of the Pancreas

Pancreatic cancer is usually rapidly fatal and is the fifth most common cause of cancer-related death in the United States. Its diagnosis is difficult because of the location of the pancreas and the lack of symptoms before extensive local spread. Even with diagnostic advances in CT and sonography, the prognosis is poor. In most cases, the tumor is well advanced before the diagnosis is made. Its incidence is greater in men than in women and in African Americans than in Caucasians. A clear-cut association with cigarette smoking has been demonstrated,

and other risk factors include alcoholism, chronic pancreatitis, diabetes mellitus, and a family history of adenocarcinoma. Most tumors (approximately 90%) arise as epithelial tumors of the duct (adenocarcinoma) and cause pancreatic obstruction (Fig. 6.40). In addition, the majority (60%–70%) of these neoplasms arise in the head of the pancreas, followed by the body (10%–15%),

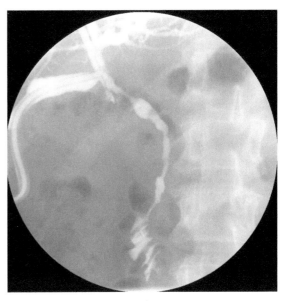

FIG. 6.39 Spot image from a T-tube cholangiogram study. Note the irregular contour of the common hepatic duct and the common bile duct with scattered areas of narrowing and variance in contrast density throughout.

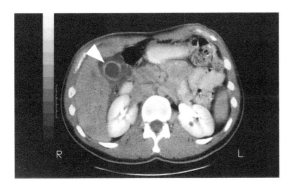

FIG. 6.38 Gallbladder carcinoma resulting in metastasis to surrounding structures, as seen on this computed tomography scan of a 23-year-old man. The gallbladder (*arrow*) is surrounded by metastasis, with significant metastasis into the pancreas area and right kidney.

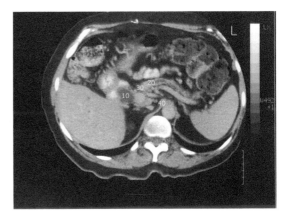

FIG. 6.40 Pancreatic carcinoma in the head of the pancreas, as indicated by atrophy of the pancreatic body and tail. Numbers shown are for density sampling, with 10, 20, and 30 in the pancreas.

and then the tail (5%–10%). The rich supply of nerves to the pancreas results in pain as a prominent feature of this carcinoma. The tumor infiltrates and replaces normal tissue without significant hemorrhage, necrosis, or calcification. Signs and symptoms are nonspecific and include pain, weight loss, jaundice, fatigue, nausea, vomiting, and onset of diabetes mellitus.

Carcinomas of the pancreatic head may be visible on barium studies of the stomach and small bowel because the head of the pancreas lies within the duodenal C-loop. Carcinomas of the body and tail may affect the duodenojejunal junction and cause distortion on a barium-filled

small-bowel study. When sonography is used to evaluate the biliary tree, the sequence of images begins with the right and left branches of the common hepatic duct within the liver and ends with the common bile duct to its termination at the hepatopancreatic ampulla. Tumors of the pancreatic head cause enlargement and may result in compression of the duodenum (Fig. 6.41). With the compression of the duodenum, the hepatopancreatic ampulla is also compressed, causing a dilation of the distal common bile duct. Sonographic images of a common bile duct that begins coursing normally but increases in size distally to more than 1 cm in diameter should suggest the possibility

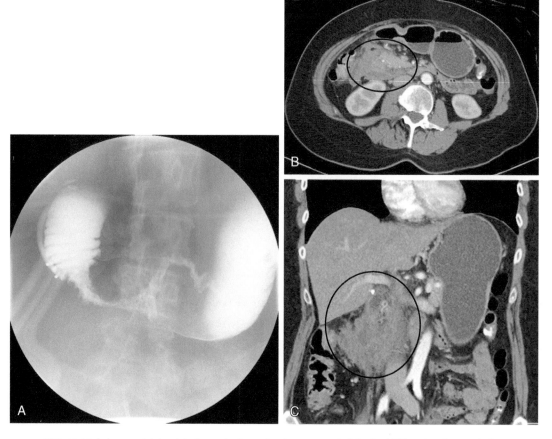

FIG. 6.41 A, Image obtained during a single contrast upper gastrointestinal (GI) series demonstrates a contour change beginning in the second portion of the duodenum and extending through the remainder of the duodenum and proximal jejunum. There is a long segment of narrowing with a markedly irregular and nodular mucosal pattern. The stomach is also dilated and fluid filled, as demonstrated by the hazy dilution of the contrast in the gastric body. B, Axial computed tomography (CT) image demonstrating a large pancreatic mass enveloping the duodenum that has a thickened lumen as a result of tumor invasion. C, CT image showing the large size of the same pancreatic mass as seen in the coronal plane. Fluid distension of the gastric body, similar to the upper GI image in A, is also visible.

of a pancreatic head mass. The ACR highly recommends CT of the abdomen, with and without contrast, as the best method of imaging the pancreas, the most common finding being a mass deforming the pancreas. The use of sonography and MRI, with and without contrast, is also recommended for patients who have been experiencing weight loss, fatigue, anorexia, and symptoms for more than 3 months. However, in most cases, by the time the mass is visible on the CT image, the tumor is not resectable because of its size. If the lesion is not resectable, a percutaneous needle aspiration under CT guidance is performed to obtain a biopsy of the tissue. In cases where the tumor is resectable, CT helps stage the disease. Radical surgery as a treatment mode is about the only hope for remission, but it carries a high mortality rate. Radiation therapy is difficult because of the proximity of the pancreas to highly radiosensitive structures such as the spinal cord, and chemotherapy also produces poor results. The prognosis for pancreatic carcinoma is very poor, demonstrating a 5-year survival rate of only 2%.

Pathologic Summary of the Hepatobiliary System

Pathology	Imaging Modality of Choice
Fatty infiltration	CT and sonography
Cirrhosis	CT
Ascites	CT and sonography
Hepatitis	CT, MRI, nuclear medicine, and sonography
Cholecystitis	Sonography and CT
Cholelithiasis	Sonography and CT
Pancreatitis	CT, ERCP, and sonography
Hemangioma	CT, nuclear medicine, angiography, and sonography
Hepatoma	CT and nuclear medicine
Hepatocellular adenoma	CT and sonography
Hepatocellular carcinoma	CT, MRI, and sonography
Metastatic disease of the liver	CT, MRI, and sonography
Carcinoma of the gallbladder	CT and sonography
Carcinoma of the pancreas	CT and sonography

CT, Computed tomography; ERCP, endoscopic retrograde cholangiopancreatography; MRI, magnetic resonance imaging.

Review Questions

1. Bile drains from the liver's right and left hepatic ducts directly into the:
   a. Common bile duct
   b. Common hepatic duct
   c. Cystic duct
   d. Duodenum
2. The noninvasive modality of choice that does not employ ionizing radiation for visualization of gallbladder disease is:
   a. Computed tomography
   b. Diagnostic medical sonography
   c. Nuclear medicine
   d. All of the above

3. Impairment of normal liver function might result in:
   a. Cirrhosis
   b. Jaundice
   c. Milk of calcium
   d. Viral hepatitis type A
4. Patients with liver cirrhosis have a tendency to develop:
   1. Ascites
   2. Esophageal varices
   3. Jaundice
   a. 1 and 2
   b. 1 and 3
   c. 2 and 3
   d. 1, 2, and 3

5. Which types of viral hepatitis may be transmitted via blood or blood products?
   a. Type A
   b. Type B
   c. Type C
   d. Type E
   e. Both a and d
   f. Both b and c

6. Liver condition commonly associated with alcohol abuse is:
   a. Biliary obstruction
   b. Cholelithiasis
   c. Cirrhosis
   d. Hemangioma

7. The yellowish discoloration of the skin associated with jaundice is caused by:
   a. Accumulation of milk of calcium
   b. Transmission of infected fecal material
   c. Paralysis of small-bowel wall
   d. Presence of bilirubin in blood
   e. None of the above

8. Gallstone ileus refers to impaction of a gallstone in the:
   a. Biliary tree
   b. Gallbladder
   c. Liver
   d. Small bowel

9. The diagnostic imaging modalities of choice for following the progress of a liver malignancy are:
   1. Computed tomography
   2. Radiography
   3. Sonography
   a. 1 and 2
   b. 1 and 3
   c. 2 and 3
   d. 1, 2, and 3

10. A malignant liver tumor is a:
    a. Hepatitis
    b. Hemangioma
    c. Hepatocellular carcinoma
    d. Jaundice

11. Compare and contrast medical *versus* surgical jaundice.

12. Explain the process by which alcoholism results in fatty infiltration of the liver.

13. What are the advantages of imaging the biliary ductal system antegrade with percutaneous transhepatic cholangiogram (PTC) *versus* retrograde with endoscopic retrograde cholangiopancreatogram (ERCP)? What are the disadvantages of PTC?

14. Explain why cancers of the gallbladder and pancreas carry a poor prognosis.

15. Describe the physiologic cause of esophageal varices in conjunction with cirrhosis of the liver.

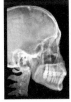
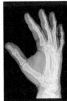
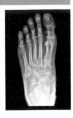

Urinary System

ⓔ http://evolve.elsevier.com/Kowalczyk/pathology/

LEARNING OBJECTIVES

On completion of Chapter 7, the reader should be able to do the following:

1. Describe the anatomic components of the urinary system and their functions.
2. Discuss the role of other modalities in imaging the urinary system, particularly sonography and computed tomography.
3. Discuss common congenital anomalies of the urinary system.
4. Characterize a given condition as inflammatory or neoplastic.
5. Identify the pathogenesis of the diseases cited and the typical treatments for each.
6. Describe, in general, the radiographic appearance of each of the given pathologies.

OUTLINE

Anatomy and Physiology
Imaging Considerations
KUB Radiography
   Intravenous Urography
   Cystography
   Retrograde Pyelography
   Sonography
   Computed Tomography
   Renal Angiography
   Magnetic Resonance Imaging
   Interventional Procedures and Techniques
   Urinary Tubes and Catheters

Congenital and Hereditary Diseases
   Number and Size
   Anomalies of the Kidney
   Fusion Anomalies of the Kidney
   Position Anomalies of the Kidney
   Renal Pelvis and Ureter Anomalies
   Lower Urinary Tract Anomalies
   Polycystic Kidney Disease
   Medullary Sponge Kidney
Inflammatory Diseases

Urinary Tract Infection
   Pyelonephritis
   Acute Glomerulonephritis
   Cystitis
Urinary System Calcifications
Degenerative Diseases
   Nephrosclerosis
   Renal Failure
   Hydronephrosis
Neoplastic Diseases
   Renal Cysts
   Renal Cell Carcinoma
   Nephroblastoma (Wilms Tumor)
   Bladder Carcinoma

KEY TERMS

Acute glomerulonephritis
Adenocarcinoma
Bladder carcinoma
Bladder diverticula
Bladder trabeculae

Bright disease
Crossed ectopy
Cystitis
Ectopic kidney
Foley catheter
Horseshoe kidney

Hydronephrosis
Hyperplasia
Hypoplasia
Malrotation
Medullary sponge kidney

Nephroblastoma	Radiofrequency ablation	Uremia
Nephroptosis	Renal agenesis	Ureteral diverticula
Nephrosclerosis	Renal calculi	Ureteral stents
Nephrostomy tube	Renal colic	Ureterocele
Neurogenic bladder	Renal cysts	Urethral valves
Polycystic kidney disease	Renal failure	Urinary meatus
Pyelonephritis	Staghorn calculus	Urinary tract infection
Pyuria	Supernumerary kidney	Vesicoureteral reflux
	Suprapubic catheter	

Anatomy and Physiology

The urinary system typically consists of two kidneys, two ureters, a urinary bladder, and a urethra (Fig. 7.1). Its main function is to remove waste from the bloodstream for excretion by forming urine. The kidneys are the site where urine is formed and excreted through the remarkable processes of filtration and reabsorption, involving up to 180 L of blood per day. Urine formed by this process amounts to approximately 1 L to 1.5 L per day and passes from the kidneys to the bladder through the ureters. Stored in the bladder, it is eventually excreted through the urethra.

The kidneys are retroperitoneal, normally located between the twelfth thoracic vertebra and the third lumbar vertebra. The right kidney lies slightly lower

because of the presence of the liver superiorly. The notch located on the medial surface of each kidney is the hilus, the area where structures enter and leave the kidney. These structures include the renal artery and vein, lymphatics, and a nerve plexus. Microscopically, the nephron is the functional unit of the kidney responsible for forming and excreting urine (Fig. 7.2). The nephron unit is composed of the glomerulus, Bowman's capsule, and numerous convoluted tubules. Blood flowing through the glomerulus, a ball-like cluster of specialized capillaries, is filtered and cleaned of impurities. Fluid moves out of the glomerulus into Bowman's capsule and through the various convoluted tubules, resulting in the production of urine. The nephron unit terminates into a collecting tubule, which forms a tube opening at the

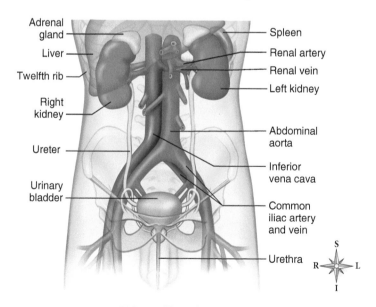

FIG. 7.1 The urinary system.

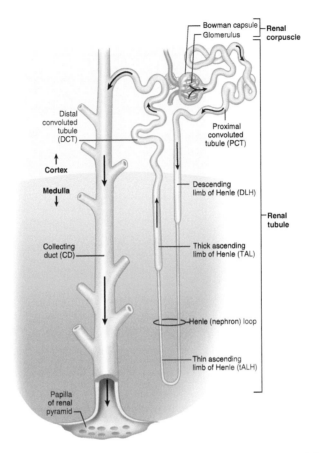

FIG. 7.2 Components of the Nephron. (*From Patton & Thibodeu,* Anatomy & Physiology, *ed. 8, 2013.*)

renal papilla into a minor calyx. Minor calyces terminate in the major calyces, which, in turn, terminate at the renal pelvis (Fig. 7.3). This is often referred to as the renal collecting system.

The ureters extend from the kidneys to the urinary bladder and are approximately 10 inches in length (Fig. 7.4). They normally enter the bladder obliquely, in the posterolateral portion, equidistant from the urethral orifice in a triangular fashion. A number of variations of this exist. The function of the ureters is to drain the urine from the kidneys into the bladder.

The bladder is located posterior to the symphysis pubis. It serves as a reservoir for urine before urine is expelled from the body. The bladder is very muscular and capable of distension. Valves located at the junction

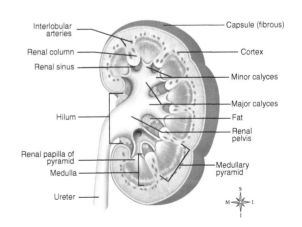

FIG. 7.3 The structure of a kidney.

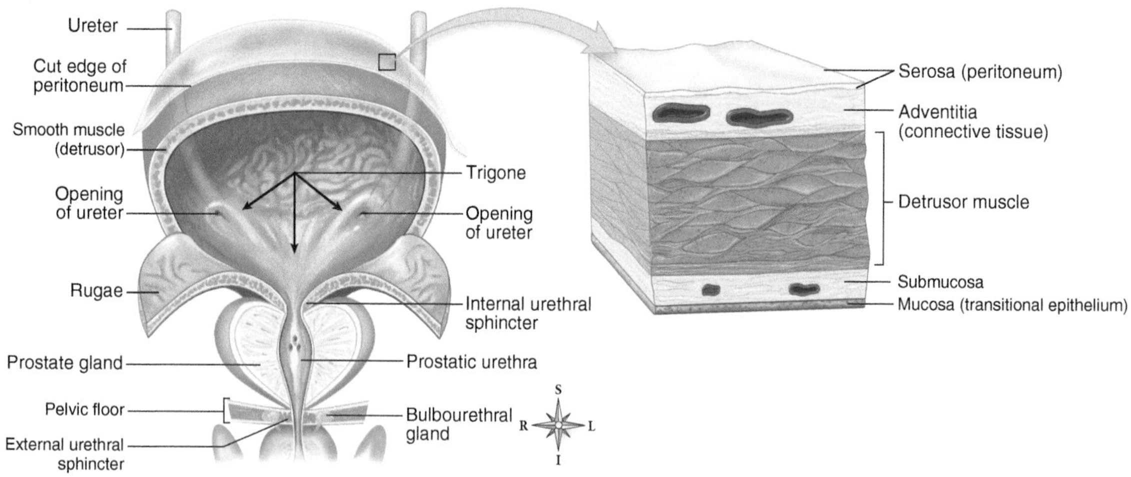
Ureter
Cut edge of peritoneum
Smooth muscle (detrusor)
Opening of ureter
Rugae
Prostate gland
Pelvic floor
External urethral sphincter
Trigone
Opening of ureter
Internal urethral sphincter
Prostatic urethra
Bulbourethral gland
S
R
L
I
Serosa (peritoneum)
Adventitia (connective tissue)
Detrusor muscle
Submucosa
Mucosa (transitional epithelium)

FIG. 7.4 An anterior cutaway view of the bladder.

of the ureters and bladder prevent the backflow of urine. The superior portion of the bladder is often referred to as the dome. The normal adult bladder can store up to 600 mL of urine with the urge to void typically triggered at a volume of 400 mL.

The urethra is a tube leading from the urinary bladder to the exterior of the body. The female urethra is approximately 1 to 1½ inches in length, whereas the male urethra is approximately 8 inches in length. In men, the urethra passes through the prostate gland and also serves as a part of the reproductive system by receiving seminal fluid via the ejaculatory ducts, which open into the urethra from the prostate. The male urethra is classified by three separate portions: (1) the prostatic portion, (2) the membranous portion, and (3) the cavernous portion. The cavernous portion may also be referred to as the spongy, penile, or pendulous urethra. Some sources will also include a bulbous portion of the urethra between the membranous and cavernous portions. The urethra opens to the exterior of the body via the **urinary meatus**. In females, the urinary meatus is located just anterior to the vagina.

Imaging Considerations

Urinary disorders may be suggested by abnormal laboratory or clinical findings. Clinical findings include frequent urination, polyuria, oliguria, dysuria, or obstructive symptoms. The urine may also have an abnormal color, resulting from a variety of factors. Kidney pain is generally located in the flank or back around the level of the twelfth thoracic vertebra, whereas bladder pain resulting from cystitis is usually limited to the urinary bladder.

Patient renal function should be assessed before administering intravenous (IV) contrast agents in radiology. The most common laboratory tests conducted include serum creatinine, blood urea nitrogen (BUN), and glomerular filtration rate (GFR). In a normal adult, serum creatinine production and excretion are constant. Creatinine is a waste product derived from a breakdown of a compound normally found in muscle tissue. BUN levels are influenced by urine flow and the production and metabolism of urea. BUN designates the ability of the urinary system to break down nitrogenous compounds from proteins to produce urea nitrogen. Individuals with significant kidney function impairment often have raised blood levels of creatinine, urea nitrogen, or both because the glomerulus cannot adequately filter substances, the tubular system is not functioning properly, or both. The GFR may be estimated (eGFR) by using the serum creatinine value in combination with the patient's age, race, and gender. Normally, the GFR should be 90 mL per minute per 1.73 m^2 (mL/min/1.73 m^2) or greater. IV contrast agents should not be used in patients with a BUN greater than 50 mg/dL or a serum creatinine greater than 3 mg/dL. The exact GFR threshold contraindicating the administration of IV contrast medium has not been established at this time. However, literature provided by the ACR suggests that current evidence demonstrates a greater risk for kidney injury in persons with an eGFR ≤30 mL/min/1.73m².

KUB Radiography

Kidneys, ureters, and bladder (KUB) radiography is useful in demonstrating the size and location of the kidneys. These organs may be visible radiographically because of the perirenal fat capsule that surrounds them. The kidneys are generally well fixed to the abdominal wall and are seen to move with respiratory effort. As mentioned earlier, the right kidney is usually located inferior to the left kidney because of the presence of the liver. Male kidneys are generally larger than those of a female. The kidneys lie in an oblique plane within the abdomen and tend to parallel the borders of the psoas muscle shadows. Evaluation of the kidneys using only a KUB image is limited because the kidney shadows may often be obscured by bowel content and are difficult to visualize because of the inherent low subject contrast in the abdomen. However, KUB radiography is the usual beginning for intravenous urography (IVU), sometimes referred to as intravenous pyelography (IVP) (Fig. 7.5). In this case its primary purposes are to (1) determine whether adequate bowel preparation has been accomplished and (2) visualize radiopaque calculi of the KUB that may otherwise be hidden by the presence of contrast media. The radiologist also examines areas unrelated to the urinary tract because they may hold clues to diagnosis and may also assist in differentiating between gastrointestinal (GI) and genitourinary (GU) disorders.

Intravenous Urography

One procedure used to assess the urinary system is the IVU (or IVP). The indications for performing IVU include flank pain, calculus disease, suspected urinary tract obstruction, abnormal urinary sediment (especially hematuria), systemic hypertension, urinary tract infections, screening for genitourinary anomalies, or, frequently in men, symptoms of prostatism. The IVU may also be performed if

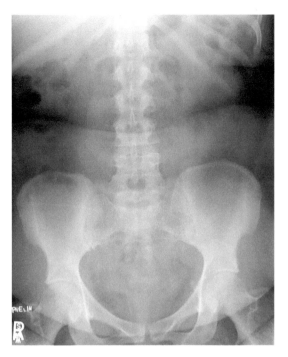

FIG. 7.5 A preliminary or scout image before injection of intravenous contrast for an intravenous urogram. The image demonstrates the renal and psoas major muscle shadows.

there is concern of injury to the GU tract related to trauma or abdominal or pelvic surgery. The IVU has largely been replaced by a CT examination of the GU tract known as the CT urogram, which provides cross-sectional imaging of the GU tract before and after contrast administration as well as allowing for three dimensional (3D) reconstruction of the urinary system.

Although few serious adverse effects typically accompany the injection of urographic contrast agents, current research indicates an increased risk of mortality in older adult Caucasian females because of renal failure and anaphylaxis. The risk of adverse reactions to an iodinated contrast agent increases because of a variety of factors, including a history of previous contrast reactions; asthma or other allergies; heart disease; dehydration; preexisting kidney disease; treatment with β-blockers, nonsteroidal antiinflammatory drugs (NSAIDs), or interleukin-2 (IL-2); a history of other pathologic diseases such as sickle cell anemia, polycythemia, and myeloma; or all of these factors.

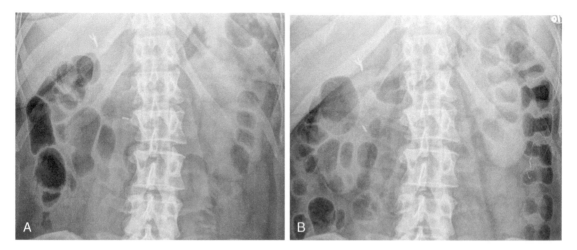

FIG. 7.6 **A**, An image of the kidneys before contrast administration. **B**, An image of the kidneys obtained approximately 30 seconds after contrast injection demonstrating the nephrogram phase of an IVU. Note how the outline of the right kidney is barely visible on image A because of overlying bowel gas. Both renal outlines are better visualized on image B as a result of contrast enhancement and proper timing of the exposure in relationship to contrast administration.

The use of nonionic, low-osmolar contrast agents significantly reduces minor and moderate reactions. These contrast agents still contain iodine, but the molecular makeup prevents them from disassociating into ions (nonionic) in the bloodstream, thus reducing the risk of an anaphylactic reaction. Visualization of the urinary system depends on the concentration of contrast material filtered by the kidneys and present in the collecting system; therefore, the patient must have fairly normal physiologic function for diagnostic images to be obtained. Other imaging techniques such as sonography and computed tomography (CT) should be considered in patients with compromised renal function.

Many IVU routines call for an image to be taken within 30 seconds to 1 minute after contrast medium injection. Because the contrast agents for most IVU examinations are injected by hand, the timing generally begins with the completion of the bolus injection and will vary from institution to institution. This is termed the *nephrogram phase* and may be used to demonstrate the contrast agent in the nephrons before it reaches the renal calyces. Ready visualization of the renal parenchyma allows for an inspection of the renal outline that appears brighter if timed correctly (Fig. 7.6, A and B). Indentations or bulges may indicate the presence of

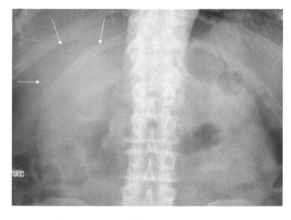

FIG. 7.7 Nephrogram of the renal parenchyma obtained 30 seconds after contrast injection during an IVU shows an abnormal contour of the upper pole of the right kidney and looks like a large rounded bulge from the top of the kidney. The left renal outline has a normal shape.

disease (Fig. 7.7). The nephrogram image is also used to check for normal kidney position, which may be altered by congenital malposition, ptosis, or the presence of a retroperitoneal mass.

Although the numbers and types of images obtained may vary from one institution to another, a series of collecting system sequence images are part

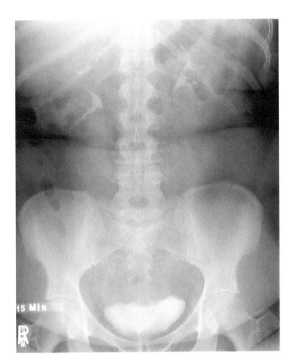

FIG. 7.8 A 15-minute post injection image during intravenous urography demonstrating the normal collecting system.

of IVU (Fig. 7.8). KUB images are usually performed at certain requested time delays from the contrast injection such as 5 minute delay, 15 minute delay and so on. Early timed images will show filling of the calyces and renal pelvis, whereas 10 to 15 minute delays are often aimed at contrast filling of the ureters. Later times will provide contrast filling of the urinary bladder. Oblique images are used to improve visualization of certain portions of the urinary tract during an IVU. Patient rotation of approximately 30 degrees profiles the renal pelvis and its communication with the ureter known as the ureteropelvic junction (UPJ) on the elevated side of a posterior oblique radiograph (Fig. 7.9, A). Rotation of approximately 45 degrees depicts the ureterovesical junction (UVJ), where the ureter inserts into the posterolateral and inferior bladder of the elevated side of a posterior oblique image (Fig. 7.9, B). The UVJ is not well seen on an anteroposterior (AP) KUB because of its location. Prone positioning of the patient may augment contrast distension of the renal pelvis and upper ureters (Fig. 7.10, A and B). Upright positioning can be performed to evaluate the distal ureters or suspected obstruction. Upright images are often performed last in the IVU series as the contrast will progress to the bladder quickly if there is no urinary tract obstruction. Lateral positioning may also be requested especially in cases where trauma to the GU tract is a concern. A "postvoid" KUB is the final step in an IVU examination (Fig. 7.11). The postvoid image provides information regarding decompression of the urinary tract after emptying of the bladder. Residual dilation of any portion of the collecting system after voiding can indicate some level of obstruction. Residual contrast stasis within the bladder may indicate voiding or bladder outlet problems however, bladder emptying is better assessed with a cystogram study that utilizes a higher volume of contrast.

The renal pelvis, calyces, ureters, and bladder are examined for any abnormalities. The calyces should be evenly distributed and reasonably symmetric. When normal, they appear as buttercup-shaped projections, the side edges of which should appear conical and sharp, surrounding the renal papillae. When abnormal, usually as a result of dilation, the calyces become less conical and more rounded at the edges, which is commonly referred to as "blunting" (Fig. 7.12). Calyceal dilation may be demonstrated as a result of acute or chronic urinary tract obstruction, obstructive uropathy, or reflux. Dilation secondary to destruction of the renal pyramids is less common. When the calyces and renal pelvis are dilated, this is referred to as pelvocaliectasis. Dilated renal pelvis and calyces as a result of an obstructive process is termed hydronephrosis. Because of the peristaltic activity of ureters, only part of their length in a collecting system sequence may be demonstrated (Fig. 7.13). Nonopaque ureteral calculi sometimes cause filling defects and an obstructive dilation of the ureter called hydroureter. The majority of all urinary tract calculi are found at the UVJ. Any pronounced deviation of the ureter suggests the presence of a retroperitoneal mass. Various filling defects may be demonstrated in the contrast agent–filled ureter during IVU, including tumors, blood clots, and nonradiopaque calculi. Common bladder defects visualized during IVU include urinary catheter balloons, normal uterus and colon, prostate enlargement and extrinsic deformities such as uterine or sigmoid colon tumors.

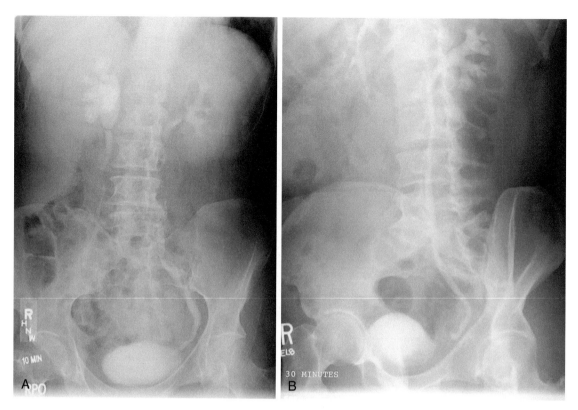

FIG. 7.9 **A,** Radiograph obtained during an intravenous urography (IVU) examination with the patient rotated into a 30 degree right posterior oblique position to profile the left ureteropelvic junction (UPJ). Note how the ureter is still overlapping with the bladder obscuring the ureterovesical junction (UVJ). **B,** Right posterior oblique projection with the patient in 45 degrees of rotation resolves the overlap of the bladder and the distal ureter and profiles the left-sided UVJ.

Cystography

Cystography is a common radiographic examination for studying the lower urinary tract. This involves insertion of a urinary catheter through the urethra into the bladder to facilitate retrograde filling of the bladder with iodinated water-soluble contrast material (Fig. 7.14). The contrast media may be instilled into the bladder via gravity or injected by hand. Renal function impairment is not a contraindication to cystography as the contrast is injected into the bladder and not the vascular system. Images are typically obtained at various volume intervals with the final volume determined by a patient's sensation of fullness. Imaging may be performed as conventional radiographs, utilizing fluoroscopy or a combination of both methods. Desired projections traditionally include AP, left posterior oblique (LPO), right posterior

(RPO), and lateral. These may also be acquired with a combination of supine and upright positioning depending on patient status and the indication for the study.

A frequent indication for this procedure is to identify **vesicoureteral reflux** (VUR). In the normal bladder, increased pressure as the bladder fills effectively shuts down any chance of reflux. Bladder infection, however, may render the ureteral "valve" incompetent, refluxing the infection into the kidney. Cystography may also be used to evaluate for congenital bladder anomalies, tumors, diverticula (Fig. 7.15), calculi, bladder injury, fistula, urinary retention, or neurogenic bladder. Cystography is often performed postoperatively to evaluate anatomy after a kidney and/or pancreas transplant or to evaluate for bladder injury that may occur during such surgical procedures as prostatectomies, cesarean sections, or other abdominopelvic surgeries.

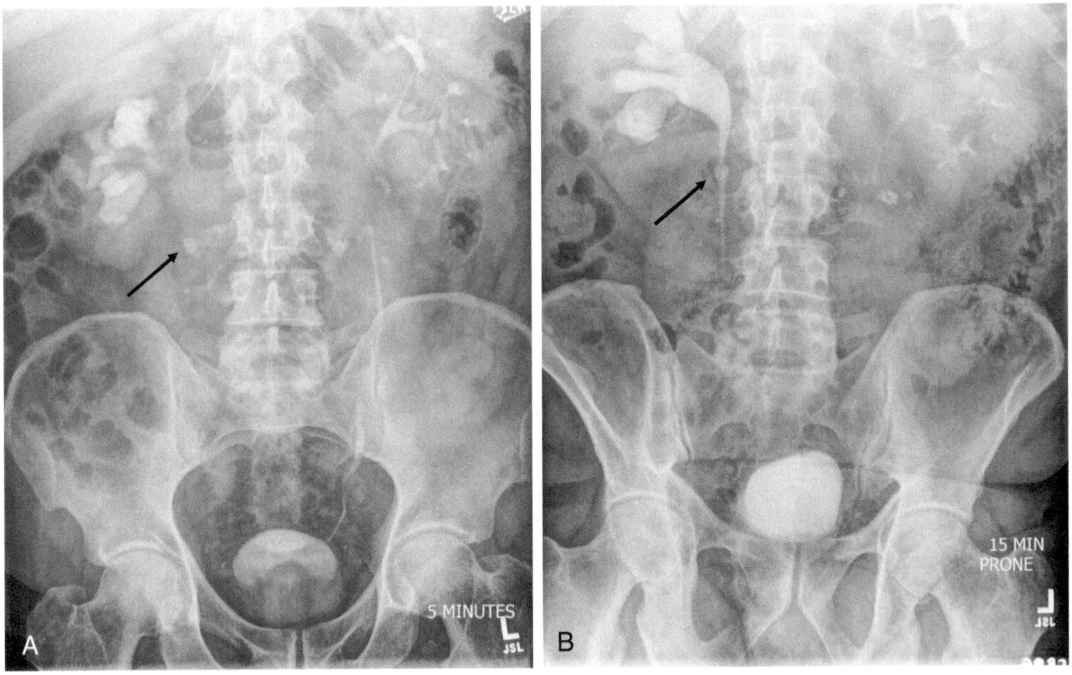

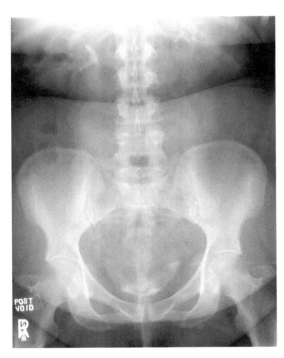

FIG. 7.10 **A,** During and intravenous urography (IVU) examination the right renal pelvis was not filling in this 5 minute kidneys, ureters, bladder (KUB) radiograph. Also can be seen is the right-sided hydronephrosis with dilation of the calyces and a large calcification (*black arrow*) where the proximal ureter should be. **B,** Radiograph obtained at the 15 minute time interval using a prone positioning strategy. Note how the renal pelvis and proximal ureter are opacified with contrast. The change in position allows for the radiologist to determine if the ureter is only partially obstructed, as contrast is seen distal to the stone (*black arrow*).

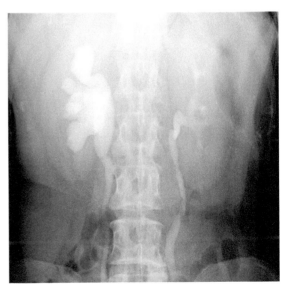

FIG. 7.11 A postvoid image after an intravenous urography examination.

FIG. 7.12 Radiograph of the kidneys obtained during an intravenous urography (IVU) examination shows normal calyces with sharp edges on the left side, whereas the calyces on the right side are dilated resulting in a more rounded contour with blunting of the edges.

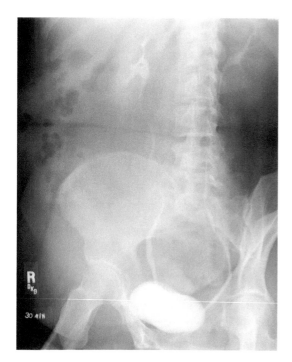

FIG. 7.13 A right posterior oblique projection after contrast injection for intravenous urography demonstrating the correct entrance of the ureters into the posterior bladder wall.

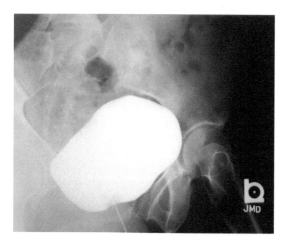

FIG. 7.14 A normal cystogram without reflux, as seen in this oblique projection of the bladder in a 56-year-old woman.

Voiding (micturition) cystourethrography (VCUG) is sometimes used in conjunction with retrograde cystography to allow visualization of the urethra during voiding (Fig. 7.16 A and B). A VCUG examination is also frequently used to assess for VUR, especially among the

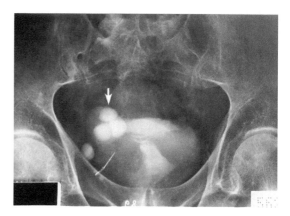

FIG. 7.15 Bladder diverticula in an 88-year-old man demonstrate the presence of numerous calculi within them.

pediatric population. Urethrography may be accomplished using the antegrade approach, as with voiding cystourethrography, or retrograde when cystography is not necessary. The retrograde approach is known as a retrograde urethrogram (RUG). The antegrade approach is frequently used to study the short female urethra and the proximal urethra in the male patient. The retrograde approach is helpful in studying the distal urethra in males (Fig. 7.17). Urethrography, whether antegrade or retrograde, can assess for strictures or urethral diverticula (Fig. 7.18). A RUG is usually the method of choice when looking for urethral trauma in males. The male urethra may also require examination with a RUG to assess for urethral injury following a pancreas transplant. The pancreas is transplanted with the donor duodenum, which is anastomosed to the recipient bladder (Fig. 7.19 A and B). This results in excretion of pancreatic enzymes directly into the bladder. These enzymes can be corrosive to urethral mucosa over time resulting in erosions or tears (Fig. 7.20).

Retrograde Pyelography

Retrograde pyelography requires the placement of a catheter into the ureteric orifice in a retrograde fashion. This is usually performed by a urologist during cystoscopy so that injection of the contrast medium is directly into the ureter to opacify the renal collecting system (Fig. 7.21). The approach is termed *retrograde* because the contrast agent is injected through the ureter into the affected kidney, opposite the normal direction of urine flow. Indications for this study may include hematuria of unknown cause, hydronephrosis, and, in cases of a nonfunctioning kidney, the determination of further information about possible obstruction.

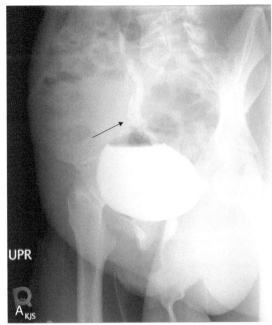

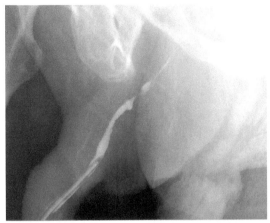

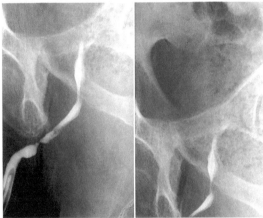

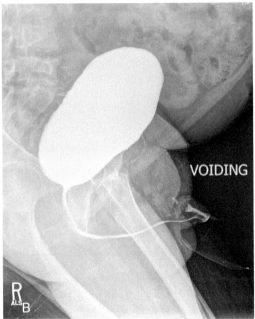

FIG. 7.17 Retrograde urethrography procedure demonstrating a urethral stricture in a male patient. The location of the stricture is confirmed by its consistent appearance on all three images.

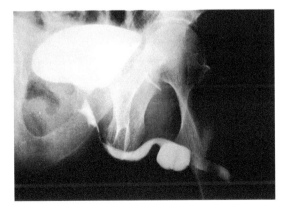

FIG. 7.16 **A,** An oblique projection captured during the voiding phase of a voiding cystourethrogram (VCUG) on a female patient shows a normal appearing female urethra. The image also captures vesicoureteral reflux (*black arrow*) on the right side with visualization of duplicated ureters. **B,** An oblique projection captured during the voiding phase of a VCUG on a male patient shows a normal male urethra.

FIG. 7.18 A voiding cystourethrogram demonstrates a urethral diverticula. The mucosal margin of the prostatic urethra is ragged as a result of scarring after transurethral resection.

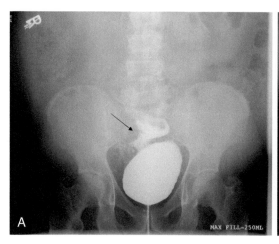 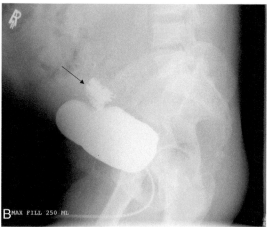

FIG. 7.19 **A,** anteroposterior (AP) and **B,** lateral projections during cystography capturing the anastomosis between the bladder and the transplanted duodenum associated with this method of pancreas transplantation. The donor duodenum (*black arrows*) is partially filled with contrast.

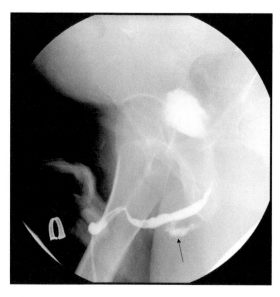

FIG. 7.20 Retrograde urethrogram (RUG) examination of a male urethra in a patient who has had a kidney and pancreas transplant and now has a tear in the urethral mucosa. Contrast extravasation (*black arrow*) can be seen from the penile segment of the urethra.

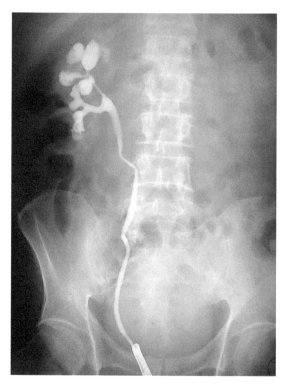

FIG. 7.21 Kidneys, ureters, bladder (KUB) radiograph taken during retrograde pyelography examination. Note the metallic cystoscope device, which is providing direct access to the ureter for retrograde injection of contrast.

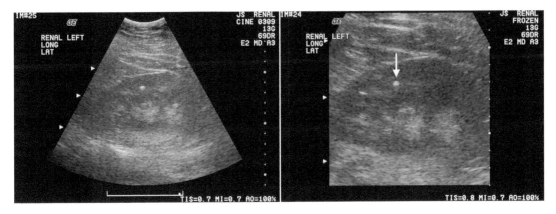

FIG. 7.22 A sonogram demonstrating a renal stone in the cortex of the kidney.

Sonography

Sonography is a noninvasive method of imaging both functioning and nonfunctioning kidneys. Because sonography can clearly demonstrate the parenchymal structure of the kidney and the renal pelvis without the use of contrast agents, it is becoming the primary method of visualizing the kidneys and evaluating most renal disorders. It is useful in evaluating kidney stones (Fig. 7.22), calcifications, hydronephrosis (Fig. 7.23), abscesses, renal masses, and renal cysts (Fig. 7.24) and to assess renal size, atrophy, or both. Sonography is the modality of choice for evaluating individuals after kidney transplantation. Doppler techniques are helpful in assessing blood flow in the renal arteries and veins for both transplant recipients and individuals with suspected renal artery stenosis. Sonography is also used to visualize abnormalities of the urinary system present in the fetus.

Computed Tomography

CT is an excellent modality for imaging the kidneys because it can detect small differences in tissue densities within the body. Kidneys can be visualized on CT with or without the use of a contrast agent; sometimes CT examination of the urinary tract includes scans without and with contrast as part of the same study. Abdominal CT is particularly important in determining the nature of renal masses, either solid or cystic, which may not be visible on a KUB radiograph because of the presence of gas in the bowel. CT evaluation of the urinary system generally requires the use of an IV contrast agent to differentiate renal cysts from solid masses and to evaluate

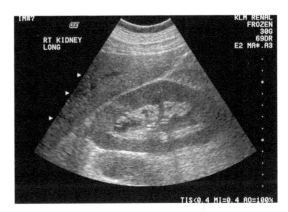

FIG. 7.23 A sonogram confirming hydronephrosis of the kidney and proper placement of a ureteral stent to assist in allowing the kidney to drain properly into the urinary bladder.

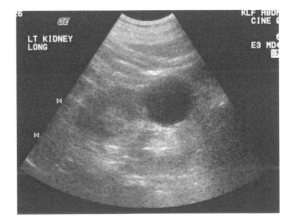

FIG. 7.24 A sonogram showing a renal cyst.

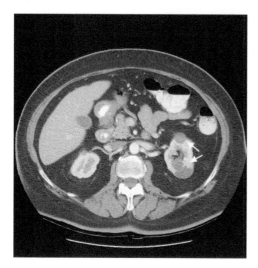 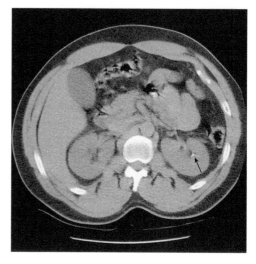

FIG. 7.25 A computed tomography image of a complex cystic structure of the left kidney after contrast injection during the nephrogram phase.

FIG. 7.26 A computed tomography image demonstrating a calcification in the left kidney indicative of a renal stone without the use of a contrast agent.

the extent of the lesion (Fig. 7.25). Because most institutions use an automatic injector in CT, scanning may begin when the bolus of contrast medium is injected or shortly after injection, and a delay is programmed into the scanner to allow the contrast medium to reach the bladder before the pelvis is imaged.

CT is also useful for looking for sites of obstruction caused by **renal calculi** or retroperitoneal masses, which may distort the urinary tract; assessing renal infection or trauma; and staging tumors of the lymph nodes. A CT renal stone study is considered the imaging modality of choice by the American College of Radiology (ACR) when patients present with an acute onset of flank pain or when other symptoms suggest the presence of renal calculi. Because CT displays excellent contrast resolution, stones are identified more easily than with conventional radiography, and without the use of an IV contrast agent (Fig. 7.26). In addition, pelvic CT is the imaging modality of choice for the evaluation of bladder tumors or masses.

Renal Angiography

Renal angiography is one of the most invasive imaging procedures performed on the urinary system. It is usually indicated to further evaluate a renal mass suspected of being malignant, to embolize blood flow to a renal mass, or to assess renal artery stenosis that may cause hypertension. It is also used to assess other vascular

disorders such as aneurysms, thrombus (Fig. 7.27 A and B), or congenital anomalies. It is also performed on kidney donors before surgical removal of the kidney to serve as a "road map" of vascular anatomy for the surgeon. In renal angiography, a catheter is introduced peripherally, most commonly into the femoral artery. The catheter tip may be advanced into the specific renal artery of interest or into the abdominal aorta just superior to the renal arteries. The contrast agent is injected via the catheter to image the vasculature of the kidney or kidneys.

Magnetic Resonance Imaging

The role of magnetic resonance imaging (MRI) has greatly improved as a result of breath-hold imaging sequences and bolus injections of gadolinium contrast agents. Abdominal MRI is a useful follow-up study in patients with known renal cell carcinoma or invasive bladder cancers and adrenal masses. Additionally, magnetic resonance angiography (MRA) is now highly recommended by the ACR in the diagnosis of renovascular hypertension (Fig. 7.28). Contrast-enhanced 3D MRA obtains coronal images of the renal arteries in as little as 20 seconds. The images can then be rotated for better visualization. MRA is also an excellent modality for demonstrating other vascular anomalies such as thrombosis, aneurysms, and arteriovenous malformations (AVMs). Because it

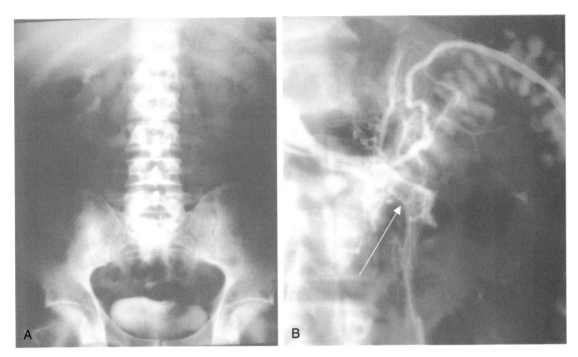

FIG. 7.27 **A,** Kidneys, ureters, bladder (KUB) radiograph obtained at a 15 minute delay shows contrast within the right collecting system but no contrast within the left collecting system. **B,** Follow-up renal angiography demonstrates thrombus (*white arrow*) within the right renal artery, which is occluding blood flow into the left kidney.

allows for imaging of the urinary system in all three planes, it is also used in conjunction with CT for the evaluation of renal masses and their extensions. In cases of renal cyst evaluation, MRI is capable of differentiating between fluid accumulation from hemorrhage and infection. Pelvic MRI is used to readily demonstrate the seminal vesicles and prostate gland in men as well as masses within the urinary bladder. Because of its ability to clearly image soft tissue, pelvic MRI allows for thorough evaluation of invasive cancers within the urinary bladder.

Interventional Procedures and Techniques

Percutaneous nephrostography is an antegrade study in which the contrast medium is injected directly into the renal pelvis. It involves posterolateral insertion of a needle or catheter into the renal pelvis using medical sonography, fluoroscopy, or sometimes a combination of both modalities (Fig. 7.29). The nephrostomy tube may be left in place to provide drainage of an obstructed kidney

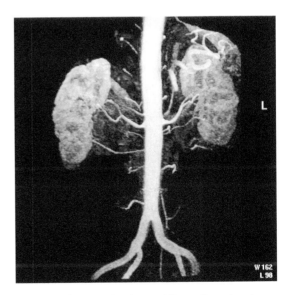

FIG. 7.28 A contrast-enhanced three-dimensional magnetic resonance angiography image of the renal arteries demonstrating normal renal artery patency.

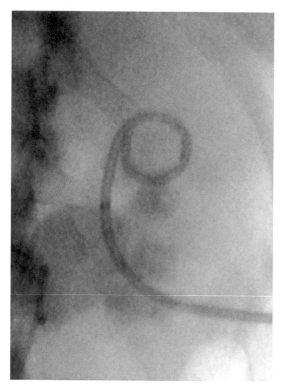

FIG. 7.29 Placement of a right percutaneous renal drainage tube under fluoroscopic guidance.

or to allow for retrieval of the calculus with a basket catheter. Sometimes the procedure is used to relieve obstruction in patients for whom immediate surgery is not possible. A nephrostomy tube also provides a means for diverting urine in cases where there is leakage from the ureters or the bladder (Fig. 7.30 A and B), which requires time to resolve. This tube type can also be used to divert urine away from a urinary tract anastomosis, which also needs time to heal. The injection of contrast into an existing nephrostomy tube, usually performed in fluoroscopy, is known as a nephrostogram or antegrade nephrostogram study.

Extracorporeal shock wave lithotripsy (SWL) is a method used to locate and treat renal calculi. After the location of the stone is determined radiographically, fluoroscopy or sonography aids in alignment of a high-frequency shock wave directed at the stone. If the treatment is successful, the stone disintegrates into fragments and is excreted via urination, thus helping the patient avoid surgery and a much lengthier recovery period (Fig. 7.31 A and B).

Percutaneous renal biopsy or drainage may be performed under fluoroscopy, sonography, or CT guidance. Biopsies help in the evaluation of the histologic origin of renal masses. Percutaneous drainage may be used to aspirate renal cysts or abscesses.

Percutaneous radiofrequency ablation and percutaneous **cryoablation** are minimally invasive alternative treatments for patients who are poor candidates for a major surgery. Percutaneous ablative therapy is a treatment option for patients with renal cell carcinoma because these procedures not only preserve renal function, but also decrease postoperative morbidity and recovery time. Percutaneous radiofrequency ablation involves insertion of a probe into the tumor site and induction of a high electrical current that heats up the tumor and eventually destroys it. The process of cryoablative therapy is the exact opposite. Probes are inserted into the tumor and high pressure argon and nitrogen gases are circulated throughout the probes. This allows the core temperature of the tumor to reach as low as $-190°$ C, causing ice crystallization, which necrotizes the tumor. With this procedure, the tumor goes through multiple freeze-and-thaw cycles.

Urinary Tubes and Catheters

When certain types of pathologies, such as tumors or stone formation, inhibit the normal flow of urine through the urinary system, several types of tubes may be used to allow drainage of urine. A **nephrostomy tube** connects the renal pelvis to the outside of the body (see Fig. 7.29). It is inserted percutaneously through the renal cortex and medulla into the renal pelvis to allow urine to drain outside of the body directly from the renal pelvis. Special care must be taken, as patients are readily prone to infections because of the direct opening into the urinary system.

Ureteral stents may also be placed in cases of ureteral obstruction. Unlike nephrostomy tubes, ureteral stents do not connect the urinary system to the outside of the patient's body (Fig. 7.32). **Ureteral stents** are placed surgically or via cystoscopy, with the upper portion of the stent in the renal pelvis and the lower portion within the urinary bladder. The stent maintains patency of the diseased ureter and enables urine to flow normally. These stents are visible on plain abdominal radiographs and on CT scans of the abdomen (Fig. 7.33).

Urinary catheterization is performed to obtain urine specimens, relieve urinary retention, monitor renal

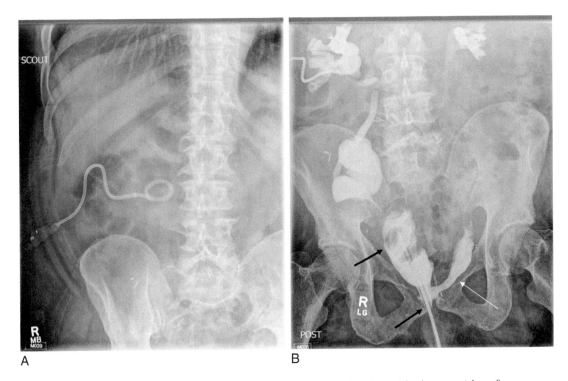

FIG. 7.30 A, Preliminary radiograph shows a right-sided nephrostomy tube is present for a fluoroscopy nephrostogram study. **B,** Postcontrast radiograph reveals postoperative changes related to a total cystectomy and the use of small intestine to create a neobladder. Contrast extravasation (*white arrow*) is visualized where there is a leak between the anastomosis of the neobladder and the urethra. A Foley catheter with inflated balloon (*black arrows*) is visible within the neobladder.

function, and manage urinary incontinence. A **Foley catheter** is the most common indwelling urinary catheter. It is placed within the urinary bladder using sterile technique. Once the catheter is placed through the urethra and the urinary sphincter, a small balloon is inflated to keep the catheter in place within the urinary bladder (see Fig. 7.30). This catheter is generally connected to a bag that collects urine as it flows through the catheter to the outside of the body. Care must be taken to ensure that the catheter is not displaced during a radiographic procedure, and at all times the urine collection bag must be placed at a level lower than that of the patient's bladder to prevent the reflux of urine back into the bladder, which could result in a **urinary tract infection** (UTI). A Foley catheter must be placed in the patient before cystography or cystourethrography is performed to allow for installation of contrast material into the bladder. Again, the importance of proper sterile technique cannot be overemphasized. For patients

such as those with quadriplegia who require long-term catheterization, a **suprapubic catheter** may be used instead of a Foley catheter.

Congenital and Hereditary Diseases

Anomalies of the kidneys and ureters are caused by errors in development. They can be classified as anomalies of number, size and form, fusion, and position. About 10% of all persons have some sort of congenital malformation of the urinary system, and these congenital anomalies often result in impaired renal function leading to infection and stone formation. At least half of those with kidney anomalies have malformations elsewhere in the urinary system or in other systems, most commonly the reproductive system, which may result in sexual dysfunction or infertility. Surgical correction may be required for complications associated with the anomaly.

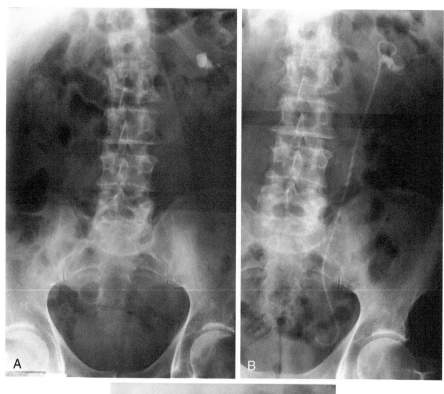

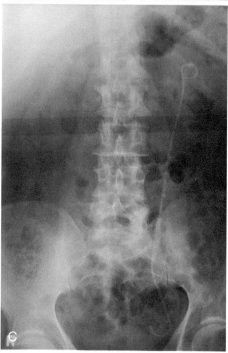

FIG. 7.31 **A,** Scout film taken before lithotripsy demonstrates a large, solid renal stone in the left kidney. **B,** Two months after lithotripsy, the stone is clearly seen to be fragmented and beginning to descend the left ureter. A stent has been placed in the left ureter to aid in draining urine. **C,** A film taken 2 months later demonstrates further movement of stone fragments down the ureter. The stent is still in place.

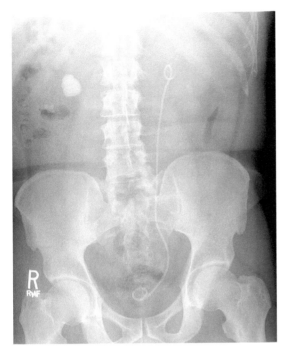

FIG. 7.32 An abdominal radiograph demonstrating bilateral renal calculi with a left ureteral stent properly placed to allow drainage of urine into the urinary bladder.

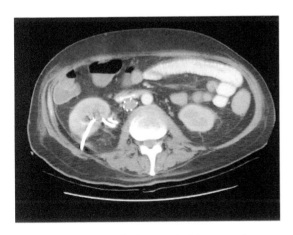

FIG. 7.33 An abdominal computed tomography scan demonstrating a right percutaneous nephrostomy placement and ureteral stent.

Number and Size Anomalies of the Kidney

In an embryo, the urinary system develops in three stages with the formation of the kidneys beginning from growth of the ureteric duct and the development of

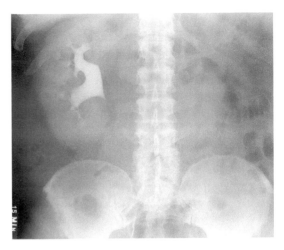

FIG. 7.34 An intravenous urogram demonstrating agenesis of the left kidney accompanied by a large, functioning right kidney.

metanephric tissue. If proper growth does not occur, the kidney does not form in the normal manner. **Renal agenesis** or **aplasia** is a relatively rare anomaly occurring in approximately 1 in 1000 live births and is more common in males than females. This anomaly can be detected by prenatal sonography, and it generally manifests as absence of a kidney on one side (unilaterally) and an associated unusually large kidney on the other side (Fig. 7.34). This condition is known as *compensatory hypertrophy*. In instances of unilateral renal agenesis, more frequently the left kidney is absent. The single hypertrophic kidney is more subject to trauma because of its enlarged size. In an individual with only one kidney, protection against disease is very important. The absence of both kidneys, termed *Potter syndrome* or *bilateral agenesis*, is more common in males and is incompatible with life. Almost half of the infants with this problem are stillborn and those who are born alive die within the first 4 hours of birth.

A **supernumerary kidney**, which is also relatively rare, involves the presence of a third, small, rudimentary kidney. It has no parenchymal attachment to a kidney, and in about half the cases, the supernumerary kidney drains from an independent renal pelvis into the ureter on that side. It often becomes symptomatic as a result of infection.

Hypoplasia is a rare anomaly of size involving a kidney that has developed less than normal in size but contains normal nephrons (Fig. 7.35). Usually, hypoplasia is

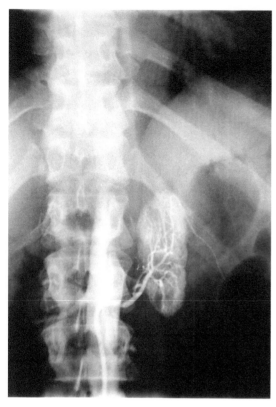

FIG. 7.35 The normal vasculature of this small kidney demonstrates renal hypoplasia.

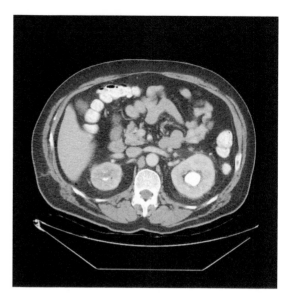

FIG. 7.36 An abdominal computed tomography image of an atrophic right kidney.

associated with hyperplasia of the other kidney. It requires renal arteriography to differentiate congenital hypertrophic changes from atrophy caused by acquired vascular disease (Fig. 7.36). The clinical significance of hypoplasia depends on the volume of the functioning kidney; however, hypertension often accompanies this anomaly. **Hyperplasia** is the opposite condition; it involves overdevelopment of a kidney. Again, this is often associated with renal agenesis or hypoplasia of the other kidney.

Fusion Anomalies of the Kidney

Fusion anomalies of the kidneys are often distinguishable on plain radiographs (Fig. 7.37). **Horseshoe kidney**, the most common fusion anomaly, is a condition affecting approximately 0.25% of the population in the United

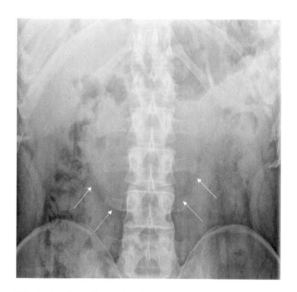

FIG. 7.37 A radiograph of the upper abdomen demonstrating a horseshoe kidney fusion anomaly. Note how the renal shadows are very close to the spine and the bilateral inferior poles can be followed to where they overlap with the spine.

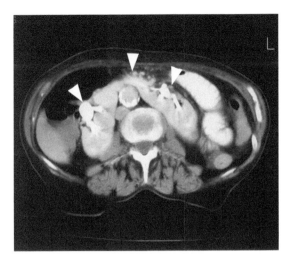

FIG. 7.38 Horseshoe kidney with apparent obstruction on a computed tomography scan of a 72-year-old woman.

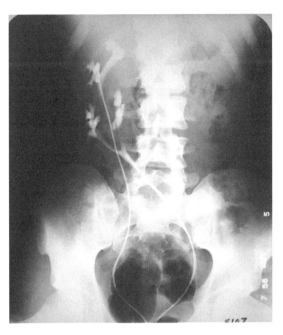

FIG. 7.39 A retrograde pyelogram demonstrates the left ureter crossing midline to connect with the lower pelvis of an anomalous right kidney, as consistent with crossed fused renal ectopy.

States, with men affected twice as frequently as women. In this condition, the lower poles of the kidneys are joined across the midline by a band of soft tissue, causing a rotation anomaly on one side or both sides. The ureters exit the kidneys anteriorly instead of medially, and the lower pole calyces point medially rather than laterally (Fig. 7.38). Kidney function is generally unimpaired in this condition; however, if obstruction is present because of the abnormal location of the ureters, pyeloplastic surgery may be required. The lower bridge frequently lies on a sacral promontory, where it is susceptible to trauma and may be palpated as an abdominal mass.

In **crossed ectopy**, one kidney lies across the midline and is fused with the other kidney (Fig. 7.39). This is the second most common fusion anomaly. Both kidneys demonstrate various anomalies of position, shape, fusion, and rotation with crossed ectopy. The crossed kidney generally lies inferior to the uncrossed one, and its ureter crosses the midline to enter the bladder on the proper side. Its drainage may be impaired by malposition of its ureter within the renal pelvis, which may require surgical repair with pyeloplasty.

Position Anomalies of the Kidney

Anomalies of position are relatively common. **Malrotation** consists of incomplete or excessive rotation of the kidneys as they ascend from the pelvis in utero. This is generally of little clinical significance unless an obstruction is created. An **ectopic kidney** is one that is out of its normal position, a condition found in approximately 1 in 800 urologic examinations. Most patients are asymptomatic throughout their lives; however, the incidence of ureteropelvic junction obstruction or VUR is increasing. Ectopic kidneys are usually lower than normal, often in a pelvic location (Fig. 7.40) or a sacral location. In rare cases, the ectopic kidney may be in an intrathoracic location. In severe cases of ectopy, surgical intervention may be necessary. In some lean and athletic persons, the kidney is mobile and may drop toward the pelvis when the person is in the erect position. This is termed *kidney prolapse* or **nephroptosis**.

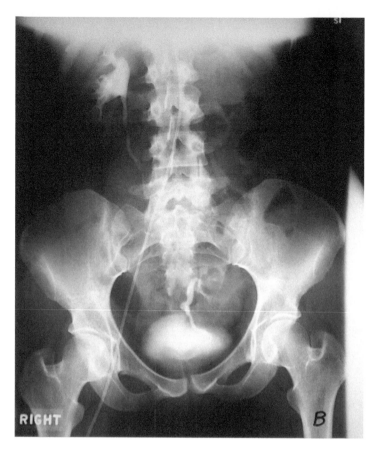

FIG. 7.40 An ectopic kidney, indicated by a urogram taken at the end of angiography, demonstrates the left kidney with a shortened ureter in the left pelvis.

Nephroptosis is distinguished from a pelvic kidney by the length of the ureter; if the ureter is short, it is a congenital pelvic kidney.

Renal Pelvis and Ureter Anomalies

Renal pelvis and ureter anomalies are frequent. They may be unilateral or bilateral, and they have a tendency to be asymmetric. Such anomalies may occur as a double renal pelvis, either in isolation or in combination with a double ureter (Figs. 7.41 and 7.42). The problem with these and other upper urinary tract anomalies is that they may impair renal drainage, predisposing the patient to infection and calculi formation.

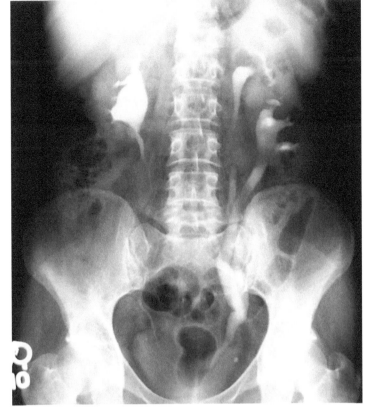

FIG. 7.41 A congenital double ureter is clearly seen on the left side.

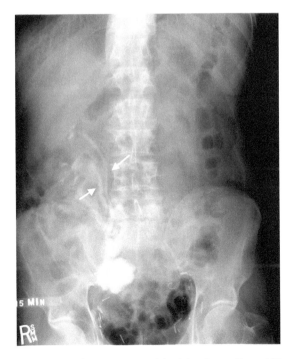

FIG. 7.42 A duplicated right collecting system emptying into a loop of bowel. The urinary bladder has been surgically removed because of bladder carcinoma and replaced with a loop of small intestines.

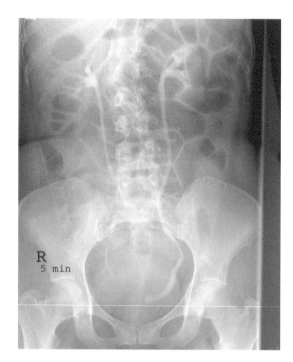

FIG. 7.43 A 5-minute kidneys, ureters, bladder (KUB) radiograph during an intravenous urography (IVU) examination captures a left-sided simple ureterocele. The left ureter has a rounded contour at the ureterovesical junction (UVJ), whereas the right ureter has a tapered and normal contour.

Lower Urinary Tract Anomalies

A simple **ureterocele** is a cyst-like dilation of a ureter near its opening into the bladder (Fig. 7.43). Ureteroceles usually result from congenital stenosis of the ureteral orifice. Radiographically, a ureterocele appears as a filling defect in the bladder with a characteristic "cobra head" appearance. A ureterocele that appears with ureteral duplication is an "ectopic" ureterocele; it often causes substantial obstruction, primarily of the upper pole, and kidney infection. It may also lead to **renal failure**. Treatment in this situation involves endoscopic or open surgical repair to allow for increased flow of urine into the bladder.

Ureteral diverticula are probably a congenital anomaly and may actually represent a dilated, branched ureteric remnant. The appearance of ureteral diverticula is the same as that of any other diverticula and is best demonstrated by retrograde urography (Fig. 7.44). **Bladder diverticula** (Fig. 7.45) may occur as a congenital anomaly or be caused by chronic bladder outlet obstruction and resultant infection. They usually occur in

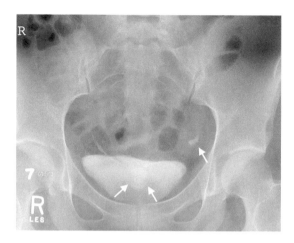

FIG. 7.44 The left ureteric diverticula, visible as double densities superimposed on the posterior bladder, is seen on this intravenous urogram of a female patient with recurrent urinary tract infections.

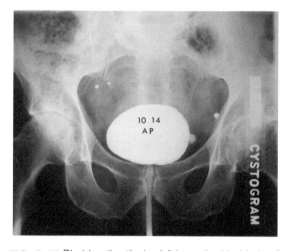

FIG. 7.45 Bladder diverticula visible on the bladder's left margin in this cystogram.

middle-aged men and may be diagnosed via cystography or cystoscopy. In severe cases, the bladder may have to be surgically reconstructed.

Urethral valves, also known as posterior urethral valves, are mucosal folds that protrude into the posterior (prostatic) urethra as a congenital condition. These may cause significant obstruction to urine flow (Fig. 7.46). Such "valves" occur in males, are usually discovered during infancy or early childhood, and are commonly diagnosed by using voiding cystourethrography. The condition is corrected by endoscopic surgery at an early age to prevent renal damage.

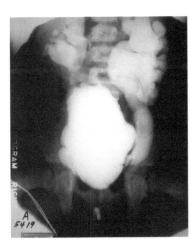

Large, trabeculated bladder and large tortuous ureters and renal pelves seen on this cystogram of a 15-year-old boy, consistent with bladder outflow obstruction secondary to congenital posterior urethral valves.

Polycystic Kidney Disease

Polycystic kidney disease (PKD) is a congenital, familial kidney disorder that may be classified as either autosomal recessive or autosomal dominant. This anomaly results from mutations of the *PKD-1* and *PKD-2* genes and occurs in 1 in 1000 live births. Innumerable tiny cysts within the nephron unit are present at birth and may be discovered with in utero ultrasonography. Autosomal recessive PKD is a rare condition causing childhood cystic disease and ultimately resulting in childhood renal failure. Without a family history of autosomal recessive PKD, diagnosis is often difficult. Sonography plays an important role in demonstrating renal and hepatic cysts and is also used for obtaining a tissue sample via percutaneous biopsy.

Autosomal dominant PKD is often asymptomatic in childhood, although it may be visible sonographically. The cysts gradually enlarge as the patient ages, and clinical symptoms become apparent in adulthood. It is the cause of approximately 10% of all end-stage renal disease cases in adults. This enlargement compresses and eventually destroys normal tissues. The late presentation of the condition occurs because the cysts are initially very small and do not cause problems until tissue destruction becomes significant. Symptoms include lower back pain, UTIs, and stone formation. In addition, approximately 30% to 35% of affected individuals have cysts in the liver, which do not affect liver function, and 50% are diagnosed with renal hypertension.

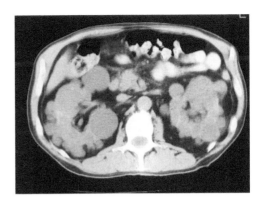

Polycystic kidney disease visible as multiple masses in the kidneys in this computed tomography scan of a 64-year-old man.

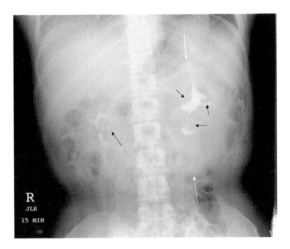

Intravenous urography (IVU) examination of a patient with polycystic kidney disease shows enlarged renal size (*white arrows*) on the left side. Also seen are areas of distortion and displacement of the calyces (*black arrows*).

The diagnosis of multiple cysts is readily confirmed with ultrasonography, which reveals multiple echo-free areas in both kidneys, or with CT evaluation (Fig. 7.47) demonstrating a moth-eaten appearance of the functional renal tissue. Both ultrasonography and CT have the advantage of demonstrating the disease in its early stages, before it may be visible on conventional radiographs. IVU images of PKD show bilateral enlargement of the kidneys with poorly visualized outlines (from the presence of cysts) and calyceal stretching and distortion (Fig. 7.48). Over half the individuals with PKD eventually develop uremia in their mid to

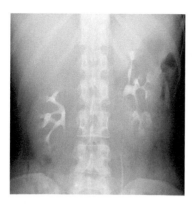

FIG. 7.49 Medullary sponge kidney demonstrated by large bilateral papillae and dilated tubules visible within the papillae.

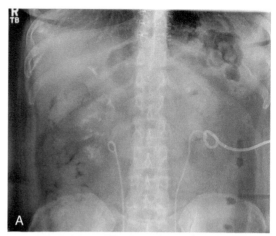

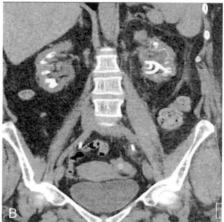

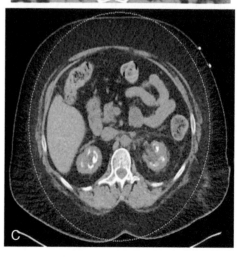

late 50s and require dialysis or kidney transplantation. Therapy for this condition consists of good management of UTI, basic fluid and electrolyte management, hypertension management, avoidance of physical activities that could cause trauma to the abdomen, and management of pain caused by the occasional rupture of a cyst.

Medullary Sponge Kidney

Medullary sponge kidney involves congenital dilation of the renal tubules leading to urinary stasis and increased levels of calcium phosphate (nephrocalcinosis). The diagnosis is not usually made until the fourth or fifth decade of life, when infective complications emerge. The only visible abnormality is the dilation of the medullary and papillary portions of the collecting ducts, usually bilaterally (Fig. 7.49). Calculi are contained in about 60% of symptomatic patients (Fig. 7.50 A, B, C), and infection and intrarenal obstruction are common. IVU reveals linear markings in the papillae or cystic collections of contrast medium in the enlarged collecting ducts. However, this anomaly is often difficult to differentiate from renal cystic disease, tuberculosis, or other disorders resulting in nephrocalcinosis (deposits of calcium phosphates in the renal tubules). Diagnostic sonography is generally unable to demonstrate the cysts, as they are very small and generally lie deep within the medulla of the kidney. Therapy for this condition consists of treatment for the infection and, if possible, resolution of nephrolithiasis with lithotripsy.

FIG. 7.50 **A,** Supine radiograph of the upper abdomen showing extensive bilateral nephrocalcinosis in a person with medullary sponge kidney. Bilateral ureteral stents and a left-sided nephrostomy tube are also present. **B,** coronal and **C,** axial computed tomography (CT) images on the same patient redemonstrating nephrocalcinosis.

Inflammatory Diseases

Urinary Tract Infection

UTIs are the most common of all bacterial infections. They occur in individuals of all ages and both genders. They are more common in boys during infancy, generally resulting from a congenital anomaly. The incidence increases in girls around the age of 10 years, and by the age of 20 years, women are twice as likely to develop UTIs as men. Up to 35% of all women experience a UTI at least once in their lifetime. A quantitative urine culture is essential in the treatment approach for UTI because the causes are broad. In most cases of UTI, the infecting organism is a gram-negative bacillus that invades the urinary system by an ascending route through the urethra to the bladder and to the kidney. Some authors believe that the offending bacteria ascend during micturition, possibly related to a turbulent stream or reflux on completion of voiding. Research also suggests that compared with women who are not sexually active, those who are sexually active tend to experience UTIs more frequently, especially when they use a diaphragm and spermicide as forms of birth control. It is believed that the spermicide inhibits the normal flora of the vagina and allows overgrowth of *Escherichia coli*. The only clearly demonstrated mechanism, however, is by instrumentation of the urethra and bladder by cystoscopy, urologic surgery, or Foley catheter placement. Antibiotics are used to treat the bacterial infection.

Pyelonephritis

Acute **pyelonephritis,** considered the most common renal disease, is a bacterial infection of the calyces and renal pelvis. Any stagnation or obstruction to urine flow in any part of the urinary tract predisposes the patient

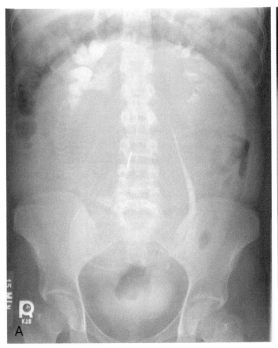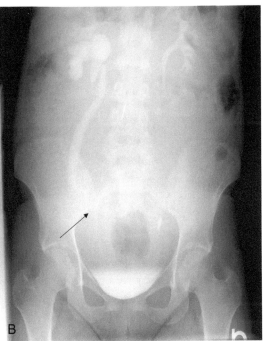

FIG. 7-51 **A,** A limited intravenous urogram (IVU) protocol was performed on a female with recurrent urinary tract infections (UTIs) and right-sided flank pain during pregnancy, after right-sided hydronephrosis was discovered on a sonogram, to determine whether the hydronephrosis was related to pregnancy or another cause such as an obstructing calculus. **B,** The 15 minute kidneys, ureters, bladder (KUB) radiograph shows dilation and blunting of the right calyces, but no contrast within the right ureter. The upright KUB demonstrates that the ureter is not obstructed as the entirety of the ureter is visible. However, there is hydronephrosis and hydroureter to the pelvis level (*black arrow*) where the ureter then resumes a normal caliber. This is a result of external compression by the uterus and was determined to be the cause of her UTIs.

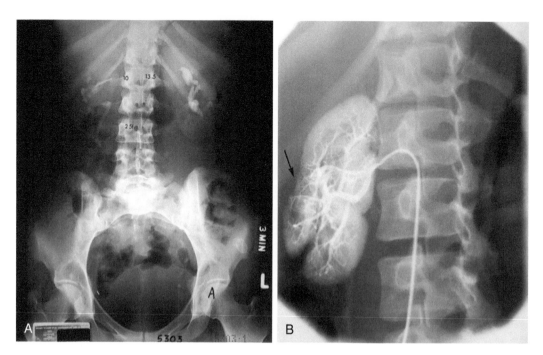

FIG. 7.52 **A,** The right kidney is small and has a scarred surface, as seen on this intravenous urogram of a 25-year-old woman with recurrent urinary tract infections. **B,** Selective renal angiography demonstrates a thinned cortex caused by scarring and bunching of the renal vessels, as consistent with chronic pyelonephritis.

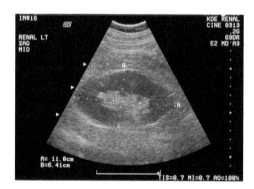

FIG. 7.53 A diagnostic medical sonogram demonstrating the echogenic texture of a normal kidney.

to kidney infection. The microorganisms involved are generally *E. coli, Proteus,* or *Pseudomonas,* which reach the kidney by ascending the ureters or via the bloodstream. Acute pyelonephritis is rare in men with a normal urinary tract but is common in women, especially pregnant women after urinary catheterization or as the increased size of the uterus compresses the ureter and decreases urinary clearance of bacteria (Fig. 7.51 A and B).

Pyelonephritis is a problem for women who have had recurrent UTIs and as a result have *E. coli* bacteria (80%) that have progressed up the ureter and infected portions of the kidney. Patients with acute pyelonephritis have fever, flank pain, and general malaise. Urinalysis demonstrates **pyuria**, the presence of pus (white cells) created by the body's reaction to the infection. Reactions include renal inflammation and edema in combination with purulent urine. Abscesses may form in the kidneys and create a flow of pus into the collecting tubules. Diagnosis of the condition is usually made on the basis of laboratory results, as radiographic findings are often nonspecific. In most cases, IVU is normal even during an acute attack. The calyces may be blunted, and collecting structures may be less well visualized because of interstitial edema. Treatment consists of administering antibiotics to eliminate the infectious bacteria.

Recurrent or persistent infection of the kidneys, such as that caused by chronic reflux of infected urine from the bladder into the renal pelvis, may result in chronic pyelonephritis. It generally has no relation to acute pyelonephritis and is seen sometimes in patients with a major anatomic abnormality (e.g., an obstruction) or more commonly in children with VUR. Chronic pyelonephritis is often bilateral and leads to destruction and scarring of the renal tissue, with marked dilation of the calyces. The eventual result is an overall reduction in kidney size, readily seen on IVU (Fig. 7.52, A). The renal pyramids atrophy, giving the calyces a clubbed appearance. Scars may also be seen and appear as indentations of the renal cortex on the kidney outline in the nephrogram phase (see Fig. 7.52, B). Chronic pyelonephritis may be caused by a congenital duplication of ureters that allows a chronic reflux of urine, by an obstruction of the urinary tract, or by a neurogenic bladder. Hypertension may result from chronic pyelonephritis. Sonography is useful in assessing and grading medical renal disease, including pyelonephritis and renal hypertension. One of the subjective sonographic techniques includes comparing the echogenicity of the kidney with that of the liver because the liver has a homogeneous sonographic texture. For a normal grading, the cortical area of the kidney should be less echogenic than the liver (Fig. 7.53). As the disease breaks down the cortical tissue, the echogenicity becomes equal to that of the liver. In the final phases of renal disease, the kidney exhibits greater echogenicity than the liver. Treatment of pyelonephritis in a chronic stage centers on control of hypertension, removal of any cause for obstruction, and use of antibiotics to control infection.

Acute Glomerulonephritis

An antigen–antibody reaction in the glomeruli causes an inflammatory reaction of the renal parenchyma known as **acute glomerulonephritis** or **Bright disease**. This inflammation begins in the cortex of the kidney and in the tiny arcuate arteries that infuse the glomeruli. The major characteristic of the glomeruli is that they allow for extraordinarily high levels of water and small solutes to flow through the system. Although the kidney has an incredible capacity to cleanse blood, glomeruli can be damaged by vascular pressure, metabolic diseases such as diabetes, and immune disorders such as systemic lupus erythematosus (SLE). Acute glomerulonephritis is an immunologic reaction that may follow streptococcal infection of the upper respiratory tract or the middle ear. It differs from acute pyelonephritis, which primarily affects the interstitial tissue rather than the nephrons. Often a renal biopsy procedure is conducted to get a sample of the glomeruli to ascertain the level of disease

or erosion within them. CT or sonographic guidance helps the physician obtain samples of renal tissue and send them to the laboratory for inspection. The biopsy samples allow the pathologist to look for the level of disease or erosion. A granular pattern develops within the glomeruli from deposits of antigens and the resulting antibodies. These microscopic deposits in the glomerulus are the gold standard for diagnosing glomerulonephritis. This condition occurs mainly in children after streptococcal infection, with most patients recovering completely. Radiographically, the kidneys appear larger, particularly during the nephrogram phase of IVU, because of edematous accumulation. Treatment may include diuretic therapy to reduce the edema and its resultant pressure on the glomeruli, as well as antiinflammatory medications and steroid therapy. Renal dialysis may be used for severe, chronic cases.

Cystitis

Cystitis, which is an acute or chronic inflammation of the bladder, is a fairly common infection that is generally caused by bacteria such as *E. coli* and *Staphylococcus saprophyticus*. Cystitis is more prevalent in women than in men because the short urethra in women allows bacteria easier access into the bladder. The bladder lining's natural resistance to inflammation, however, serves as a protective mechanism. Inflammation and congestion of the bladder mucosa cause the patient to experience burning pain during urination or the urge to urinate frequently. Although cystitis is not a serious infection, it may cause further problems by spreading into the upper urinary passages, including the renal pelvis and the kidney.

VUR, the backward flow of urine out of the bladder and into the ureters, may be seen in cases of cystitis. In the normal urinary tract, VUR is prevented by compression of the bladder musculature on the ureters during micturition. Failure of this valve mechanism usually results from a shortening of the intravesical portion of the ureter caused by abnormal embryologic development, leading to ureteric orifices that are displaced laterally. As this portion of the ureter lengthens with growth, this type of VUR may disappear completely with age. Congenital VUR is also seen in duplication of collecting systems and ureters with reflux into an ectopically placed ureter serving the upper pole of the kidney. VUR may also result from a **neurogenic bladder**, a bladder dysfunction caused by interference with the

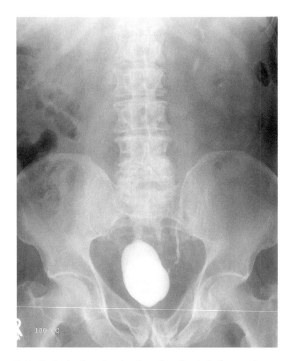

Left ureteral reflux visualized during cystography. The patient also has a pelvic fracture.

nerve impulses concerned with urination. Cystography may demonstrate the presence of reflux (Fig. 7.54) and grade its severity. It may show a roughening of the normally smooth bladder wall, a radiographic appearance referred to as **bladder trabeculae** (Fig. 7.55). Bladder trabeculae are also seen with neurogenic bladder in cases of chronic bladder outlet obstruction. Treatment of cystitis includes antibiotic therapy and an abundance of fluids. Prevention of pyelonephritis is paramount.

Urinary System Calcifications

With the exception of the gallbladder, more calculi are found in the urinary tract than anywhere else in the body. Renal calculi are stones that develop from urine and precipitate crystalline materials, especially calcium and its salts. If the body's normal equilibrium is upset, these products may precipitate out of the solution. Factors that cause this precipitation include metabolic disorders such as hyperparathyroidism, excessive intake of calcium, and a metabolic rate that causes high urine concentration. Chronic UTI is also related to stone formation.

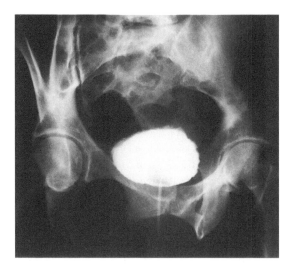

Mildly trabeculated bladder as seen in this 34-year-old woman with a small-capacity bladder.

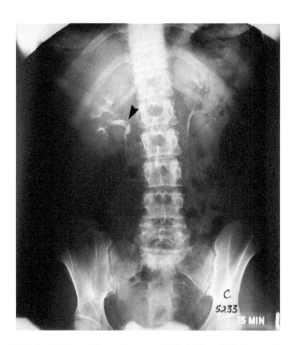

Smooth, oval, noncalcified filling defect seen in the right renal pelvis, suggestive of a radiolucent uric acid stone in this 40-year-old woman with hematuria.

Men develop calculi more often than women do, especially after the age of 30 years. Nearly all urinary tract calculi are calcified to some extent; however, approximately 5% of stones do not calcify (Fig. 7.56). These are generally made of pure uric acid and present

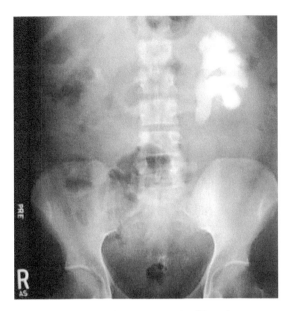

An abdominal radiograph without intravenous contrast demonstrating a large staghorn calculus.

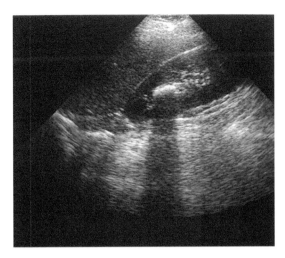

Large calculi seen on this ultrasonogram of the kidney of a young woman. Note the absence of sound transmission beyond the stone as indicated by the dark pathway beneath it.

a more difficult diagnosis to the physician because they are one of several filling defects, including blood clots and tumors. Most stones are formed in the calyces or renal pelvis. A **staghorn calculus** is a large calculus that assumes the shape of the pelvicalyceal junction (Fig. 7.57). Because of the calcium content in renal calculi, most are visible during abdominal radiography, IVU, or retrograde pyelography. Sonography (Fig. 7.58) and noncontrast CT of the abdomen (Fig. 7.59) are often used to demonstrate stones. In many institutions, a CT stone study is the first modality of choice because it does not require contrast administration and is highly sensitive for detecting small calculi that could be difficult to see on a KUB with bowel overlapping the GU tract. It is an excellent method for differentiating abdominal or flank pain caused by renal calculi *versus* appendicitis or an abdominal aortic aneurysm. In addition, it can be used to detect the location of the stone and the degree of obstruction present.

Stones tend to be asymptomatic until they begin to descend or cause an obstruction. Renal stones generally do not have a smooth texture and often have multiple jagged edges, causing pain as they move through the ureter. The most common site for a calculus to lodge and create an obstruction is the ureterovesical junction (Fig. 7.60). Obstructions may also occur in the ureter at

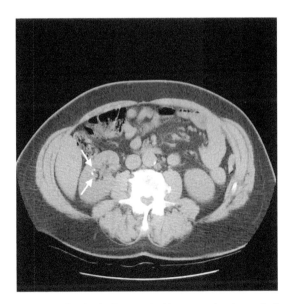

Abdominal computed tomography stone study without contrast enhancement demonstrating a right renal stone without hydronephrosis.

the pelvic brim. Movement of stones or acute obstruction results in severe, intermittent pain, which is known as **renal colic**. As the stone moves along the course of the ureter toward the flank or genital regions, it is highlighted by sudden, periodic (paroxysmal) attacks, between which a constant low-grade pain is felt. Renal

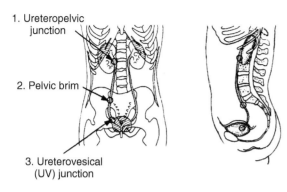

1. Ureteropelvic junction

2. Pelvic brim

3. Ureterovesical (UV) junction

FIG. 7.60 The three points at which kidney stones usually become lodged.

calculi may also cause bleeding (hematuria), fever, chills, frequent urination, and secondary infection. The physician is generally able to distinguish between biliary colic and renal colic because biliary colic usually causes referred pain to the subscapular area or the epigastrium. The probability for recurrent calculus formation is increased by as much as 50% in individuals who develop an initial renal stone; therefore, many patients are placed on a prophylactic regimen such as diuretics, potassium alkali, and increased fluid intake to help reduce their chance of developing further stones.

In most instances, the first treatment is to wait for the stone to pass normally through the urinary system in combination with the administration of antibiotics for the presence of any infection. If the stone is not passed, either lithotripsy of the stone or surgical excision of the cause of obstruction is necessary. SWL is often used to crush calculi less than 2 cm in diameter located in the renal pelvis or ureter. A percutaneous nephrolithotomy may be used to remove larger renal calculi, and ureteroscopy is necessary to remove larger stones within the ureter. Depending on the size of the stone, it may be removed with a special basket catheter, or it may be crushed into smaller pieces by using laser or pneumatic lithotripsy. All of these methods use fluoroscopic guidance.

In addition to the kidneys, other sites of calcification in the urinary tract include the wall of the bladder and, in men, the prostate gland. Calcification of the bladder wall is very rare and is usually caused by calcium deposition in a tumor extrinsic to the bladder, such as a tumor in the ovary or the rectum. Rarely, it may also be on the surface of a bladder tumor. Bladder calculi often cause suprapubic pain. Prostatic calcification (Fig. 7.61 A and B) appears as numerous flecks of calcium of varying

size below the bladder. It does not, however, correlate with either prostatic hypertrophy or carcinoma and usually is of no real significance.

Urinary tract calcifications are sometimes difficult to distinguish from other abnormal calcifications such as gallstones, vascular calcifications, and calcified costal cartilages. To be in the kidney, the calcification must remain within the outline of the kidney on both frontal and oblique projections. In the case of gallstones, oblique projections of the abdomen help demonstrate whether the calculus in question is anterior to the kidney. The pancreas may also demonstrate calcification that usually conforms to its shape (Fig. 7.62).

Degenerative Diseases

Nephrosclerosis

Nephrosclerosis involves intimal thickening of predominantly the small vessels of the kidney. It may occur as a part of the normal aging process and/or in younger patients in association with hypertension and diabetes. Reduced blood flow caused by arteriosclerosis of the renal vasculature causes atrophy of the renal parenchyma. Local infarction may occur, appearing as an irregularity of the cortical margin, usually an indentation. The collecting system of the affected kidney is usually normal, but the kidney itself is decreased in size. Laboratory tests will also demonstrate a gradual increase in BUN and creatinine levels. Other conditions that cause the kidneys to appear smaller than normal include hypoplasia, atrophy after obstruction, and ischemia from large vessel obstruction. Treatment of nephrosclerosis consists of managing the associated hypertension, administration of diuretic agents, and use of proper dietary restrictions (e.g., low-sodium diet).

Renal Failure

Although it can arise acutely, renal failure usually represents the end result of a chronic process such as chronic glomerulonephritis or PKD that gradually results in diminished kidney function. The kidney's normal regulatory and excretory functions become impaired because of loss of glomerular filtration and subsequent deterioration of the renal parenchyma. **Uremia**, which is characteristic of renal failure,

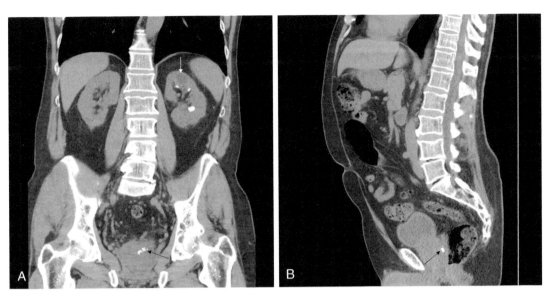

FIG. 7.61 **A,** coronal **B,** sagittal images obtained during a computed tomography (CT stone study protocol show calcifications (*black arrows*) within the prostate gland. There are also renal calculi and a renal cyst (*white arrow*) visible in the left kidney.

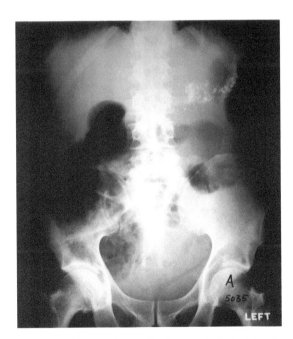

FIG. 7.62 Pancreatic calcification as indicated by the masses of calcium in the left-upper quadrant that conform neatly to the shape of the pancreas.

consists of retention of urea in blood. Although not toxic in itself, urea is normally excreted by the kidneys. Its blood level correlates with retention of other waste products and is thus a measure of the severity of renal failure. Common laboratory findings include a progressive increase in serum creatinine and BUN and a decrease of eGFR. Medical imaging may be requested to locate the cause in cases of acute renal failure. This includes abdominal radiography to rule out urinary calculi and medical sonography or abdominal CT to assess hydronephrosis and kidney size. Renal angiography or radionuclide renal scanning may also be indicated when clinical evaluation suggests a vascular anomaly. A renal biopsy may be necessary if the cause cannot be identified by other, less invasive means. Contrast enhanced studies are contraindicated in patients with renal failure as the contrast media will most likely result in further decline of renal function. However, they are not impossible and can be performed, if medically necessary, using prehydration strategies and/or dialysis after contrast administration. With IVU examination, acute renal failure would manifest as a delayed nephrogram because of markedly delayed excretion of contrast (Fig 7.63). This would likely never be requested in the modern imaging era of readily

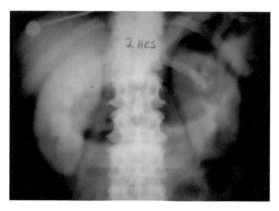

FIG. 7.63 Upper abdominal radiograph obtained 2 hours after IV contrast injection for an intravenous urography (IVU) examination reveals bilateral delayed nephrograms with minimal contrast excretion in the calyces.

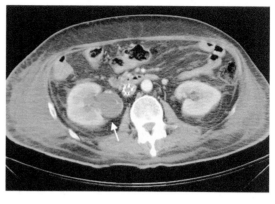

FIG. 7.65 A large hydronephrosis of the right kidney easily identified with computed tomography without the use of a contrast agent.

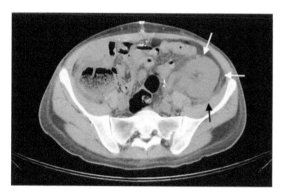

FIG. 7.64 Pelvic computed tomography without contrast enhancement demonstrating the position of a transplanted kidney in the left pelvis.

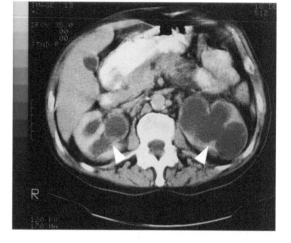

FIG. 7.66 Gross bilateral hydronephrosis as caused by pyelonephritis in this 64-year-old man.

available advanced modalities for renal imaging and routine evaluation of eGFR and creatinine before contrast administration.

The gradual deterioration of renal function brings with it a host of changes in other body systems. The patient experiences moderate anemia, hypertension, heart arrhythmia, congestive heart failure, and other problems related to the body's severe electrolyte and acid–base imbalances. Treatment consists of dialysis and possible transplantation (Fig. 7.64).

Hydronephrosis

Hydronephrosis is an obstructive disorder of the urinary system that causes dilation of the renal pelvis and calyces with urine. In case of longstanding hydronephrosis, the resultant increase in intrarenal pressure

causes ischemia, parenchymal atrophy, and loss of renal function. Although the most common cause of hydronephrosis is a calculus (Fig. 7.65), it may also occur as a congenital defect or because of a blockage of the system by a tumor, stricture, blood clot, or inflammation (Fig. 7.66). Patients with hydronephrosis often complain of pain in their flanks, and their urine may contain blood (hematuria) or pus (pyuria). The long-term changes of hydronephrosis are reversible if the cause of obstruction is relieved early in the process. As in most urinary system pathologies, abdominal sonography is the initial examination of choice because the kidneys do not have to be functioning properly and IV contrast agents are not necessary for the kidneys to be visualized by

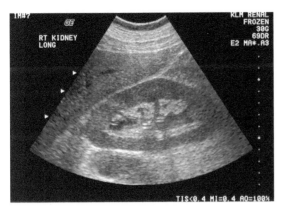

FIG. 7.67 A sonogram of the kidney demonstrating hydronephrosis.

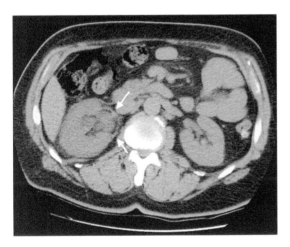

FIG. 7.68 Hydronephrosis of the right kidney demonstrated without contrast enhancement.

sonography (Fig. 7.67). Additional information regarding increased vascular resistance can be obtained using Doppler ultrasonography. Abdominal CT (Fig. 7.68) allows diagnosis of obstruction more than 90% of the time and is the most highly recommended imaging modality when an obstruction is suspected.

Neoplastic Diseases

Masses can cause filling defects in the urinary tract, becoming visible when they stretch and displace the collecting system or form an evident mass. Almost all solitary masses are either malignant tumors or simple cysts. Profuse hematuria resulting from a blood clot also causes a filling defect. The diagnosis of the condition

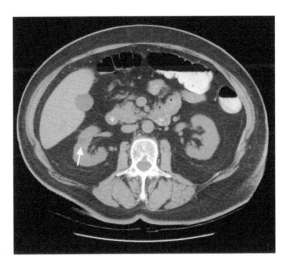

FIG. 7.69 A small, simple cyst on the right kidney demonstrated by an abdominal computed tomography scan without contrast enhancement.

depends on the radiologist's awareness of a history of hematuria. Distinguishing between a blood clot and a tumor is difficult for the physician. However, blood clots tend to have a smooth outline and show change with repeat examinations after treatment.

Renal Cysts

Renal cysts are an acquired abnormality common in adults. It is estimated that more than half of people at age 50 years have renal cysts. Simple cysts may be solitary or multiple and bilateral. They are usually asymptomatic and do not impair renal function, but they may cause symptoms from rupture, hemorrhage, infection, or obstruction. Their pathogenesis is unknown, but obstruction of nephrons by an acquired disease may have a relationship. They are commonly found in a lower pole of the kidney and are readily demonstrated with CT (Fig. 7.69), MRI (Fig. 7.70), and sonography (see Fig. 7.24).

Radiographically, cysts have sharply defined margins and show calyceal spreading, but they can be distinguished from tumors by nephrotomography, in which a cyst shows an absence of a nephrogram phase after contrast medium injection (Fig. 7.71). In contrast, tumors, the majority of which have vascularity, may show irregular opacification during the nephrogram phase. Treatment, if needed, consists of aspiration of the cyst contents. Most cysts are asymptomatic and no treatment is needed.

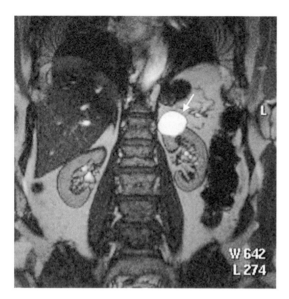

FIG. 7.70 A T2-weighted true fast imaging with steady state precession (True Fisp) magnetic resonance scan of the abdomen demonstrating a renal cyst of the left kidney.

Renal Cell Carcinoma

The most common malignant tumor of the kidney is renal cell carcinoma (RCC), an adenocarcinoma arising from the proximal convoluted tubule. It occurs two to three times more frequently in men than in women, with an increased incidence after age 50 years, and accounts for approximately 2% of adult cancer-related deaths. Its cause is unknown, but chronic inflammation from obstruction, cigarette smoking, obesity, and hypertension are thought to contribute to the development of renal cell carcinoma. The affected patient often first reports hematuria but may also experience flank pain, fever, or a palpable mass. RCC may be an incidental finding on abdominal sonography or abdominal CT.

CT is most useful in demonstrating the density of the renal carcinoma and its degree of metastasis, including extension to adjacent areas and lymph nodes, as well as venous involvement (Fig. 7.72). The ACR recommends abdominal CT with and without contrast or abdominal MRI with and without contrast, for staging and follow-up of renal cell carcinomas (Fig. 7.73). Confirmation of a mass may also be accomplished with IVU. Radiographically, the space-occupying lesion may be evident and may distort, stretch, and displace the kidney's collecting system, as visualized on IVU.

If the carcinoma is caught early, surgical excision of the kidney in combination with chemotherapy provides a significant cure rate. The use of radiofrequency ablation and **cryoablation** therapies in interventional radiology

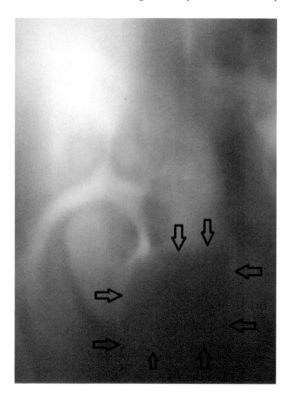

FIG. 7.71 A radiograph of the kidneys obtained utilizing tomography shows a renal cyst in the lower pole of the left kidney. Note the lack of contrast excretion (*black arrows*) in the region of the cyst.

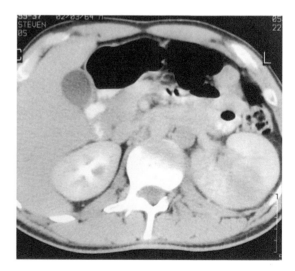

FIG. 7.72 Computed tomography demonstrating a large metastatic lesion in the left kidney of this 25-year-old man with renal adenocarcinoma.

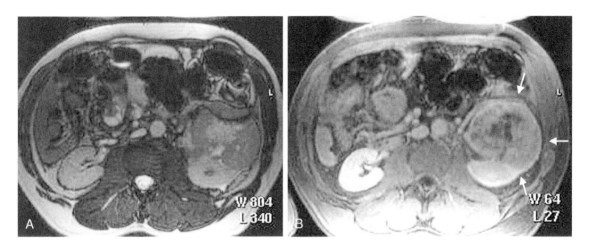

FIG. 7.73 **A,** Axial T2-weighted true fast imaging with steady state precession (True Fisp) magnetic resonance scan of the abdomen demonstrates a mass involving a large portion of the left kidney. **B,** Axial T1-weighted postcontrast image shows the same mass, consistent with renal cell carcinoma. Note the internal necrosis (*arrows*).

TABLE 7.1
Staging of Renal Cell Carcinoma

Stage	Metastasis
I	Tumor confined within kidney capsule ≤7 cm in size
II	Invasion through renal capsule and renal vein but within surrounding fascia ≥7 cm in size
III	Involvement of adrenal glands and vena cava and one nearby lymph node: **T3a–T3c, N0, M0:** The main tumor has reached the adrenal gland, the fatty tissue around the kidney, the renal vein, the large vein (vena cava) leading from the kidney to the heart, or all of these. It has not spread beyond Gerota fascia. No spread to lymph nodes or distant organs has occurred. **T1a–T3c, N1, M0:** The main tumor may be any size and may be located outside of the kidney, but it has not spread beyond Gerota fascia. The cancer has spread to one nearby lymph node but has not spread to distant lymph nodes or other organs.
IV	Distant metastases (e.g., liver and lung) and more than one lymph node: **T4, N0–N1, M0:** The main tumor has invaded beyond Gerota fascia. It has spread to no more than one nearby lymph node. It has not spread to distant lymph nodes or other organs. **Any T, N2, M0:** The main tumor may be any size and may be located outside of the kidney. The cancer has spread to more than one nearby lymph node but has not spread to distant lymph nodes or other organs. **Any T, any N, M1:** The main tumor can be any size and may be located outside of the kidney. It may or may not have spread to nearby lymph nodes. It has spread to distant lymph nodes, other organs, or both.

T, Tumor; *N,* node; *M,* metastasis.
Data from American Cancer Society. Available at http://www.cancer.org/cancer/kidneycancer/detailedguide/kidney-cancer-adult-staging.

is increasing as an alternative to nephrectomy is some patients. In addition, targeted immunotherapies such as interferon and IL-2 are also currently being tested. The tendency of adenocarcinoma to metastasize early from the kidneys poses a serious threat. Staging of the tumor is critical (Table 7.1), as survival is highly dependent on the tumor grade, cell type, and the extent of metastasis. The most common sites of metastasis are the lungs,

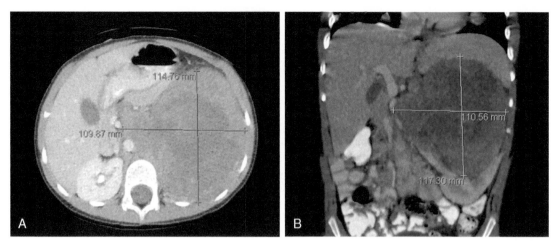

FIG. 7.74 Computed tomography examination of a 3-year-old male with a stage IV Wilms tumor of the left kidney demonstrates a large growth on the **A,** axial and **B,** coronal images.

brain, liver, and bone. Because pulmonary metastases are common, chest radiography should be performed immediately upon discovering a renal carcinoma.

Nephroblastoma (Wilms Tumor)

Nephroblastoma is a malignant renal tumor found in approximately 500 children per year. It is an embryonal tumor that is almost invariably diagnosed before 5 years of age. It is associated with the deletion or inactivation of the *WT1* or *WTX* (X chromosome) tumor suppressor gene and may be inherited or sporadic in origin. Wilms tumor is more common in African Americans than in Caucasians and Asians, and slightly more common in girls than in boys. Children with nephroblastoma often have no symptoms but may have the tumor discovered by a parent or physician who feels a large, palpable abdominal mass. The relative firmness and immobility help distinguish Wilms tumor from hydronephrosis and renal cysts. Diagnostic sonography is also used extensively to differentiate a cystic mass from a solid mass. During urography, the kidneys appear quite enlarged, with marked calyceal spreading—an indication nearly diagnostic of the condition when seen in children. Abdominal CT is the modality of choice for assessing the extent and spread of the tumor (Figs. 7.74, A and B, and 7.75) and has replaced IVU because CT can demonstrate spread to the lymphatics, liver, and the contralateral kidney.

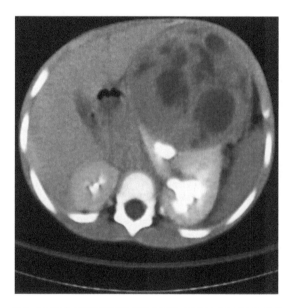

FIG. 7.75 A computed tomography image demonstrates a huge, noncalcified mass arising from the left kidney, as seen in Wilms tumor.

Staging of the tumor is very important (Table 7.2), as the cure rate is very high (95%) for stage I to stage III disease. Left untreated, widespread metastases to the lungs, liver, adrenal glands, and bone occur. Early surgical excision, combined with radiation therapy and chemotherapy, is the most effective treatment.

TABLE 7.2
Staging of Wilms Tumor

Stage	Tumor Characteristics
Stage I (40%–45%)	Tumor limited to the kidney, completely resected
Stage II (20%–25%)	Tumor ascending beyond the kidney or into vessels of renal sinus, but appearing to be totally resected
Stage III (20%–25%)	Residual nonhematogenous tumor confined to the abdomen, positive lymph node in renal hila
Stage IV (10%)	Hematogenous metastases (e.g., lung, liver, bone, brain)
Stage V (5%)	Bilateral disease either at diagnosis or later, but need to stage each kidney

Note: Staging system of the Third National Wilms Tumor Study Group (NWTS-3).
Data from American Cancer Association. Available at http://www.cancer.org/cancer/wilmstumor/detailedguide/wilms-tumor-staging.

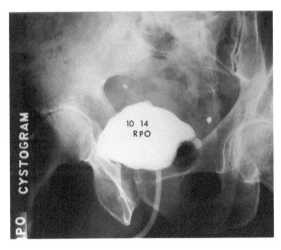

FIG. 7.76 Urothelial carcinoma of the bladder, seen as a space-occupying lesion on this right posterior oblique view of the bladder on a cystogram of a 67-year-old man.

Bladder Carcinoma

Bladder carcinoma is usually seen three times more often in men than in women, particularly after age 60 years. Its cause is clearly related to cigarette smoking and certain industrial chemicals. Bladder carcinoma may be classified as urothelial carcinoma, formerly known as *transitional cell carcinoma* (most frequent), *squamous cell carcinoma* (usually resulting from chronic irritation), or *adenocarcinoma*. Painless hematuria is the main symptom. Tumors are generally small and located in the area of the trigone. IVU or cystography may reveal a filling defect in the bladder (Fig. 7.76), but it is often difficult to distinguish among tumor, stone, and blood clot. Therefore cystoscopy is the method of choice for

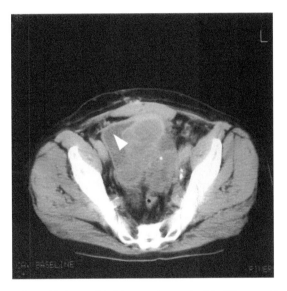

FIG. 7.77 Large bladder carcinoma in this 65-year-old man as seen on computed tomography.

investigation of bladder carcinoma, and diagnosis is made via biopsy or resection. CT (Figs. 7.77 and 7.78), sonography, and MRI are useful in staging the disease once the diagnosis is confirmed.

Treatment depends on the invasiveness of the tumor. Superficial tumors may be treated with transurethral resection or ablation, in combination with chemotherapy and immunotherapy, whereas invasive tumors require resection or total cystectomy with adjuvant chemotherapy, radiation therapy, or a combination of both, depending on the amount of involvement and extent of metastasis. Radiation therapy may also be used for palliative care. With bladder carcinoma, distant metastases usually develop late.

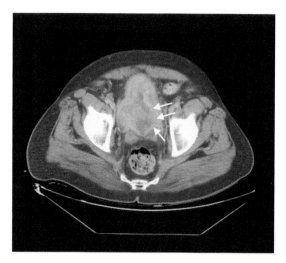

FIG. 7.78 Pelvic computed tomography examination demonstrates an extensive mass in the urinary bladder representing bladder carcinoma.

In the case of total cystectomy, the distal ureters are generally attached into a loop of the bowel (Fig. 7.79), most frequently the ileum (ileal conduit), although cecum or a combination of ileum and cecum may be used. The loop of bowel may be connected to the native urethra (see Fig. 7.30), however, it is usually brought to a stoma at the skin surface known as a urostomy. Some urostomies are incontinent, meaning that the urine drains into an ostomy bag, whereas others are continent and require regular self-catheterization and drainage. A fluoroscopic injection study of this type of anatomy is called a loopogram and it is a retrograde contrast study requiring catheterization of the urostomy and bowel segment (Fig. 7.80). A loopogram may be requested to evaluate for patency of the anastomoses between the ureters and the bowel segment, rule out obstruction, evaluate for postoperative urine leaks or assess for tumor recurrence.

Pathologic Summary of the Urinary System

Pathology	Imaging Modality of Choice
Congenital anomalies	Sonography in the fetus
Lower urinary tract anomalies	Cystography and sonography
Polycystic kidney disease	Sonography, CT with and without contrast, MRI with and without contrast
Medullary sponge kidney	Sonography
Pyelonephritis	IVU, CT with and without contrast, sonography
Cystitis	Abdominal and pelvic CT without contrast, cystography and sonography
Nephrosclerosis	Angiography and sonography
Nephrocalcinosis	Sonography, CT, and KUB
Renal failure	Sonography, CT, and angiography
Calcifications	CT, sonography, KUB
Hydronephrosis	Sonography, CT, and IVU
Renal cyst	Sonography, CT with and without contrast, MRI with and without contrast
Renal cell carcinoma	CT, MRI, and chest radiography
Nephroblastoma	Sonography
	Sonography
Bladder carcinoma	Sonography, MRI, CT, FDG-PET, and cystography

CT, Computed tomography; *FDG-PET,* 18F-fluorodeoxyglucose positron emission tomography; *IVU,* intravenous urography; *KUB,* kidney, ureter, bladder radiography; *MRI,* magnetic resonance imaging.

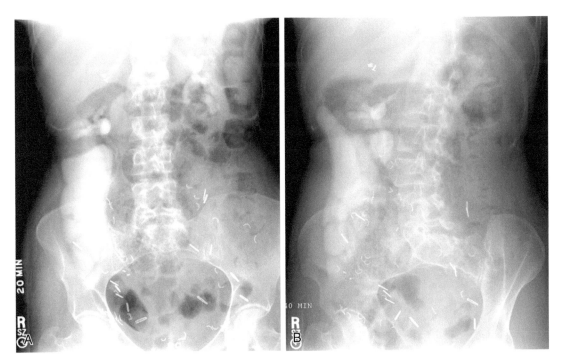

FIG. 7.79 An intravenous urogram of a patient after cystectomy. A portion of the cecum has been formed into a pouch to allow for the collection of urine.

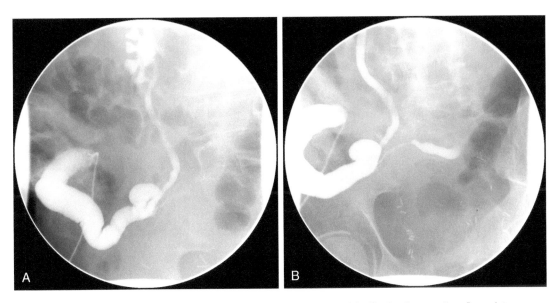

FIG. 7.80 **A,** A loopogram study on a patient with an ileal conduit. Contrast promptly refluxes into the right ureter but not as easily into the left ureter. **B,** A more delayed image demonstrates reflux into the left ureter, which has a long-segment distal stricture.

1. A malignant tumor of the kidney generally occurring in children under 5 years of age is:
   a. Adenocarcinoma
   b. Hypernephroma
   c. Fibroadenoma
   d. Nephroblastoma

2. Which of the following statements are true regarding the anatomy and function of the urinary system?
   1. The amount of urine formed in a typical day is about 1 L to 1.5 L.
   2. Urine is formed and excreted in the nephron, the microscopic unit of the kidney.
   3. The left kidney lies lower than the right because of the spleen's presence above it.
      a. 1 and 2
      b. 1 and 3
      c. 2 and 3
      d. 1, 2, and 3

3. Urinary system disorders may be suggested by an abnormal:
   1. Blood urea nitrogen level
   2. Creatinine blood level
   3. Coloration of urine
      a. 1 and 2
      b. 1 and 3
      c. 2 and 3
      d. 1, 2, and 3

4. Horseshoe kidney is an anomaly of:
   a. Fusion
   b. Number
   c. Position
   d. Size

5. Which of the following statements are true of urinary system anomalies?
   1. Crossed ectopy exists when one kidney lies across the midline, fused to the other.
   2. Nephroptosis and a pelvic kidney are identical conditions.
   3. Ureteroceles are ureteral dilatations near the ureter's termination.
      a. 1 and 2
      b. 1 and 3
      c. 2 and 3
      d. 1, 2, and 3

6. *Vesicoureteral reflux* refers to the backward flow of urine into the:
   a. Bladder
   b. Major calyx
   c. Urethra
   d. Any of the above

7. Arterial and venous renal blood flow in a patient who has received a kidney transplant is best assessed by using:
   a. Computed tomography
   b. Conventional urography
   c. Doppler sonography
   d. Magnetic resonance imaging

8. Which of the following conditions can make the kidneys appear smaller than normal?
   1. Atrophy following obstruction
   2. Chronic pyelonephritis
   3. Hypoplasia
      a. 1 and 2
      b. 1 and 3
      c. 2 and 3
      d. 1, 2, and 3

9. Which of the following procedures would most likely be performed to image a nonfunctioning kidney?
   1. Computed tomography (CT)
   2. Intravenous urography (IVU)
   3. Renal sonography
      a. 1 and 2
      b. 1 and 3
      c. 2 and 3
      d. 1, 2, and 3

10. Gradual and chronic deterioration of the renal parenchyma eventually results in:
    a. Glomerulonephritis
    b. Polycystic kidney disease
    c. Renal calculi
    d. Renal failure

11. Renal failure is characterized by the abnormal retention one of the following substances in blood. Which is it?
    a. Bilirubin
    b. Calcium
    c. Pus
    d. Urea

12. Which of the following statements are true of renal calculi?

    1. Precipitation of solutes out of urine is the pathogenesis of renal calculi.

    2. Renal colic causes referred pain into the subscapular area or epigastrium.

    3. Stones tend to be asymptomatic until they move or cause an obstruction.

        a. 1 and 2

        b. 1 and 3

        c. 2 and 3

        d. 1, 2, and 3

13. Significant dilation of the renal pelvis and calyces as a result of an obstruction from a stone is characteristic of:

    a. Hydronephrosis

    b. Renal failure

    c. Nephroblastoma

    d. Vesicoureteral reflux

14. Which of the following statements are true of neoplastic diseases of the urinary system?

    1. Chronic inflammation from obstruction may result in adenocarcinoma.

    2. Wilms tumor is generally associated with older patients in renal failure.

    3. Early excision of nephroblastoma has shown a very high cure rate.

        a. 1 and 2

        b. 1 and 3

        c. 2 and 3

        d. 1, 2, and 3

15. A patient arrives in the CT department for a contrast-enhanced abdominal examination. What blood laboratory values must be checked before the patient is injected, and what are the maximum values allowed for contrast administration?

16. A delayed image of the abdomen in an IVU routine demonstrates only a portion of the ureters. Is this cause for concern? Why, or why not?

17. How can nephroptosis and a pelvic kidney be differentiated?

18. Identify at least three mechanisms through which bacteria can enter the urinary tract.

19. A 30-year-old pregnant woman presents with fever, flank pain, and general malaise. Although the IVU image looks normal, urinalysis demonstrates pyuria. What might you suspect?

20. In renal failure, what causes the kidney to lose its normal regulatory and excretory functions?

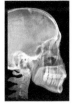
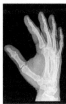
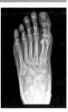

CHAPTER 8

Central Nervous System

e http://evolve.elsevier.com/Kowalczyk/pathology/

KEY TERMS

Acoustic neuroma

Alzheimer's disease

Annulus fibrosus

Astrocytomas

Atherothrombotic brain
  infarction

Blood-brain barrier

Brain abscess

Cervical spondylosis

Craniopharyngioma

Encephalitis

Ependymoma

Glioblastoma multiforme

Gliomas

Anatomy and Physiology

The central nervous system (CNS) includes the brain and the spinal cord. The CNS is composed of neurons (nerve cells) and neuroglia (the interstitial tissue). It extends peripherally through the nerves that carry motor messages via efferent nerves to muscles and sensory messages from the skin and elsewhere back to the spinal cord and brain through the afferent nerves. This chapter concentrates on conditions involving the brain and the spinal cord.

The brain consists of the cerebrum (right and left hemispheres), cerebellum, diencephalon (including the hypothalamus), and brainstem. The brainstem, composed of the midbrain, pons, and medulla oblongata, connects the cerebrum with the spinal cord. The innumerable motor and sensory nerves pass through the brainstem into the spinal cord. The spinal cord originates as an extension of the medulla oblongata at the foramen magnum in the base of the skull. It extends to approximately the level of the first or second lumbar vertebra and terminates with a cone-shaped area called the *conus medullaris* (Fig. 8.1). Spinal nerves beyond this point are referred to as the *cauda equina*.

Both the brain and the spinal cord are covered by the meninges, which consist of three distinct layers (Fig. 8.2). The dura mater is the outermost and is tough and fibrous. It has three major extensions: (1) the falx cerebri,

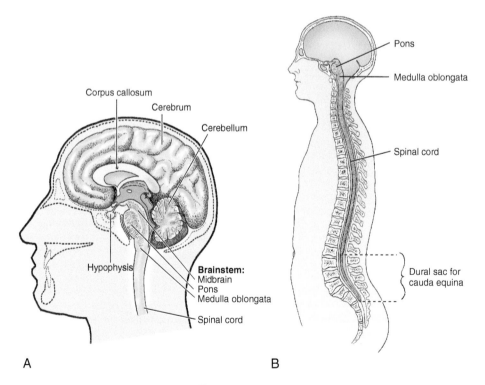

Corpus callosum
Cerebrum
Cerebellum
Hypophysis
Brainstem:
Midbrain
Pons
Medulla oblongata
Spinal cord

Pons
Medulla oblongata
Spinal cord
Dural sac for
cauda equina

A   B

FIG. 8.1 The central nervous system.

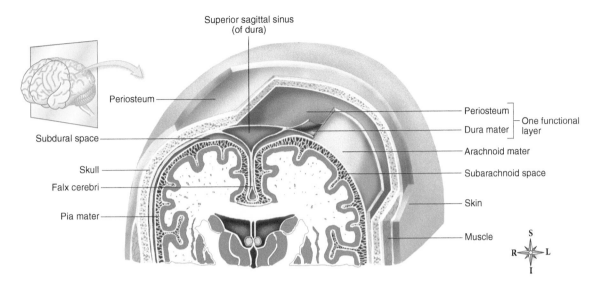

FIG. 8.2 Coronal perspective of meninges and meningeal spaces.

which divides the cerebral hemispheres; (2) the falx cerebelli, which similarly divides the cerebellar hemispheres; and (3) the tentorium cerebelli, which separates the occipital lobe of the cerebrum from the cerebellum. The arachnoid is the middle layer of the meninges and has the appearance of cobwebs. The pia mater is innermost and adheres directly to the cortex of the brain and the spinal cord. The subarachnoid space, at its deepest at the base of the brain, is located between the arachnoid and the pia mater. It is filled with cerebrospinal fluid (CSF) to continuously bathe the brain and the spinal cord with nutrients and to cushion them against shocks and blows. CSF is secreted by the choroid plexus, a network of capillaries located in the brain's ventricles.

The ventricles are four interconnected cavities within the brain. As noted earlier, they house the choroid plexus, which secretes CSF. The right and left lateral ventricles are located in their respective cerebral hemispheres (Fig. 8.3, A and B). They may be further divided into anterior, posterior, and inferior horns, as well as a body and a trigone. CSF flows from the lateral ventricles into the third ventricle via the interventricular foramina (of Monro). The third and fourth ventricles are midline structures connected to each other by the cerebral aqueduct (see Fig. 8.3, C). From there, CSF flows through a median and two lateral foramina (Magendie and Luschka, respectively) into the subarachnoid space surrounding the brain and the spinal cord.

Most of the brain's blood is supplied anteriorly via the bilateral internal carotid arteries and posteriorly via the bilateral vertebral arteries. After entering the cranial vault through the foramen magnum, the vertebral arteries converge to form the basilar artery. The basilar artery and the internal carotid arteries form the circle of Willis (Fig. 8.4) to distribute oxygenated, arterial blood through various branches to all parts of the brain. Venous blood is returned to large venous sinuses in the dura mater, which ultimately drain into the internal jugular veins (Fig. 8.5).

The capillaries that connect the arteries and veins function somewhat differently in the brain than in other organs. In the brain, they prevent passage of unwanted substances into the brain through a special function called the **blood-brain barrier**. This is accomplished in a number of ways, but especially as a result of these capillary cells having a very tight junction that prevents macromolecules and fluids from leaking out into the brain parenchyma. This protects the brain by keeping toxins out, yet it allows for removal of waste products resulting from brain metabolism. These specialized capillaries are found everywhere in the brain except in the pineal and pituitary glands and the choroid plexus. The significance of the blood-brain barrier in terms of imaging is that enhancement of contrast media occurs in the brain where the barrier breaks down from inflammation, ischemia, or neoplastic growth (with its new

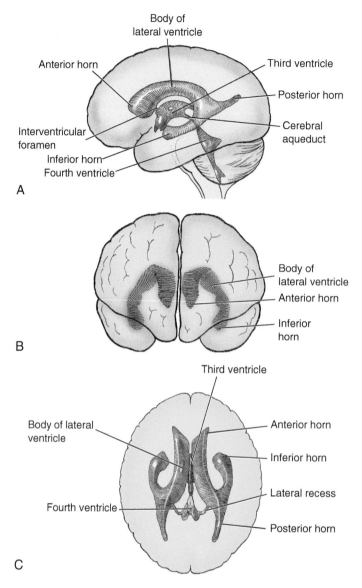

FIG. 8.3 **A,** Lateral and superior views of the lateral ventricles. **B,** A lateral view of the ventricular system. **C,** A superior view of the ventricular system.

vascularity). Also, glucose readily passes over this barrier and is the primary agent used in positron emission tomography (PET).

Neurons are the primary tissue comprising the nervous system, and they may vary greatly in size. At birth, the human body has an excess of neurons, which begin to die if they are not used. The three basic components of a neuron are the cell body, or soma, which is located within the CNS; dendrites, which carry nerve impulses toward the soma; and axons, responsible for carrying impulses away from the cell body. Most neurons have only one axon, which is covered by a delicate web of connective tissue of Schwann cells covered by a myelin sheath. Myelin is a lipid substance that acts as an insulator and assists in nerve impulse transmission. Neuroglia or supporting cells also play a major role in the nervous system

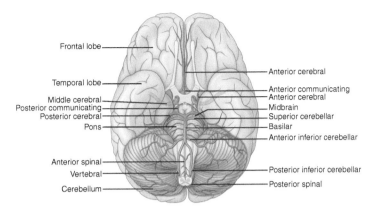

FIG. 8.4 The circle of Willis.

Frontal lobe

Temporal lobe

Middle cerebral
Posterior communicating
Posterior cerebral
Pons

Anterior cerebral
Anterior communicating
Anterior cerebral
Midbrain
Superior cerebellar
Basilar
Anterior inferior cerebellar

Anterior spinal
Vertebral
Cerebellum

Posterior inferior cerebellar
Posterior spinal

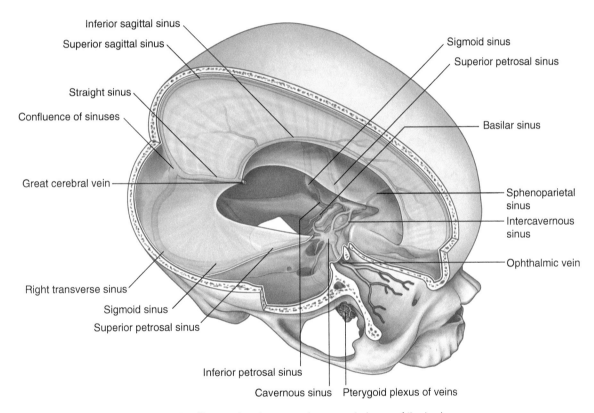

FIG. 8.5 Dura mater sinuses and venous drainage of the brain.

Inferior sagittal sinus
Superior sagittal sinus

Sigmoid sinus
Superior petrosal sinus

Straight sinus

Confluence of sinuses

Basilar sinus

Great cerebral vein

Sphenoparietal sinus
Intercavernous sinus

Ophthalmic vein

Right transverse sinus

Sigmoid sinus
Superior petrosal sinus

Inferior petrosal sinus

Cavernous sinus   Pterygoid plexus of veins

and are much more numerous than neurons. In addition to Schwann cells, neuroglias include astrocytes, oligodendrocytes, ependymal cells, and microglia (Table 8.1).

Although the intervertebral disks are not a part of the CNS, they may come into contact with it when they herniate and impinge on adjacent spinal nerves. Disks cushion the movement of the vertebral column. They are composed of a tough outer covering, known as the **annulus fibrosus**, and a pulpy center called the **nucleus pulposus** (Fig. 8.6).

TABLE 8.1
Support Cells of the Nervous System

Cell Type	Primary Functions
Astrocytes	Form specialized contacts
	Provide rapid transport for nutrients and metabolites
	Believed to form an essential component of the blood-brain barrier
	Appear to be the scar-forming cells of the CNS, which may be the foci for seizures
	Appear to work with neurons in processing information and memory storage
Oligodendroglia (oligodendrocytes)	Formation of myelin sheath and neurilemma in the CNS
Schwann cells (neurolemmocytes)	Formation of myelin sheath and neurilemma in the PNS
Microglia	Responsible for clearing cellular debris (phagocytic properties)
Ependymal cells	Serve as a lining for ventricles and choroid plexuses involved in production of cerebrospinal fluid

CNS, Central nervous system; *PNS,* peripheral nervous system.
From: McCance, K. L., Huether, S. E.: *Pathophysiology: The biologic basis for disease in adults and children,* ed 5, St. Louis, MO, 2006, Mosby.

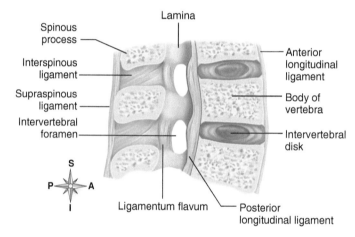

FIG. 8.6 An intervertebral disk.

Imaging Considerations

Radiography

Conventional radiography has largely been reduced in the evaluation of cranial trauma and disease processes because of the increased use of magnetic resonance imaging (MRI) and computed tomography (CT). However, the role of radiography in the evaluation of the spine is considered a common procedure, as described in Chapter 2. A number of conditions that affect the spinal cord can also be readily demonstrated through the use of radiography (Fig. 8.7). The fluoroscopic procedure of myelography has been a staple of radiology for years, allowing visualization of conditions (such as herniated disks) that impinge on the spinal cord. Its role, however, is diminishing because of the significant specificity of MRI in providing detailed images of the spine and spinal cord. When myelography is still performed, it is often followed by a CT myelographic examination of the spine.

Magnetic Resonance Imaging

For a wide variety of conditions related to the CNS, MRI is the modality of choice (Fig. 8.8). Its sensitivity

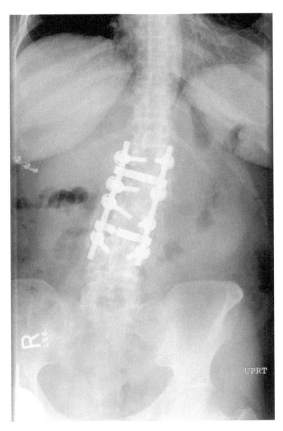

FIG. 8.7 An anteroposterior lumbar spine radiograph showing L1 through L4 fusion with stable hardware in place.

is excellent for the evaluation of all types of spinal diseases, including tumors, abscesses, and disk disease. The ability of MRI to evaluate brain tumors and conditions such as stroke, cranial tumors, and infection surpasses that of CT. Because MRI does not image the dense petrous bone, it is excellent for evaluating the brainstem and anomalies of the posterior fossa (Fig. 8.9). Evaluation of demyelinating disease such as **multiple sclerosis** (MS) is substantively enhanced by MRI. It is, however, important to note that the high sensitivity associated with MRI in the diagnosis of myelopathy may also prove to be a limitation at times. The ease with which MRI studies depict expansion and compression of the spinal cord may potentially lead to false-positive examinations and inappropriately aggressive therapies. These issues can be minimized by experienced observers meticulously correlating clinical and radiologic findings. Despite rapid evolution in technology, MRI

currently has a small role in the evaluation of trauma, mainly limited to evaluation of spinal cord compression and, in some instances, vertebral fractures.

Magnetic resonance angiography (MRA) is used to evaluate the vascular anatomy of the head and neck (Fig. 8.10). It has been proven to accurately locate vascular occlusions within the large arteries of the brain that may lead to a stroke. Magnetic resonance venography (MRV) also demonstrates the major veins and dural sinuses within the brain and plays a large role in the diagnosis and treatment of cerebral venous thrombosis. To date, it has not replaced conventional cerebral angiography, but is often used as an adjunct modality.

Functional MRI (fMRI) may be used to correlate and map motor functions to specific locations in the brain. This procedure identifies neural activation on the basis of hemodynamic changes within the brain. It provides useful information in demonstrating alterations in normal CNS function caused by structural changes in individuals with MS. fMRI is also helpful in identifying the regions of the cortex affected by neoplastic lesions within the brain and in assessing patients with a history of seizures and epilepsy. Currently, researchers are also using this modality to achieve a better understanding of the physiologic basis of autism by seeking information about neuroanatomic and physiologic changes resulting from this disorder.

Diffusion-weighted imaging (DWI) involves monitoring the extent to which water can freely move in any volume element (voxel). When the motion of water molecules within a voxel is restricted, greater magnetization will result, and the associated voxels will appear brighter. Reduced water diffusivity has been correlated with more aggressive tumor behavior and is sometimes seen with high cellular density and tumor recurrence, as well as ischemic stroke (Fig. 8.11). Diffusion-tensor imaging (DTI) capitalizes on the expected relative increase in restricted water molecules among neurologic fiber tracts by acquiring a three-dimensional map of the fiber tracts with a postprocessing technique referred to as *tractography*. The higher information content of the voxels makes DTI extremely sensitive to subtle pathology in the brain, which may be preventing the natural movement of water in the brain.

Perfusion-weighted imaging (PWI) involves the use of paramagnetic contrast agents to assess the cerebral hemodynamic status of a patient. By utilizing acquisition times that are short enough to capture the changes

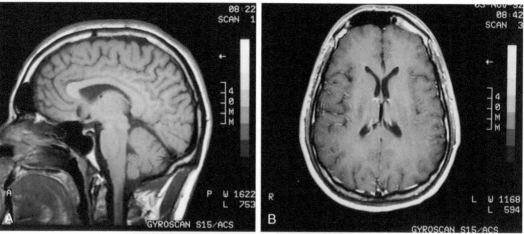

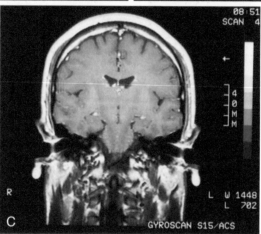

FIG. 8.8 **A,** A normal magnetic resonance image of a young woman with a history of seizures as seen in a sagittal, T1-weighted view without gadolinium contrast. **B,** A normal T1-weighted axial view with gadolinium contrast of the same patient. **C,** A normal T1-weighted coronal view with gadolinium contrast of the same patient.

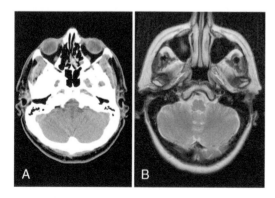

FIG. 8.9 **A,** A computed tomography scan of the posterior fossa region demonstrating the dense petrous portion of the temporal bone and associated artifacts. **B,** A magnetic resonance imaging scan of the posterior fossa region; note how the brain structures are visualized because the bone is not visible.

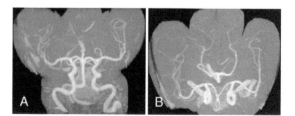

FIG. 8.10 A, A magnetic resonance angiogram (MRA) without contrast enhancement readily showing vasculature within the head and neck. B, An MRA without contrast enhancement demonstrating the circle of Willis within the brain.

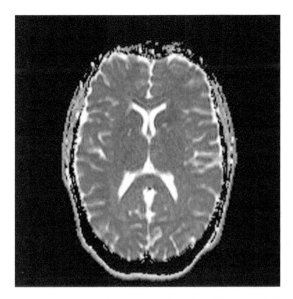

FIG. 8.11 A magnetic resonance imaging diffusion-weighted apparent diffusion coefficient map image of the brain.

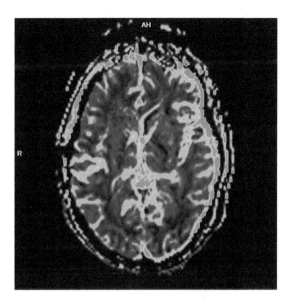

FIG. 8.12 A magnetic resonance imaging perfusion scan of the brain.

in signal intensity as a bolus of contrast material passes through the brain, PWI provides useful information on the vascular supply of various tumors, which is only implied from conventional MRI. The relative cerebral blood volume (rCBV) within a tumor can also be measured and compared with the contralateral normal white matter, typically displayed on color maps. The perfusion curves that are generated provide additional prognostic information by distinguishing between the characteristics of benign and malignant tumors. Investigative studies that are now under way indicate that intraarterial MRI perfusion methods could be useful in better understanding the perfusion characteristics of some tumors and may also be useful in monitoring the delivery of therapeutics (Fig. 8.12).

Computed Tomography

CT continues to play a significant role in the evaluation of the CNS. It is rapid, noninvasive, and reasonably accurate. Because CT has excellent contrast resolution, it readily differentiates among the sulci, ventricles, and the gray and white matter within the brain (Fig. 8.13). It is particularly useful in evaluating cerebral bleeding after trauma because it readily reveals the extent of hematomas, if present. In many institutions, it is common practice to routinely perform CT examinations of the head and neck after significant trauma. CT of

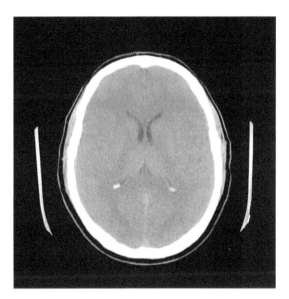

FIG. 8.13 An axial computed tomography scan of a normal brain distinguishing between white and gray matter and demonstrating ventricular anatomy.

the brain is also performed to evaluate the ventricles, as in the case of hydrocephalus; to demonstrate cortical atrophy, as in the case of dementia; and to identify neoplasms within the brain, which may or may not create a mass effect or shifting of the midline of the brain. In

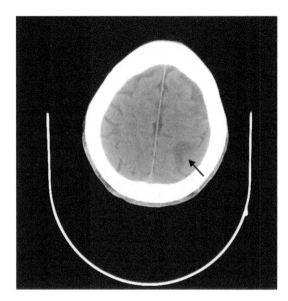

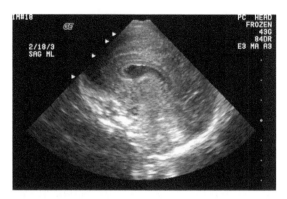

FIG. 8.15 A sonogram of a normal premature neonate head with no evidence of periventricular hemorrhage.

FIG. 8.14 A computed tomography scan of the brain showing a decreased density in brain tissue as a result of infarction.

cases of infarction, edema, abscess, or cyst formation, tissue density is decreased (Fig. 8.14). Tissue density is increased by fresh blood or recent hemorrhage and calcifications within the brain. Other related roles include routine anatomic evaluation such as assessment of shunt (an artificial passageway) functioning and assessment of the bony cerebral and visceral skull. Contrast-enhanced CT of the brain is used to demonstrate anomalies in the cerebral vasculature and to delineate neoplastic growth within the cranial vault. It should be noted, however, that CT-related artifacts that may occur in association with bone at the margins of the posterior fossa often require the use of MRI to optimally evaluate pathology in this region of the brain. As discussed earlier, postmyelographic CT of the spine is also fairly prevalent. CT myelograms demonstrate encroachments of the spinal cord and nerve roots, as does MRI, but bone detail is best visualized with CT. CT is also used to evaluate vertebral fractures, as discussed in Chapter 2.

Sonography

Sonography is useful in evaluating the brains of neonates before closure of the fontanels because the fibrous tissue covering the fontanels provides a ready window into the brain (Fig. 8.15). Sonography readily detects cerebral hemorrhage and hydrocephalus. In premature

infants, brain tissue around the ventricles (periventricular germinal matrix) is prone to hemorrhage, often resulting in intraventricular hemorrhage. In addition, premature infants are at an increased risk for periventricular white matter infarction. Portable sonography is a noninvasive method of evaluating cerebral anatomy and can be performed in the neonatal intensive care unit (NICU) to evaluate the status of affected infants.

Duplex Doppler sonography is a noninvasive modality useful in evaluating carotid blood flow. It demonstrates vascular occlusion and ulceration within the carotid arteries, most commonly at the point of bifurcation. Although it cannot provide the same level of detail compared with traditional angiography or CTA, it is a cost-effective and radiation-free alternative that is useful for evaluating patients experiencing carotid artery transient ischemic attacks (TIAs).

Nuclear Medicine

In nuclear medicine, radionuclide brain scans are primarily used to confirm brain death in patients with the appropriate clinical signs, generally after trauma or an intracranial bleed (Fig. 8.16). Technetium-labeled flow agents in combination with single photon emission computed tomography (SPECT) may be used experimentally to assess tumors, areas of stroke and ischemia, and Alzheimer disease. To complement the more traditional anatomic evaluation of other modalities, PET scanning allows imaging of the body's normal chemical processes and provides physiologic evaluation (Fig. 8.17). In high-risk patients with identified intracranial pathology, PET and SPECT both assist in differentiating tumors from infections.

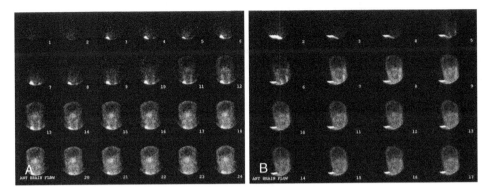

FIG. 8.16 **A,** A portable radionuclide brain scan confirming brain death by the absence of intracranial blood flow. The brain death occurred after an intracranial hemorrhage from preeclampsia in a postpartum woman. **B,** A portable brain scan also confirming brain death in a patient after a subarachnoid hemorrhage.

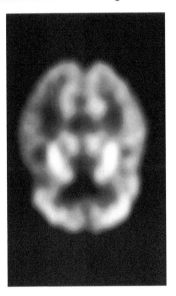

FIG. 8.17 An axial image from a positron emission tomography scan demonstrating an infarct in the posterior left parietotemporal region, with shunting of blood to hypermetabolic basal ganglia.

Vascular and Interventional Radiology

Cerebral angiography is used to demonstrate vessel anatomy within the neck and brain (Fig. 8.18). Because of the increased use of MRA and CT angiography (CTA) vascular studies, conventional angiography is most frequently utilized when an interventional therapeutic procedure is warranted. It is used to diagnose and treat neoplastic lesions, stenosis, aneurysms, arteriovenous malformations (AVMs), and congenital anomalies

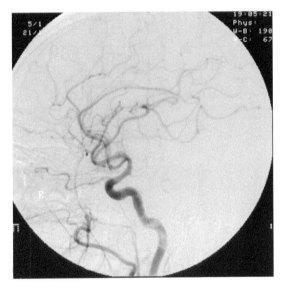

FIG. 8.18 Carotid arteriogram showing vasculature of the head and neck.

of the CNS. Cerebral blood flow may be visualized by placing the catheter in the aortic arch or in selected vessels such as the carotid or vertebral arteries. Therapeutic devices such as stents and shunts and therapeutic medications are also placed by the interventionalist via catheters, often eliminating the need for a more invasive surgical intervention.

Interventional techniques include angioplasty, stent or shunt placement, thrombolysis, or embolization. Percutaneous transluminal angioplasty (PTA) and intraarterial thrombolysis are used to open stenotic vessels and improve blood flow within the vessel treated.

Laser-tipped angioplasty and percutaneous atherectomy may also be performed to open stenotic vessels, especially in the neck. Spheres, coils, or beads are used to embolize or occlude cerebral vasculature, as in the case of aneurysms or AVMs. If an AVM is suspected, contrast-enhanced MRI, MRA, and CTA, as well as traditional myelography images can be utilized to initially identify abnormal spinal vasculature and guide spinal arteriography and intervention, potentially limiting the number of direct vascular injections required.

Congenital and Hereditary Diseases

Meningomyelocele (Spina Bifida)

As mentioned in Chapter 2, spina bifida is a condition in which the bony neural arch that encloses and protects the spinal cord is not completely closed (Fig. 8.19). It most commonly occurs in the lumbar region, and the spinal cord and its meninges may or may not herniate through the resultant opening. Elevated α-fetoprotein (AFP) levels in the mother's blood and during amniocentesis may allow spina bifida to be diagnosed prenatally. The defect and soft tissue sac are confirmed with fetal sonography. Complications depend on the extent of protrusion and range from treatable to life-threatening. Any opening of the sac to the exterior of the body risks meningeal infection, so surgical closure is critical. If only the meninges protrude, the condition is termed a **meningocele** (Fig. 8.20). These are treated surgically without difficulty and usually have an excellent prognosis. A **myelocele** is a protrusion of the spinal cord, minus its meningeal coverings, which may also be treatable surgically. A **meningomyelocele** is the most common and most serious of possible conditions, affecting approximately one in every 800 infants and

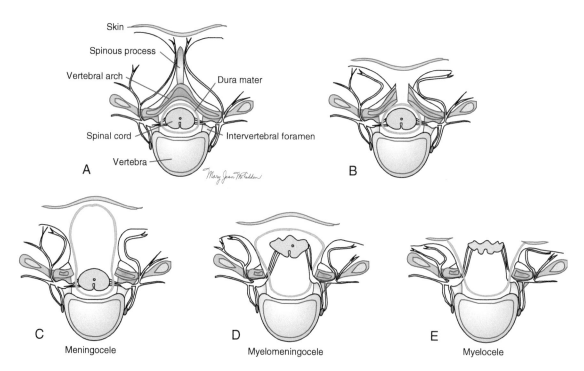

FIG. 8.19 **A normal neural arch in comparison with congenital defects. A,** Normal. **B,** Spina bifida occulta. The median segment of the vertebral arch is missing and covered by skin. **C,** Meningocele. The arch is mostly absent with a bulging dura; however, the spinal cord remains in the vertebral canal. **D,** Myelomeningocele with a deformed spinal cord within the protruding dural sac. **E,** Myelocele: the area is totally exposed.

consisting of a protrusion of both the meninges and the spinal cord into the skin of the back (Figs. 8.21 and 8.22). Affected patients often have severe neurologic deficits, the extent of which depends on the level of herniation. Associated neurologic difficulties include paraplegia and diminished control of the lower limbs, bladder, and bowel. Hydrocephalus may affect as many as 90% of children diagnosed with meningomyelocele.

Some structural anomalies of the brain have been associated with the presence of meningomyelocele, in which MRI techniques have proven useful for further evaluation. One such example is the use of DTI to demonstrate the compromised integrity of some specific white matter pathways. Other structural anomalies that may be identified with MRI include cerebellar hyperplasia and altered development of the corpus callosum and posterior fossa.

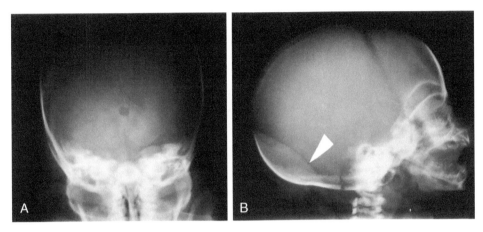

FIG. 8.20 **A,** The circular defect seen in the middle of the occipital bone of this newborn is the site of a meningocele. **B,** A lateral skull radiograph demonstrates the soft tissue density associated with the meningocele superimposed over the occipital bone.

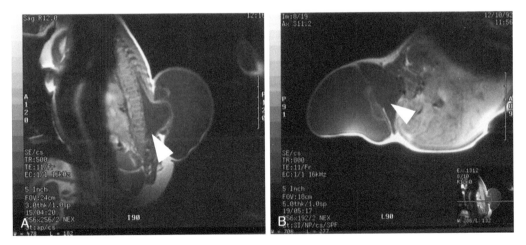

FIG. 8.21 **A,** A T1-weighted sagittal magnetic resonance imaging (MRI) view without gadolinium in this newborn readily demonstrates a meningomyelocele, with the arrow indicating the herniated spinal cord. **B,** A T1-weighted axial MRI view without gadolinium in the same patient similarly demonstrates the meningomyelocele, with the arrow indicating the herniated spinal cord.

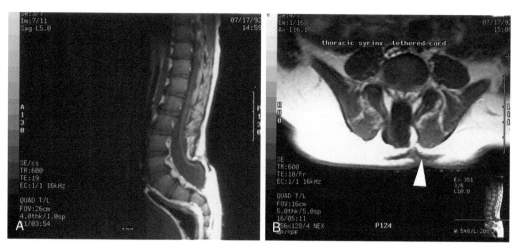

FIG. 8.22 **A,** A T1-weighted sagittal magnetic resonance imaging (MRI) view without gadolinium in this infant demonstrates a surgically repaired meningomyelocele. **B,** A T1-weighted axial MRI view without gadolinium similarly demonstrates the surgically repaired meningomyelocele, with the arrow pointing to the surgical site.

Hydrocephalus

Normally CSF flows around the spinal cord and over the convexity of the brain before reabsorption into the venous sinuses. This normal circulation may be interrupted by causes such as an obstruction to flow (noncommunicating hydrocephalus) and impaired absorption (communicating hydrocephalus); increased CSF production may also disturb normal circulation. The ventricles then distend proximal to the site of obstruction, which results in compression atrophy of the brain tissue around the dilated ventricles. In such cases, the sulci are obliterated and the gyri are flattened. **Hydrocephalus** refers to an excessive accumulation of CSF within the ventricles and can be either congenital or acquired.

In noncommunicating hydrocephalus, an obstruction may occur congenitally or result from tumor growth, trauma (hemorrhage), or inflammation. It interferes with or blocks normal CSF circulation from the ventricles to the subarachnoid space. It is also commonly associated with malformations of the posterior fossa such as Arnold-Chiari malformation, which is a congenital defect in which the cerebellar tonsils are displaced downward below the level of the foramen magnum and are clearly visible on a sagittal T1-weighted image during an MRI examination of the brain.

Poor reabsorption of CSF by arachnoid villi results in communicating hydrocephalus. It may arise from a number of factors, including increased ICP caused by tumor compression, raised intrathoracic pressure impairing venous drainage, inflammation from meningitis, or subarachnoid hemorrhage. Hydrocephalus may also occur from overproduction of CSF, although this is the least common cause.

CT and MRI provide excellent visualization of hydrocephalus (Fig. 8.23). In neonates, sonography is used to demonstrate the ventricular system through the infant's fontanels, which permit passage of the beam until their eventual closure. Treatment may consist of surgery. In some cases, a shunt is surgically inserted to divert excess fluids. Placed between the ventricles and the internal jugular vein, the heart, or the peritoneum, it drains excess CSF. The shunt contains a one-way valve to prevent the backflow of blood into the ventricles. Radiographs are taken to demonstrate shunt placement after insertion (Fig. 8.24) and CT is used for periodic follow-up to evaluate ventricular size, which indirectly allows for the assessment of shunt function.

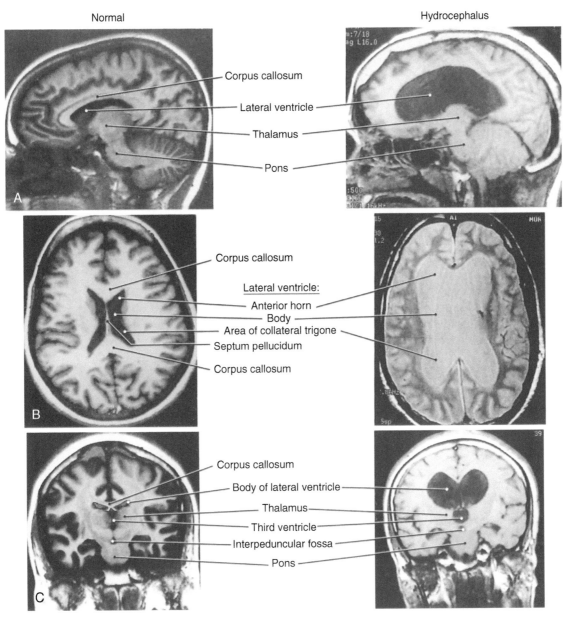

Normal · Hydrocephalus

Corpus callosum

Lateral ventricle

Thalamus

Pons

A

Corpus callosum

Lateral ventricle:

Anterior horn

Body

Area of collateral trigone

Septum pellucidum

Corpus callosum

B

Corpus callosum

Body of lateral ventricle

Thalamus

Third ventricle

Interpeduncular fossa

Pons

C

FIG. 8.23 Comparison of normal and hydrocephalic brains. **A,** sagittal image. **B,** axial image. **C,** coronal image.

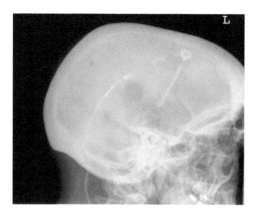

FIG. 8.24 A lateral projection of the skull showing ventriculojugular shunt placement.

Inflammatory and Infectious Diseases

Meningitis

An inflammation of the meningeal coverings of the brain and spinal cord is termed **meningitis**. It may be caused by bacteria, viruses, or other organisms that reach the meninges from elsewhere in the body via blood or lymph, or it may occur as a result of trauma and penetrating wounds, or from adjacent structures (e.g., the mastoids) that become infected. Bacterial infection is the most common cause of meningitis (Fig. 8.25). Pathogens responsible for acute bacterial meningitis include meningococci, streptococci, and pneumococci.

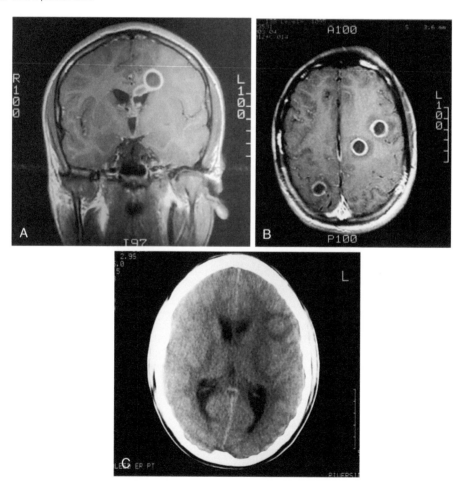

FIG. 8.25 **A,** A T1-weighted coronal magnetic resonance imaging (MRI) view with gadolinium demonstrates a ring lesion that communicates with the left lateral ventricle in this 17-year-old boy, creating meningitis as a result of transplantation into the brain of a bacterial (*Staphylococcus*) infection. **B,** A T1-weighted axial MRI view with gadolinium of the same patient demonstrates the presence of multiple infectious lesions. **C,** An axial computed tomography view of the same patient demonstrates the presence of an infectious lesion and slightly widened ventricles, as characteristic of meningitis.

These are pus-forming (pyogenic) types of bacteria and they may be carried to the meninges via the middle ear or the frontal sinus. Meningococcal meningitis is most common in infants, streptococcal meningitis in children, and pneumococcal meningitis in the adult population. In addition, a few cases result from infection by the tubercle bacillus *Mycobacterium tuberculosis*, which is not a pus-forming pathogen. This type of bacterial meningitis is more difficult to diagnose because it does not have the same acute symptoms as those of the other types of bacterial meningitis. Tuberculous meningitis is usually spread from the lung in association with miliary tuberculosis.

In cases of bacterial meningitis, CSF is under increased pressure and may contribute to hydrocephalus. Acute bacterial meningitis may follow an upper respiratory infection or a sore throat. Symptoms include fever, headache, stiff neck, vomiting, and changes in consciousness, with the patient becoming severely ill within 24 hours. Because bacterial meningitis can become lethal within a short period, accurate and immediate diagnosis and treatment are imperative. The primary means of diagnosing meningitis is the increased ICP detectable via the results of a lumbar puncture (spinal tap) procedure. During laboratory examination, CSF contains both bacteria responsible for the infection and a large number of polymorphonuclear leukocytes (pus cells).

A brain CT or MRI may be performed before the lumbar puncture to rule out the presence of abnormalities such as a midline shift of the central brain structures secondary to a brain mass or intracranial hemorrhage. If a mass or hemorrhage is present, it should be assumed that an increase in ICP exists; therefore, a lumbar puncture is contraindicated because of the risk of subsequent further CNS pressure changes and potential herniation of brain tissue. Antibiotics, in particular, have been very successful against many forms of meningitis and antibiotic therapy may begin before a definite diagnosis has been established. If antibiotic therapy is started early, the mortality rate from bacterial meningitis is less than 10%. Contrast-enhanced MRI scans help identify subarachnoid inflammation and inflammation of the mastoids or sinuses. CT scans may also be helpful in assessing the presence of pathologic skull fractures or a brain abscess.

Chronic meningitis is most commonly caused by fungi and is often seen in patients with acquired immunodeficiency syndrome (AIDS) or in individuals undergoing immunosuppressant drug therapy. The symptoms are similar to those associated with acute meningitis; however, unlike in acute meningitis, the symptoms of chronic meningitis occur over weeks rather than days. Treatment depends on the infecting agent, with amphotericin B being the preferred drug for all fungal infections. Although the disease may progress at a slower rate, the outcome may still be fatal.

Encephalitis

An infection of the brain tissue is termed encephalitis. In contrast to meningitis, which is most frequently a bacterial infection, encephalitis is usually viral in nature (Fig. 8.26) and may also occur subsequent to conditions such as chickenpox, smallpox, influenza, and measles. Primary viral encephalitis may be caused by the arbovirus transmitted by mosquitoes during warm weather or by herpes simplex virus. The symptoms and signs most commonly associated with encephalitis are headache, malaise, and coma. This condition is more serious than meningitis because individuals who acquire encephalitis more frequently develop permanent neurologic disabilities. The viral infection results in cerebral edema with numerous hemorrhagic spots scattered throughout the cerebral hemispheres, brainstem, and cerebellum.

MRI is especially valuable because it can detect brain inflammation earlier compared with CT, nuclear medicine studies, or electroencephalography (EEG). MRI can also rule out other anomalies such as a brain abscess or a subdural empyema or hematoma, which may mimic the clinical signs associated with viral encephalitis.

Herpes simplex encephalitis is treated with the antiviral medication acyclovir. Survival rates depend on the cause of the disease. In some instances, it may be fatal.

Brain Abscess

A brain abscess is an encapsulated accumulation of pus within the cranium resulting from a cranial infection, a penetrating head wound, or an infection spread through the bloodstream. A brain abscess may also result from the direct spread of organisms associated with a complicated case of sinusitis, chronic otitis, or mastoiditis. The symptoms are similar to those of encephalitis and include fever, headache, nausea and vomiting, seizures, and personality changes. An early diagnosis of a brain abscess or of cerebritis, which is

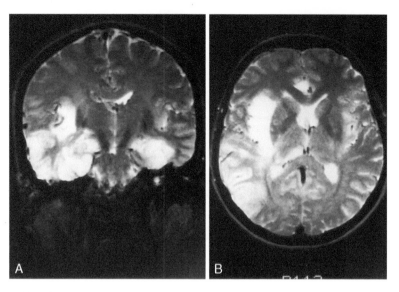

FIG. 8.26 A, A T2-weighted coronal magnetic resonance imaging (MRI) view demonstrates the infectious response in the brain of this boy with herpes encephalitis. **B,** A T2-weighted axial MRI view demonstrates the extent of the infectious process in the same patient with herpes encephalitis.

its earlier stage, guides appropriate treatment, including careful selection of antibiotics, drainage of the abscess cavity, and correction of the original source of the infection, particularly if the abscess is secondary to a sinus or middle ear infection. Brain abscesses are fatal unless they are treated with antibiotic therapy. The specific antibiotic agent depends on the infecting organism and treatment lasts approximately 4 to 8 weeks (Fig. 8.27).

The diagnosis of a brain abscess is usually made by CT or MRI evaluation of the brain. Since the introduction of CT, the overall mortality rate from abscesses has decreased from more than 40% to less than 5%. Serial CT examinations are often performed during antibiotic therapy to assess the progression of treatment. Although it is less sensitive than CT for detecting small calcifications related to brain abscesses, MRI provides greater sensitivity in the assessment of intracranial abscesses and may be more specific. The demonstration of a mature abscess seen by MRI includes shortening of the T1 and T2 relaxation times in the abscess wall, which results in hyperintensity on T1-weighted and hypointensity on T2-weighted images. However, the CT or MRI appearance of such a lesion is not specific enough to preclude histologic confirmation before initiation of treatment.

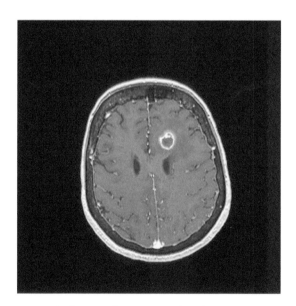

FIG. 8.27 A magnetic resonance imaging scan demonstrating a brain abscess.

If pus associated with the abscess accumulates within the meningeal layers between the dura mater and the arachnoid, it is termed a **subdural empyema**. Like brain abscesses, subdural empyemas are diagnosed with CT or MRI of the brain. Symptoms are the same as those of a brain abscess; however, subdural empyemas require immediate drainage. After drainage, the patient is treated with antibiotic therapy similar to that used for brain abscesses.

Degenerative Diseases

Degenerative Disk Disease and Herniated Nucleus Pulposus

A **herniated nucleus pulposus**, or herniated disk, may result from either degenerative disease (Fig. 8.28) or trauma. A weakened or torn annulus fibrosus is subject to rupture, which allows the nucleus pulposus to protrude and compress spinal nerve roots. The disk may prolapse in any direction and, in some instances, may not produce pain. However, pressure may be placed on the spinal cord as the nucleus pulposus spreads beyond its normal confines posteriorly (Fig. 8.29), resulting in pain along the course of adjacent nerve roots and a weakening of the muscles supplied by these nerves. The most common locations for disk herniation are in the lower cervical and lower lumbar regions. In the lumbar region, over 80% occur at the L5–S1 nerve roots, and in the cervical region, C6–C7 herniations are most common.

Symptoms may include a sudden and severe onset of pain in the distribution of the compressed nerve root, in combination with weakened muscles, although at times symptoms may be more insidious. Compression of the nerve roots in the cervical area causes pain in the neck and upper extremities, whereas compression in the lumbar area results in pain of the hip, posterior thigh, calf, and foot. The extent of nerve root compression may be demonstrated through myelography, CT, and MRI, with MRI remaining the imaging modality of choice (Fig. 8.30). Patients with complicated lower back pain can be evaluated for edema associated with facet arthropathy through the use of short-tau inversion recovery (STIR) and fat-saturated T2 spin-echo pulse sequences. In postoperative patients, contrast-enhanced MRI studies allow for a distinction between vertebral disks and scar tissue that extends beyond the vertebral interspace. It should also be noted that with normal aging, the nucleus pulposus tends to dehydrate, and the change in water content is well demonstrated on the basis of subsequent alteration in MRI relaxation times.

CT scans provide superior bone detail but are not as useful in depicting extradural soft tissue pathologies such as disk disease compared with multiplanar MRI. Myelography examinations are usually combined with postmyelography CT. The combined study serves as a complement to standard CT or MRI and occasionally leads to a more accurate diagnosis of disk herniation. Myelography may also be useful in surgical planning, with weight-bearing and flexion-extension views aiding in a comprehensive image-guided assessment.

Diskography is a radiographic technique that evaluates the vertebral column after injection of radiopaque material into an intervertebral disk of interest. This examination may have a role in localizing the source of back pain that cannot be defined with other less invasive studies, as well as in patients with multifocal abnormalities seen by MRI. Although radiography, MRI, and postinjection CT may depict nonspecific aging or degenerative changes, the diskography injection itself may reproduce or provoke the patient's pain, which can be of diagnostic value. Used alone, diskography has limited specificity in disease diagnosis; however, recent research indicates that certain signal intensity changes seen by MRI may have a high positive predictive value in identifying pain generation during the diskography examination.

Physical therapy and analgesics are used as treatment, with 95% of patients recovering within 3 months without surgical intervention. If these fail to relieve pain, microscopic diskectomy, surgical decompression, or laminectomy with spinal fusion may be performed.

Cervical Spondylosis

Osteoarthritic conditions may also affect the vertebral column, leading to nerve disorders caused by chronic nerve root compression. These osteoarthritic changes of the neck are referred to as **cervical spondylosis** and are well demonstrated radiographically, most notably on an oblique projection of the cervical spine. Osteophytes (bone spurs) form in the articular facets of the cervical vertebrae and compress the nerves located in the intervertebral foramina. They may also compress the spinal cord (Fig. 8.31).

The ability of MRI to depict the spinal cord directly and assess its contour and internal signal characteristics reliably and noninvasively has resulted in general acceptance of MRI as the study of choice in evaluating cervical myelopathy, especially in cases of suspected

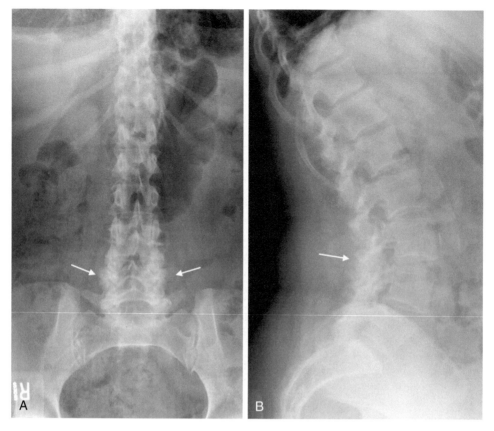

FIG. 8.28 **A,** An anteroposterior projection of the lumbar spine demonstrating degenerative joint disease of the lower lumbar spine. **B,** A lateral lumbar projection of the same patient as in *A*.

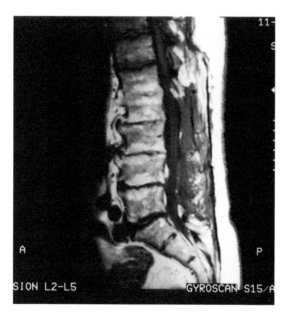

FIG. 8.29 A T1-weighted sagittal magnetic resonance imaging view of the spine in this 75-year-old man readily demonstrates severe degenerative disk disease as well as fusion of L1 and L2.

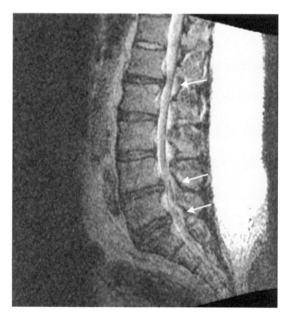

FIG. 8.30 A sagittal magnetic resonance image demonstrating degenerative disk disease in the lumbar vertebral column.

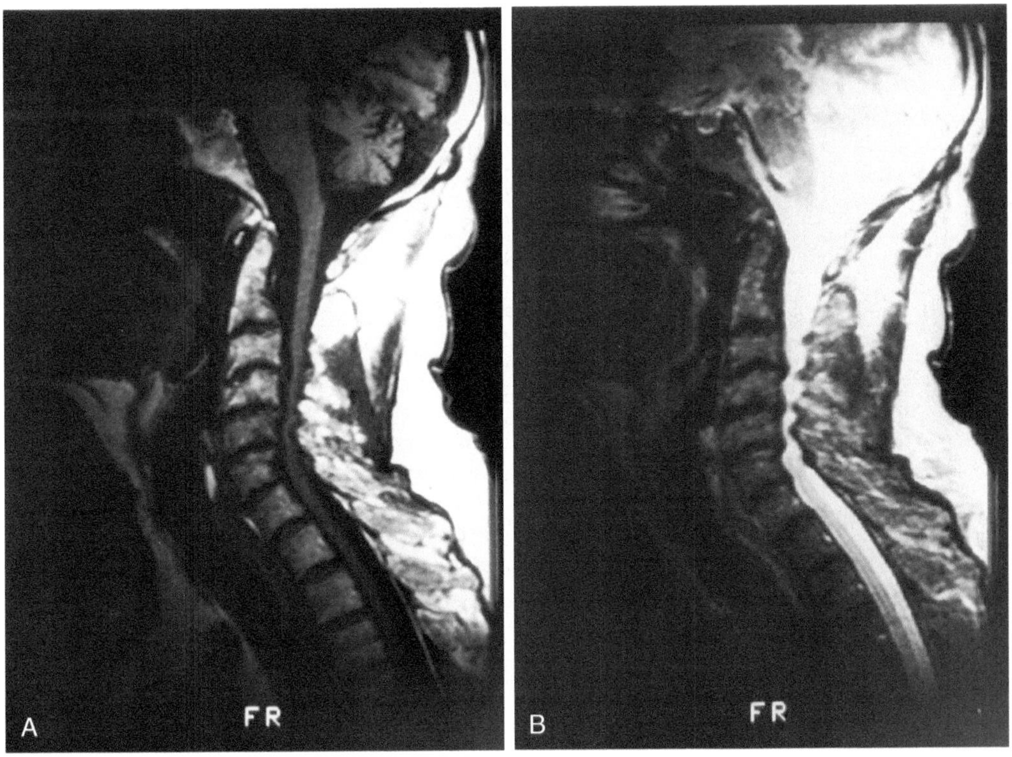

FIG. 8.31 **A,** A T1-weighted sagittal magnetic resonance imaging (MRI) view demonstrates compression of the spinal cord in this older man with cervical spondylosis. Cerebrospinal fluid (CSF) is dark adjacent to the gray spinal cord. **B,** A T2-weighted sagittal MRI image indicates the constriction of CSF flow (white) at C2 through C5.

spondylosis. Current research indicates that bone scintigraphy SPECT imaging, followed by a limited CT if scintigraphy is positive, has been found to be more sensitive than MRI; however, this imaging protocol has yet to be adopted in routine clinical practice. When MRI is contraindicated, or is unavailable, or to answer specific questions before surgical intervention, cervical myelography and CT myelography may be useful. Standard CT imaging, with multiplanar reformatted sagittal and coronal planes, is also useful in depicting bone structural problems related to spondylosis and in the postsurgical evaluation process.

As with degenerative disk disease, treatment is conservative at first but may include laminectomy and decompression procedures.

Multiple Sclerosis

MS, a chronic, progressive disease of the nervous system, most commonly affects individuals between the ages of 20 and 40 years. It affects women more often than men. The etiology of this disease is unknown, but research indicates that it may result from a latent herpesvirus or retrovirus infection. It also appears more often in individuals living in a temperate climate than in those living in a tropical environment. Although the disorder does not exhibit a defined inheritance pattern, 15% of individuals diagnosed with MS have an affected relative. Furthermore, a single gene, *DR2*, is implicated in this potential genetic susceptibility. MS involves the degeneration of the myelin sheath covering the nervous tissue of the spinal cord and the white matter within the brain. This demyelination impairs nerve conduction, beginning with muscle impairment and loss of balance and coordination. As MS progresses, tremors, vision impairment, and urinary bladder dysfunction develop, along with continued weakening of muscles. Numerous patchy areas of demyelinated nerves develop, forming scar tissue or sclerotic lesions throughout the nervous

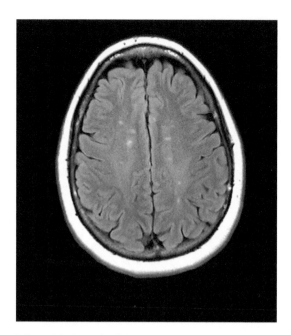

FIG. 8.32 An axial fluid-attenuated inversion recovery (FLAIR) magnetic resonance imaging (MRI) scan from a patient with known multiple sclerosis (MS). The examination demonstrates MS plaques on the white matter of the brain.

system. These scars are called *MS plaques* and present as multiple oval periventricular regions of increased T2 signal intensity, making MRI the modality of choice for evaluating individuals with suspected MS (Fig. 8.32). In cases of established MS diagnoses, contrast-enhanced MRI aids in differentiating new onset of active inflammation from older brain plaques by demonstrating ring enhancement of the newer lesions. Other MRI features of MS include generalized cerebral volume loss and lesions involving the corpus callosum and the optic nerve. On occasion, the use of advanced MRI techniques such as diffusion imaging, spectroscopy, perfusion imaging, and magnetization transfer imaging may be useful in supporting, though not establishing, a diagnosis of MS. fMRI may also be used to assess alterations in normal CNS function resulting from structural changes within the brain.

MS runs a long and unpredictable course, eventually leading to permanent neurologic disabilities. Except in severe cases, however, the patient's life span is not shortened by MS. Patients may be placed on corticosteroids to shorten the symptomatic periods, but

long-term use of corticosteroids is contraindicated. Interferon-β is a more promising drug that has also been used to reduce the frequency of symptomatic periods, and it may actually delay the progression of the disease. Most patients benefit from regular exercise, alterations in diet, and physical therapy in conjunction with medications to reduce muscle spasticity and improve range of motion.

Dementia

Dementia is a disease of impairment of several higher cortical functions in the brain as a result of anatomic changes within the brain. Forms of dementia include Alzheimer's disease (AD), vascular dementia, dementia with Lewy bodies, and frontotemporal dementia (Table 8.2).

The most prevalent of these is **Alzheimer's disease**, which the sixth leading cause of death in the United States. The number of people with the Alzheimer's disease doubles every 5 years in individuals aged 65 years or more and it is more common in females than males. Involving the prefrontal cortex and medial temporal lobe, Alzheimer's is a progressive neurodegenerative disorder beginning with mild memory loss and progressing to the loss of an individual's ability to respond to his/her surroundings. The etiology of Alzheimer's disease is unknown and most cases in adults over the age of 65 years are sporadic. However, 15% of cases in individuals under the age of 65 years with early-onset Alzheimer's disease are autosomal dominant caused by known genetic mutations. Mutations have been identified in the amyloid precursor proteins (APP) on chromosome 21, presenilin I and presenilin II located on chromosome 14 and chromosome 1, respectively. Alterations in chromosome 19 that influence β-amyloid deposition, cytoskeletal integrity, and efficiency of neuronal repair have also been identified in individuals with late onset Alzheimer's disease. The pathology associated with Alzheimer's disease results in the development of extracellular deposits of β-amyloid, referred to as senile plaques, and neurofibrillary tangles in the cerebral cortex and subcortical gray matter. As the development of these plaques and tangles progress, synapses and neurons are destroyed, which decreases acetylcholine and other neurotransmitters. These changes lead to a decline in memory and cognitive function. Anatomically, the affected parts of the brain demonstrate widening the sulci and thinning

TABLE 8.2
Common Types of Degenerative Dementia

Type	Molecular Mechanism	Pathology	Mental Status	Neurobehavior
Alzheimer's Disease	Amyloid β protein (AB)	Amyloid plaques, neurofibrillary tangles; neural and synaptic loss in the brain	Memory loss, disorientation to place and time; loss of facial recognition	Initially normal; progressive cognitive, language, abstraction, and judgment impairment
Vascular dementia	Not applicable	Single or multiple infarcts or cerebral bleeds	Frontal/executive, cognitive slowing; memory can be intact	Often, but not always sudden, usually within 3 months of a stroke; variable apathy, falls, focal weakness, delusions, anxiety
Lewy body dementia	Autosomal dominant: α-synuclein	Neuronal degeneration, α-synuclein inclusions (Lewy bodies)	Initially affects concentration and attention, followed by memory and cognition loss; unpredictable levels of ability, attention, and alertness; delirium prone	Visual hallucinations, depression, sleep disorder, delusions, transient loss of consciousness
Frontotemporal dementia	Abnormal tau protein; mutation of chromosome 17q 21 to chromosome 22	Tauopathy; gene mutations affecting the microtubule binding tau proteins	Language loss including speech and loss of understanding of language, often preceding memory loss	Loss of empathy; apathy; increases inappropriate social conduct; loss of judgment and resonating; euphoria; depression

Adapted from Table 17.13 The Molecular Basis for Degenerative and Table 17.14 Clinical Differentiation of the Major Degenerative Dementias. McCance, K. L., Huether, S. E.: *Pathophysiology: The biologic basis for disease in adults and children,* ed 7, St. Louis, MO, 2014, Mosby.

the gyri, eventually leading to atrophy. The most common areas affected by Alzheimer's disease include the frontal and temporal lobes of the cerebrum. Biomarkers for Alzheimer's disease include a low level of β-amyloid in the cerebrospinal fluid and β-amyloid deposits identified by an amyloid PET scan, which use radioactive tracers that specifically bind to β-amyloid. The cognitive decline with Alzheimer's disease is not reversible with a progressive worsening of memory and other cognitive functions. The average survival time from diagnosis is 7 years.

Vascular dementia is caused by a disruption of blood flow to the brain. It may result from multiple, small cerebral infarcts or bleeds, or from a single cerebral episode. Those occurring from multiple episodes tend to progress in distinct steps, unlike other types of dementia. The 5 year mortality rate of 65% associated with vascular dementia is much higher than those associated with other forms of dementia, in part because of other existing vascular pathologies.

Lewy body dementia is associated with late stage Parkinson's disease. **Parkinson's disease** is a complex neurologic disease resulting from degeneration of the basal ganglia and dopamine-secreting pathways affecting both motor and nonmotor neurologic functions. **Lewy bodies** are abnormal cellular inclusions in the cytoplasm of cortical neurons composed of aggregates of a synaptic protein with an unknown function called α-synuclein. This protein naturally occurs in the healthy brain and helps with neurotransmission. However, with this disorder, an abnormal mutation of α-synuclein forms in clumps within particular areas of the brain eventually killing the affected neurons. Approximately 40% of late stage Parkinson's disease patients over the age of 70 years develop this type of dementia, affecting over 1 million patients in the United States. Symptoms include fluctuating cognitive function primarily affecting alertness more than memory. Individuals with Lewy body dementia often stare into space for long periods of time, are excessively drowsy, often have vivid visual hallucinations, and demonstrate behavioral disturbances. Most individuals live an average of 5 to 7 years following diagnosis, but some individuals may live up to 20 years following the development of this disease. Definitive diagnosis of Lewy body dementia requires autopsy samples of brain tissues.

Frontotemporal dementia, also known as Pick disease, affects individuals under the age of 60 years and results from degeneration of the frontal and temporal lobes of the cerebrum. Approximately 50% of patients diagnosed with frontotemporal dementia have an inherited mutation of chromosome 17q 21 to chromosome 22 causing an abnormality in tau proteins. Common symptoms include social, behavioral, and personality changes, as well as language function disorders that are significant enough to interfere with daily activities.

Dementia disorders are imaged with structural and functional imaging modalities to evaluate anatomic change, blood flow, and metabolic response. Although CT and MRI do not demonstrate characteristic changes in patients with Lewy body dementia, they do help rule out other types of dementia. MRI is the preferred method of imaging for Alzheimer's dementia, detecting atrophy or volume loss in the lobes of the brain, particularly the hippocampus (Fig. 8.33). Following MRI, CT provides structural imaging, includes the presence of cerebral atrophy, and excludes other neurologic conditions, such as hematoma, tumor, or hydrocephalus. Volumetric or Functional imaging, fMRI, SPECT, and amyloid or FDG-PET assist in understanding blood flow, metabolism, and amyloid deposition in demented patients and are not routinely used in the diagnosis or differentiation of forms of dementia. Individuals with frontotemporal dementia often demonstrate brain atrophy upon brain CT and MR examination. However the extreme thinning of the gyri within the temporal and frontal lobes is often not visible until the dementia has progressed to late stage.

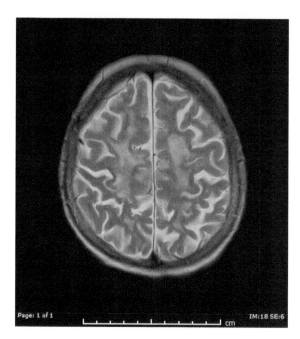

FIG. 8.33 Brain atrophy as a result of late stage Alzheimer's disease

Vascular Diseases

Cerebrovascular Accident

Atherosclerotic disease affecting the blood supply to the brain may eventually result in a cerebrovascular accident (CVA), commonly referred to as a *stroke*. About 795,000 strokes per a year occur in the United States, resulting in an average of 1 per 40 seconds, with 185,000 cases being recurrent attacks. Stroke is the fifth leading cause of death in the United States, killing 130,000 Americans each year. A stroke can occur in essentially two ways and is classified as either *ischemic* or *hemorrhagic*. Ischemic strokes make up 87% of all strokes and are caused when a blood clot blocks a blood vessel in the brain. In contrast, hemorrhagic strokes, 10% being intracerebral in nature and 3% classified as subarachnoid, occur when a blood vessel in the brain ruptures and bleeds into the adjacent brain tissues and structures. Hemorrhagic strokes generally have a more sudden onset compared with ischemic strokes. Both CT and MRI (Fig. 8.34) examinations of the brain distinguish between ischemic and hemorrhagic causes.

Carotid duplex sonography and contrast-enhanced magnetic resonance angiography (CE-MRA) are also

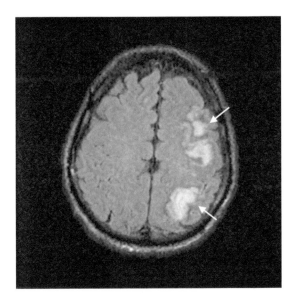

FIG. 8.34 An axial fluid-attenuated inversion recovery magnetic resonance imaging scan of the brain demonstrating an infarct in the left parietal lobe.

useful in the diagnosis of a stroke when carotid stenosis is believed to be the cause of the reduced cerebral blood flow. Although CTA, CE-MRA, and duplex sonography exhibit an accuracy ranging from 70% to 99% in diagnosing internal carotid artery (ICA) stenosis, only sonography offers a cost-effective method of initial screening in a large patient population. However, dependency on sonographer performance, presence of calcified plaque artifact, and difficulty distinguishing subtotal occlusion from total occlusion preclude endorsement of its routine use as the sole examination before treatment. For this reason, combined use of sonography and CE-MRA is becoming an increasingly common practice.

Ischemic Strokes

Under normal circumstances, the natural blood clotting cascade slows and eventually stops the bleeding and is beneficial. In an ischemic stroke, however, blood clots are dangerous because they may block blood flow and cause vessel occlusion. An ischemic stroke may occur in two ways: (1) infarction caused by thrombosis of a cerebral artery or (2) embolism to the brain from a thrombus elsewhere in the body. A *thrombus* is a blood clot that obstructs a blood vessel, and an *embolus* is a mass of undissolved matter (solid, liquid, or gas) present in a blood vessel brought there by blood current.

Vessel occlusion or ischemia lasting over 1 hour usually results in the development of an infarct and permanent neurologic damage. Infarcts are often diagnosed with CT or MRI. However, angiography may be performed if the diagnosis with these imaging modalities is questionable. Two types of thromboses may cause stroke: (1) large vessel thrombosis and (2) small vessel disease, also known as **lacunar infarction**. Large vessel thrombosis most often occurs in the large arteries as a result of long-term atherosclerosis followed by rapid blood clot formation. Typical sites are the bifurcation of the common carotid artery, within the carotid sinus, or the termination of the internal carotid artery, giving rise to the cerebral arteries (Figs. 8.35 and 8.36). An infarct caused by thrombosis of a cerebral artery is termed an **atherothrombotic brain infarction** (ABI). Symptoms associated with ABI develop slowly over a period of hours or days and include confusion, hemiplegia, and aphasia. This type of CVA may be preceded by a temporary episode of neurologic dysfunction, termed **transient ischemic attack** (TIA), and includes hemiparesis, hemiparesthesia, or monocular blindness. In 70% of cases, these symptoms should clear within 2 hours or less. Furthermore, patients with TIA will exhibit positive signs for ischemic injury during MRI-based DWI in 30% to 50% of cases. This calls for an evaluation of stroke risk arising from a 10% to 15% increase in the likelihood that these patients will eventually suffer a debilitating stroke. Patients with a thrombotic stroke are also likely to have coronary artery disease, and heart attack is a frequent cause of death in those who have a thrombotic stroke.

Small vessel disease, or lacunar infarction, occurs when blood flow to a very small arterial vessel is blocked. *Lacune* is the French term for "hole" and describes the small cavity that remains after products of a deep infarct have been removed by other cells. Although little is known about small vessel disease, it is closely linked to hypertension. About 20% of all strokes are caused by small vessel disease.

An embolism may also cause infarction in the brain from a thrombus elsewhere in the body, most commonly from the left side of the heart. CVAs resulting from cerebral embolism have a sudden onset of symptoms without warning. The mortality rate associated with ischemic stroke is approximately 20%. The prognosis depends on the location and extent of the stroke in addition to the patient's age and general health.

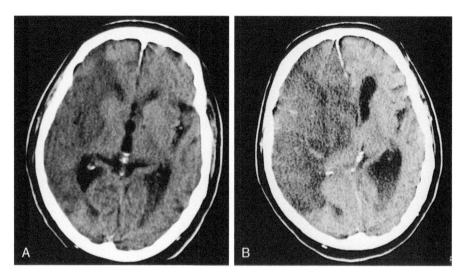

FIG. 8.35 **A,** An unenhanced computed tomography (CT) scan of the brain of an 83-year-old woman reveals a large infarct along the distribution of the middle cerebral artery on the right side. **B,** A similar unenhanced CT scan taken 4 days later reveals worsening of the edema with early shift of the right lateral and third ventricles to the left.

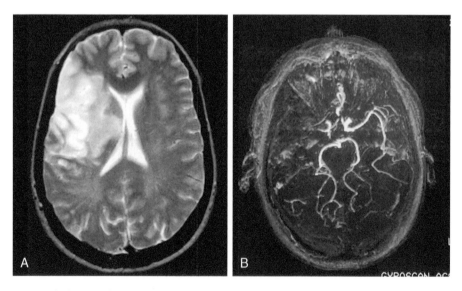

FIG. 8.36 **A,** A magnetic resonance imaging scan of the head of a 54-year-old woman who experienced sudden left facial paralysis and slumped forward while shopping reveals a large infarct along the distribution of the middle cerebral artery. **B,** A magnetic resonance angiogram of the same patient demonstrates occlusion of the middle cerebral artery, thought to be secondary to an embolus from carotid artery disease.

Complete recovery is very rare, and deficits that are present 6 months following the stroke incident most likely are permanent neurologic changes. Between 50% and 70% of stroke survivors eventually regain functional independence, but 15% to 30% become permanently disabled, and 20% require institutional care at 3 months after onset. One of the most common treatments involves the administration of recombinant tissue plasminogen activator (rtPA) within 3 hours of the onset of symptoms.

Noncontrast brain CT is most commonly used to diagnose patients with stroke-like symptoms, especially before treatment with thrombolytic agents. This is primarily because of its wide availability and high sensitivity to acute hemorrhage, although it is relatively insensitive to acute ischemia and infarction with only one third to two thirds of such lesions being detected. According to the latest stroke management guidelines from the American Heart Association (AHA), ischemic stroke victims treated with thrombolytic agents (rtPA) have the best success if the CT examination is completed and results interpreted within 45 minutes from the onset of the stroke. Perfusion CT techniques may be used to diagnose the stroke subtype and to guide other management decisions. According to the ACR appropriateness criteria, for cerebrovascular disease within 24 hours, CT brain perfusion scan with contrast enhancement ranks 6 out of 9. It has become the adopted technique in accrediting stroke network organizations. With advancements in technology, garnering this additional diagnostic information does not result in a delay of rtPA in patients for whom it is needed. Follow-up brain CT or transcranial Doppler sonography is used after the administration of rtPA to monitor the success of thrombolysis. Although traditional T1- or T2-weighted MRI is of limited value, DWI-MRI is a highly sensitive tool for imaging the onset of an acute ischemic stroke, and in many cases, it is more accurate than CT in identifying early infarct signs. DWI can be used in combination with PWI to identify potentially salvageable ischemic tissue, especially 3 hours after symptom onset.

CTA, MRA, and sonography may offer information about vessel patency in the brain and carotid arteries. In the future, PET may also prove to be a valuable asset in managing patients who have suffered an ischemic stroke, as the use of oxygen-15 PET shows promise in its ability to identify regions of decreased blood flow and to demonstrate oxygen consumption within the brain.

Hemorrhagic Strokes

In a hemorrhagic stroke, brain hemorrhage results from a weakening in the diseased vessel wall. Typically, the ruptured vessel has been weakened by arteriosclerosis from hypertension; however, hemorrhage may also result from congenital aneurysms or vascular anomalies. The onset of this type of CVA is sudden and often lethal because it expands rapidly. Brain hemorrhages account for approximately 10% to 15% of all CVAs and are of two types: (1) subarachnoid or (2) intracerebral. Most bleeds occur in the cerebrum and bleed into the lateral ventricle. Most commonly they are preceded by an intense headache that is often accompanied by vomiting. Loss of consciousness follows within minutes and leads to total contralateral hemiplegia or death. CT of the brain is often used in the case of a hemorrhagic stroke because fresh blood appears denser than surrounding brain tissue, which makes this imaging modality highly specific for this particular condition. However, if CT is negative but a hemorrhage is still suspected, a lumbar puncture may be performed to confirm the negative result. MRI identification of acute intracranial hemorrhage may be variable and nonspecific. For this reason, although MRI is potentially more sensitive than CT, it is not generally used as a substitute for CT to detect acute intracranial hemorrhage.

Surgical intervention is necessary when the bleed causes brain displacement (midline shift) or when an aneurysm must be clipped to prevent fatal bleeding. The prognosis of this type of CVA is very poor, with approximately 35% of patients dying after the stroke and another 15% dying within a few weeks, usually from a subsequent vessel rupture.

Neoplastic Diseases

Research has revealed more than 100 histologically distinct types of primary brain and central nervous system tumors and survival varies significantly based upon the histology of the neoplasm, the associated molecular markers, and age of the individual. Over 75,000 new cases of primary brain tumors are diagnosed in the United States each year, one third of which are classified as malignant neoplasms. Primary brain tumors are often difficult to classify as purely benign or malignant. In many cases the location of the brain neoplasm is of equal or greater importance than its malignancy or benignancy. Neoplasms within the brain can

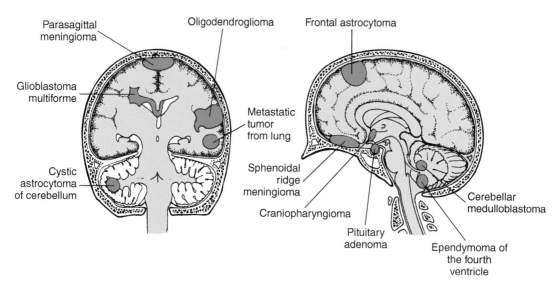

FIG. 8.37 Common sites of intracranial tumors.

create complications produced by mass effect (Fig. 8.37). Edema accompanying a tumor causes an increase in ICP, which, in turn, causes headache, vomiting, blurred vision, and seizure. Hemorrhage and brainstem herniation may also occur resulting in death as brainstem function (e.g., control of respiration) fails.

Other characteristics of primary brain tumors include a greater incidence in children through young adults, and in the older adult population. In fact, primary brain tumors are the most common cancer occurring in people aged 0 to 19 years and are the second leading cause of cancer deaths in individuals under the age of 20 years. Brain tumors often tend to occur in the posterior fossa of children, whereas the anterior portion of the cerebrum is a more prevalent site in adults. Primary brain tumors have a low frequency of metastasis, but metastases to the brain from other primary areas are more common in adults.

Primary brain tumors may be classified according to the site, such as the specific lobe of the brain or according to histologic composition. The two categories of brain tumors based on histologic type are *glial* and *nonglial* neoplasms. Glial tumors generate from the supporting tissues of the brain and spinal cord. **Gliomas** account for about half of all primary brain tumors. Their growth occurs through infiltration, making them difficult to treat surgically through resection. Nonglial tumors grow through

expansion and are more treatable surgically. Meningiomas are the most frequently occurring nonglial tumors, accounting for over 36% of all primary brain neoplasms.

The modalities of choice in imaging brain tumors of all types are MRI and CT. As mentioned earlier, because optimal details of the posterior fossa structures may be obscured by beam-hardening artifact associated with CT, MRI is usually the initial modality of choice for evaluating patients of all ages unless an apparent contraindication exists. CT imaging, PET imaging, or both are indicated when an underlying primary is not evident with MRI examination. In addition to surgical intervention, radiation therapy and chemotherapy also play an important role in the treatment of brain tumors. fMRI and DTI may be used for mapping of the neural pathways to delineate motor and speech areas and assess any tumor-induced deflection of nerve fibers, subsequently contributing to surgical and radiation treatment planning.

When patients previously treated for brain neoplasms present with new neurologic complaints, distinguishing between radiation necrosis and tumor recurrence may be a diagnostic challenge. These lesions, which may have a similar appearance during contrast-enhanced MRI, call for significantly different clinical management. Nuclear medicine SPECT imaging, PET, MR spectroscopy, and dynamic PWI-MRI studies may

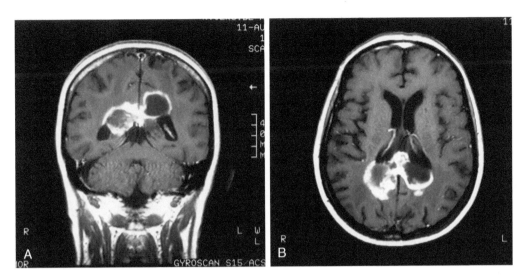

FIG. 8.38 **A,** A "butterfly" glioma seen in this T1-weighted coronal magnetic resonance imaging (MRI) view with gadolinium in a 54-year-old woman. **B,** A T1-weighted axial MRI view with gadolinium of the same "butterfly" glioma.

provide some improved specificity in making the differential diagnosis. Catheter angiography may also play a role in the treatment planning process by providing information related to tumor vascularity.

Gliomas

The most common type of primary intracranial brain tumor is the glioma (Fig. 8.38), accounting for approximately 45% of all intracranial tumors. Although derived from glial (supporting) cells, their precise classification is still being debated. However, several growth factors and their receptors have been identified and are associated with the development of gliomas. These tumors may contain different types of cells in the same tumor, but one commonality is loss of genetic information from chromosome 17p. Gliomas commonly occur in the cerebral hemispheres and the posterior fossa, with nearly half of all gliomas classified as the malignant glioblastoma variety (Fig. 8.39). The most significant risk factor associated with gliomas is exposure to ionizing radiation. Survival varies by the type and grade of the glioma. Glioblastomas carry the lowest survival rate with less than 5% of patients surviving 5 years. Other types of gliomas include benign astrocytomas, oligodendrogliomas, and ependymomas.

In terms of MRI results, gliomas are evaluated on the basis of associated edema (Fig. 8.40), mass effect, and

amount of contrast enhancement. An association exists between the aggressiveness of the tumor and these three factors. Malignant gliomas may be extremely vascular, demonstrating pathologic vessels during angiographic examination. Low-grade malignant gliomas, however, are relatively avascular. CT images generally demonstrate an ill-defined area of decreased density (attenuation) with displacement of the midline structures and ventricular compression. Without contrast enhancement, it is difficult to differentiate the surrounding edema from the actual tumor, so the use of an iodinated intravenous (IV) contrast agent is necessary to enhance the lesion. Surgical biopsy generally provides the final diagnosis of the exact type of glioma. As described earlier, signs and symptoms include severe headaches, vision impairment, personality changes, and seizures as a result of increased ICP.

Astrocytomas account for about a third of all gliomas and are the most common childhood brain tumors. They are composed of astrocytes, which are star-shaped neuroglial cells with many branching processes (Fig. 8.41). Astrocytomas are white, usually slow-growing, infiltrative tumors with a low grade of malignancy. Although their etiology remains unconfirmed, multiple genetic deletions, additions, duplications, mutations, and amplifications of specific genes have been linked with these tumors in different stages

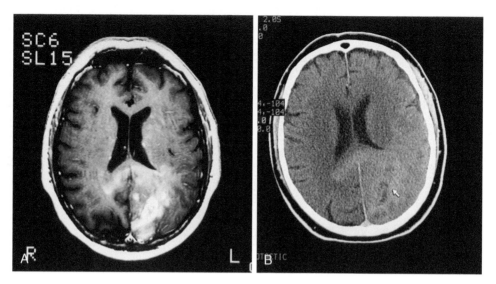

FIG. 8.39 **A,** A T1-weighted axial magnetic resonance imaging view with gadolinium demonstrates a glioblastoma multiforme in a 70-year-old man. **B,** Computed tomography study of the brain without contrast demonstrates an intraparenchymal hemorrhage after biopsy in the same patient with the glioblastoma multiforme.

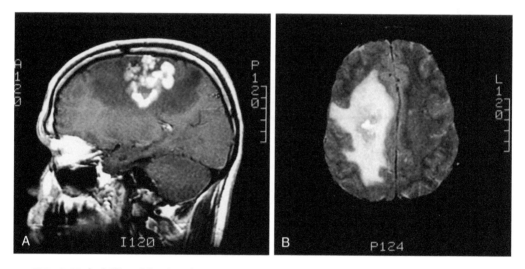

FIG. 8.40 **A,** A T1-weighted sagittal magnetic resonance imaging (MRI) view with gadolinium of a large glioma with surrounding edema in a 25-year-old man. **B,** A T2-weighted axial MRI view without gadolinium of the same glioma in the right parietal region, again with edema (white on T2) surrounding the tumor.

of malignant progression. Early detection leads to a good prognosis. A **glioblastoma multiforme** (an advanced astrocytoma) is highly malignant. An **oligodendroglioma** is a slow-growing astrocytic tumor, and histologically, it is often relatively benign (Fig. 8.42). It typically calcifies so that its appearance in a punctate or stippled pattern on a skull radiograph is virtually diagnostic. **Ependymoma** is a firm, whitish tumor that arises from the ependyma, the lining of the ventricles (Fig. 8.43). Typically, it derives from the roof of the fourth ventricle, but it may also appear from the central canal of the spinal cord.

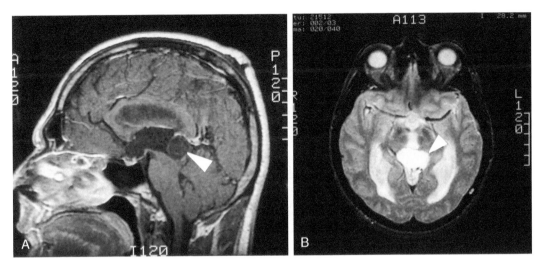

FIG. 8.41 A, A T1-weighted sagittal magnetic resonance imaging (MRI) view with gadolinium demonstrates a pineal gland astrocytoma in this 32-year-old man. **B,** A T2-weighted axial MRI view demonstrates the same pineal gland astrocytoma.

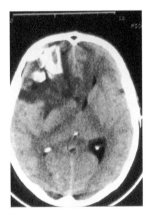

FIG. 8.42 An axial computed tomography view without contrast demonstrates the presence of an oligodendroglioma and surrounding edema.

Contrast-enhanced MRI is the imaging modality of choice as it clearly demonstrates the extent of the disease and any recurrence. Stereotactic biopsy of the brain lesion is generally used to confirm the type and grade of the glioma. Surgical resection is the primary treatment of low grade tumors and most children with low grade astrocytomas are cured. Radiation therapy may be used in patients aged 10 years or older and chemotherapy may be used in patients under 10 years of age in situations where the tumor is not resectable, the resection is incomplete, or in cases

of recurrence. High grade astrocytomas are treated with a combination of surgery, followed by radiation therapy and chemotherapy. However, the prognosis is very poor, with only 20% to 30% of patients surviving after 3 years. Glioblastomas are routinely treated by surgical resection followed by conformal radiation therapy in combination with chemotherapy, most commonly temozolomide. Investigational therapies such as radiosurgery, gene therapy, and immune therapy may also be used. The prognosis for glioblastomas remains poor with about a 50% 1 year survival rate and 10% to 15% survival at 5 years.

Medulloblastoma

Like astrocytic tumors, **medulloblastomas** are soft, infiltrating tumors of neuroepithelial tissue. These rapidly growing tumors are highly malignant and most often occur in the cerebellum of children and young adults (Fig. 8.44) and usually extend from the roof of the fourth ventricle. They are more common in boys and rarely seen in adults. Because MRI does not image bone or demonstrate artifacts associated with the dense bone within the base of the skull, it is an excellent modality for the demonstration of a medulloblastoma during both enhanced and nonenhanced examination. These tumors may also be demonstrated by CT, with the medulloblastoma visible as a midline lesion that is denser than normal brain tissue and surrounded by edema. In addition, tumor dissemination

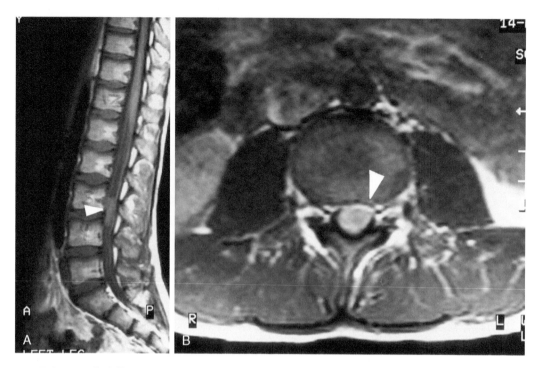

FIG. 8.43 **A,** A T1-weighted sagittal magnetic resonance imaging (MRI) view of the lumbosacral spine demonstrates an ependymoma at the L3–L4 interspace in this young man. **B,** A T1-weighted axial MRI view with gadolinium demonstrates the same ependymoma.

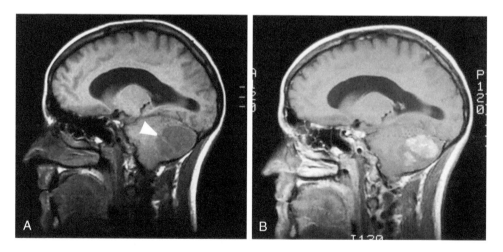

FIG. 8.44 **A,** A T1-weighted sagittal magnetic resonance imaging (MRI) view without gadolinium demonstrates a medulloblastoma in the cerebellum of this 25-year-old man. **B,** A T1-weighted sagittal MRI view with gadolinium demonstrates the medulloblastoma, illustrating more of its actual size.

throughout the subarachnoid space often blocks the flow of CSF, causing hydrocephalus. Shunting is used to relieve the hydrocephalus. Surgical excision of the tumor as much as possible and radiation to the entire CNS (brain and spinal cord) have improved the 5-year survival rate to over 50% and the 10-year survival rate to about 40%. Unfortunately, recurrence is common with this tumor and chemotherapy regimens have not been found to be consistently effective in controlling the recurrence.

Meningioma

A **meningioma** is a slow-growing, generally benign tumor that originates in the arachnoid tissue. It is the most common nonglial tumor, accounting for about 15% of all intracranial tumors. Meningiomas are more frequent in women than in men, and although meningiomas may affect individuals at any age, they usually arise in adults between the ages of 40 and 60 years. Furthermore, a loss of chromosome 22 has been isolated as a possible genetic etiology of this tumor type. Meningiomas are most often found adhering to the dura in relation to the intracranial venous sinuses. These tumors do not invade the brain but compress it with their growth. Resultant neurologic deficits are generally less in proportion to the tumor size compared with gliomas.

In some instances, the skull may thicken over the site of the meningioma, with the increased calcification visible on conventional skull radiographs. This area of hyperostosis may be palpable during a physical examination. Because these tumors are fed by the meningeal arteries, plain skull radiography may also demonstrate an enlarged foramen spinosum and increased meningeal vascular markings on the inner table of the skull. Catheter angiography, when performed during preoperative embolization of the meningioma, is useful in identifying the feeding arteries of the tumor. Reports of the use of nuclear medicine imaging with radiolabeled agents such as ^{111}In-octreotide, which have an affinity for somatostatin receptors, can be useful in detecting and localizing meningiomas. This benefit is diminished, however, by the lack of specificity in differentiating meningiomas from other lesions such as high-grade gliomas or pituitary adenomas. PET is attractive for investigating the metabolic activity of tumors, but its role in the evaluation of meningiomas is complicated by variable metabolic presentations in different meningioma types. In general, nuclear medicine techniques provide capabilities that are sensitive for meningiomas but have relatively low specificity.

During MRI and CT, meningiomas show a typical yet variable appearance. For this reason, these modern imaging tools usually suggest the histologic diagnosis, but usually not the grade of the tumor. CT studies of patients with a diagnosis of meningioma demonstrate a well-defined mass of increased attenuation, with calcifications visible in approximately 20% of the lesions. The extent of the meningioma is clearly visible on enhancement with an IV contrast agent. In comparison, nonenhanced MRI is not as sensitive as CT in detecting meningiomas because a significant inherent contrast difference does not exist between these tumors and the normal brain tissue. However, an IV gadolinium contrast agent clearly demonstrates meningiomas during MRI examination (Fig. 8.45). Perfusion and diffusion imaging have also been useful tools for diagnosis, especially in suggesting alternative histologies and predicting aggressive histologic features.

Surgical removal is the method of treatment for a symptomatic meningioma. However, if the meningioma is surgically inaccessible, stereotactic radiosurgery using a gamma knife may be required.

Pituitary Adenoma

A **pituitary adenoma** is usually a benign tumor of the pituitary gland, and these tumors comprise about 15% of all intracranial tumors. Anatomically, these tumors are classified according to size, based on radiologic findings, as either microadenomas (less than <10 mm) or macroadenomas (≥10 mm). Hormones produced by the pituitary are affected, with one type of adenoma of the anterior pituitary resulting in gigantism if it develops before puberty and acromegaly if it occurs in adults because of excessive production of growth hormone (GH). Prolactin-secreting adenomas cause amenorrhea–galactorrhea syndrome, in which the breasts spontaneously secrete milk and menstrual periods cease. Pituitary adenomas may grow out of the sella turcica. As they grow, they compress structures such as the optic chiasm, resulting in vision problems.

A common radiographic demonstration of this growth is an enlargement and erosion of the sella turcica on a lateral skull radiograph. Angiography

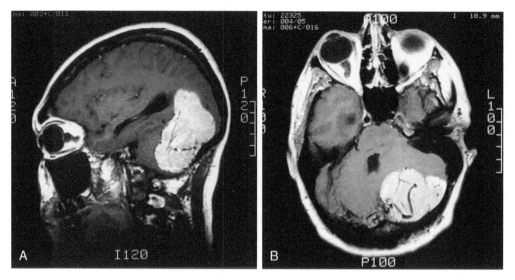

FIG. 8.45 A, A T1-weighted sagittal magnetic resonance imaging (MRI) view with gadolinium of a large meningioma in the posterior occipital area with marked hydrocephalus in this 31-year-old woman. **B,** A T1-weighted axial MRI view with gadolinium of the same meningioma. Displacement of the fourth ventricle is seen, including a distortion of the vascular structures within the meningioma.

might demonstrate a displacement of the Sylvian triangle, but generally only after the adenoma has assumed a considerable size. The **Sylvian triangle** is an anatomic landmark created by the middle cerebral artery and its branches. A brain CT is useful to confirm the diagnosis of pituitary adenomas and to detect the extent of these lesions, especially when the tumor extends above the sella turcica. Enlargement of the sella turcica and suprasellar extension into the optic chiasm are generally demonstrated. These neoplasms are generally slightly denser than the surrounding brain tissue and show obvious enhancement on IV injection of contrast medium. Small microadenomas are best demonstrated on thin slice, contrast-enhanced MRI images (Figs. 8.46 and 8.47) or high-resolution CT.

Generally, pituitary adenomas are treatable through surgical extraction, possibly followed by radiation therapy. Small adenomas may also be treated medically by drugs such as bromocriptine, which increase prolactin inhibitory factor (PIF) and suppress tumor growth.

Craniopharyngioma

A **craniopharyngioma** is a cystic, benign tumor growing from remnants of the development of the pituitary gland. It is thought to be developmental in origin and most commonly manifests in childhood. Craniopharyngiomas usually arise above the sella and extend upward into the third ventricle (Fig. 8.48). Occasionally, they are seen within the sella, causing erosion of the sella turcica. Although traditional radiography of the skull has been superseded by newer imaging techniques, it still may be useful in cases of tumor wall calcification. Furthermore, it has been reported that in 46% to 87% of cases, skull radiography may show an abnormal sella with widening of its outlet, uniform expansion, and shortening or erosion of the dorsum sellae.

The CT appearance of craniopharyngiomas depends on the proportion of the solid and cystic components of the tumor. They are usually of mixed attenuation, with the cyst fluid having a low density and the contrast medium enhancing any solid portion, as well as the cyst capsule. For this reason, pre- and postcontrast enhanced images in the axial plane followed by postcontrast coronal images are typically recommended.

MRI, especially after contrast administration, is valuable for topographic and structural analyses of craniopharyngiomas. Similar to CT, the appearance of the craniopharyngioma during MRI will depend on

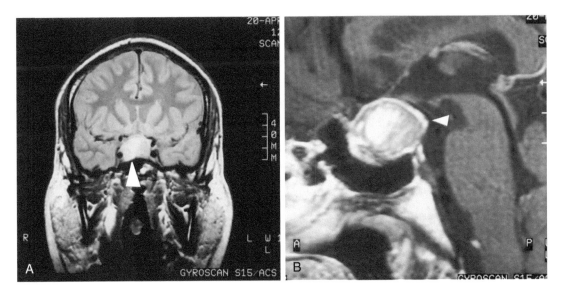

FIG. 8.46 **A,** A T1-weighted coronal magnetic resonance imaging (MRI) view demonstrates a suprasellar macroadenoma of the pituitary in this 37-year-old man. **B,** A T1-weighted sagittal MRI high-resolution scan with gadolinium demonstrates the same suprasellar macroadenoma of the pituitary.

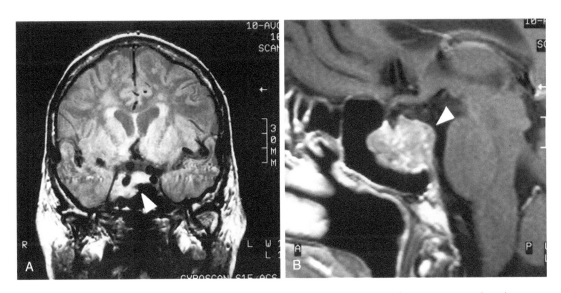

FIG. 8.47 **A,** Large pituitary adenoma extending downward into the right cavernous sinus in a 79-year-old woman as seen on this magnetic resonance imaging (MRI) T2-weighted coronal scan. **B,** A high-resolution T1-weighted sagittal MRI view of the same pituitary adenoma with gadolinium.

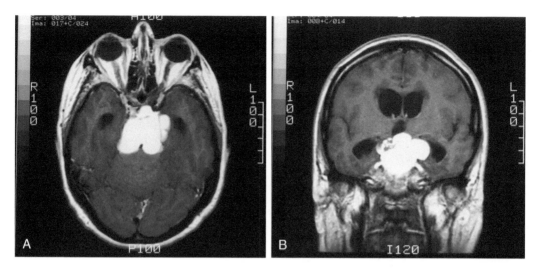

FIG. 8.48 **A,** A T1-weighted axial magnetic resonance imaging (MRI) view with gadolinium demonstrates a mass, later confirmed by biopsy to be a craniopharyngioma, in this 53-year-old woman. **B,** A T1-weighted coronal MRI view with gadolinium demonstrates the relative size of the craniopharyngioma in the same patient.

the proportion of the solid and cystic components, the content of the cyst (cholesterol, keratin, hemorrhage), and the amount of calcification present. The signal of a solid tumor is isointense or hypointense relative to the surrounding brain tissue on precontrast T1-weighted sequences, showing enhancement after gadolinium, whereas it is usually of mixed hypointensity or hyperintensity on T2-weighted sequences. The cystic component is usually hypointense on T1-weighted sequences and hyperintense on T2-weighted sequences. Postcontrast T1-weighted images demonstrate the thin peripheral contrast-enhancing rim of the cyst. Additionally, edema in the adjacent brain parenchyma, either from a reaction to the craniopharyngioma itself or an associated disturbance in CSF flow caused by the tumor, may be present and provide useful information for distinguishing craniopharyngiomas from other common parasellar tumors.

Cerebral angiography may be useful for clarifying the anatomic relationship between the tumor and blood vessels. Occasionally, images revealing displacement of the Sylvian triangle, as caused by a pituitary adenoma, can be visualized if the tumor is large. Furthermore, in cases of craniopharyngioma in which angiography was performed; displacement or encasement of the carotid artery was identified in 54% of the cases, with an additional

22% involving the basilar artery. Although craniopharyngiomas are treated surgically, excision is often difficult because of their location and proximity to structures such as the third ventricle and the optic nerves. Radiation therapy is used to enhance the effects of surgery.

Tumors of Central Nerve Sheath Cells

Two tumors of the peripheral nerve sheath are the **acoustic neuroma** (Fig. 8.49), and **schwannoma** (Fig. 8.50). They account for up to 10% of all intracranial tumors and are most common in middle-aged and older adults. The most common site is the eighth cranial (vestibulocochlear or acoustic) nerve. At this location, the tumor compresses the adjacent brain tissue and erodes the temporal bone. Symptoms of acoustic neuromas include facial paralysis, tinnitus, and partial hearing loss on the affected side. Nerve sheath tumors may also be found on other cranial nerves, especially the fifth cranial nerve (trigeminal), and on spinal nerve roots and peripheral nerves. The imaging method of choice for acoustic neuromas is MRI. In general, high-field strength magnets (1.5T to 3.0T) are preferred to low-field strength units because of the optimal signal-to-noise ratios, gradient strength, and spatial resolution that are achievable. In extreme cases, erosion and expansion of the internal auditory canal may be visible

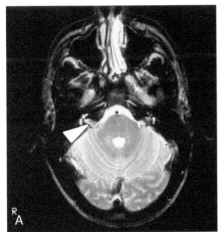

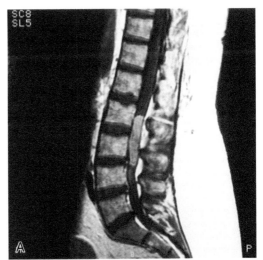

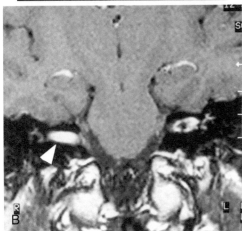

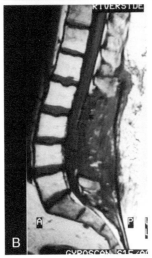

FIG. 8.49 **A,** A T2-weighted axial magnetic resonance imaging (MRI) view of a right acoustic neuroma that is not readily visible without gadolinium in this 24-year-old man. **B,** A high-resolution T1-weighted coronal MRI view with gadolinium readily reveals the acoustic neuroma. Compare the appearance of the tumor with the appearance of the normal vasculature and anatomy on the left side.

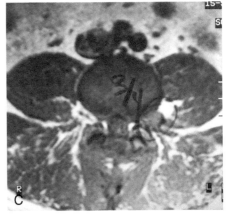

FIG. 8.50 **A,** A T1-weighted sagittal magnetic resonance imaging (MRI) view of the lumbar spine with gadolinium shows a schwannoma at L3–L4 before surgery in this 27-year-old woman. **B,** A T1-weighted sagittal MRI view of the same lumbar spine without gadolinium after surgery demonstrates that apparent total excision of the tumor has been accomplished. Note also the excision of the spinous processes from the surgical site. **C,** A T1-weighted axial MRI view with gadolinium of the L3–L4 interspace demonstrates that some residual tumor is present in the left neural foramina.

on an anteroposterior (AP) axial projection of the skull. The use of CT is primarily indicated in relation to tumors involving the skull base foramina and for evaluating calcific matrices within lesions and tumor-related osseous erosions. Stereotactic radiosurgery or conventional surgical excision of the tumor is the method of treatment.

Metastases from Other Sites

Secondary metastases from another site can involve any intracranial structure and account for about 10% of all brain tumors (Fig. 8.51). The metastatic lesions may be solitary or multiple. Brain metastasis usually arises from lung carcinoma. Other significant causes include adenocarcinoma of the breast, bronchogenic carcinoma, and malignant melanoma. Signs and symptoms of brain metastasis are similar to those of other brain tumors. Patients with metastases from other sites usually have signs of increased ICP, especially headache and ataxia; those with primary brain tumors are more likely to have seizures. Diagnosis and follow-up are done with MRI and CT. Treatment includes resection using either conventional surgical techniques or radiosurgery followed by radiation therapy. Prognosis depends on the number of metastatic lesions and the primary type of malignant disease.

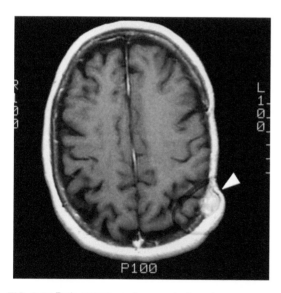

FIG. 8.51 Brain metastases from renal cell carcinoma as seen in this T1-weighted axial magnetic resonance imaging view with gadolinium after craniotomy in this 59-year-old woman.

Spinal Tumors

Primary tumors of the spinal cord are even less common than those of the brain. They are commonly divided into extradural and intradural groups, with the latter further divided into extramedullary (outside the spinal cord) and intramedullary (within the spinal cord) (Fig. 8.52). The most common types (>60%) of primary spinal neoplasms are **meningiomas** (Fig. 8.53) and **neurofibromas** (Fig. 8.54), both of which are extramedullary tumors. Neurofibromatosis is an inherited autosomal dominant disorder, and the gene for type 1 is located on chromosome 17, whereas the gene for type 2 is on chromosome 22. The most common intramedullary tumors are **astrocytoma** and **ependymoma**.

Symptoms of extramedullary tumors may be similar to those of a herniated nucleus pulposus in

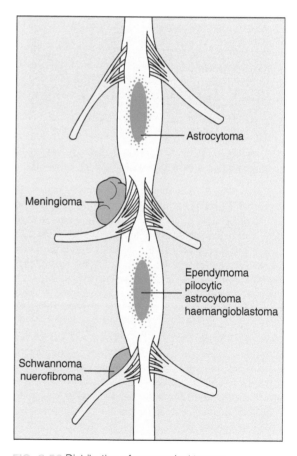

FIG. 8.52 Distribution of some spinal tumors.

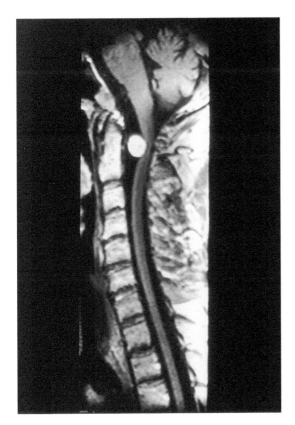

that spinal tumors also compress the nerve roots, leading to pain and muscular weakness. In contrast, intramedullary tumors cause progressive paraparesis and sensory loss. In terms of imaging, CT myelography may be necessary to identify extradural tumors. Enlargement of the spinal cord by intramedullary masses may also be well depicted with myelography, but this is possible only in cases where large masses are present. For this reason, when evaluating spinal cord tumors, contrast-enhanced MRI is the examination of choice and has essentially replaced myelography. Differentiating syrinx from tumor, location of tumor nodules, and extent of cystic pathology, and differentiating nodules and cysts from edema are all factors that are crucial to the treatment planning process for intramedullary disease, so MRI becomes a practical necessity. Conventional spine radiography is primarily reserved for demonstrating bone destruction and for the widening of the vertebral pedicles related to tumor growth.

Both intramedullary and extramedullary tumors may be surgically resected, depending on the location and degree of damage. Approximately 50% of patients undergoing surgery experience a reversal of clinical anomalies resulting from the neoplasm. In cases in which surgery is not a viable alternative, radiation therapy is the primary means of treating the tumor.

FIG. 8.53 A T1-weighted sagittal magnetic resonance imaging view of the spine with gadolinium demonstrates the presence of a meningioma in this 45-year-old woman with ataxia.

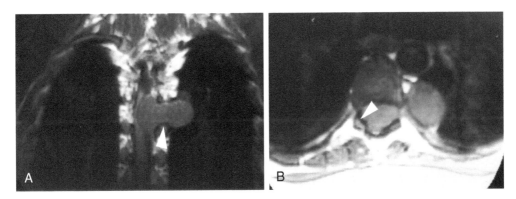

FIG. 8.54 **A,** A T1-weighted coronal magnetic resonance imaging (MRI) view demonstrates the presence of a "dumbbell" neurofibroma showing clear compression of the spinal cord of this young female patient with back pain and leg weakness. **B,** An axial T1-weighted MRI image similarly demonstrates the lesion and compression of the spinal cord (*arrow*) into a narrow space.

Pathologic Summary of the Central Nervous System

Pathology	Imaging Modality of Choice
Hydrocephalus	CT, MRI, sonography in the neonate
Meningitis	MRI, CT without contrast
Encephalitis	MRI, CT without contrast
Brain abscess	CT, MRI
Herniated nucleus pulposus	MRI, CT without contrast, myelography, and postmyelography CT
Cervical spondylosis	Radiography
Multiple sclerosis	MRI
CVA	MRI, CT, sonography with Doppler, CTA, MRA
Glioma	MRI, CT
Medulloblastoma	MRI, CT
Meningioma	CT, MRI
Pituitary adenoma	CT, MRI
Craniopharyngioma	CT
Acoustic neuroma	MRI
Spinal tumor	MRI, radiography, CT, myelography
Metastases from other sites	MRI, radiography, CT

CT, Computed tomography; *CTA,* computed tomographic angiography; *CVA,* cerebrovascular accident; *MRA,* magnetic resonance angiography; *MRI,* magnetic resonance imaging.

Review Questions

1. Under normal conditions, the central nervous system (CNS) within the cranial vault is well protected from damage by all of the following except:
   a. The cauda equina
   b. Cerebrospinal fluid (CSF)
   c. The diploë
   d. The dura mater

2. The correct order of meninges from outermost to innermost is:
   a. Arachnoid, pia, dura
   b. Dura, arachnoid, pia
   c. Dura, pia, arachnoid
   d. Pia, arachnoid, dura

3. The blood-brain barrier prevents passage of unwanted substances into the CNS through the cerebral:
   a. Arteries
   b. Capillaries
   c. Dura mater
   d. Veins

4. "Protrusion of both the spinal cord and the meninges into the skin of the back" describes a:
   f. Meningocele
   g. Meningomyelocele
   h. Myelocele
   i. Spinal hydrocephalus

5. The most typical cause of meningitis is:
   a. Bacterial infection
   b. Trauma
   c. Tumor compression
   d. Viral infection

6. The imaging modality of choice for demonstration of herniated nucleus pulposus is:
   a. Computed tomography (CT)
   b. Magnetic resonance imaging (MRI)
   c. Conventional myelography
   d. Sonography

7. Which of the following results from the development amyloid plaques, neurofibrillary tangles?
   a. Alzheimer's dementia
   b. Frontotemporal dementia
   c. Lewy body dementia
   d. Vascular dementia

8. The term atherothrombotic brain infarction denotes:
   a. Brain hemorrhage caused by atherosclerosis
   b. Infarction caused by thrombosis of a cerebral artery
   c. An embolism to the brain from a left heart thrombus
   d. None of the above
9. Which of the following neoplastic conditions is highly malignant and often occurs in the cerebellum of children?
   a. Astrocytoma
   b. Medulloblastoma
   c. Meningioma
   d. Pituitary adenoma
10. Which cranial nerve is the most common site for tumors of the peripheral nerve sheath (e.g., schwannoma)?
    a. 4
    b. 6
    c. 7
    d. 8
11. Where is CSF manufactured and absorbed? Explain the physiologic basis for the development of hydrocephalus.
12. Why is MRI the modality of choice for demonstrating diseases in the posterior fossa?
13. What is the most common cause for a cerebrovascular accident, and what is its most common site?
14. What are the major differences between meningitis and encephalitis?
15. Explain the differences between glial and nonglial tumors, and give an example of each type.

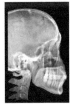
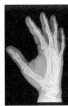
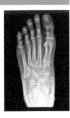

Hematopoietic System

ⓔ http://evolve.elsevier.com/Kowalczyk/pathology/

LEARNING OBJECTIVES

On completion of Chapter 9, the reader should be able to:

1. Identify the major constituents of blood and describe the function of each constituent.
2. Specify the various blood types.
3. Explain the role of the lymphatic system in terms of immunity.
4. Describe the pathogenesis, prognosis, and signs and symptoms of the disease processes discussed in this chapter.
5. Identify the various imaging modalities used in diagnosing hematopoietic disorders.

OUTLINE

Anatomy and Physiology
Imaging Considerations
Human Immunodeficiency
Virus (HIV) Infection
Congenital and Hereditary
Diseases

Sickle Cell Disease
Thalassemias
Hemophilias
von Willebrand Disease
Neoplastic Diseases

Multiple Myeloma
Leukemia
Non-Hodgkin Lymphoma
Hodgkin Lymphoma

KEY TERMS

Acquired
  immunodeficiency
  syndrome
Acute lymphocytic
  leukemia
Acute monoblastic
  leukemia
Acute myelocytic
  leukemia
Agglutination
Anemia
Chronic lymphocytic
  leukemia
Chronic myelocytic
  leukemia

Erythrocytes
Hematocrit
Hemocytoblasts
Hemophilia A
Hemophilia B
Hemophilia C
HIV protease
Hodgkin lymphoma
Human
  immunodeficiency
  virus
Kaposi sarcoma
Leukemia
Leukocytes

Lymph
Lymph nodes
Lymphocytes
Multiple myeloma
Myeloid tissue
Non-Hodgkin lymphoma
Pneumocystis carinii
  pneumonia
Reed-Sternberg cells
Reticuloendothelial
  system
Reverse transcriptase
Rh factor
Rh-negative

Anatomy and Physiology

The hematopoietic system consists of blood, lymphatic tissue, bone marrow, and the spleen. Circulating blood contains both plasma and blood cells, with the plasma constituting approximately 55% of the total blood volume (Fig. 9.1). The plasma is about 90% water and 10% solutes such as proteins, glucose, amino acids, and lipids. Plasma proteins are classified as globulins, albumins, and clotting factors. With the exception of immunoglobulins (Igs), all of these proteins are synthesized by the liver. Immunoglobulins are synthesized by the lymphatic system, specifically by mature lymphocytes termed *plasma cells*. Immunoglobulins are responsible for fighting infectious organisms and include IgA, IgB, IgM, IgD, and IgE. Albumins regulate the passage of water and solutes through the capillaries. Fibrinogen, the precursor of the fibrin clot, is the primary clotting factor found within the plasma.

Three basic types of blood cells—erythrocytes, leukocytes, and thrombocytes (Table 9.1)—make up the remaining 45% of total blood volume.

Erythrocytes, or red blood cells (RBCs), are very small in relation to the other blood cells. They do not possess a nucleus and are shaped like biconcave disks. Erythrocytes are responsible for transporting oxygen and carbon dioxide to and from the various organs of the body. This is accomplished via the hemoglobin in erythrocytes, which allows oxygen or carbon dioxide molecules to attach to the cell for transport. Individuals with a hemoglobin level of less than 12 g/100 mL of blood have **anemia** and are considered "anemic" because less than normal oxygen or carbon dioxide transportation occurs in them. The total percentage of RBCs in blood volume is determined by a laboratory test termed **hematocrit**.

Erythrocytes are formed by specialized cells called **hemocytoblasts**, which are located in the myeloid tissue found within red bone marrow. These cells live approximately 120 days and are phagocytosed by the **reticuloendothelial system**, which consists of specialized cells in the liver, spleen, and bone marrow. During phagocytosis, the iron within the hemoglobin is released and bilirubin is formed. The released iron is used again in the development of new erythrocytes, and bilirubin is excreted in bile.

Erythrocytes may contain various antigens that determine blood type. This is especially critical for blood transfusions because blood type incompatibility could have fatal results. Erythrocytes may contain no antigens, either the A or B antigen, or both the A and B antigens. The resulting blood types are O (no antigen), A, B, and AB. If incompatible blood types are mixed (e.g., a type O patient receives type AB blood), erythrocytes from the donor clump together in the serum of the recipient. Because the type O recipient does not possess the A or B antigen, antibodies are formed to fight against the foreign RBCs. This is termed **agglutination**. Eventually, donor erythrocytes are destroyed, and the rejection possibly results in immediate shock. In some cases, the reaction may be delayed and may result in fever, pain, and ultimate renal failure as the kidneys try to excrete the byproducts from the destruction of the donor erythrocytes. Cross-matching of blood types to eliminate the risk of transfusion of incompatible blood is essential.

The person with type O blood is considered the universal donor because this type does not contain any antigens and can be given to anyone regardless of the recipient's blood type. The person with type AB blood is considered the universal recipient because this type of blood possesses both antigens, which enables the person to receive any type of blood (Table 9.2). In addition, the Rh blood factor should be considered. The **Rh factor** is termed such because it was first discovered in the blood of the rhesus monkey. Approximately 85% of the human population has this factor; these people are classified as **Rh-positive**. Individuals not possessing the Rh factor are **Rh-negative**. The Rh factor becomes a problem if an Rh-positive father transmits the Rh factor to a fetus carried by an Rh-negative mother. The first pregnancy generally progresses normally, but in subsequent pregnancies, the mother's anti-Rh antibodies, made during the first pregnancy, attack the Rh-positive fetal blood. This scenario can be avoided by Rh-immunization of the mother before pregnancy.

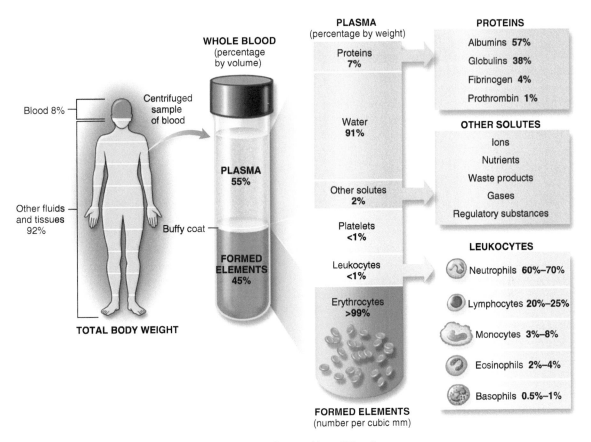

FIG. 9.1 Composition of Blood.

TABLE 9.1
Blood Cell Types

Type	Formed By	Function	Life Span
Erythrocyte	Myeloid tissue within red bone marrow	Transporting oxygen and carbon dioxide	120 days
Leukocyte			
Granular	Red bone marrow	Body defense	2 weeks
Nongranular	Lymphatic tissue	Immunity	Years
Thrombocyte	Myeloid tissue within red bone marrow	Blood clotting	10 days

   Leukocytes, or white blood cells (WBCs), may be classified as *granular* or *nongranular*. Granular leukocytes contain cytoplasmic granules and irregular nuclei. They are formed within the red bone marrow and include basophils, neutrophils, and eosinophils. The names of these cells correspond to the manner in which they respond to certain dyes for microscopic inspection. Nongranular leukocytes do not contain cytoplasmic granules, and they possess regular nuclei. They are mainly formed in the lymphatic tissue of the spleen and include lymphocytes and monocytes. Leukocytes play an important role in the body's defense system. They are able to move out of capillaries into tissue to "attack" and phagocytose foreign substances. The life span of leukocytes varies, depending on the type of cell. Granular leukocytes live for only about 2 weeks, whereas lymphocytes may live for years. Normal blood contains between 5000 and 9000 leukocytes per milliliter. Changes in the number of leukocytes often indicate the presence of disease.

The third major type of blood cells is the **thrombocytes**, or platelets. These cells are necessary for blood to clot properly and respond within seconds to initiate the coagulation process. Thrombocytes are also formed

in the myeloid tissue within the red bone marrow and have a life span of approximately 10 days. The normal platelet count is $140,000/mm^3$ to $340,000/mm^3$. Platelet activation is increased by an inflammatory response. Vascular damage results in a physiologic response to maintain homeostasis, including vasoconstriction, the development of a platelet plug, the activation of blood coagulation (thrombin), and the formation of a blood clot. This process is critical in preventing hemorrhage and is dependent on the availability of the proper number of platelets (Fig. 9.2).

The lymphoid system is closely integrated with the circulatory system and includes the lymphatic system, thymus, bone marrow, spleen, tonsils, and lymphoid follicles within the mucosa of the ileum termed Peyer's patches. The major function of the lymphoid system is ensuring immunity through production of lymphocytes and antibodies, but it is also responsible for absorbing fat from the intestinal tract and for manufacturing blood under certain circumstances.

The lymphatic system is composed of both lymphatic vessels and nodes. Lymphatic vessels contain a milky liquid substance termed **lymph**. **Lymph nodes** are small ovoid bodies attached in a chain-like pattern along the vessels. They filter out particles and foreign materials from blood. Major areas of lymph node chains include the neck, the mediastinum, and the axillary, retroperitoneal, pelvic, and inguinal regions. These

TABLE 9.2
Cross-Matching of Blood Types

Recipient Blood Type	Acceptable Donor Type			
	A	B	AB*	OE†
A	Yes	No	No	Yes
B	No	Yes	No	Yes
AB*	Yes	Yes	Yes	Yes
O†	No	No	No	Yes

*AB, Universal recipient.
†O, Universal donor.

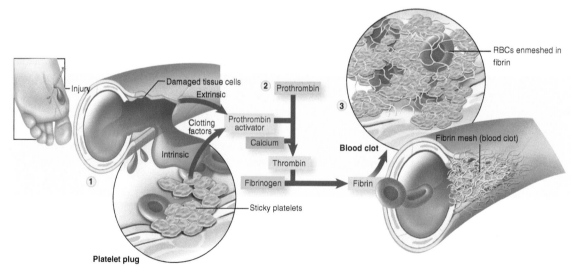

FIG. 9.2 The blood clotting mechanism involves the release of platelet factors at the injury site, formation of thrombin, and trapping of red blood cells in fibrin to form a clot.

lymph nodes often become enlarged when the body is invaded by an infectious agent and in cases of neoplastic disease.

Mature **lymphocytes** are the most important cells in the development of immunity. T lymphocytes are derived from lymphatic tissue of the thymus gland, and B lymphocytes are derived from bone marrow. These two types of lymphocytes work together with macrophages to ingest foreign substances and process specific foreign antigens. Through a complex process, an antibody that is capable of attacking the foreign antigen is formed. An *antibody* is an immunoglobulin produced by plasma cells and is categorized into one of five classifications: IgG, IgM, IgA, IgD, and IgE. The formation of antibodies is the systemic response that could have a negative effect on tissue grafts and organ transplants. The human body sees the transplant as foreign, so the lymphocytes and macrophages try to destroy the foreign antigens, which results in rejection of the graft or transplant.

Although the risk of whole-body radiation exposure is of little concern in diagnostic radiology, it is important for the radiographer to remember that exposure to x-rays or gamma-rays can have a harmful effect on blood marrow and lymphoid tissue. It takes a whole-body dose of approximately 0.5 Gy to 0.75 Gy (50–75 rad) to cause a detectable change in blood cells. The most radiosensitive blood cells are lymphocytes, followed by leukocytes and thrombocytes.

The **spleen** is the largest lymphoid organ and is located in the upper left quadrant of the abdomen. Its chief function is production of lymphocytes and plasma cells. It serves as a reservoir for blood and contains mononuclear phagocytes that cleanse the blood and lymphocytes to fight infectious blood-borne microorganisms. The splenic artery arises from the trifurcation of the celiac trunk off the abdominal aorta and supplies fresh blood to the spleen. This blood is cleansed by macrophages, which remove old or defective blood cells and microorganisms. The splenic vein empties into the portal vein. The spleen is occasionally ruptured in abdominal trauma and can be removed without detrimental effects.

Myeloid tissue, or bone marrow, is located within the spongy bone cavities formed by the outer layer of compact bone and may be classified as red or yellow marrow. This tissue contains blood vessels, nerves, stem cells, blood cells, mononuclear phagocytes, and fatty tissue. Red marrow is myeloid tissue that is still active in the production of blood cells, whereas yellow marrow is inactive tissue that is primarily composed of fatty tissue. Red bone marrow is predominantly found in flat bones (cranium, ribs, pelvis, and vertebrae) and in the proximal end of long bones, such as the humerus and femur.

Imaging Considerations

Radiography plays a limited role in the diagnosis and treatment of hematopoietic disorders. Skeletal survey radiography may be used in cases of multiple myeloma, a neoplastic disease of plasma cells, and for some types of leukemia. Chest radiography is helpful in identifying lymphatic changes within the mediastinum often associated with lymphomas. Chest radiography is also warranted in diagnosing various opportunistic infections resulting in acute respiratory infections in immunocompromised patients, such as those with **human immunodeficiency virus** (**HIV**).

Although abdominal computed tomography (CT) is useful in the assessment of lymph node enlargement (Fig. 9.3) and to further determine the location and extent of neoplastic diseases of the lymphatic system, positron emission tomography (PET) is now considered the modality of choice in the follow-up treatment for patients with Hodgkin lymphoma. Compared with CT, PET has been shown to have a higher specificity in demonstrating relapses of the disease. CT of the brain, without contrast enhancement, and magnetic resonance imaging (MRI) of the brain, with or without contrast enhancement, are highly recommended by the American College

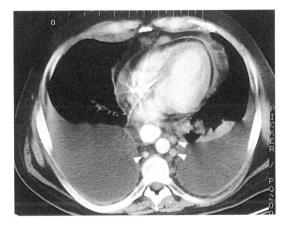

FIG. 9.3 Computed tomography of the lower chest and upper abdomen demonstrates enlargement of lymph nodes on a 27-year-old man with lymphoma.

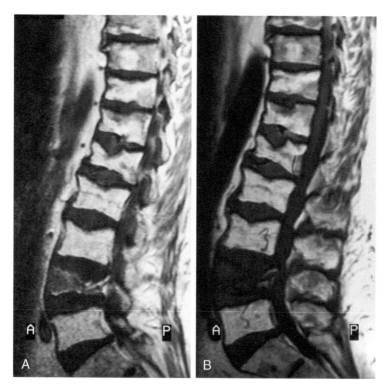

FIG. 9.4 **A,** A T2-weighted sagittal magnetic resonance imaging (MRI) view without gadolinium demonstrates an obvious L4 lesion. **B,** A T2-weighted sagittal MRI view with gadolinium demonstrates L4 destruction consistent with multiple myeloma in this 55-year-old man.

of Radiology (ACR) in assessing focal neurologic deficits associated with HIV infection. CT of the chest without contrast enhancement is also appropriate in evaluating acute respiratory infections associated with HIV.

MRI is useful in imaging bone marrow and the diseases that affect the marrow. Although MRI produces a signal void in areas of compact bone, changes in the marrow pattern are visible and useful in the diagnosis of many disorders (Fig. 9.4).

Nuclear medicine technetium-99m (^{99m}Tc) bone scans are indicated for metastatic bone disease such as multiple myeloma, and follow-up radiography after a positive bone scan may be appropriate. As previously mentioned, PET is increasingly used in the initial staging and follow-up of patients with Hodgkin lymphoma and has been deemed highly predictive of patient outcomes by the ACR. In addition, PET or CT is used in the radiation treatment planning process and posttreatment follow-up of patients undergoing radiation therapy for Hodgkin lymphoma.

Many blood-borne pathogens may be transmitted from patients to health care workers. Therefore it is of utmost importance that radiographers always practice standard precautions in terms of blood and bodily fluids. Gloves should be worn when performing venipuncture or whenever the possibility of contamination with blood or other bodily fluids exists. Additional protective apparel may be necessary if large amounts of bodily fluids may be encountered. Needles should not be recapped; they should be placed in puncture-proof containers for hazardous waste disposal. The importance of hand washing cannot be overemphasized because it is a vital part of infection control practices. It is the single most significant factor in infection control.

Human Immunodeficiency Virus (HIV) Infection

HIV is a blood-borne pathogen that is found in blood and body fluids. It is often transmitted through blood and blood products, vaginal fluid, semen, saliva; and it can be transmitted from an infected mother to her child in utero across the placenta, during childbirth through contact with blood and body fluids, or through breast milk during breast-feeding. An HIV infection affects the immune system by destroying CD4 cells, thus weakening the body's defenses against infections and other diseases. HIV is caused by one of two related **human immunodeficiency retroviruses**, HIV-1 and HIV-2. HIV-1 was identified in 1984 and it is responsible for most cases of HIV in the Western hemisphere. In late 2012, the Centers for Disease Control and Prevention (CDC) estimated that 1.2 million individuals aged 13 years and older in the United States had an HIV infection. Less virulent than HIV-1, HIV-2 is the principal agent of HIV in Sub-Saharan Africa. Although the annual number of HIV diagnoses in the United States has steadily declined since 2005, scientists estimate that worldwide, there were approximately 36.9 million people living with HIV in 2015. It continues to be a serious health issue throughout Africa, Asia, Latin America, the Caribbean, the Pacific, and Eastern Europe.

Retroviruses contain reverse transcriptase, an enzyme that converts viral ribonucleic acid (RNA) into a deoxyribonucleic acid (DNA) copy that becomes integrated into the host cell DNA. Each time the cell divides, the retroviral DNA is duplicated. Both types of HIV also contain HIV protease, an enzyme that converts immature, noninfectious HIV to its infectious state within the cell. HIV infects a part of the T lymphocyte, termed *T4* or *CD4*, responsible for immune response to infection, as well as nonlymphoid cells such as macrophages. Infected individuals experience a brief antibody-negative period immediately after infection, during which time the virus rapidly reproduces until the immune system begins to react to the infectious agent. If left untreated, the infection will progress through three stages of disease. Stage 1 is the acute phase, occurring 2 to 4 weeks following the initial infection. During stage 1, individuals may exhibit flu-like symptoms and are extremely contagious. The best method for diagnosing stage 1 HIV is to conduct one of the following laboratory tests: a fourth generation antibody/antigen test that identifies HIV antibodies and antigens within the blood or a nucleic acid test, which looks for the actual presence of HIV in the blood. Stage 2 is the latent period; although the individual may not exhibit symptoms of the viral infection, the virus is still replicating.

As the viral load increases during stage 2, the CD4 cell count begins to drop as the infected individual transitions into stage 3. Stage 3 is the development of acquired immunodeficiency syndrome (AIDS).

Because HIV inhibits the body's defensive response to the presence of a variety of diseases, one major sign of AIDS is the presence of unusual opportunistic infections (Box 9.1) such as *Pneumocystis carinii*,

---

BOX 9.1 AIDS-Defining Opportunistic Infections and Neoplasms Found in Individuals with Human Immunodeficiency Virus Infection

Infections

Protozoal and Helminthic Infections

Cryptosporidiosis or isosporiasis (enteritis)
Pneumocystosis (pneumonia or disseminated infection)
Toxoplasmosis (pneumonia or CNS infection)
Fungal infections
Candidiasis (esophageal, tracheal, or pulmonary)
Cryptococcosis (CNS infection)
Coccidiomycosis (disseminated)
Histoplasmosis (disseminated)

Bacterial Infections

Mycobacteriosis (atypical, e.g., *Mycobacterium avium-intracellulare,* disseminated or extra-pulmonary; *Mycobacterium tuberculosis,* pulmonary or extrapulmonary)
Nocardiosis (pneumonia, meningitis, disseminated)
Salmonella infections (disseminated)

Viral Infections

Cytomegalovirus (pulmonary, intestinal, retinitis, or CNS infections)
Herpes simplex virus (localized or disseminated)
Varicella-zoster virus (localized or disseminated)
Progressive multifocal leukoencephalopathy

Neoplasms

Kaposi sarcoma
B-cell non-Hodgkin lymphomas
Primary lymphoma of the brain
Invasive cancer of the uterine cervix

AIDS, Acquired immunodeficiency syndrome; *CNS,* central nervous system.
From: Kumar, V., Abbas, A., Aster, J.: *Robbins and Cotran pathologic basis for disease,* ed 9, Philadelphia, PA, 2013, Elsevier.

Toxoplasma gondii, cryptococci, *Mycobacterium avium,* and the herpes simplex virus. AIDS is also directly linked to an increased incidence of malignancies such as Kaposi sarcoma, **non-Hodgkin lymphoma** (NHL), Hodgkin lymphoma, and primary central nervous system (CNS) lymphoma. It is the most common disease associated with lymphocytopenia, or the depletion of lymphocytes. This occurs through the destruction of CD4+ T-cells infected by the virus. Anemia, thrombocytopenia, and leukopenia also commonly occur in HIV-infected patients (Fig. 9.5).

Signs and symptoms associated with HIV and AIDS are broad and may mimic those of other diseases. Symptoms of HIV infection include generalized lymphadenopathy, malaise, fever, and joint pain within 1 to 4 weeks after infection. These early-stage HIV symptoms may last up to 10 years before progressing to AIDS. Left untreated, approximately 99% of HIV infections progress to AIDS. As this progression takes place, weight loss may occur as a result of nausea, vomiting, and diarrhea. As mentioned earlier, leukopenia, anemia, and thrombocytopenia also occur. AIDS

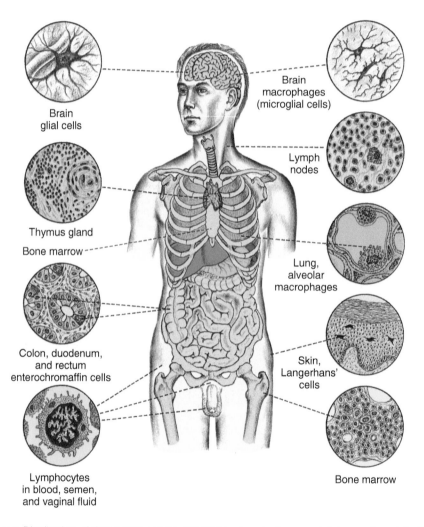

FIG. 9.5 Distribution of tissue that can be infected by human immunodeficiency virus. Infection is closely linked to the presence of CD4 receptors or chemokine coreceptors on the host tissue, particularly T-cells and macrophages.

may affect the CNS, which results in apathy, memory loss, inability to concentrate, and dementia. Headache, fever, or photophobia associated with acute aseptic meningitis, encephalopathy with seizure, or motor, sensory, or gait deficits may be the first manifestations of the disease. Atrophy of the brain cortex is commonly demonstrated by brain CT and MRI studies in patients with subacute encephalitis related to AIDS. In cases of toxoplasmic encephalitis, CT and MRI will demonstrate contrast-enhanced lesions within the basal ganglia.

With no known cure, AIDS remains a major health crisis and places a burden on the health care system in the United States and throughout the world. As a result of advances in the production and use of antiretroviral therapy (ART) in the United States, the number of individuals diagnosed with AIDS and the number of deaths associated with AIDS have continually declined since 1996. In 2014 the CDC's cumulative estimated number of individuals in the United States that had been diagnosed with stage 3 HIV (AIDS) was over 1,200,000. ART has reduced the incidence of opportunistic infections and extended the lives of individuals infected with HIV. However, the use of antiviral drugs in the treatment of HIV infection is continually being reevaluated because the use of only one drug results in mutation of the virus, resistance to the drug, and a loss of efficacy of the therapy. HIV infection must be staged before placing an individual on an ART regimen. Staging includes HIV antibody testing, CD4 T-cell count, viral load, a complete blood cell (CBC) count and chemistry profile, as well as genotypic resistance testing. The CD4 T-cell count is the primary indicator of immune function, and the CDC recommends that CD4 T-cell counts should be monitored quarterly. Current ART regimens may reduce HIV-associated morbidity and improve the quality of life. Currently, the most common therapy calls for an individualized two- or three-drug regimen of a combination of 20 antiretroviral drugs that have been approved by the U.S. Food and Drug Administration (FDA) and categorized into six mechanistic drug classifications. Guidelines for preventing opportunistic infections in persons with HIV infection were updated in 2009 by the CDC, the National Institutes of Health, and the HIV Medicine Association of the Infectious Diseases Society of America. Additional information can be accessed at the CDC website. Bone marrow evaluation is common in HIV-positive individuals. This diagnostic tool is used to evaluate decreased blood cell counts, stage malignancies, and obtain cultures for determining associated infections.

Although it can affect anyone regardless of age or sexual orientation, in the United States, HIV most frequently affects homosexual and bisexual men and intravenous (IV) drug users. The virus is transmitted through sexual contact and exposure to infected blood and bodily fluids.

One of the most common lung infections associated with HIV is tuberculosis (TB). TB may be the first indication of HIV infection in areas of the world where TB is prevalent. In developed countries such as the United States, HIV has caused an increase in the rates of TB. The lungs are also a common site for opportunistic infections associated with AIDS, such as **Pneumocystis carinii pneumonia**, often in combination with a cytomegalovirus. In the early stages of disease, the small multifocal infiltrates of the lungs associated with this pneumonia are often termed *ground glass lesions*. This fungal infection occurs in over half of all patients with AIDS; however, in developed countries, the risk of these infections has been reduced through the use of effective prophylactic treatment. Bacterial pneumonias are also common in IV drug users infected with HIV. Chest radiography demonstrates localized consolidation, which usually indicates a bacterial infection (Fig. 9.6). *P. carinii* infections (Fig. 9.7) generally reveal bilateral perihilar reticular–interstitial infiltrates that rapidly progress within 3 to 5 days to diffuse consolidation.

Kaposi sarcoma is the most common malignancy in patients with AIDS, especially in homosexual or bisexual men who are often coinfected with herpesvirus 8. It is present in approximately 25% to 30% of patients with AIDS and may affect connective tissue in various sites of the body. It most often affects the skin, lymph nodes, and the gastrointestinal system. About 20% of patients with Kaposi sarcoma also demonstrate pulmonary involvement. Radiographically, hilar adenopathy, nodular pulmonary infiltrates, and pleural effusion are demonstrated (Fig. 9.8). Endobronchial Kaposi sarcoma is common among patients with AIDS and may result in atelectasis or postobstruction pneumonia.

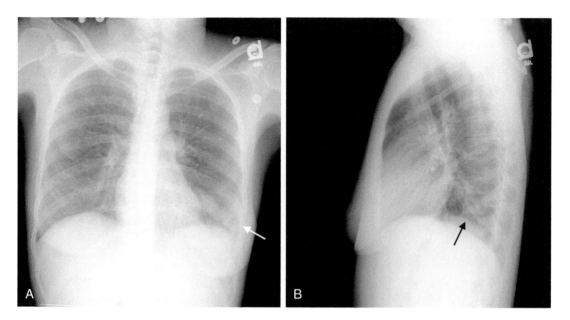

FIG. 9.6 **A,** Posteroanterior and **B,** left lateral chest radiographs of a patient with known acquired immunodeficiency syndrome demonstrate a left lower lobe infiltrate.

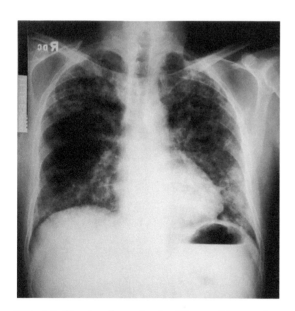

FIG. 9.7 Chest radiograph of a 53-year-old man diagnosed with acquired immunodeficiency syndrome. The radiograph demonstrates *Pneumocystis carinii* pneumonia with diffuse bilateral airspace parenchymal infiltrative densities.

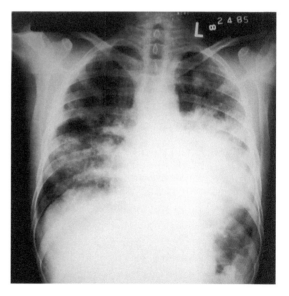

FIG. 9.8 Chest radiograph of a 27-year-old man with Kaposi sarcoma of the skin including pulmonary involvement. The radiograph shows nodular diffuse patchy parenchymal infiltration with nodular densities in the upper lobes.

Congenital and Hereditary Diseases

Sickle Cell Disease

Sickle cell disease is a group of hereditary autosomal recessive disorders resulting from an abnormal type of hemoglobin with the RBC. The abnormal hemoglobin, hemoglobin S (HbS), is caused by a mutation in the β-chain of the hemoglobin molecule (Fig. 9.9). In its most severe form, termed **sickle cell anemia**, it may lead to chronic hemolytic anemia progressing to organ failure. The sickle cell trait is present during infancy and is most common in individuals of African, Near Eastern, Mediterranean, or Indian descent.

Deoxygenation causes the erythrocyte to stiffen and elongate to a crescent or sickle shape, prohibiting the normal movement of the blood cell through the circulatory system. This results in acute pain from poorly oxygenated tissue as a result of vessel occlusion, atypical pneumonias caused by pulmonary vessel infarction, and the development of a variety of infectious diseases. Sickle cell disease generally affects the abdomen, the chest, and the skeletal system. Early clinical manifestations occur 6 to 12 months following birth, as the normal hemoglobin is replaced with HbS. The clinical course of sickle cell disease is highly variable, and medical imaging plays a small role in its diagnosis and management. Treatment is often limited to supportive care to prevent anemia and infection, but the most definitive treatment requires stem cell transplantation to permanently alter the hemoglobin phenotype. Genetic counseling and psychological support are also an important component of the treatment.

Thalassemias

Thalassemias are inherited disorders caused by a mutation on the α-chain or β-chain of the hemoglobin molecule. Like sickle cell disease, this disorder tends to occur most frequently in individuals of Mediterranean or African descent. Thalassemias are classified as α-major, α-minor, β-major, and β-minor. The effects of the disorder vary, depending on the number of defective genes and the mode of inheritance. As with sickle cell anemia, evaluation is based on family history and

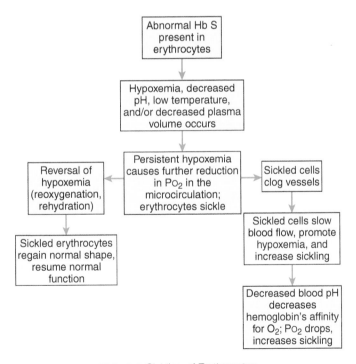

FIG. 9.9 Sickling of Erythrocytes.

laboratory tests. Radiography does not play a role in the diagnosis and treatment of these disorders.

Hemophilias

Hemophilias are inherited hemorrhagic diseases that involve a congenital deficiency of three plasma clotting factors. **Hemophilia A** results from a deficiency in plasma clotting factor VIII and is the most common type of hemophilia. This disorder only affects males, but it is transmitted by females. **Hemophilia B** results from a deficiency in plasma clotting factor IX and is clinically indistinguishable from hemophilia A. These hemophiliac conditions may be mild, moderate, or severe. **Hemophilia C** results from a deficiency in plasma clotting factor XI and occurs equally in both males and females. The severity of this deficiency is less than that of either hemophilia A or B.

In individuals with hemophilia, clinical manifestations begin to appear before the age of 4 years, and these patients experience persistent bleeding from minor injuries. As with other hereditary hematopoietic diseases, radiography does not play a role in the diagnosis and treatment of hemophilia. Evaluation is based on family history and laboratory tests. Common laboratory tests include thrombin time, prothrombin time (PT), and activated partial thromboplastin time (aPTT).

von Willebrand Disease

von Willebrand disease, the fourth type of hereditary bleeding disorder, is relatively common in both males and females. This disorder results from a defect in the plasma clotting factor termed *von Willebrand factor* (vWF) and is not diagnosed in adulthood. Many variants of this disorder exist, but the most common clinical signs include spontaneous bleeding from the nose, mouth, and gastrointestinal tract. The bleeding episodes are not as severe as those associated with hemophilia A, hemophilia B, or hemophilia C; usually the only treatment is prevention and includes the avoidance of aspirin ingestion.

Neoplastic Diseases

Multiple Myeloma

Multiple myeloma (**MM**), a neoplastic disease of B-cells in plasma, results in cell proliferation as a result of an abnormally large amount of immunoglobulin, most commonly IgG. This disorder results from chromosomal translocations primarily involving the immunoglobulin heavy chain on chromosome 14 relocating to chromosome 6 (p21), chromosome 11 (q13), and chromosome 12 (q13) affecting the cell cycle (cyclins); chromosome 8 (q24), chromosome 16 (q23), and chromosome 20 affecting the oncogenes; and chromosome 4 (p16) affecting the fibroblast growth factor receptor. Further genetic alterations secondary to these translocations lead to the development of aggressive MM. MM is usually confined to the bone marrow and forms discrete osteolytic tumors that weaken the affected bone. It most frequently affects the pelvis, spine, ribs, and skull, which results in multiple osteolytic lesions, renal insufficiency, and hypercalcemia. It is typically seen in persons over the age of 60 years and its signs and symptoms include progressive bone pain, especially in the back and thorax, anemia, fatigue, bleeding disorders, renal insufficiency or failure, hypercalcemia, and recurrent bacterial infections, especially pneumococcal pneumonia. The incidence of MM is slightly more common in men than in women and in African Americans than in Caucasians.

The abnormal plasma cells produce large amounts of monoclonal paraprotein (*M protein*), specifically IgG, IgA, IgD, and IgE, which create a variety of problems in addition to skeletal involvement. This protein is excreted via urine and disrupts normal renal function. M protein can be detected in both blood and urine. Blood tests for hypercalcemia, elevated erythrocyte sediment rate (ESR), and renal failure, as well as bone marrow biopsies, are most commonly used in the diagnosis of MM. Radiography plays a vital role in the diagnosis and treatment of MM because about 90% of these patients have bone involvement. Skeletal survey radiography demonstrates diffuse osteoporosis with discrete punched-out, osteolytic regions (Figs. 9.10 and 9.11). These patients are at risk for pathologic fractures and vertebral compression fractures because MM primarily affects the axial skeleton. A 30% bone loss should have occurred before the disease can be visualized with conventional radiography, but MRI is useful in the diagnosis and management of early-stage MM. In addition, approximately 90% of patients exhibit proteinuria and 50% of patients develop renal

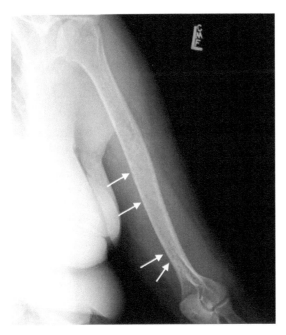

FIG. 9.10 Humerus radiograph of a patient with multiple myeloma. The radiograph demonstrates the presence of discrete, lytic, well-circumscribed skeletal defects.

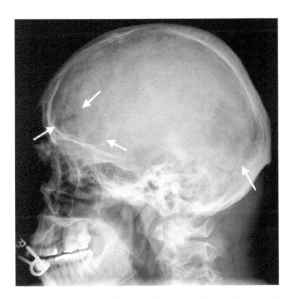

FIG. 9.11 Lateral skull radiograph of a patient with multiple myeloma. The radiograph demonstrates the presence of discrete, lytic, well-circumscribed skeletal defects.

insufficiency. High levels of protein in blood increase the viscosity of blood, thus affecting circulation to the brain, kidneys, and extremities.

Treatment involves the use of chemotherapy, radiation therapy, plasmapheresis, and bone marrow transplantation. Thalidomide drugs in combination with a corticosteroid may be used to disrupt the stromal marrow – MM cell interaction and inhibiting angiogenesis. Stem cell transplantation is often employed following chemotherapy and using autologous cells or a donor's stem cells. Survival may be prolonged by performing a second stem cell transplant within 6 to 12 months following the first transplant. The prognosis for MM is poor, the median survival rate being approximately 3 years.

Leukemia

Leukemia is a term associated with neoplastic disease of leukocytes that result in an overproduction of WBCs. This increase in leukocytes interferes with normal blood cell production and may lead to anemia, bleeding, and infection. Leukemias may infiltrate lymphatic tissue and organs such as the liver and spleen. The causes of leukemia are unknown and most likely vary according to the type of leukemia. However, exposure to radiation and to certain chemicals (especially benzene) and genetic defects such as Down syndrome seem to predispose individuals to developing these disorders. Current research also indicates an association between leukemia and two viruses: (1) the Epstein-Barr virus and (2) the human T-cell leukemia and lymphoma virus. Structural molecular changes disrupting the genes that regulate normal blood cell development have been observed. Most frequently, these disruptions include the translocation of chromosomes, the inversion of chromosome 16, and the deletion of part of chromosome 6.

Leukemias are classified according to cell type and cell maturity. *Myelocytic leukemias* develop from primitive or stem cells. *Monocytic leukemias* develop from precursor cells (the cells from which leukocytes are derived) and are the least common type of leukemia. *Lymphocytic leukemias* arise from lymphoid cells. In addition, leukemias are classified as either acute or chronic. *Acute leukemias* have an abrupt onset and may manifest as a hemorrhagic episode. They generally are associated with primitive or poorly differentiated cells. *Chronic leukemias* progress at a relatively slow pace with nonspecific signs such as fatigue and weakness. They are associated with mature or well-differentiated cells. All of the above-mentioned terms are used in combination to describe the specific type of leukemia.

Acute lymphocytic leukemia (ALL) affects both children and adults. **Chronic lymphocytic leukemia** (CLL) predominantly affects individuals over the age of 60 years. **Chronic myelocytic leukemia** (CML) most often affects older adults. **Acute myelocytic leukemia** (AML) and **acute monoblastic leukemia** (AMOL) affect anyone at any age. Leukemias, in general, account for approximately 33% of all cancer-related deaths in children under the age of 15 years. Radiography plays a limited role in the diagnosis and treatment of most leukemias.

Common symptoms and signs associated with acute leukemia include fatigue, anemia, low-grade fever, night sweats, weight loss, bruising as a result of a decreased platelet count, and bone pain caused by the expansion of the bone marrow. Patients with ALL may also present with an enlarged spleen and liver, whereas patients with AML often exhibit infiltration of the malignant cells to the skin and other soft tissues within the body. In some instances, the leukemic cells may pass the blood-brain barrier, causing cranial nerve palsies, headaches, lethargy, confusion, and seizures. The definitive diagnoses of acute leukemias are primarily established through blood tests, bone marrow biopsies, and cytogenetic studies used to determine chromosomal abnormalities. CT of the chest, abdomen, and pelvis are frequently performed to identify sites of the disease. Additionally, lumbar puncture under fluoroscopic guidance is also common for analysis of the cerebrospinal fluid to assess involvement of the CNS. The primary treatment of acute leukemia is chemotherapy, although stem cell transplantation and bone marrow transfusions may also be used in patients under the age of 50 years. Most patients with acute leukemias die within 6 months without treatment. ALL therapies carry a 5-year survival rate of 80% or better in children and 40% in adults. AML carries a 5 year survival rate of 24% and continued improvements in induced remissions and survival are attributed to more effective chemotherapeutic agents and bone marrow transplants. In all cases, survival depends on complete remission.

Individuals with CLL are often asymptomatic and the disease is often discovered during routine blood counts. With progression of the disease, lymph node involvement, which leads to an enlarged spleen and liver, becomes evident. Symptoms at this stage of the disease include fever, abdominal pain, and weight loss. These patients will also present with anemia and susceptibility to other infectious pathogens such as *Streptococcus pneumoniae, Staphylococcus aureus,* and *Haemophilus influenzae.* The treatment for individuals with CLL varies, as many patients may remain stable for years, whereas others may require chemotherapy or bone marrow irradiation and stem cell transplantation.

Patients with CML present with a slow chronic phase of variable length. During this phase, these individuals are asymptomatic, but as the disease progresses to the short accelerated stage, they present with weakness, weight loss, splenomegaly, low-grade fever, bone pain, dysfunctional platelets, and anemia. The final stage of CML is the blast crisis stage, in which the number of myeloid precursor blast cells increases dramatically (>100,000 cells/μL). CML is progressive, with an average survival of about 3 to 4 years after the onset of the disease and a 5-year survival rate of approximately 20%. Patients reaching the blast crisis stage only survive an average of 3 months. Treatment for CML is constantly evolving; however, the only curative treatment currently available is bone marrow or stem cell transplantation.

Non-Hodgkin Lymphoma

Non-Hodgkin Lymphoma is a malignancy of the lymphoid cells found in the lymph nodes, bone marrow, spleen, liver, and gastrointestinal system. It is the most common type of lymphoma and its incidence increases with age, most commonly occurring in individuals aged 50 years or older. Some patients tolerate NHL very well, and others die very quickly from the disease. Although its etiology is unknown, it is believed to result from chromosomal translocation alterations. Research indicates that the chance of developing NHL increases with exposure to certain chemicals; an impaired immune system, as occurs with HIV or in immunosuppressed patients following organ transplantation; or chronic *Helicobacter pylori* infection. Most cases arise from B-cells (80%–85%), and approximately 15% arise from T-cells. Currently, multiple methods of classifying NHLs exist, with approximately 40 types of lymphomas identified. The most common classification system has been established by the World Health Organization (WHO), and in this system, lymphomas are designated by cell type, cell maturation, and anatomic site. B-cell lymphomas include both precursor B-cell lymphoma and a multitude of mature B-cell lymphomas, whereas T-cell lymphomas include one precursor T-cell lymphoma and two mature T-cell lymphomas.

The signs and symptoms of NHL are varied. In a few cases, the patient manifests general lymphadenopathy before developing lymphoma. Many patients also have anemia. Diagnosis is made from histologic examination of the diseased tissue via lymph node biopsy to differentiate NHL from Hodgkin lymphoma, leukemia, and metastatic disease. CT scans of the neck, chest, abdomen, and pelvis are commonly used to stage the disease and to demonstrate the extent of disease in the lymphatic system around the aorta and mesentery (Figs. 9.12 and 9.13). PET or CT is gaining popularity, and MRI of the chest and abdomen may also be indicated. A bone marrow biopsy may also be performed, as bone marrow involvement and organ infiltration are more common with NHL than with Hodgkin lymphoma. Treatment of NHL depends on the stage of the disease. It consists of chemotherapy and radiation therapy, either independently or in combination. In some advanced cases, radiolabeled antibody therapy may also be used.

Hodgkin Lymphoma

Hodgkin lymphoma is another neoplastic disease that affects lymphoid tissue. Its cause is unknown and it commonly affects individuals between the ages of 20 and 40 years and those over 60 years of age. It tends to affect men slightly more often than women and Caucasians more than African Americans. The presence of **Reed-Sternberg cells** differentiates Hodgkin lymphoma from other types of lymphatic diseases. Reed-Sternberg cells are believed to be mutant B-cells that secrete and release cytokines, which leads to an inflammatory cellular response. However, the genetic etiology of Hodgkin lymphoma is unknown.

Common signs and symptoms associated with Hodgkin lymphoma are general malaise, fever, night sweats, weight loss, splenomegaly, and enlarged lymph nodes (Fig. 9.14). Mediastinal and hilar lymph nodes are often visible on a chest radiograph, although a definitive diagnosis is made via biopsy of the lymphatic tissue. As with other neoplastic disorders, Hodgkin lymphoma is staged according to the extent of the disease.

Hodgkin lymphoma and NHL generally have different nodal distributions as seen by CT, as Hodgkin disease is generally retroperitoneal with less mesenteric involvement compared with NHL. CT examinations of the chest, abdomen, and pelvis, which are used to stage the disease, commonly demonstrate enlarged

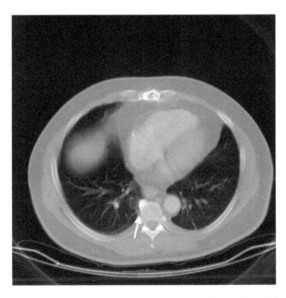

FIG. 9.12 Chest computed tomography of a patient with non-Hodgkin lymphoma. The scan demonstrates a necrotic lymph node in the cardiophrenic angle.

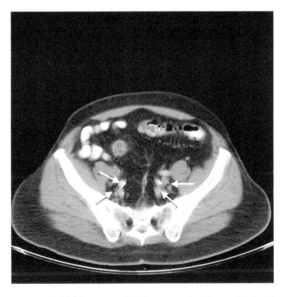

FIG. 9.13 Pelvic computed tomography of a patient with non-Hodgkin lymphoma. The scan demonstrates enlarged inguinal lymph nodes.

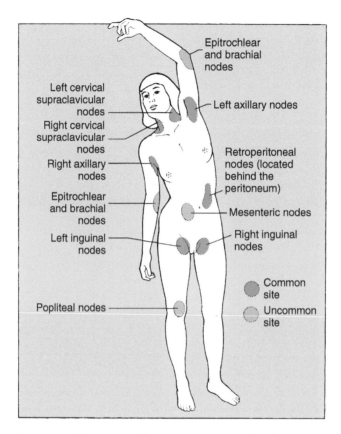

FIG. 9.14 Common and uncommonly involved lymph node sites for Hodgkin lymphoma.

retroperitoneal nodes. FDG-PET/CT whole body scans are also useful in staging Hodgkin lymphoma. In some cases, a laparotomy, including splenectomy, may also be indicated. Stage I denotes one anatomic node location, and stage IV denotes extranodal spread to bone marrow, the lungs, or the liver. The ACR suggests FDG-PET/CT whole body imaging every 6 months for 2 years, then yearly for 3 years as the most appropriate follow-up to patients with Hodgkin lymphoma.

Hodgkin disease is most commonly treated and cured with a combination of radiotherapy, bone marrow and stem cell transplantation, and chemotherapy. Stage I and stage IIA Hodgkin lymphoma may be treated with radiation therapy alone and is associated with a 5-year survival rate of 85% to 90%. Stage IV Hodgkin lymphoma has approximately a 70% to 80% complete remission rate, with more than 50% of patients remaining disease-free for up to 15 years.

Pathologic Summary of the Hematopoietic System

Pathology	Imaging Modality of Choice
HIV infection	CT and MRI
Multiple myeloma	MRI, skeletal radiography, and nuclear medicine bone scan
Non-Hodgkin lymphoma	CT, PET, and MRI
Hodgkin lymphoma	Chest radiography, PET, CT, and MRI

CT, Computed tomography; *MRI,* magnetic resonance imaging; *PET,* positron emission tomography.

Review Questions

1. The majority of blood volume is composed of:
   a. Erythrocytes
   b. Leukocytes
   c. Plasma
   d. Thrombocytes

2. Bilirubin is formed during the destruction of:
   a. Erythrocytes
   b. Leukocytes
   c. Plastocytes
   d. Thrombocytes

3. Which of the following is considered the universal donor type of blood?
   a. A
   b. B
   c. AB
   d. O

4. Which cells are most important in the development of immunity?
   a. Erythrocytes
   b. Lymphocytes
   c. Platelets
   d. Thrombocytes

5. The most common pulmonary complication resulting from acquired immunodeficiency syndrome is:
   a. Pneumocystis carinii pneumonia
   b. Pneumococcal pneumonia
   c. Legionnaire pneumonia
   d. Tuberculosis

6. Kaposi sarcoma is frequently associated with AIDS, and it may affect:
   a. The gastrointestinal system
   b. Lymph nodes
   c. Skin
   d. All of the above

7. A neoplastic disease of the plasma is called:
   a. Hodgkin lymphoma
   b. Leukemia
   c. Non-Hodgkin lymphoma
   d. Multiple myeloma

8. Which type of leukemia predominantly affects children?
   a. Acute lymphocytic
   b. Chronic lymphocytic
   c. Chronic myelocytic
   d. Acute myelocytic

9. With what type of neoplastic disease are Reed-Sternberg cells associated?
   a. Leukemia
   b. Hodgkin lymphoma
   c. Multiple myeloma
   d. Non-Hodgkin lymphoma

10. What blood cells are affected by non-Hodgkin lymphoma?
    a. Erythrocytes
    b. Lymphocytes
    c. Plastocytes
    d. Thrombocytes

11. Explain why researchers currently believe that an association exists between viral agents and the development of lymphomas.

12. Identify two means of transmission of human immunodeficiency virus (HIV) infection.

13. What is the difference in cellular origin between multiple myeloma and leukemia?

14. What is the risk of using radiation or antileukemic drug therapy in treating leukemias?

15. Identify at least three signs and symptoms of Hodgkin lymphoma.

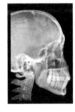
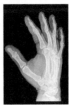
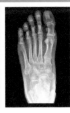

Reproductive System

ⓔ http://evolve.elsevier.com/Kowalczyk/pathology/

LEARNING OBJECTIVES

On completion of Chapter 10, the reader should be able to:

1. Discuss the basic anatomic structures associated with the male and female reproductive systems.
2. Briefly explain the role of general radiography, mammography, diagnostic medical sonography, computed tomography, and magnetic resonance imaging in the diagnosis and treatment of reproductive system disorders.
3. Compare and contrast breast imaging modalities, including diagnostic *versus* screening mammography, localization techniques, and sonography.
4. Differentiate among the major congenital anomalies of the female reproductive system.
5. Describe the various neoplastic diseases of both the female and male reproductive systems in terms of etiology, incidence, signs and symptoms, treatment, and prognosis.
6. Differentiate among the common disorders during pregnancy and explain the role of diagnostic medical sonography in the management of the gravid female.

OUTLINE

Female Reproductive System
  Anatomy and Physiology
  Imaging Considerations
  Congenital Anomalies
  Inflammatory Diseases
  Neoplastic Diseases

Uterine Masses
Breast Masses
Disorders during Pregnancy
Male Reproductive System
  Anatomy and Physiology

Imaging Considerations
Congenital Anomalies
  Cryptorchidism
Neoplastic Diseases
  Benign Prostatic Hyperplasia

KEY TERMS

Adenocarcinoma of the prostate
Benign prostatic hyperplasia
Bicornuate uterus
Breast carcinoma
Cervical carcinoma
Cervical dysplasia

Corpus luteum ovarian cysts
Cryptorchidism
Cystic teratomas
Dermoid cysts
Ectopic pregnancy
Endometrial carcinoma
Endometriosis

Epididymo-orchitis
Fibroadenoma
Fibrocystic breasts
Follicular ovarian cysts
Hydatidiform mole
Hydroceles
Hysterosalpingography
Leiomyomas

Female Reproductive System

Anatomy and Physiology

The female reproductive system consists of one pair of ovaries, which are the primary sex organs, and the secondary sex organs, which include one pair of fallopian tubes, the uterus, the vagina (Fig. 10.1), and two breasts. The primary function of the system is to provide a female reproductive cell (the ovum), hormones, and a site for the development of the zygote.

The external genitalia (the vulva) include the mons pubis, the labia majora and minora, the clitoris, the openings of the urethra and vagina, and the perineum. The vagina connects the external genitalia with the uterus and is the mode of exit for menstrual fluids and conception products.

The uterus is a pear-shaped organ and its primary purpose is to provide an environment for fetal growth and development. Located within the pelvic cavity, it can be divided into the upper portion, termed the *fundus*; the midportion, termed the *body*; and the lower portion, termed the *cervix*. The cervix connects the uterine cavity with the upper vagina. Anatomically, the uterus is flexed so that the cervix and lower portion of the body lie anterior to the rectum. The body of the uterus follows the contour of the posterior urinary bladder wall. The fundus normally lies superior to the bladder. The walls of the uterus include an inner, endometrial layer; a middle, muscular, myometrial layer; and an outer layer, termed the *parietal peritoneum*. In actuality, the parietal peritoneum drapes over the fundus and the upper three fourths of the body but does not enclose the lower fourth

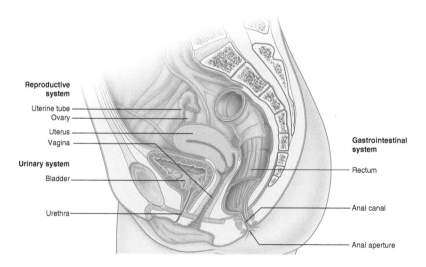

FIG. 10.1 Female pelvic organs.

of the body or the cervix. The actual cavity within the uterus is fairly small and can be well visualized with ultrasonography. It is divided into the *internal os*, leading to the cervical canal, and the *external os*, which opens into the vagina. The uterus is held in place within the pelvic cavity via eight ligaments.

Occasionally a lack of proper uterine support is present, resulting in a condition known as **pelvic organ prolapse** that affects approximately 50% of women over 50 years of age. A device known as the **pessary** (Fig. 10.2) is inserted into the vagina to provide proper support. Current research has demonstrated that the majority of women who use the pessary are very satisfied, as the device relieves the majority of urinary symptoms. Some women report that although the use of a pessary helps improve urinary symptoms, stress incontinence remains an ongoing problem. Although some patient reluctance as a result of inconvenience exists, the general consensus is that pessaries are an effective

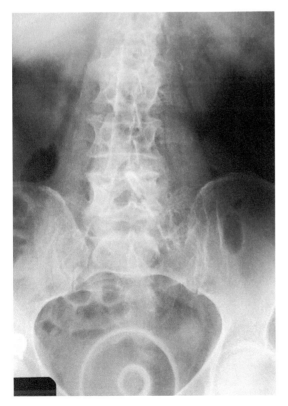

FIG. 10.2 A pessary, inserted into the vagina for uterine support, is readily visible on this abdominal radiograph of an 88-year-old woman.

and simple solution to alleviating symptoms of pelvic organ prolapse and associated pelvic organ dysfunction.

The fallopian tubes extend from the upper, outer edges of the uterus and expand distally into the infundibulum located close to, but not attached to, the ovaries. Suspended in place by the broad ligament, they are 8 to 12 cm long and tend to fall behind the uterus. These tubes serve as a passageway for the mature ova and are the normal site of fertilization. In a normal pregnancy, the fertilized ovum continues to travel through the fallopian tube and implants itself into the endometrium of the uterus.

The ovaries are the primary reproductive glands and are responsible for ovulation and secretion of estrogen and progesterone. Attached to the broad ligament and the posterior uterine wall, each ovary contains numerous graafian follicles enclosing ova. After puberty, several graafian follicles and ova grow and develop each month. Normally only one follicle matures, migrates to the surface of the ovary, and degenerates, thus expelling a mature ovum, which is the hallmark of the *ovulation* process.

Breasts—like the fallopian tubes, uterus, and vagina—are considered secondary sex organs. Breast parenchyma differs according to age and parity. Women in their 20s and 30s, especially nulliparous women, have dense, fibroglandular parenchyma that may conceal breast masses during a clinical breast examination and imaging. However with advancing age, decline in estrogen and progesterone causes breast tissue to undergo what is known as *involutional change*. Involution is the conversion of glandular breast tissue into adipose and also refers to the loss of the supportive tissue. As a result of this slow process, the breast changes its architecture, and fibroglandular tissue is replaced by fat. This process is variable, but it typically begins at the back of the breast and progresses forward to the nipple. The term **mastalgia** applies to conditions that result in pain in one or both breasts. Many patients fear that mastalgia is indicative of breast cancer; however, it is more closely related to architectural changes in breast tissue. Involution aids the imaging professional and the interpreting physician because fatty tissue is radiolucent and enhances the radiographic visibility of many breast masses.

Anatomically, breasts are attached via Cooper ligaments to the pectoral muscles and this gives the breast its contour and shape. The breast consists of about 12 lobes separated by connective tissue, much like the spokes of a wheel. The lobes are further divided into lobules clustered

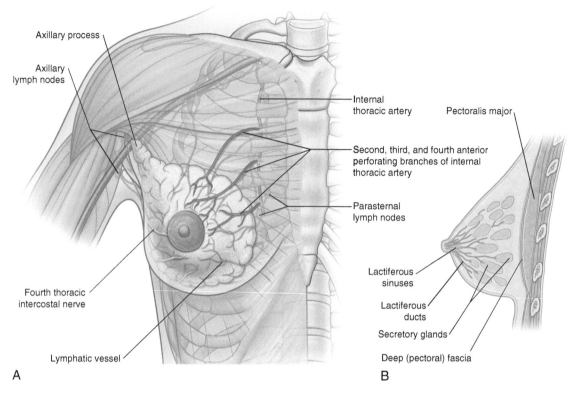

A, Anterior and B, lateral breast anatomy.

around small ducts. These small ducts join to form larger ducts, which terminate at the nipple (Fig. 10.3). Breasts function as accessory reproductive glands to secrete milk for the newborn. During pregnancy, changes in estrogen and progesterone levels prepare breasts for lactation. Approximately 3 days after delivery, a lactogenic hormone stimulates the secretion of milk.

Imaging Considerations

Hysterosalpingography

One of the most common radiographic studies of the female reproductive system is the **hysterosalpingography** (HSG). The procedure involves radiographic imaging of the cervical canal, uterine cavity, fallopian tubes, and peritoneal cavity during injection of contrast media with fluoroscopic visualization. HSG is performed for screening of the **nongravid** (nonpregnant) woman, especially in cases of suspected infertility. A common finding in cases of infertility is nonpatent fallopian tubes (Fig. 10.4). In addition,

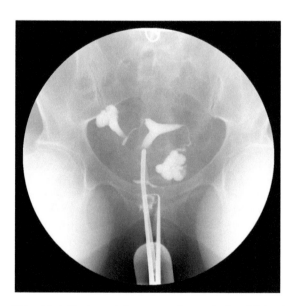

FIG. 10.4 Hysterosalpingogram demonstrating bilateral tubal obstruction and hydrosalpinx.

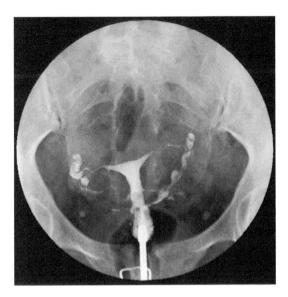

FIG. 10.5 Free spillage of contrast medium bilaterally, as seen in this hysterosalpingogram, in a 38-year-old woman indicates that the uterine tubes are open.

although HSG does not define the extent of certain conditions such as endometriosis, it is useful in revealing the shape of the uterus and certain characteristics of the fallopian tubes other than their patency. The practice guideline of the American College of Radiology (ACR) for the performance of HSG is to inject approximately 10 mL to 30 mL of contrast medium into the uterine cavity done slowly to avoid causing spasms and discomfort. Minimum radiation exposure settings that provide sufficient anatomy detail for diagnosis should be used. Spillage of the contrast medium from the fallopian tubes indicates the patency of the tubes (Fig. 10.5). Typically, HSG is used for diagnostic purposes, but it can also be used therapeutically for restoring tubal patency or to dilate or stretch the fallopian tubes.

An adjunct procedure that has the potential to replace the conventional HSG is known as sonohysterography (SHG). This examination is similar to hysterosalpingography in procedural approach; however, with SHG, normal saline, instead of an iodinated contrast agent, is injected into the uterus. Because saline is devoid of the complications associated with iodinated contrast agents, the procedure may be better tolerated by the patient. In the current application of SHG, saline is used to pry apart the layers of the endometrium to reveal abnormalities within the uterus. The saline fluid is expelled via the fallopian tubes, and this may also indicate their patency. This procedure is viewed via a transvaginal sonographic probe as the physician injects the saline. With real-time images, the dynamics of the reproductive system can be assessed without radiation to the patient.

In a study of a group of 100 patients with infertility, HSG was compared with SHG. These patients' HSG results were matched to their laparoscopic results. In this small group of women, HSG and SHG were equally effective in the evaluation of tubal disease. However, a study conducted in 2011 found that SHG has greater sensitivity, positive predictive value, and accuracy than HSG for detecting intrauterine lesions. HSG remains a reliable screening tool for infertility because of its ability to assess architecture and patency of fallopian tubes, but SHG is a more accurate diagnostic tool for evaluation of intrauterine masses.

Mammography

The use of mammography as a diagnostic procedure for symptomatic patients is well documented. Mammography provides important information about specific clinical problems such as a breast mass, pain, nipple discharge, and abnormalities of the skin and lymph nodes. With modern mammographic equipment and techniques, radiation exposure is minimal, and evidence does not suggest significant risk to women over 35 years of age. If a risk does exist, it is thought to be so minimal that it has never been observed, but only inferred scientifically.

The use of mammography in asymptomatic patients for screening purposes is based on its ability to detect nonpalpable breast lesions at an early stage when they are too small to be identified by physical examination. Current literature suggests that mammography can detect some cancers 2 years before they are palpable; survival depends on tumor size and lymph node involvement. According to the American Cancer Society, women aged 45 to 54 years should get yearly screening mammograms. In this age group, breast tissue is less sensitive to radiation and the incidence of breast cancer increases with age. This also takes advantage of the involutional process, making occult lesions easier to identify on a radiograph. The benefits far outweigh the associated risks from radiation exposure. Women aged 55 years and older should switch to mammograms every 2 years and continue as long as they are in good health and have a life expectancy of 10 or more years.

Mammography is also a valuable examination tool in the detection and evaluation of breast disease in individuals with augmentation prostheses. Although experience with patients who have undergone augmentation mammoplasty is limited, current research indicates that mammography can demonstrate both palpable and nonpalpable breast lesions. For mammographic screening of these patients, it is important to displace the implant so that the native breast tissue can be imaged and assessed for disease. To demonstrate the underlying breast parenchyma in these individuals, implant-displaced views are required. Technologists are encouraged to use the Eckland maneuver to displace the implant from the native breast tissue to radiograph as much of the native breast tissue as possible. The Eckland maneuver is accomplished by the technologist applying pressure at the area of the nipple and then carefully rolling the native breast tissue away from the implant. The implant-displaced view is performed for both craniocaudal and mediolateral projections of the breast. Once the implant is pushed upward and away from the native breast tissue, the compression paddle is used to continue to hold the implant so that the native breast tissue can be more fully imaged. Because of the variations in patients' breast tissue and their implants, manual exposure techniques are commonly used.

Needle guidewire localization is a specialized procedure to identify nonpalpable, mammographically detected abnormalities of the breast. It helps direct the surgeon to the lesion in question and allows excision of the suspect tissue for biopsy. Needle guidewire localizations cause minimal morbidity, with complications including hematoma formation, intraoperative wire dislodgement, and wire breakage. The development and refinement of localization techniques have greatly increased the percentage of positive findings on surgical biopsy and allow more accurate diagnosis and treatment of early-stage carcinoma of the breast. Fine-needle and large-core biopsy techniques offer an alternative to surgical biopsy as an initial step in the investigation of breast masses. These procedures are performed on an outpatient basis by the mammographer and the radiologist, or by the surgeon in the mammography area using a specially designed

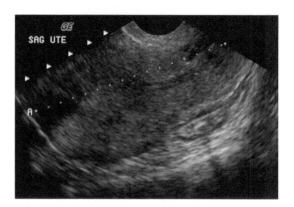

FIG. 10.6 A sagittal sonographic image of the normal uterus.

stereotactic localization unit. Ductal lavage of the breast may also be performed in cases of suspected intraductal disease to obtain a specimen for laboratory analysis. Use of sonography-guided aspiration and biopsy is also common because sonography provides the ability to visualize the area in question and note whether the area has been completely removed while the needle or biopsy gun is still *in situ*. This may prevent additional punctures into the patient's skin during the biopsy procedure.

In patients who have a positive finding during screening mammography, according to the ACR Appropriateness Criteria, diagnostic mammography is rated as highly appropriate as the next step in a patient's diagnostic workup. The only finding seen by screening mammography that would not result in the use of diagnostic mammography is a mass that has circumscribed margins, no additional malignant qualities, and has not enlarged compared with the last mammogram. In this case the use of breast sonography would be highly appropriate.

Sonography

Sonography is the primary modality for examining the gravid or nongravid female reproductive system because of its excellent accuracy and because it presents no radiation hazards to the fetus or the mother (Fig. 10.6). Not only is sonography applicable in pregnancy, but it is also useful in normal gynecologic examinations to visualize the reproductive organs or to monitor the progress of a medical fertility regimen.

Transabdominal pelvic sonography requires a distended urinary bladder to serve as an "acoustic window" for good visualization of the pelvic organs. In addition, the fluid within the urinary bladder displaces bowel gas away from the area of interest. Sonography of the uterus and ovaries has been greatly enhanced by the use of the transvaginal transducer, which provides more accurate clinical information with magnification of the images of internal pelvic structures. The most common indications for sonography in the nongravid female include evaluation of pelvic, uterine, and ovarian masses because sonography can provide information about mass size, location, internal characteristics, and effect on surrounding organs. Obstetrically, sonography is the method of choice for visualizing the position of the placenta, multiple gestations, or ectopic pregnancies and for determining gestational age. It is used to assist and guide the physician during amniocentesis and is invaluable in assessing fetal abnormalities such as anencephaly, hydrocephaly, congenital heart defects, polycystic kidney disease, urinary tract obstructions, and gastrointestinal (GI) tract obstructions and in determining fetal death.

The use of sonography to assess the pregnant uterus for determining fetal growth, any disturbances, or risk of growth restriction is recommended by the ACR. Sonography is the best imaging modality to assess the fetus, growth, the amniotic fluid, and for an overall survey of fetal well-being.

Sonography is an excellent modality for differentiating cystic masses from solid masses within the breast. However, sonography has limitations in the diagnosis of malignant breast disease because of the solid nature of most breast cancers. Recently researchers and clinicians have made great strides in the use of sonography to evaluate the dense breast for disease. To reduce the radiation dose to young patients, research continues to strive to perfect an accurate and safe screening modality. However, currently, breast sonography is not advocated as a screening modality for breast cancer because of the difficulty in consistently differentiating between a solid benign mass and malignant disease.

Magnetic Resonance Imaging

Magnetic resonance imaging (MRI) is now often used in conjunction with sonography in the evaluation of the female pelvis (Fig. 10.7). MRI, like sonography, uses no ionizing radiation and is noninvasive. MRI provides detailed information on pelvic, uterine, and ovarian masses (Fig. 10.8). In cases of ovarian cancer, MRI

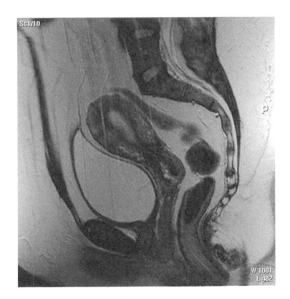

FIG. 10.7 A sagittal T2-weighted magnetic resonance image of a normal female pelvis demonstrating the bladder and the uterus.

accurately demonstrates proliferation into other pelvic structures. In addition, multiple leiomyomas can be detected and localized in a short period.

MRI is increasingly being used to assist with differentiating between malignant and benign solid lesions within the breast. Fat suppression imaging is used before and after contrast enhancement. This technique suppresses the normal, fatty tissue of the breast, allowing for easier identification of malignant masses through contrast enhancement (Fig. 10.9). MRI is also used to detect faulty or leaking breast implants. Again, fat suppression imaging is used to suppress the normal breast tissue and detect the presence of silicone in surrounding tissue.

A review of published studies on the value of adding MRI as a screening tool for breast cancer found that it was better for screening patients compared with mammography alone or a combination of mammography, sonography, and clinical breast examination. One concern about using MRI as a screening tool for breast cancer was that it raised the return rate for additional imaging; therefore, it has been suggested that MRI be used as an adjunct to mammography. MRI has also proven to be a safe, more effective screening tool in women who have a family history of breast cancer and are positive for the *BRCA* oncogene, for whom early screening is recommended.

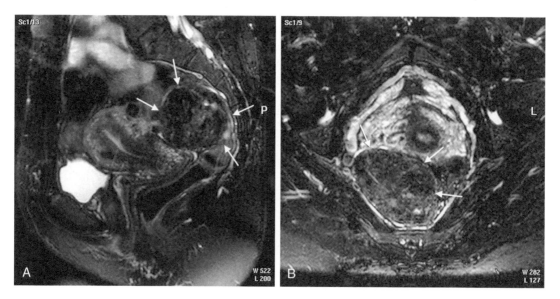

FIG. 10.8 A, A sagittal T2-weighted fat-suppressed magnetic resonance imaging (MRI) scan demonstrating a large mass, most likely a subserosal fibroid, posterior to the endocervical junction. B, An axial T2-weighted fat-suppressed MRI image depicting the large subserosal fibroid shown in A.

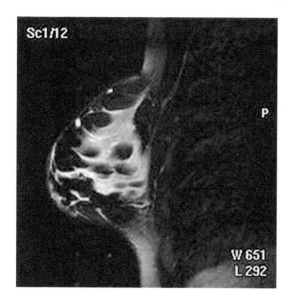

FIG. 10.9 A sagittal T2-weighted fat-suppressed magnetic resonance imaging scan of the left breast.

Computed Tomography

Computed tomography (CT) of the pelvis and abdomen is often performed to diagnose diseases of the female and male reproductive systems. It is quite helpful in assessing neoplastic growth and abscess formation resulting from inflammatory processes. It is often used in conjunction with transvaginal sonography to evaluate ovarian lesions, especially cystic teratomas in females, and is used extensively in staging cancers of the female reproductive system. In the male patient, CT is also used in conjunction with sonography to demonstrate anomalies of the seminal vesicles and prostate gland. CT and positron emission tomography (PET) fusion studies (CT-PET) are also of value in the diagnosis and staging of neoplastic disease of the reproductive system, as well as for the assessment of disease progression.

Sonography is highly recommended by the ACR for suspected gynecologic adnexal masses (masses of the uterus, ovaries, fallopian tubes, or surrounding connective tissue). However, CT of the pelvis, with or without contrast, is also equally indicated for nongravid women in the reproductive age group who have a complex or solid mass that is growing in the short term.

Congenital Anomalies

Congenital anomalies of the female reproductive system occur in approximately 5.5% of the unselected population as diagnosed by optimal tests. They are a result of the abnormal fusion or formation of the Müllerian ducts during gestation. The most common anomaly is the **bicornuate uterus**, in which paired uterine horns extend into the fallopian tubes (Figs. 10.10 and 10.11).

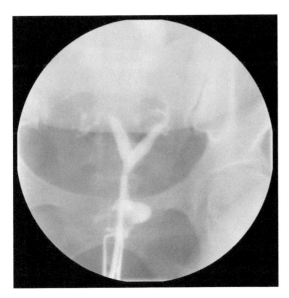

FIG. 10.10 A hysterosalpingogram demonstrating bicornuate uterus.

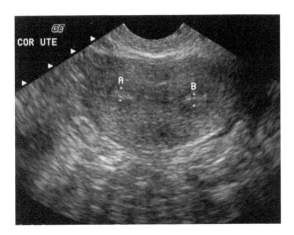

FIG. 10.11 A transverse sonographic image of a bicornuate uterus.

A **unicornuate uterus** occurs when the uterine cavity is elongated and has a single fallopian tube emerging from it (Fig. 10.12). Often, the kidney on the side of the missing fallopian tube is also absent. **Uterus didelphys** is a rare congenital anomaly with complete duplication of the uterus, cervix, and vagina. The most serious complication of these anomalies involves problems with reproduction, although various surgical corrections can be performed.

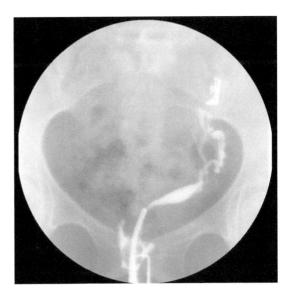

FIG. 10.12 A hysterosalpingogram demonstrating a unicornuate uterus

In the normal female reproductive system, the fundus of the uterus lies anterior to the cervix and away from the rectum and is said to be *anteverted*. Occasionally, the normal uterus may lie in an abnormal position. If the uterus is more vertical than normal and points backward toward the bowel, it is said to be *retroverted*. If the uterus is completely bent back and lies against the rectosigmoid region of the bowel, it is said to be *retroflexed*. A uterus that is tilted vertically forward is *anteflexed*, and it lies on top of the urinary bladder. Although neither position is normal, this is generally of little clinical significance.

Inflammatory Diseases

Pelvic Inflammatory Disease

Pelvic inflammatory disease (PID) is a bacterial infection of the upper female reproductive system, including the fallopian tubes, endometrium, ovaries, or pelvic peritoneum. One third of cases is caused by *Gonococcus*, one third is caused by a mixture of infections, and the last third of cases is caused by *Staphylococcus* or *Streptococcus*. The disease may result from an unsterile abortion or introduction of a pathogen from other sources. This inflammation is generally bilateral, and without treatment, the infection spreads to the peritoneum, resulting in bacteremia. Tubo-ovarian abscess formation may also occur with PID, often resulting in sterility. The clinical presentation of this entity involves pelvic

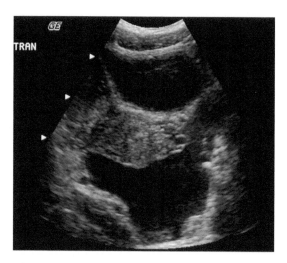

FIG. 10.13 A transverse sonographic image of bacterial fluid in the posterior cul-de-sac.

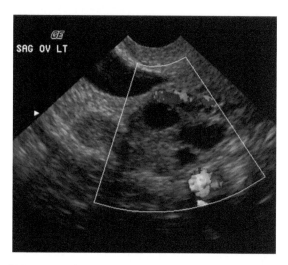

FIG. 10.14 A transvaginal sonographic image of a follicular cyst on an ovary.

pain and tenderness, guarding, rebound tenderness, or both. Patients often have fever and chills, elevated white blood cell (WBC) count, nausea and vomiting, and purulent cervical discharge.

The most common treatment for PID is aggressive antibiotic therapy, but healing often results in scarring and obstruction of the fallopian tubes, which predisposes the individual to ectopic pregnancy because of tubal narrowing. Rupture of the fallopian tubes because of infection results in septic shock and can be a life-threatening situation. Sonography is commonly indicated as an imaging method for determining the presence of infection and the extent of the disease (Fig. 10.13). Transvaginal ultrasonography and MRI may reveal thickened, fluid-filled tubes highly suggestive of PID. Severe cases with abscess formation may also require surgical intervention.

Mastitis

Inflammation of the breast, or **mastitis**, is most often caused by *Staphylococcus aureus*, though fungal infections are possible as well. Acute mastitis begins when bacteria gain access to breast tissue via the ducts. This bacterial route of infection occurs because of cracks or fissures in the nipple that may develop during the first weeks of lactation and the subsequent nursing of an infant. Common signs and symptoms of mastitis include pain, redness, and swelling of the affected breast, elevated temperature, and, in severe cases, abscess formation. Mastitis is treated medically with antibiotic therapy and

heat application to the affected breast. Risk factors for lactational mastitis are diabetes mellitus, steroid use, cigarette smoking, and inverted nipples. Mammography is difficult to perform on these patients because of the substantial engorgement of breast tissue. Mammographic imaging to document mastitis may result in higher doses owing to the thickness of the tissue and is of little value in the diagnosis and treatment of mastitis. Diagnosis is often based upon physical examination.

Neoplastic Diseases

Ovarian Cystic Masses

Simple ovarian cysts are fairly common in women in the reproductive age group. They are frequently asymptomatic but may cause abdominal aching and pressure. Acute, sharp abdominal pain may indicate rupture or hemorrhage of the cyst. They include follicular ovarian cysts and corpus luteum ovarian cysts. Follicular and corpus luteum cysts form as part of the normal menstrual cycle. **Follicular ovarian cysts** result from faulty reabsorption of the fluid from incompletely developed follicles (Fig. 10.14). **Corpus luteum ovarian cysts** occur when reabsorption of any blood leaked into the cavity after ovulation leaves a small cyst behind. Changes in the sizes of follicular and corpus luteum cysts occur quickly and vary with the menstrual cycle. These cysts may occasionally increase in size and cause pelvic discomfort or abnormal pressure on

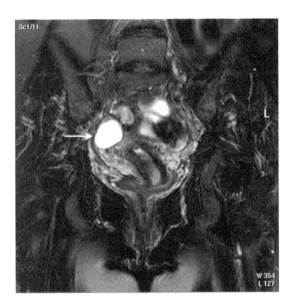

FIG. 10.15 A coronal T2-weighted fat-suppressed magnetic resonance imaging scan of the female pelvis demonstrating a cyst of the right ovary (*arrow*).

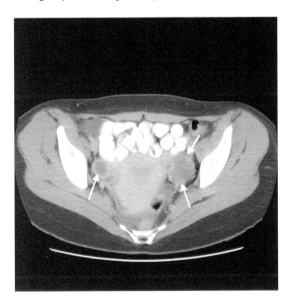

FIG. 10.16 A computed tomography scan of a female pelvis demonstrating bilateral cysts. The patient is currently taking fertility drugs.

the urinary bladder. These cysts are readily visible with sonography, MRI (Fig. 10.15), and CT (Fig. 10.16) of the pelvis. Treatment is generally not necessary because these cysts often disappear completely without medical intervention. Cysts larger than 3 cm may become symptomatic and require surgical resection.

Multiple cystic masses may indicate **endometriosis**, a disease caused by the presence of endometrial tissue or glands outside the uterus in abnormal locations within the pelvis. It has a prevalence of 5% to 10% in women of childbearing age, most commonly between 25 and 35 years. External endometriosis commonly involves the ovaries, the uterine ligaments, the rectovaginal septum, and the pelvic peritoneum; however, it may also attach to the rectal wall, the ureters, or the urinary bladder. Endometriosis is believed to arise from lymphatic spread, seeding from retrograde menstruation, or from direct surgical spread. The endometrial implants appear to respond to normal hormonal stimuli and are clinically significant in women between the ages of 20 and 40 years. The external endometrial tissue implants contain normal functioning endometrium. Responsive to hormonal changes, it continues to bleed cyclically. These blood-filled cysts (also referred to as *chocolate cysts*) are often visible during ultrasonographic examination. Longstanding endometriosis results in the development of fibrosis, adhesions, scarring, and eventually sterility. Common signs and symptoms include pelvic and low back pain, dysmenorrhea, intermittent constipation and diarrhea, and infertility. Transvaginal sonography is the primary imaging modality for the evaluation of endometriosis. An endometrioma will often appear as a unilocular, thick-walled, homogenous cyst with low-level echogenicity. MRI is also useful in distinguishing endometriosis from dermoids as endometriomas present as thick-walled masses with hyperintense T1 signal. However, laparoscopy is considered the gold standard to confirm diagnosis. Mild cases of endometriosis may be treated with hormone therapy; severe cases generally require surgical therapy.

Polycystic ovaries consist of enlarged ovaries containing multiple small cysts. The ovaries are bilaterally enlarged and have a smooth exterior surface, with multiple cysts lying just below the outer surface. Polycystic ovaries are often associated with Stein-Leventhal syndrome, a fairly rare disease. Women with Stein-Leventhal syndrome rarely ovulate because of an endocrine abnormality that inhibits maturation and release of the ovarian follicle. In addition, these individuals may experience amenorrhea and sterility. Primary treatment involves medication to induce ovulation.

Benign **cystic teratomas** of the ovary, often referred to as **dermoid cysts**, account for approximately 10% to 20% of ovarian tumors and are the most common type of germ cell tumor containing mature tissue. It is also the most common ovarian tumor in adolescents and women of reproductive age. These masses arise from an unfertilized ovum that undergoes neoplastic change. Cystic teratomas are composed of tissue derived from the ectoderm, endoderm, and mesoderm, and they often contain hair, thyroid tissue, keratin, sebaceous secretions, and occasionally teeth (Fig. 10.17). Cystic teratomas have only a 0.17% to 3% chance of undergoing malignant transformation. Although most are asymptomatic, some of the complications associated with a cystic teratoma are torsion of the mass and, in some cases, bleeding that may result in rupture and severe peritonitis. The treatment for cystic teratomas is surgical removal of the mass.

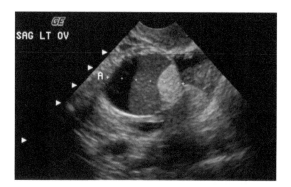

FIG. 10.17 A transvaginal sonographic image of a dermoid mass.

Ovarian Cancers

Ovarian cancers are malignant tumors of the ovary accounting for 3% of all cancers in females (Figs. 10.18 and 10.19). These cancers are the eighth most common cancer in females and the fifth most common cause of death from cancer in women in the United States. Ovarian cancers are histologically diverse and classified as either an epithelial ovarian neoplasms or germ cell neoplasms (Table 10.1). Approximately 80% of ovarian cancers are epithelial neoplasms, with 75% further classified as serous cystadenocarcinomas. The remaining 20% of ovarian cancers originate in the germ cells. Epithelial ovarian cancers primarily occur in women over age 40 years, whereas ovarian germ cell cancers primarily affect females under the age of 30 years. Ovarian cancers are the most lethal gynecologic malignancy because they tend to be asymptomatic in the early stages and the prognosis depends on the stage at which the tumor is discovered. Late stage tumors that have broken through the capsule of the ovary carry a very poor prognosis.

The cause of ovarian cancer is unknown. Known risk factors include a history of late childbearing or nulliparity, delayed menopause, a family history of cancers of the endometrium, breast, or colon, and the presence of an inherited autosomal dominant gene known as the *BRCA1 I* or *BRCA2* gene. Epithelial ovarian and breast tumors are also believed to be linked to mutations in the following genes: *TP53*,

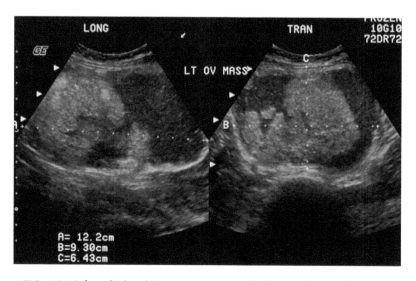

FIG. 10.18 A sagittal and transverse sonographic image of an ovarian mass.

PTEN, STK11/LKB1, CDH1, CHEK2, ATM, MLH1 and *MSH2*. Germ cell ovarian tumors have been associated with XY gonadal dysgenesis.

The signs and symptoms of ovarian cancer are very vague and include urinary bladder or rectal pressure, back pain, unexpected weight loss, change in bowel habits, abdominal pain and bloating. In many cases, the disease is completely asymptomatic and discovered only during routine pelvic examination. This tends to delay diagnosis and treatment, thus reducing the chance for cure. As a woman's age increases, the probability of an enlarged ovary testing positive for ovarian cancer increases proportionately.

According to the most recent literature, the laboratory test, CA 125, is the best noninvasive technique to detect ovarian cancers, as it provides the most specific diagnosis. Sonography, CT, and MR are useful in the diagnosis and staging of ovarian cancers. Sonography is most commonly employed for suspected early stage cancers. Sonographic evaluation demonstrates a rough, irregular ovarian surface, with the tumor often containing both cystic and solid areas. Serous tumors are frequently bilateral, whereas mucinous tumors are more likely to be unilateral. Pelvic CT and MR may be used in advanced stages of the disease. Additionally, PET-CT is also highly sensitive in the detection of ovarian cancer and it may be used in patients with an abnormal CA 125 laboratory test or questionable results from other imaging studies.

Staging of ovarian cancers is generally confirmed by surgery. The cancers are histologically graded as low-grade (1) or high-grade (2–3); and staged I to IV depending on whether the tumor remains local to the ovaries (I), has spread to other pelvic areas (II), or has metastasized beyond the pelvic region (III and IV). These tumors often spread to other pelvic organs, the small intestines, the omentum, and the stomach and less frequently to the liver and lungs, resulting in associated ascites and pleural effusions.

Common treatment of ovarian cancers includes a hysterectomy and bilateral salpingo-oopherectomy in combination with chemotherapy. Radiation therapy is an infrequent treatment and is generally only used against stage IV ovarian cancers. With treatment, the current 5 year survival rates are: stage I = 70% to 100%; stage II = 50% to 70%; stage III = 20% to 50%; and stage IV = 10% to 20%.

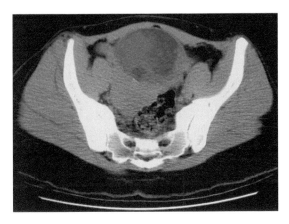

FIG. 10.19 Computed tomography scan of an ovarian mass in the female pelvis that confirms the mass seen on the sonogram.

TABLE 10.1
Types of Ovarian Cancers

Epithelial Origin	Germ Cell Origin
Brenner tumor	Choriocarcinomas
Clear cell carcinomas	Dysgerminomas
Endometriod carcinomas	Embryonal carcinomas
Mucinous carcinomas	Endodermal sinus tumors
Serous cystadenocacinomas	Immature teratomas
Transitional cell carcinomas	Polyembryomas
Unclassified carninomas	

2016 Merck Sharp & Dohme Corp., a subsidiary of Merck & Co., Inc., Kenilworth, NJ, USA. Available at http://www.merckmanuals.com/professional/gynecology-and-obstetrics/gynecologic-tumors/ovarian-cancer#Etiology

Carcinoma of the Cervix

Cervical carcinoma or dysplasia is a common malignancy of the female reproductive system caused by an abnormal growth pattern of epithelial cells around the neck of the uterus. It is the third most common carcinoma of the female genital organs and the eighth most common malignancy in American women, accounting for 10% to 15% of cancer-related deaths in women worldwide. Cervical intraepithelial neoplasias (CINs) are classified or staged as mild (I), moderate (II), or severe (III) and are generally diagnosed with a Papanicolaou (Pap) test and confirmed with surgical biopsy. Cervical cancer is essentially a sexually transmitted disease, as a history of multiple sexual partners or prior sexually transmitted infections predisposes women to this disease. The development of cervical cancer is strongly associated with infection with human papillomavirus (HPV) type 16, 18, 31, 33, 45, 52, and 58. HPV types 16 and 18 are responsible for approximately 70% of all cervical cancers, with types 31, 33, 45, 52, and 58 accounting for another 20%. Associated risk factors include cigarette smoking and immunodeficiency. Multiple clinical trials are ongoing to investigate vaccines against the different strains of the virus. To date, the U.S. Food and Drug Administration (FDA) has approved three vaccines against HPV. Gardasil (Quadrivalent Human Papillomavirus Recombinant Vaccine) is effective in preventing HPV types 6, 11, 16, and 18 and Cervarix protects against types 16 and 18. As a result of recent clinical trials, a third vaccine, Gardasil 9, was approved to protect against infection with types 6, 11, 16, 18, 31, 33, 45, 52, and 58. Gardasil and Gardasil 9 are currently available to young females aged 9 to 26 years for vaccination against HPV and cervical cancer. The National Cancer Institute is also supportive of programs that are attempting to develop a therapeutic vaccine for those already infected with HPV. Current clinical trials are being conducted to test the efficacy of topical microbicides in the prevention of genital HPV infection (Fig. 10.20).

Symptoms commonly associated with **cervical dysplasia** include abnormal bleeding, especially postcoital bleeding. In addition, impaired renal function resulting from ureteral obstruction is often seen. If the cancer is invasive, radiography of the chest, urinary system, and skeletal system, in combination with CT or MRI of the abdomen and pelvis, is performed to assist in staging the disease. MRI has been proven an excellent modality in assessing the extent of the primary neoplasm. The treatment of cervical dysplasia varies according to the classification. The

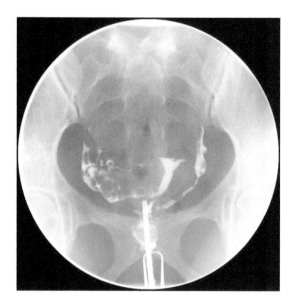

FIG. 10.20 Hysterosalpingogram demonstrating scarring of the uterine cavity (synechiae) in a patient with a history of human papillomavirus (HPV).

Pap test allows early detection of this disease, thus improving the chance of cure and survival. According to statistics from the National Cancer Institute, the 5-year survival rate ranges from approximately 90% for stage I dysplasia to 16% for advanced disease. The primary treatments are radiation therapy and surgical intervention. Chemotherapy may also be administered in combination with radiation therapy to act as a radiosensitizer.

Postoperative radiation therapy planning is essential to minimize the adverse effects of the treatment and also to prevent extension of extracervical disease. The ACR recommends the use of several techniques to spare radiation exposure to the small bowel, including displacement of the small bowel from the radiation treatment field.

Uterine Masses

Leiomyomas (Uterine Fibroids)

Leiomyomas are benign, solid masses of the uterus, which develop from an overgrowth of the uterine smooth muscle tissue. The lifetime prevalence of fibroids is 70% in Caucasian women and 80% in African American women. Uterine fibroids are the most common benign tumors of the female reproductive system. Many fibroids remain asymptomatic, but more severe cases may cause uterine enlargement and distortion, low back pain, pressure on the bowel

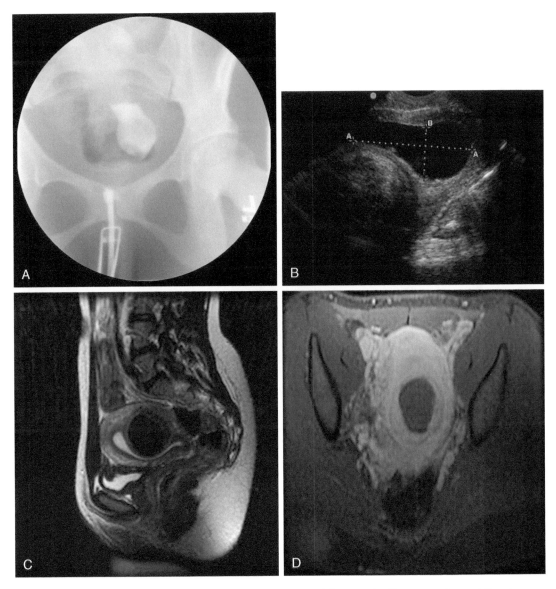

FIG. 10.21 Fibroid with image comparisons. A, Hysetosalpingography, B, sonography, and C and D, magnetic resonance imaging (MR).

and the bladder, intermenstrual bleeding, and acute pain. They may also result in heavy or prolonged menstrual bleeding resulting in anemia. The cause of this neoplasm is unknown; however, leiomyomas tend to grow under the influence of estrogen, may enlarge during pregnancy, and stop growing at menopause. After menopause, leiomyomas are replaced largely by fibrous scar tissue, which has led to the misnomer **uterine fibroids**. In addition, they often contain radiographically visible calcifications. The tumors

vary in size and number (usually occurring in multiples). About 70% to 80% of uterine fibroids are located in the wall of the uterus. They may remain asymptomatic until they grow large enough to place pressure on surrounding structures, and they are usually detected during a pelvic examination. Hysterosalpingography, sonography, CT, and MRI are all useful in confirming the presence of leiomyomas (Figs. 10.21 and 10.22). Sonographically, fibroids appear as sharply circumscribed, encapsulated lesions and may

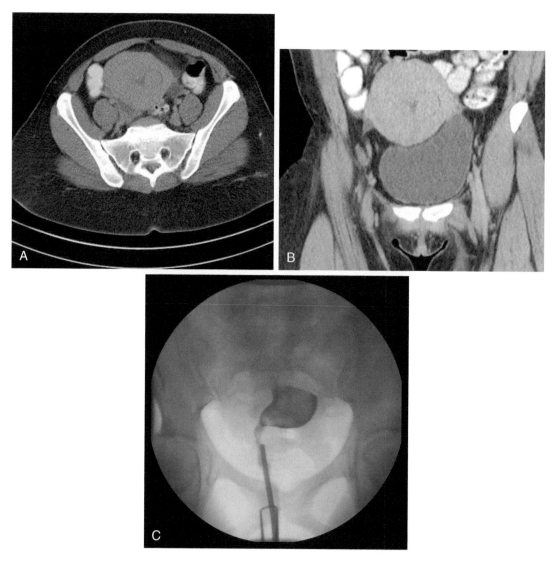

FIG. 10.22 Fibroid comparisons. A and B, Computed tomography (CT), and C, Hysterosalpingography.

contain cystic areas (Fig. 10.23). Malignant transformation is rare and treatment depends on the severity of the patient's symptoms, ranging from no treatment to complete hysterectomy. Uterine artery embolization is a successful, minimally invasive interventional radiologic technique for uterine leiomyoma treatment. MRI-guided focused ultrasound is a newer, minimally invasive treatment approved by the FDA that involves targeting fibroids with ultrasound thermal ablation under MRI visualization.

Adenocarcinoma of the Endometrium

Adenocarcinoma of the endometrium is, by far, the most common malignancy of the uterus, accounting for more than 80% of all endometrial cancers. It is often termed **endometrial carcinoma** of the uterus and it is histopathologically different from cervical carcinoma. Endometrial cancer is one of the most common cancers of the female reproductive system, second only to breast cancer. The incidence of adenocarcinoma of the endometrium has remained fairly static; the disease

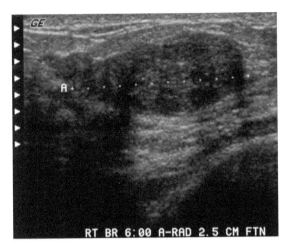

FIG. 10.23 A sagittal sonographic image of a uterus with fibroids that are located in the fundus of the uterus.

ranks as the fourth most common malignancy occurring in women in the United States, mainly in postmenopausal women and increasing in incidence with age. The development of this neoplasm has strong ties to hormonal changes in woman and is more common in nulliparous women. Obesity is a major risk factor, as are tamoxifen use, late menopause, a family history of breast or ovarian cancer, diabetes mellitus, or a history of previous pelvic radiation therapy.

Adenocarcinoma of the endometrium is usually preceded by endometrial hyperplasia. It then passes through an *in situ* stage before reaching its final invasive stage, often completely filling the uterine cavity. The cancer is graded according to cellular differentiation and staged according to the extent of the disease. The most frequent symptom is irregular or postmenopausal bleeding and pelvic pain. Endometrial cancer can be diagnosed via endometrial biopsy, dilation and curettage, and sometimes transvaginal ultrasound. Treatment varies with the stage of the disease. Stage I is contained in the uterus only and is often curable via hysterectomy. Stage II has spread to connective tissue of the cervix and is usually treated with a combination of surgery and radiation therapy, with the 5-year survival rate ranging from 70% to 95%. Stage III has spread beyond the uterus and cervix but remains in the pelvis, and stage IV has spread beyond the pelvis. Both stages III and IV often require various combinations of surgery, radiation therapy, chemotherapy, and hormone therapy.

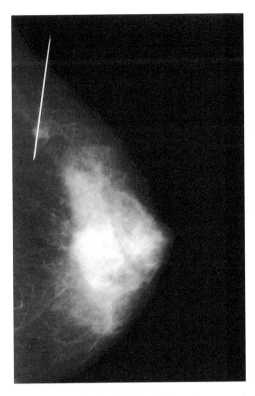

FIG. 10.24 Needle localization of fibroadenoma of the breast pinpoints the location of the mass for surgical biopsy.

Breast Masses

Fibroadenoma

A **fibroadenoma** is a common benign breast tumor. It is estimated that 10% of all women will experience a fibroadenoma in their lifetime. They are usually unilateral consisting of a solid, well-defined mass that does not invade surrounding tissue. The neoplasm is formed by an overgrowth of fibrous and glandular tissues and is commonly located in the upper, outer quadrant of the breast. Fibroadenomas almost always occur in women under 30 years of age and most frequently in those 21 to 25 years of age. Fibroadenomas appear to be estrogen-dependent and may grow rapidly during pregnancy. These lesions are often painless and can usually be moved about within the breast. Mammography, in conjunction with physical breast examination and sonography, plays a vital role in the detection of fibroadenomas (Figs. 10.24 and 10.25) and is useful in distinguishing them from mammary

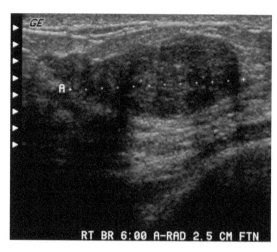

FIG. 10.25 A sonographic image of a juvenile fibroadenoma.

dysplasia (fibrocystic breast disease) and breast carcinoma. Surgical removal of the lesion is curative. Ultrasound-guided cryoablation is a new technique that has proven successful in localized detection and destruction of fibroadenomatous tissue.

Fibrocystic Breasts

An overgrowth of fibrous tissue or cystic hyperplasia results in **fibrocystic breasts**. This is the most common disorder of the female breast and occurs to some degree in 60% to 75% of all women. This condition is most frequently bilateral, with variably sized cysts located throughout the breasts (Figs. 10.26 and 10.27). The severity of this disorder varies greatly, and it is believed to result from fluctuations in hormone levels during the menstrual cycle. The most common sign or symptom associated with fibrocystic breasts is a mass or masses that increase in size and tenderness immediately before the onset of the menstrual period. The texture of the breast tissue is ropy and thick, especially in the upper outer quadrant of the breast. Sonography is extremely useful as a follow-up to mammography in differentiating solid masses from cystic masses in women with fibrocystic breasts (Fig. 10.28). Large cysts are commonly aspirated for cytologic evaluation of the fluid. If this evaluation does not yield definitive results, surgical biopsy is often performed. Although controversy exists about the correlation between fibrocystic breasts and an increased incidence of breast cancer,

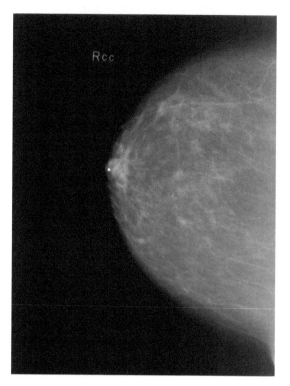

FIG. 10.26 Craniocaudad mammographic projection of a moderately fibroglandular breast.

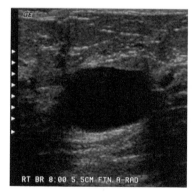

FIG. 10.27 A sonographic image of a typical breast cyst.

it is well known that a fibrocystic condition may mask a coexistent cancer. Treatment of the condition is largely symptomatic, including a monthly breast self-examination and proper support. If symptoms persist, fine-needle aspiration for fluid removal may be performed, and in some rare cases, surgical excision of the cyst is necessary.

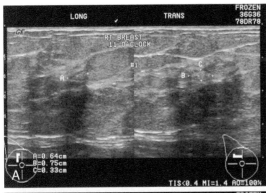

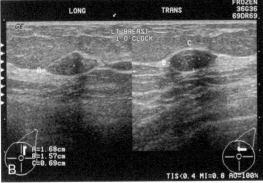

FIG. 10.28 A, A sonogram of the breast demonstrating an enlarged lymph node and cyst in the eleven o'clock axis of the right breast, right upper quadrant. B, A sonogram of a hypoechogenic solid breast mass in the left upper quadrant in the one o'clock axis.

Carcinoma of the Breast

Breast carcinoma is a very common malignancy among women in the United States and the second leading cause of cancer deaths in women, behind only lung cancer. It is the second most common cancer among American women, behind only skin cancers. Current literature suggests that 1 of every 8 women in the United States will develop invasive breast cancer during her lifetime, with an increased incidence between ages 30 and 50 years. The incidence continues to rise throughout the postmenopausal years because of changes in estrogen levels, with the mean age for breast cancer being age 60 years. Approximately 60% of all palpable lesions occur in the upper outer quadrant of the breast.

Although the exact cause of breast cancer is unknown, it is believed to be a multifactorial disorder.

Heredity, endocrine influence, oncogenic factors (such as viruses), and environmental factors (such as chemical carcinogens) appear to play a role in the development of this disease. The amount of biologically available estrogen and progesterone is a key endocrine factor in the development of breast cancer. Those individuals with an early onset of menstruation (menarche) or late menopause and women with a first pregnancy after age 30 years are at a higher risk for developing breast cancer. Women using oral contraceptives or estrogen replacement therapy over a 10-year period also have a very small increase in the risk of developing breast cancer. In terms of heredity, a family history including a parent, sibling, or child with breast cancer increases a woman's risk to two to three times that of the normal population. Approximately 5% to 10% of breast cancers are thought to be hereditary. Women who have inherited mutations in the *BRCA1* or *BRCA2* genes, the most common causes of hereditary breast cancer, have an average increased risk of 55% to 65% for developing breast cancer. Current data also indicate that hereditary ovarian cancers are caused by *BRCA1* or *BRCA2* gene mutations. This syndrome is termed *hereditary breast ovarian cancer syndrome*.

Breast cancers may be classified as *in situ* carcinoma, ductal carcinoma *in situ*, lobular carcinoma *in situ*, invasive ductal or lobular carcinoma, or inflammatory carcinoma. Breast cancers generally are discovered as a lump in the breast by the patient. With the exception of inflammatory breast cancer, which is very virulent and associated with diffuse inflammation and breast enlargement, most begin as slow-growing, relatively painless masses, but as they grow, they may infiltrate the suspensory ligaments, causing them to shorten and retract the overlying skin. Physical signs of advanced breast cancer include nipple retraction and distorted breast contour. The neoplasm may infiltrate and block the lymphatic vessels, the major route of metastases, especially to the axilla. This infiltration causes edema in the overlying skin and enlargement of the axillary or supraclavicular lymph nodes. As the infiltrating breast carcinoma blocks the lymphatic exchange, the skin pores open to allow the fluid to escape, thus causing a rough skin texture from chafing and pore enlargement. The edematous skin is described as having a **peau d'orange** (orange peel) appearance. As the tumor progresses, it may attach to surrounding fascia and ulcerate surrounding skin.

Mammography plays a very important role in the diagnosis and management of breast cancer. Routine screening mammography in asymptomatic women may lead to early detection and thus reduce breast cancer mortality by up to 30%. It has also been reported that breast cancer mortality could be reduced by as much as 50% if all women older than age 40 years received annual screening mammography. However, annual screening of women between the ages of 40 and 50 years remains controversial.

Many breast tumors commonly appear radiographically as dense, irregular, stellate masses that infiltrate surrounding tissue (Fig. 10.29). Many contain numerous microcalcifications that are radiographically visible (Fig. 10.30). In some instances, fine-needle aspiration with cytologic evaluation may be sufficient to make a definitive diagnosis. Core needle biopsy or incisional biopsy is often performed to obtain a specimen of suspect tissue for further evaluation. For patients requiring an incisional biopsy, needle localization of mammographically detected, nonpalpable cancerous breast lesions is reliable in directing the surgeon to the lesion in question and allows for excision of suspect tissue. The tissue specimen is radiographed and forwarded to a pathologist for histologic evaluation. Statistics demonstrate that this method of localization causes minimal morbidity, and the development and refinement of mammographic localization have greatly increased the percentage of positive findings during surgical biopsy. This invasive technique allows more accurate diagnosis and treatment of early-stage carcinoma of the breast. If the tumor can be removed before the lesion is palpable, the survival rate is greatly increased. Specimens are routinely analyzed for estrogen and progesterone receptors because receptor status information is useful in determining the course of therapy. Patients with estrogen-receptor–positive (ER +) tumors have a better prognosis and tend to benefit from endocrine therapy. After diagnosis, breast cancer is staged based upon the degree it has spread, ranging from stage 0 to stage IV.

As discussed earlier in this chapter, MRI may be used to detect breast cancer. PET is often used as a valuable adjunct imaging method for predicting the clinical outcome in patients who have been previously

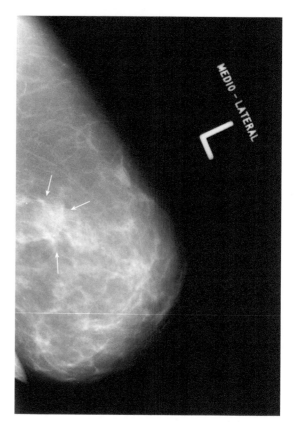

FIG. 10.29 A mammogram of the left breast of a 63-year-old woman demonstrating a stellate mass commonly associated with carcinoma of the breast. Note the irregular borders of the mass.

treated for breast cancer. Use of 18-fluorodeoxyglucose (FDG) PET provides both qualitative and quantitative information that helps detect the primary tumor and identify tumor spread via the lymphatic system, and it also has the potential to reduce the need for lymph node dissection. It is useful in assessing breast tumor metabolism and biologic behavior. Studies are currently being conducted to test a new imaging technique for breast cancer detection known as scintimammograpy (molecular breast imaging), which involves injection of a radioactive tracer that attaches to breast cancer cells.

Treatment of breast carcinoma depends on the extent of the disease. Once the carcinoma is confirmed through biopsy, an axillary lymph node resection is performed to assist in the management of the disease. The

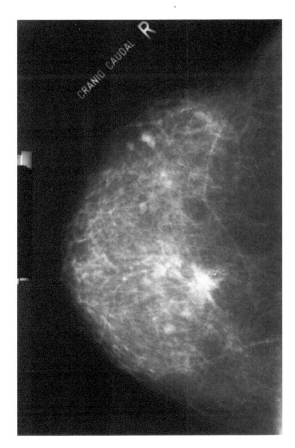

FIG. 10.30 A mammogram of the right breast in an older woman demonstrating a stellate mass containing microcalcifications commonly associated with carcinoma of the breast.

5-year survival rate for patients with localized breast cancer is 98.6%, dropping to 84.9% if the cancer is regional (spread to regional lymph nodes), and 25.9% if it is found to be distant (metastasized). Much controversy exists in terms of determining the best approach for the management and treatment of breast cancers. In the past 40 years, the 5-year survival rate for breast cancer has remained virtually unchanged. Currently, two surgical options are recommended for invasive breast cancers: (1) modified radical mastectomy and (2) breast-conserving surgery followed by radiation therapy. Both methods require axillary lymph node resection, and the difference between the survival rates of these two surgical options is insignificant. Inflammatory cancers are usually treated with a combination of chemotherapy and radiation therapy.

Treatment with an established combination of chemotherapeutic drugs is considered standard care for premenopausal women who have lymph node involvement. The chemotherapy may be continued for months or years after the primary therapy, but the adjuvant therapy may decrease the chance of death by 35% in this patient population. Breast carcinomas are also classified by a hormone receptor test. Many tumors require hormones for continued growth, and these carcinomas may undergo temporary regression if hormonal balances are altered.

Disorders during Pregnancy

Diagnostic medical sonography is often used as positive proof of pregnancy in addition to aiding in the diagnosis of multiple and ectopic pregnancies. With the use of transvaginal sonography, the sac and early fetal pole can been seen and a fetal heart detected as early as 3 weeks of gestation. Sonographic examination may be indicated if the pregnant uterus is too small or too large for the calculated delivery date. Depending on the obstetrician's policy, many pregnant women may also have sonography performed at 6 to 8 weeks of gestation to screen for fetal anomalies. Additional laboratory tests such as amniocentesis, chorionic villus sampling, and deoxyribonucleic acid (DNA) analysis are performed in cases of suspected congenital anomalies of the fetus. Infant deaths are usually attributed to congenital anomalies or prematurity. Premature delivery may be associated with many anomalies of pregnancy. Examples include multiple pregnancies, placental anomalies, preeclampsia, and eclampsia, as well as congenital anomalies of the uterus such as bicornuate uterus or cervical incompetence. Preeclampsia is the development of hypertension in combination with proteinuria or edema and usually occurs after the twentieth week of gestation. The condition in which convulsions occur in a female patient with preeclampsia is termed *eclampsia*. Cervical incompetence can be demonstrated via sonography of the cervix during the first trimester of pregnancy.

Amniotic Fluid

Amniotic fluid is produced by various physiologic functions within the mother and the fetus. The amount of amniotic fluid present varies with the stage of pregnancy. **Oligohydramnios** refers to too little amniotic

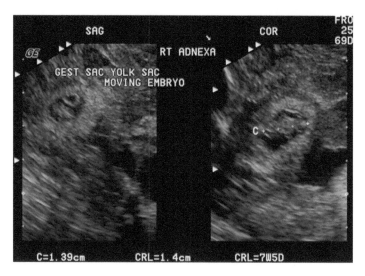

FIG. 10.31 A transvaginal sonographic image reveals a live fetus in an ectopic location.

fluid, and **polyhydramnios** refers to an excess of amniotic fluid. The normal fetus swallows several hundred milliliters of fluid per day. This fluid is absorbed by the fetal intestines, with a portion excreted via the fetal urinary system and a portion transferred across the placenta into the mother's circulatory system. The major source of amniotic fluid arises from the fetus urinating fluid once the kidneys are developed. Therefore oligohydramnios often results from poor fetal kidney function or blockage of the ureters associated with congenital anomalies of the fetal urinary system. If a fetus is unable to swallow because of anencephaly or a high GI obstruction, polyhydramnios may occur. It is also an indication of severe growth retardation and fetal death.

Ectopic Pregnancy

Ectopic pregnancy refers to the development of an embryo outside of the uterine cavity. It occurs in approximately 1 out of every 100 pregnancies. The most common site for an ectopic pregnancy is the fallopian tube (Fig. 10.31), but it may also occur in the ovary, cervix, or abdominal cavity. With tubal pregnancy, the fallopian tube distends to accommodate the growing embryo, causing blood vessels to rupture. This may produce serious internal hemorrhage and can be life-threatening. If a tubal pregnancy goes untreated, the embryo will develop and survive for only 2 to 6 weeks.

Common signs and symptoms associated with ectopic pregnancy are the same as those of early pregnancy, but distension of the tube causes acute abdominal pain and tenderness. If internal hemorrhage occurs, loss of blood may cause fainting and shock. Ectopic pregnancies are more common in women who have had damage to their fallopian tubes from a partial obstruction of the uterine tube or previous tubal surgery. The cause of tubal pregnancies is obstruction of the normal passageway for the ovum. Accurate diagnosis of ectopic pregnancy can be achieved through transvaginal ultrasonography and a quantitative serum human chorionic gonadotropin (hCG) test. Increasing evidence indicates that MRI may provide additional information on the location of an ectopic pregnancy that is located in the cervix or the interstitial area of the tube. The treatment is surgical removal of the affected uterine tube with laparoscopy as the preferred approach.

Disorders of the Placenta

The placenta is a temporary organ associated with pregnancy. Its purpose is to exchange nutrients and oxygen from mother to fetus and waste products from fetus to mother for excretion. If a woman begins to bleed during the third trimester of pregnancy, ultrasonography should be performed to evaluate the placenta because the bleeding places both mother and fetus at high risk. The most common causes of third-trimester bleeding are placenta previa and abruption of the placenta.

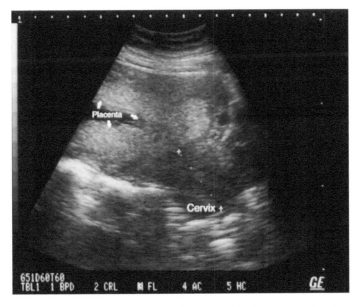

FIG. 10.32 Placenta previa seen on this sagittal sonographic view reveals the placenta covering the internal os of the cervix.

Placenta previa is a condition in which the implantation of the placenta leaves part or all of the cervical os covered. Several degrees are recognized: total, partial, marginal, and low-lying previa. These degrees of previa are related to the position of the placenta in relation to the internal cervical os. In situations of placenta previa (Fig. 10.32), the mother experiences painless vaginal bleeding during the later stages of pregnancy because of the partial separation of the placenta from the uterine wall. Hemorrhage may occur and this condition can be life-threatening to both mother and fetus. Sonography is an effective method for determining the location of the placenta in cases of suspected previa and is useful in the management of the pregnancy. Normal delivery cannot occur in patients with placenta previa, so a cesarean section is routinely performed.

Occasionally, a normally implanted placenta may prematurely separate from the uterus. This condition is termed **placental abruption** and may be life-threatening to the fetus. Predisposing factors for abruption include a history of a prior abruption, pregnancy-induced hypertension, smoking, alcohol abuse, cocaine abuse, external abuse, and multiple gestation. **Placental percreta** is a condition in which the placenta extends into the myometrium, causing an unduly firm attachment that bleeds at delivery because it will not

separate normally. In rare cases, failure of the placenta to separate after birth results in the need for an immediate hysterectomy. The use of sonography or sonography with Doppler is highly recommended to distinguish between these different pathologies within the placenta.

Hydatidiform Mole

Hydatidiform mole, or "molar pregnancy" refers to an abnormal conception in which usually no fetus is present. Instead of a fertilized egg progressing to a viable pregnancy, the placenta develops into an abnormal mass of cysts. It occurs in about 1 in 2000 pregnancies in North America, although the incidence is much greater in certain other parts of the world for unknown reasons. Often, the presenting sign is a uterine size that is inappropriate for the date. With this condition, the uterus is filled with cystically dilated chorionic villi that resemble a bunch of grapes, known as *trophoblastic tissue* (Fig. 10.33). These villi absorb fluid and become swollen, and sonography demonstrates a characteristic pattern as well as absence of heart sounds. Usually such a conception aborts spontaneously in the second trimester. If it does not, suction curettage is done, and no further treatment is required in most cases. Approximately 80% of molar pregnancies follow a benign course, but 15% to 25% may develop invasive disease. The use of sonography, clinical factors, and pelvic MRI is

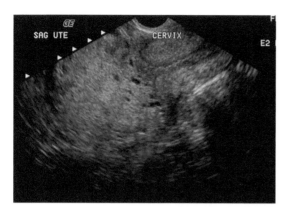

FIG. 10.33 A sagittal sonographic image of the uterus that contains molar tissue.

recommended to distinguish between an incomplete abortion and gestational trophoblastic disease.

Male Reproductive System

Anatomy and Physiology

The male reproductive system is composed of glands, ducts, and supporting structures. The glands of the male reproductive system include a pair of testes, a pair of seminal vesicles, a pair of bulbourethral glands, and one prostate gland. The testes are enclosed by a white, fibrous covering within the scrotum. They are responsible for the production of sperm and the secretion of hormones, mainly testosterone. The prostate gland lies just inferior to the bladder, and the urethra actually passes through this gland (Fig. 10.34). The prostate gland is responsible for secreting the majority of the seminal fluid and is normally about the size of a walnut.

The ducts that connect the glands include a pair of epididymides, a pair of vasa deferentia, a pair of ejaculatory ducts, and one urethra. The testes are divided into lobules that contain seminiferous tubules, which converge into larger ducts and emerge at the head of the epididymis. The epididymides lie superior and lateral to the testes and serve as a passageway for sperm. They are also responsible for secreting a portion of the seminal fluid. The vasa deferentia extend from the epididymides and pass through the inguinal canal into the pelvic cavity. They pass superior to the bladder and continue down the posterior surface of the bladder to join the ducts emerging from the seminal vesicles. This junction forms the ejaculatory ducts. These ducts eventually empty into the urethra, which is responsible for delivering the seminal fluid to the exterior of the body.

Imaging Considerations

Radiographic investigation of the male reproductive system is limited mainly to urethrography and intravenous urography. However, sonography is commonly used to evaluate testicular masses or an enlarged scrotum and to help differentiate among epididymitis, orchiditis, and testicular torsion. Nuclear medicine is also useful in distinguishing between epididymitis and testicular torsion. Prostatic sonography via a rectal probe is used to evaluate nodules and guide the physician when performing biopsy of the prostate. MRI of the male pelvis is performed to evaluate the seminal vesicles, the prostate gland, and the scrotum (Fig. 10.35). MRI is useful in detecting and staging prostate cancer in men having a positive (+ 4) prostate-specific antigen (PSA) laboratory test. A specialized rectal coil is used in examining the prostate gland; however, high-field MRI units may be able to detect pathology without the use of the rectal coil. MRI is also useful in evaluating testicular cancer and can determine whether the cancer is present in one or both testicles. This differentiation is especially important in young men who plan to have children. The use of MRI, with or without contrast, is highly rated by the ACR as a pretreatment staging for prostate cancer. The use of endorectal coil MRI (erMRI) should be considered for those patients with a high value of PSA.

Congenital Anomalies

Cryptorchidism

Near the end of gestation, the male testes normally descend through the inguinal canal into the scrotum. Cryptorchidism refers to undescended testes. It is one of the most common male endocrine pediatric disorders and is the most common genital disorder at birth. Infants born prematurely and with a low birth weight are more likely to have crytochordism. Men with this condition are at a higher risk of testicular malignancy, inguinal hernia, and infertility. Treatment involves either bringing the testicle down and fixing it surgically (orchiopexy) or removing it. More than 70% of undescended testes are palpable by physical examination, in which case imaging is not recommended. Ultrasound has limited specificity in

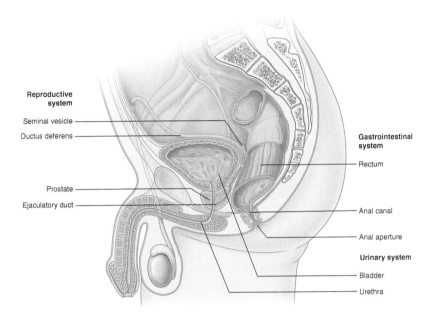

Reproductive
system

Seminal vesicle

Ductus deferens

Gastrointestinal
system

Rectum

Prostate

Ejaculatory duct

Anal canal

Anal aperture

Urinary system

Bladder

Urethra

FIG. 10.34 The male reproductive system.

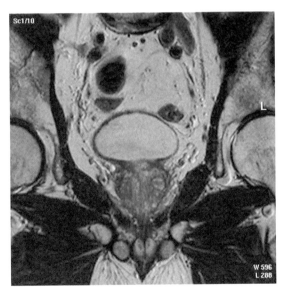

FIG. 10.35 A coronal T2-weighted magnetic resonance imaging scan of the male pelvis depicting the bladder and the prostate gland.

locating a nonpalpable testis, thus diagnostic laparoscopy is often preferred in these cases. MRI is used because of its greater sensitivity and superior soft tissue detail; however, cost may be a deterrent.

Neoplastic Diseases

Benign Prostatic Hyperplasia

Benign prostatic hyperplasia (BPH), a common benign enlargement of the prostate gland, is caused by cellular proliferation leading to the development of discrete nodules within the gland and is palpable through the rectum. Although enlargement may be determined by a digital rectal examination, results may be misleading, thus a laboratory blood test to assess serum PSA should be performed. Results may demonstrate a moderate elevation in PSA, depending on the degree of enlargement and urinary obstruction. The cause of prostatic hyperplasia is unknown, but the condition is thought to be caused by hormonal changes associated with aging, as it generally affects men after age 50 years. The benign nodules most frequently occur in the median lobe and in the central portions of the lateral lobes of the prostate gland. Because of these locations, the nodules often compress the portion of the urethra passing through the prostate gland, thus interfering with urination.

Symptoms associated with this disorder include difficulty starting, stopping, and maintaining the flow of urine and inability to completely empty the bladder.

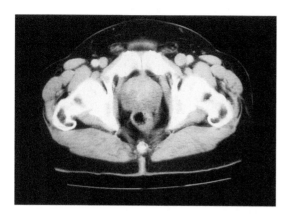

FIG. 10.36 A pelvic computed tomography image of a 68-year-old man demonstrating prostatic hyperplasia. Note the indentation into the urinary bladder.

Residual urine tends to infect the bladder and this poses a risk to the kidneys of being infected as well. In some cases, urinary tract obstructions may result from an overgrowth of the prostate gland. The most common treatment of prostatic hyperplasia is partial excision of the prostate gland, although nonsurgical treatment is available for some cases. A **transurethral resection of the prostate** (TURP) is performed by passing an endoscope through the urethra to core out the gland. Prostatic enlargement may be demonstrated on an intravenous urographic examination as a filling defect at the base of the bladder. Hyperplastic changes are also readily visible by MRI and CT examinations of the pelvic area (Fig. 10.36). Evidence does not conclusively suggest that development of prostatic hyperplasia increases an individual's risk of developing prostatic carcinoma.

Many men over age 50 years develop small, multiple calcifications within the prostate. These are termed **prostatic calculi**, which may be radiographically visible on plain abdominal or pelvic images. The development of these calculi is of no clinical significance.

Carcinoma of the Prostate

Adenocarcinoma of the prostate is a common cancer in men; it is estimated 1 in 7 will be diagnosed with the disease during his lifetime. It is the second leading cause of cancer death in American men, behind lung cancer. Prostate cancer most frequently affects older men, with the chance of developing prostate cancer rising rapidly after 50 years of age, with 6 in 10 cases occurring in men over the age of 65. The cause of prostate cancer is unknown, but there is evidence of a potential inherited

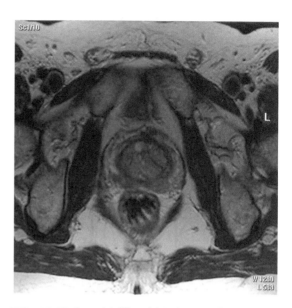

FIG. 10.37 An axial T2-weighted magnetic resonance imaging scan demonstrating enlargement of the posterior left portion of the prostate by prostate carcinoma.

or genetic link. Having a father or brother with prostate cancer more than doubles a man's risk of developing the disease. It generally affects the outer group of prostate glands and occurs more frequently in the posterior lobe of the prostate. This disease is most often diagnosed during blood tests screening for prostate-specific antigen (PSA) or digital rectal examinations. If test results come back abnormal, a transrectal ultrasound (TRUS) or MRI may be performed to determine the location and extent of the disease (Fig. 10.37). However, a prostate biopsy is necessary for disease confirmation. Common signs and symptoms associated with prostate cancer include urinary tract obstructions; a hard, enlarged prostate on rectal palpation; and low back pain, which is often caused by metastatic spread to the pelvis and lumbar spine.

Some types of prostate cancers are fairly dormant and slow growing, but others are very aggressive and yield a higher mortality rate. Prostate cancer is graded according to the Gleason system, given a number 1 to 5 based on how similar the cancerous cells are to normal prostate tissue. It is then given an overall stage of I-IV in order to determine treatment options and prognosis.

Treatment is based on the overall stage of the cancer. For stage I, active surveillance or radiation therapy is recommended. Larger cancers confined to the prostate, or stage II, require surgical removal of the prostate or radiation therapy. Radiation and hormone therapy

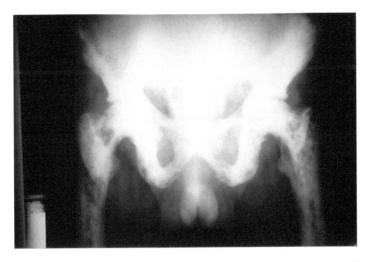

FIG. 10.38 Skeletal metastatic disease of the pelvis and spine secondary to prostate cancer.

is recommended for stage III, and finally surgery, hormone therapy, and radiation are all options for stage IV. This neoplasm is highly testosterone dependent, so in some cases the testes are removed along with the prostate. Hormone therapy may involve the administration of female hormones to control the growth of the tumor by interfering with the action of testosterone. A new treatment modality involves planting radioactive seeds in the prostate, under the guidance of ultrasonography, to destroy the tumor. Skeletal metastases occur in approximately 75% of all cases and manifest on plain radiographs as sclerotic lesions within bone (Fig. 10.38). Bone pain in an older man should particularly raise suspicion of prostate cancer. The earlier prostate cancer is diagnosed, the better the prognosis. The 5-year survival rate for localized and regional cases is 100%, falling to 28.2% for distant cancer that has metastasized. Fortunately, approximately 80% of cases are diagnosed at the local stage.

The ACR recommends a technitium-99m (^{99m}Tc) bone scan of the whole body as the most effective method for monitoring recurrence of disease after a radical prostatectomy and rising PSA levels among those men treated for prostate cancer. CT of the abdomen and pelvis with contrast is also highly recommended for monitoring for recurrence after surgery.

Testicular Torsion

Testicular torsion occurs if a testicle twists on itself, inducing severe pain and swelling. Failure to correct this surgically in an immediate fashion may result in severe compromise of testicular vascularity. The chances surgical removal of the testicle will be required increase if the blood flow is reduced for more than just 6 hours. In patients with acute pain in the scrotum, it is very important to make sure that testicular blood supply is maintained. The use of ultrasound Doppler and nuclear medicine is highly recommended by the ACR to assess these patients for adequate blood supply to the testicle. Doppler ultrasound may also be used to detect the increased vascular flow associated with inflammation, which can accompany infection. Conversely, the inability to detect vascular flow within the testicle could indicate that the vascular supply is twisted and, as a result, proximal blood supply has been lost. Power Doppler is the most sensitive sonography application for the detection of low vascular flow; therefore, it is the best imaging choice for detecting the cause of scrotal pain. Likewise, the use of a nuclear medicine scan facilitates the detection of vascular flow associated with the uptake or lack of uptake of ^{99m}Tc (Fig. 10.39). Inflammation of the epididymis, or epididymitis, may similarly lead to scrotal swelling caused by the hyperemia. This inflammatory response by the epididymis and testis (**epididymo-orchitis**) may result from a bacterial infection, such as urinary tract infection or gonorrhea, or may be secondary to the placement of an indwelling urinary catheter. In addition to scrotal edema, signs and symptoms include scrotal pain and erythema. The increased blood flow associated with or without trauma can be detected with Doppler or a nuclear medicine scan, which demonstrates increased uptake of ^{99m}Tc (Fig. 10.40).

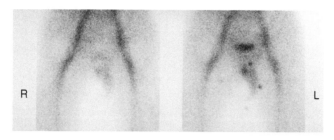

FIG. 10.39 Torsion as seen on a nuclear medicine testicular scan, which reveals a relative absence of blood flow to the right testicle.

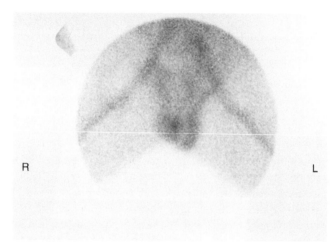

FIG. 10.40 Epididymitis as revealed on a testicular scan, which shows increased uptake in the left testicle.

Testicular Masses

Benign masses of the testes may be associated with epididymo-orchitis. Other common benign masses include hydroceles and spermatoceles. **Hydroceles** are common intrinsic scrotal masses, sometimes congenital in nature, caused by a collection of fluid in the testis or along the spermatic cord (Fig. 10.41). They may appear as a painless scrotal swelling, or they may demonstrate inflammation in combination with epididymitis and be quite painful. **Spermatoceles**, or spermatic cysts, are fluid-filled, painless scrotal masses within the testis adjacent to the epididymis (Fig. 10.42). Sonography may be used to differentiate between benign hydroceles or spermatoceles and solid, malignant neoplasms.

Malignant testicular tumors constitute approximately 1% of all cancers in males in the United States. Such tumors represent the most common malignancy among 15 to 34-year-olds, and the condition has a peak incidence around age 30 years, and a second smaller peak

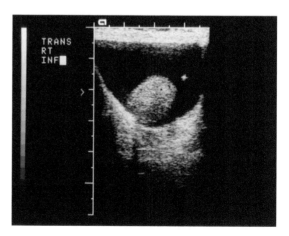

FIG. 10.41 A hydrocele is visualized as the dark collection of fluid surrounding the testicle, as seen on a sonogram of this 52-year-old man.

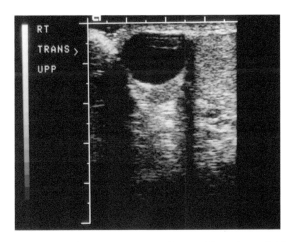

FIG. 10.42 A spermatocele, evidenced by a large fluid collection on the epididymis, as seen on a testicular sonographic scan of this 33-year-old man.

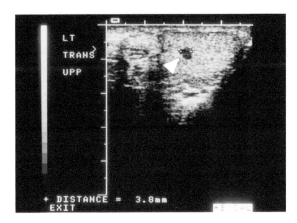

FIG. 10.43 The hypoechoic mass seen in the superior aspect of the testicle on this testicular sonogram of a 31-year-old man is strongly suggestive of a seminoma.

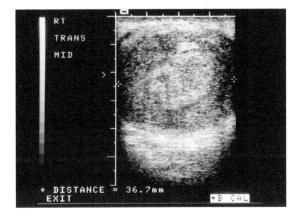

FIG. 10.44 A large, echogenic heterogeneous mass in the right testicle is highly suspicious for a teratoma in the testicular sonogram of this 27-year-old man.

around age 75 years. The cause of malignant tumors of the testes is unknown, but research has shown a strong hereditary association. The most common signs include enlargement or palpable hardness of the testis. As with other cancers, testicular tumors are staged I to III, depending on the size and extent of the disease. If cancer is suspected, an ultrasound is often the preliminary test to distinguish between benign conditions and a solid tumor. Blood tests for tumor markers are often conducted to confirm a diagnosis instead of a surgical biopsy, which increases the risk of spreading the cancer. CT scans may be conducted to determine the stage of the cancer, as well as MRI, PET, and bone scans. All types of malignant testicular neoplasms are treated with surgical resection. Chemotherapy, radiation therapy, or both may be used in conjunction with surgery, depending on the type and staging of the disease. More than 90% of testicular cancers develop from germ cells. The four types of malignant germ cell tumors are (1) seminomas, (2) embryonal carcinomas, (3) teratomas, and (4) choriocarcinomas.

Testicular seminomas arise from the seminiferous tubules and account for approximately 40% of malignant testicular tumors (Fig. 10.43). Seminomas grow rapidly but tend to remain localized for a fairly long time before metastasizing. These neoplasms have an excellent prognosis because of their extreme radiosensitivity. If treated with radiation therapy, seminomas carry a 10-year survival rate of approximately 90%.

Testicular teratomas arise from primitive germ cells and account for approximately 25% of the malignant testicular masses (Fig. 10.44). These neoplasms are composed of various cell types such as connective tissue, muscle, and thyroid glandular tissue. Teratomas are associated with a poorer prognosis compared with seminomas and carry a 10-year survival rate of approximately 50% to 75%. Like seminomas, teratomas are highly malignant, spreading to the renal hilum via the lymphatics and via hematogenous spread.

Approximately 40% of malignant testicular tumors are testicular embryonal carcinomas in some degree. They are smaller than seminomas; however, they are very invasive and metastasize fairly quickly. Embryonal carcinomas carry a 10-year survival rate of approximately 35%.

Testicular choriocarcinomas make up the smallest portion of malignant testicular tumors, accounting for only 1% of malignant neoplasms of the testes. However, choriocarcinomas are very small and aggressive neoplasms. They are often nonpalpable and metastasize very early. Choriocarcinomas carry the worst prognosis, with a 10-year survival rate of approximately 10%.

Gynecomastia. Gynecomastia is the most common male breast disorder. It is the benign proliferation of breast tissue in the male patient. This usually presents as a palpable lump under the nipple that has been detected in either young men or older men and is influenced by hormonal stimulation. For this reason, it is more common among teenage boys undergoing hormonal changes during puberty. In some cases, the nipple will produce a clear discharge associated with the proliferation of this tissue. Gynecomastia is commonly a bilateral process, with one lump dominating, but rarely is associated with breast cancer. Breast ultrasonography is the recommended imaging modality to provide diagnostic confirmation of this entity.

Breast Cancer. Breast cancer in men is rare, specifically 100 times less common than in women. The American Cancer Society estimates in the United States there will be approximately 2600 new cases diagnosed in 2016. The lifetime risk for men developing breast cancer is about 1 in 1000. Male breast cancer largely affects older men, with 68 years being the average age of diagnosis. The cause of breast cancer in men is unknown, but risk factors include: age, family history, inherited gene mutations, estrogen treatment, liver disease, and high alcohol intake. If a history and physical examination are suggestive of breast cancer, a diagnostic mammogram is often performed. Mammography is actually more accurate in males as their breasts are less dense, thus allowing better visualization. Because of the low prevalence of male breast cancer, treatment is based on experience with cancer in females and may consist of surgery, radiation therapy, chemotherapy, or hormone therapy, depending on the stage of the cancer.

Pathologic Summary of the Reproductive System

Pathology	Imaging Modality of Choice
PID (acute pelvic pain)	Sonography, MRI pelvis (with or without contrast)
Ovarian cysts (acute pelvic pain)	Sonography, MRI pelvis (with or without contrast)
Cystadenocarcinoma	Sonography
Carcinoma of the cervix	Staging: MRI pelvis (with or without contrast) and FDG-PET whole body and CT abdomen and pelvis with contrast
Leiomyoma of uterus (abnormal bleeding)	Sonography, SHG
Adenocarcinoma of endometrium (abnormal bleeding <5 mm endometrium on sonogram)	Staging: MRI pelvis (with or without contrast), CT chest (with or without contrast), CT abdomen with contrast, radiography of the chest
Fibroadenoma of breast	Mammography and sonography
Fibrocystic breast	Mammography and sonography
Carcinoma of breast	Mammography, sonography, and MRI
Pregnancy status	Sonography
Ectopic pregnancy	Sonography
Disorders of placenta	Sonography
Cryptorchidism (undescended testicle)	Sonography
Prostatic hyperplasia	Sonography of the pelvis, sonography of the kidney
Carcinoma of the prostate	MRI, ^{99m}Tc bone scan whole body
Testicular torsion	Sonography, nuclear medicine
Testicular mass	Sonography
Gynecomastia	Sonography
Breast cancer in men	Mammography

^{99m}*Tc*, Technetium-99m; *CT*, computed tomography; *FDG-PET*, 18F-fluorodeoxyglucose positron emission tomography; *MRI*, magnetic resonance imaging; *PID*, pelvic inflammatory disease; *SHG*, sonohysterography.

Review Questions

1. Imaging studies performed on a nongravid woman include:
   a. Hysterosalpingography
   b. Transvaginal pelvic sonography
   c. Transabdominal pelvic sonography
   d. All of the above

2. Regular, yearly mammographic screening should occur in women ___ years of age or older.
   a. 20
   b. 30
   c. 40
   d. 50

3. The congenital disorder resulting in a the complete duplication of the uterus, cervix, and vagina is:
   a. Bicornuate uterus
   b. Retroflexed uterus
   c. Unicornuate uterus
   d. Uterus didelphys

4. Which of the following cystic ovarian masses may form as a part of the normal menstrual cycle?
   1. Corpus luteum cysts
   2. Cystadenomas
   3. Follicular cysts
   a. 1 and 2
   b. 1 and 3
   c. 2 and 3
   d. 1, 2, and 3

5. A malignant neoplasm of the ovary is a:
   a. Cystadenocarcinoma
   b. Cystadenoma
   c. Leiomyoma
   d. Fibroadenoma

6. Which type of neoplastic disease is often diagnosed via a Pap test and confirmed by surgical biopsy?
   a. Adenocarcinoma of the endometrium
   b. Cervical carcinoma
   c. Fibroadenoma of the breast
   d. Leiomyoma of the uterus

7. In which anatomic region of the breast do the majority of breast masses occur?
   a. Lower inner quadrant
   b. Lower outer quadrant
   c. Upper inner quadrant
   d. Upper outer quadrant

8. The presence of excessive amniotic fluid is termed:
   a. Abruptio placentae
   b. Oligohydramnios
   c. Placenta previa
   d. Polyhydramnios

9. Prostatic hyperplasia most frequently occurs in men:
   a. Under age 30 years
   b. Between ages 30 and 50 years
   c. Over age 50 years
   d. None of the above; prostatic hyperplasia is a female condition

10. Benign masses of the testes include:
    1. Hydroceles
    2. Seminomas
    3. Spermatoceles
    a. 1 and 2
    b. 1 and 3
    c. 2 and 3
    d. 1, 2, and 3

11. Describe how breast parenchyma changes with age and parity and the effect these changes have on the radiographic visibility of potential masses.

12. Identify two purposes for requiring a female patient to have a full bladder for transabdominal sonographic examination.

13. Describe the benefits of routine mammography *versus* the risks of radiation exposure.

14. What would be the danger of leaving cryptorchidism untreated?

15. A 60-year-old man presents to his physician with complaints of frequent urination, particularly at night. Intravenous pyelography is ordered. The only visible abnormality is a filling defect at the base of his bladder. What is the likely cause?

CHAPTER 11

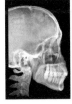
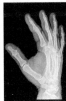
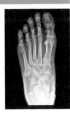

Endocrine System

ⓔ http://evolve.elsevier.com/Kowalczyk/pathology/

Anatomy and Physiology

The endocrine system is responsible for metabolic activities within the human cells through the release of hormones. Endocrine glands are ductless glands that secrete **hormones** directly into the surrounding vascular and lymphatic systems or through neuroendocrine processes. The primary endocrine glands of the body include the **pituitary gland**, **pineal gland**, **adrenal glands**, **thyroid gland**, **parathyroid gland**, and **thymus gland**. The **pancreas**, **gonads**, and **hypothalamus** also produce hormones (Fig. 11.1). Hormones are synthesized and released in response to three types of stimuli: (1) **humoral stimuli**, which involve a direct response to changes in blood chemistry; (2) **neural stimuli**, such as in the case of the adrenal glands secreting epinephrine or norepinephrine in response to the sympathetic nervous system; and (3) **hormonal stimuli**, which involve a response to other hormones secreted in the body.

The **pituitary gland** comprises three separate lobes: (1) the anterior lobe, (2) the intermediate lobe, and (3) the posterior lobe. Each lobe functions as a separate gland; however, in humans, the intermediate lobe is rudimentary, consisting of only a few cells. The pituitary is considered the "master endocrine gland," and it is located below the hypothalamus at the base of the brain within the sella turcica of the sphenoid bone (Fig. 11.2). The hypothalamus is connected to the pituitary via the pituitary stalk, and the hypothalamus is responsible for controlling the function of the pituitary gland. Each lobe of the pituitary secretes specific hormones. The anterior lobe is responsible for secreting luteinizing hormone (LH), follicle-stimulating hormone (FSH), prolactin (PRL), adrenocorticotropic hormone (ACTH), growth hormone (GH), and thyroid-stimulating hormone (TSH). The intermediate lobe secretes melanocyte-stimulating hormone (MSH), and the posterior lobe is responsible for secreting oxytocin and antidiuretic hormone (ADH). The secretion of hormones by the anterior lobe occurs through the typical endocrine control mechanism by the release of hormones directly into the blood. However, the posterior lobe of the pituitary is an extension of the nervous system, with hormone secretion occurring via a neuroendocrine mechanism, in which the hormones are synthesized within the cell bodies of neurons within the hypothalamus.

The pineal gland is also controlled by the hypothalamus. It is located within the cranium, posterior to the

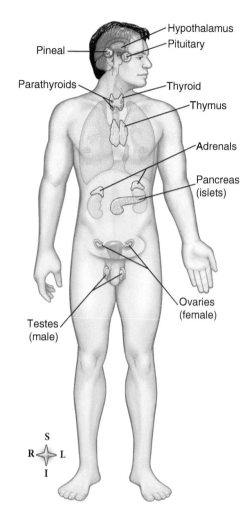

FIG. 11.1 Principal endocrine glands.

third ventricle, superior to the colliculi of the midbrain, and inferior to the splenium of the corpus callosum (Fig. 11.2). It occasionally calcifies with age and is often quite visible on computed tomography (CT) images of the brain. This small endocrine gland is responsible for the production and excretion of melatonin. Melatonin is released when light exposure is inhibited; thus, the pineal gland is responsible for regulating the circadian rhythms. This hormone is often used to treat sleep disorders. The pineal gland also secretes gonadotropin-releasing hormone (GnRH), a hormone that stimulates the release of FSH and LH and is active in the onset of puberty.

The adrenal glands are pyramid-shaped glands located on the upper poles of the kidneys (Fig. 11.3).

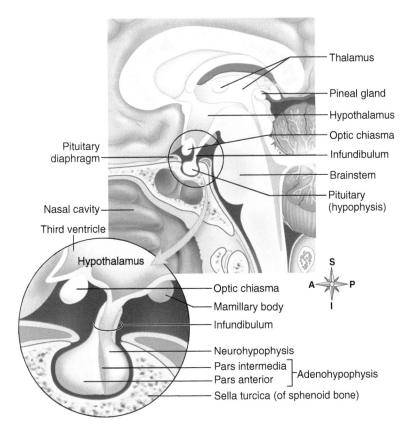

FIG. 11.2 Midsagittal section of brain demonstrating the pituitary and pineal glands.

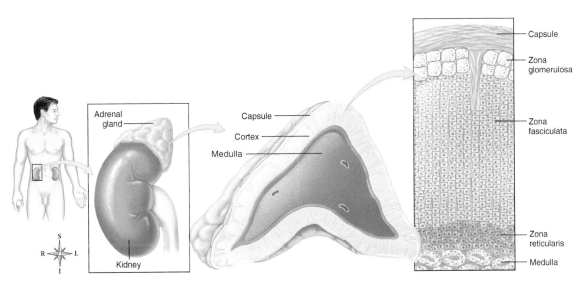

FIG. 11.3 Adrenal glands.

The inner portion of the adrenal gland, termed the *adrenal medulla*, acts as a part of the sympathetic nervous system and secretes the catecholamines epinephrine and norepinephrine. The effects of increased epinephrine production include increased cardiac output; increased heart rate; vasodilation of skeletal muscle; vasoconstriction of internal organs and skin; relaxation of smooth muscle in the gastrointestinal (GI) system, urinary bladder, and bronchial system; and increased mental alertness. Epinephrine also increases glycogenesis in the liver and lipolysis in adipose tissue, as well as affecting the pancreatic hormone secretion by decreasing insulin production and increasing glucagon secretion. The outer portion, known as the *adrenal cortex*, is responsible for corticosteroid production. The adrenal cortex activity is primarily controlled by ACTH, which is secreted by the anterior pituitary. ACTH synthesizes three major types of corticosteroids: (1) mineralocorticosteroids, which are responsible for electrolyte balance; (2) glucocorticoids, which are responsible for cell metabolism and controlling blood sugar levels; and (3) low levels of gonadocorticosteroids, or sex hormones. Mineralocorticoids such as aldosterone may affect extracellular fluid volume and blood volume, which ultimately affects blood pressure and cardiac output. Glucocorticoid secretions are greatly influenced by physical or psychological stress stimuli such as hypoglycemia, trauma, and acute or chronic anxiety. Hypoglycemia stimulates the secretion of cortisol, which, in turn, triggers a response in the liver to convert amino acids to glucose, thus increasing blood glucose levels.

The thyroid gland is located in the anterior neck just below the larynx (Fig. 11.4). It is divided into two lobes connected by an isthmus. This endocrine gland secretes two hormones: (1) thyroid hormone (TH) and (2) calcitonin. TH stimulates enzymes responsible for glucose oxidation and is actually a composition of two hormones: (1) thyroxine (T_4) and (2) triiodothyronine (T_3), both of which contain iodine as an integral part of the molecule. Unlike other hormones within the body, thyroid hormone synthesis requires the presence of iodine. Levels of T_4 and T_3 are regulated by TSH, which is synthesized and stored within the anterior lobe of the pituitary. The thyroid gland is vital to maintaining normal blood pressure and in regulating tissue growth and development. Overactivity of the thyroid gland is termed **hyperthyroidism**, and underactivity is termed **hypothyroidism**. Either

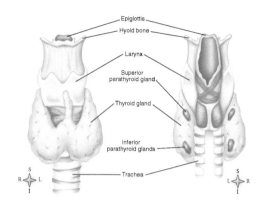

FIG. 11.4 Thyroid and parathyroid glands.

abnormal activity level may cause severe metabolic disturbances in the human body. Calcitonin is most important in childhood. It is an antagonist of parathyroid hormone (PTH) and serves to lower blood calcium levels by inhibiting osteoclast activity and stimulating calcium uptake in the bone matrix. The parathyroid glands are located on the posterior aspect of the thyroid gland. They are responsible for producing and secreting PTH, which also serves to control blood calcium levels. This hormone stimulates osteoclasts and increases calcium absorption in the kidneys and in the GI system. It is important to note that a reduction in bone density may occur and result in increased bone fragility if PTH secretion is sustained at a high level. However, new research in the use of therapeutic recombinant parathyroid hormone (rPTH) shows promise in strengthening bone and increasing bone density in patients with osteoporosis.

The pancreas is located in the midabdomen just posterior to the stomach (Fig. 11.5) and functions both as an endocrine and an exocrine organ. The tail of the pancreas ends at the spleen and the head is encircled by the duodenum. Specialized cells within the pancreas, termed the *islets of Langerhans* or *pancreatic islets*, are responsible for the production of important hormones. The α-cells are responsible for glucagon synthesis; the β-cells are responsible for balancing the secretion of insulin and glucagon, depending on food intake; and the γ-cells are responsible for secreting somatostatin, a hormone that influences α- and β-cell secretion. **Glucagon** promotes the breakdown of glycogen to glucose within the liver, and glucose is ultimately released into the bloodstream. The α-cells of

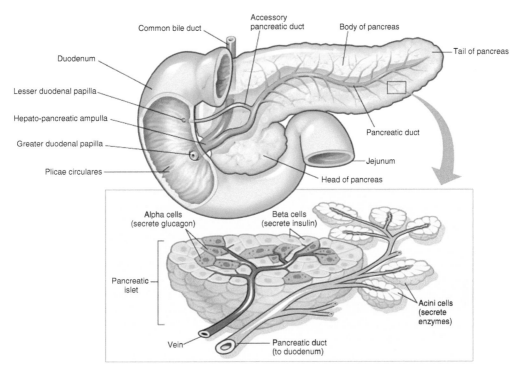

FIG. 11.5 The pancreas.

the pancreas secrete glucagon to increase blood sugar levels and these cells are driven by humeral stimuli. Insulin, whose role is the opposite of glucagon's, acts to decrease blood sugar levels. **Insulin** is produced by the β-cells to inhibit the breakdown of glycogen to glucose.

Imaging Considerations

Radiography

Radiographic examination is very helpful in diagnosing metabolic diseases of the skeletal system or endocrine disorders that ultimately affect the skeletal system, for example, Cushing disease. Skeletal disorders that result in a decrease of calcium in the bone matrix include osteoporosis and osteomalacia. Skull radiography is of limited use in evaluating metabolic disorders of the pituitary gland and is increasingly being replaced by magnetic resonance imaging (MRI), computed tomography (CT), or positron emission tomography (PET) in making a definitive diagnosis for pituitary disorders.

Bone Mineral Densitometry

Dual-energy x-ray absorptiometry (DXA) or bone mineral densitometry is an important modality in the evaluation of osteoporosis. DXA units readily show bone density by evaluating the bone mass of the distal radius, femoral neck, and lumbar spine. The results of bone densitometry are used in combination with routine laboratory tests of blood and urine to determine loss of bone mass. Bone mineral densitometry reports indicate the amount of bone mass present and compare the density of a particular individual to norms used during evaluation. A "T-score" is used to reflect standard deviations above or below the 30-year-old national reference population because it is assumed that this is the age of peak bone mass. Based on criteria established by the World Health Organization (WHO), a T-score greater than −1 is normal. T-scores less than −1 but greater than −2.49 are classified as osteopenia, and T-scores less than −2.5 reflect osteoporosis. The "Z-score" reports standard deviation above or below a population matched for age, gender, weight, and ethnicity. Z-scores less than −2 suggest bone disease.

Magnetic Resonance Imaging

MRI has largely replaced CT for imaging neuroendocrine disorders. According to the American College of Radiology (ACR), MRI is the only imaging modality that can reliably demonstrate pathologies of the hypothalamus. Pituitary disorders often result in an enlarged sella turcica, represented by the "empty sella syndrome," which can be confirmed with MRI. Gadolinium contrast-enhanced MRI is routinely used to demonstrate pituitary adenomas and is the modality of choice for visualizing microadenomas. MRI is also helpful in monitoring the progress of patients with pituitary adenomas. (See Chapter 8 for additional information on pituitary adenomas.)

Computed Tomography

Contrast-enhanced, high-resolution brain CT may also be used in the diagnosis and follow-up care of patients with pituitary disorders. It is frequently used when MRI is not available or may be contraindicated. The pineal gland is also clearly visible during CT evaluation. CT examinations of the neck are useful in the evaluation of neoplastic disease of the thyroid and parathyroid glands.

Most adrenal neoplasms in the cortex and medulla are identified with abdominal CT, and biopsies of these tumors are frequently performed with CT-guided small-needle aspiration. Abdominal CT is also used in assessing enlargement of the adrenal glands of patients with Cushing disease.

Nuclear Medicine Procedures

In the case of thyroid disorders, nuclear medicine testing for iodine-123 (^{123}I) uptake is quite valuable in diagnosing thyroid gland function. It is used to detect nonpalpable nodules and to evaluate the remaining thyroid tissue after surgical resection or ablation.

The use of nuclear medicine imaging to localize medullary tumors in the adrenal glands using iodine-131 (^{131}I)-metaiodobenzylguanidine (MIBG) is gaining popularity. Patients are scanned over a 3-day period to look for an increased uptake, which indicates the presence of a pheochromocytoma. This radioisotope may also be used to treat this tumor of the medullary portion of the adrenal gland.

Skeletal Disorders

Osteoporosis

A radiographically visible decrease in bone density is termed **osteopenia** and may occur as a result of osteoporosis or osteomalacia. Osteopenia is identified as a bone mass between 648 mg/cm^2 and 833 mg/cm^2. **Osteoporosis** is a commonly known metabolic bone disorder in which the structural integrity of the trabecular pattern of bone is destroyed and is identified as a bone mass less than 648 mg/cm^2. It may be classified as *primary osteoporosis* (type 1) or *secondary osteoporosis* (type 2). Primary osteoporosis may be further classified as *postmenopausal* or *senile*, and secondary osteoporosis is most commonly associated with an existing disease process or is the result of a medication. Osteoporosis may also be classified as *generalized* or *regional*. Postmenopausal osteoporosis is the most common form of the disease. Greater than 70% of women aged 60 years or older within the United States have osteoporosis. It is a major cause of fractures of the hip, spine, and wrist in women over the age of 50 years. It is more common in Caucasian and Asian women. Although the formation of bone is normal, the bone reabsorption rate is abnormally high in individuals with osteoporosis. Thus osteoporosis results in a thinning of cortical bone and an enlargement of the medullary canal without any change in the actual diameter of the bone. The normal equilibrium associated with osteoid production and withdrawal is quite complex and depends on a combination of dietary intake and absorption, hormonal interplay, and normal stress or muscular activity. In postmenopausal women, for example, the lack of the hormone estrogen creates a weakened bone matrix, contributing to the development of "porous" bones. As the condition becomes more severe, bones are subject to compression fractures, and they may literally cave in from the weakness. Risk factors for osteoporosis are listed in Table 11.1. As the vertebral bodies of the thoracic and lumbar spine are weakened, they collapse anteriorly, causing a kyphotic deformity of the spine, often termed "dowager's hump." These bony changes are well demonstrated by radiography of the spine (Fig. 11.6), in which decreased bone density stands out clearly against the cortex. Osteoporosis is a subtractive or destructive pathologic condition and requires a decrease in exposure technique. However, conventional radiography may be used to identify bone mass loss only

TABLE 11.1
Risk Factors for Osteoporosis

Genetic	Family history of osteoporosis
	White or Asian race
	Advanced age
	Female sex
Anthropometric	Small stature
	Fair or pale complexion
	Thin build
Hormonal and Metabolic	Early menopause (natural or surgical)
	Late menarche
	Nulliparity
	Obesity
	Hypogonadism
	Gaucher disease
	Cushing syndrome
	Weight below healthy range
	Acidosis
Dietary	Low dietary calcium and vitamin D
	Low endogenous magnesium
	Excessive protein*
	Excessive sodium intake
	High caffeine intake
	Anorexia
	Malabsorption
Lifestyle	Sedentary lifestyle
	Smoking
	Alcohol consumption (excessive)
Concurrent Disease	Hyperparathyroidism
Illness and Trauma	Renal insufficiency, hypocalciuria
	Rheumatoid arthritis
	Spinal cord injury
	Systemic lupus erythematosus
	Liver disease
	Marrow disease (myeloma, mastocytosis, thalassemia)
Drugs	Corticosteroids
	Dilantin
	Gonadotropin-releasing hormone agonists
Loop diuretics	Methotrexate
	Thyroid
	Heparin
	Cyclosporine
	Depo-medroxyprogesterone acetate
	Retinoids

*Low levels of protein intake have also been reported.
Data from: McCance KL, Huether SE, Brashers VL, etal: Pathophysiology: The biologic basis for disease in adults and children, ed 6.

when it is advanced or the bone has lost approximately 30% to 50% of its original mass. In this case a decrease in cortical thickness and loss of bony trabecula will be present. The best method for evaluating the early stages of osteoporosis is bone mineral densitometry of the hip and lumbar spine using DXA (Fig. 11.7).

Secondary osteoporosis may be caused by other diseases such as pathologies of the endocrine system, neoplastic disease, malnutrition, chronic renal failure, or hereditary diseases of the skeletal system, or it may be a result of drug therapy. Osteoporosis is, by far, the most common form of metabolic bone disease and can be differentiated from other causes of bone weakening by examining serum enzyme levels, especially alkaline phosphatase. For example, patients with osteoporosis have normal or elevated serum alkaline levels, whereas these serum levels are decreased in patients with osteomalacia. Elevated alkaline phosphatase is an indication of increased bone activity because it is found on the outside of osteoclast cells. Treatment of osteoporosis generally includes an increase in dietary intake of calcium, vitamin D, and magnesium in combination with moderate weight-bearing exercise.

Osteomalacia

Osteomalacia is a condition caused by lack of calcium in tissues and failure of bone tissue to calcify. The mature bone exhibits an abnormal bone matrix consisting of soft osteoid instead of rigid bone. This normally results from a low-serum phosphate level because of inadequate intake or absorption of vitamin D, most commonly as a consequence of intestinal malabsorption of fats. Osteomalacia may be associated with hepatic disease, chronic pancreatitis, regional ileitis, and resections of the GI system because these conditions may inhibit the body from absorbing fat-soluble vitamin D. It is often also present in individuals with chronic renal failure secondary to the loss of renal parenchyma and the kidneys' inability to convert vitamin D into a form useful to the human body. If osteomalacia occurs before growth plate closure, it is known as **Rickets** (Fig. 11.8).

With this condition, the bones are sponge-like and demonstrate osteopenia during radiographic evaluation. Radiographically, osteomalacia appears similar to osteoporosis except for the presence of bands of radiolucency within the bone, termed **pseudofractures** or Looser zones. Abnormal mineralization of bone is often most evident at the metaphysis, resulting in growth plate

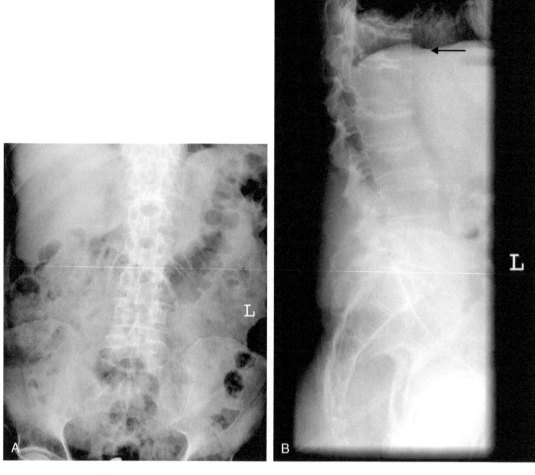

FIG. 11.6 **A,** Anteroposterior and **B,** lateral lumbar spine radiographs demonstrating osteopenia secondary to long-term steroid use.

widening and a "frayed" appearance. Common signs and symptoms include skeletal pain, muscular weakness, lower back pain, uremia, and bone fractures resulting from minimal trauma. Symptoms from low calcium levels may also occur and include: numbness around the mouth, arms, or legs, and spasms of the hands or feet. Laboratory analysis to measure blood urea nitrogen (BUN), creatinine, serum calcium levels, and serum inorganic phosphate levels, and other tests, are necessary for differential diagnosis. Bone density tests are useful in the detection of pseudofractures, bone loss, and bone softening. Bone biopsy and measurement of serum fibroblast growth factor 23 (FGF-23) levels are the definitive methods of determining the presence

of osteomalacia. This disorder may be treated by adjusting serum calcium and phosphate levels, inclusion of a dietary supplement of vitamin D, administering calcium carbonate, chelating bone aluminum, renal dialysis, and controlling other disease processes such as hyperthyroidism and renal osteodystrophy.

Paget's Disease (Osteitis Deformans)

Paget's disease is a metabolic disorder of unknown cause; however, recent research indicates a genetic link and the possible role of viral infectious agents. It is fairly common in the older adult population, with a small predominance in males. It usually begins in the fifth decade

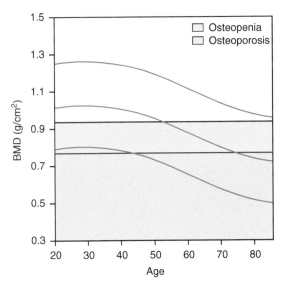

FIG. 11.7 Lumbar spine bone mass density.

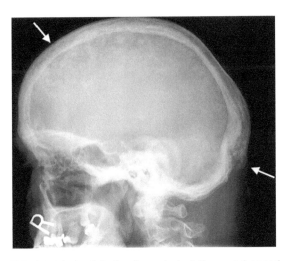

FIG. 11.9 Lateral skull radiograph depicting an advanced proliferative phase of Paget disease. Note the changes within the inner and outer tables of the skull.

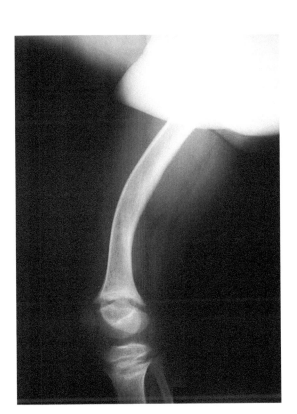

FIG. 11.8 Radiograph of a femur of a child diagnosed with vitamin D–resistant rickets. Note the bowing of the extremity.

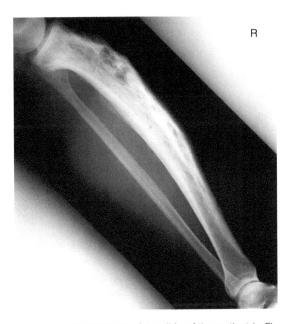

FIG. 11.10 Radiograph of the tibia of the patient in Fig. 11.8 demonstrating the effect of advanced proliferative Paget disease on the tibia.

of life with a prevalence of 2% to 3% among adults over the age of 55 years. Paget's may affect one or more bones, most commonly the pelvis, spine, skull, femur and tibia (Fig. 11.9), and long bones (Fig. 11.10). **Paget's disease** is characterized by two stages: (1) the *osteolytic stage*, in which the bone undergoes continuous destruction and (2) the *osteoblastic stage*, in which the bone is simultaneously replaced by abnormally soft and poorly mineralized material. The osteoid material that replaces normal bone tissue diminishes the trabeculae and is very bulky and porous, with exceptional vascularity. Although this osteoid matrix is thicker than normal bone, its softness often leads to weight-bearing, stress-induced deformities and fractures. This bony destruction and replacement produce a classic "cotton wool" appearance radiographically. As the skull enlarges, additional complications may occur because of impingement on the cranial nerves. These complications include hearing and vision disturbances. In addition, individuals with Paget disease have an increased risk of developing osteogenic sarcoma, a malignant neoplastic disease of the skeletal system. Radionuclide bone scans readily detect Paget disease, even in its very early stages. Radiographically, affected bones typically demonstrate cortical thickening, with a coarse, thickened trabecular pattern. Mixed areas of radiolucent osteolysis and radiopaque osteosclerosis may be seen, with earlier lesions appearing osteolytic until osteoblastic activity transforms them into bone. Sclerosis that is visible radiographically is typically sufficient for diagnosis and a bone biopsy is rarely required. Blood chemistry results indicate very high alkaline phosphatase levels with normal serum calcium and phosphorus. After diagnosis, skeletal radionuclide imaging is recommended as the standard to assess the extent of skeletal involvement and detect localized increases in bone cell activity that may not yet be visible on radiographs. No known cure exists for this disease. Most cases are mild and asymptomatic; no treatment is necessary. In symptomatic cases, bisphosphonate medications are administered to decrease bone reabsorption.

Pituitary Gland Disorders

Acromegaly

Acromegaly is an endocrine disorder caused by a disturbance in the function of the pituitary gland; this disorder primarily affects the skeletal system. It is more common in females than in males and most frequently occurs in individuals over the age of 40 years. This disorder is caused by excessive secretion of GH in adults, which is often the result of a pituitary adenoma. In fact, in more than 95% of patients with acromegaly, a GH-secreting pituitary adenoma is present. Although small pituitary adenomas are not uncommon, affecting approximately

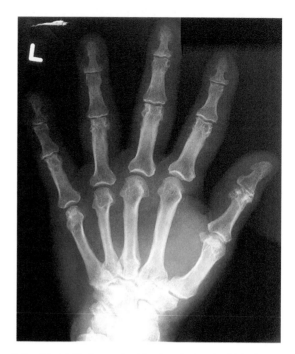

FIG. 11.11 Radiograph of the hand of an individual diagnosed with acromegaly. Note the spade-like appearance of the hand.

17% of the population, they are often asymptomatic. It is estimated that three to four out of every million people develop acromegaly each year. Acromegaly is a slowly progressive disease that may be diagnosed years after the individual has symptoms. For this reason, clinical diagnoses are commonly missed, leading to an underestimate in statistics projecting disease frequency. In adults, an increase in GH produces a thickening and coarsening of bone because the epiphyses have closed and bone cannot grow in length. Radiographic studies demonstrate an enlarged sella turcica and changes in the skull, often obliterating the diploë found between the inner and outer tables of cortical bone. A blood test may reveal increased levels of GH. However, MRI of the brain, with or without contrast enhancement, is the primary modality recommended by the ACR to evaluate the pituitary. Individuals with acromegaly have a prominent forehead and jaw, widened teeth, and abnormally large, spade-like hands (Fig. 11.11), and a coarsening of facial features (Fig. 11.12). This disorder is frequently treated with a combination of surgery and radiotherapy to eradicate the adenoma. Although this is a slowly progressing disease, it may lead to premature death from associated cardiovascular and renal complications if it is not treated.

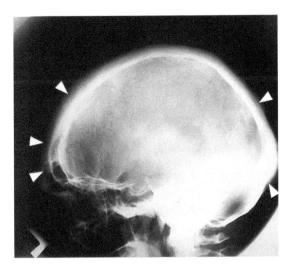

FIG. 11.12 Skull radiograph depicting the changes caused by acromegaly.

Diabetes Insipidus

Central **diabetes insipidus** (DI), the most common and serious form of diabetes insipidus, results from damage to the pituitary gland causing a disruption in the secretion of antidiuretic hormone (ADH), also known as vasopressin. In central DI, this can be the result of head trauma, genetic disorders, or neurosurgery affecting the hypothalamus, pituitary stalk, or posterior pituitary gland. Insufficient levels of ADH secretion by the posterior pituitary cause frequent urination (polyuria) and dehydration. Other symptoms include low urine osmolality in combination with high-normal plasma osmolality. Treatment involves administration of the synthetic hormone desmopressin.

In cases of nephrogenic DI, in which the kidneys are unable to respond to ADH because of the presence of drugs or chronic kidney disorders, combination drug therapy is required for treatment. MRI of the brain, with or without contrast, is helpful in demonstrating the presence of a lesion disturbing the balance of ADH. However, urinalysis and fluid deprivation tests are often used for diagnosis.

Hypopituitarism

Hypopituitarism is the decreased level or absence of pituitary hormones originating from the anterior pituitary gland. The most common causes of this disorder are embryonic mutations of the prophet of pituitary transcription factor gene (*PROP-1*) or pituitary infarction, which may be caused by ischemic pituitary

necrosis. It may also be associated with infarction caused by pregnancy (Sheehan syndrome), postpartum hemorrhage, shock, sickle cell disease, meningitis, syphilis, or head trauma. Signs and symptoms vary with the severity and types of hormones involved, and treatment includes the replacement of the hormone or hormones that are deficient. The ACR recommends enhanced and nonenhanced multiplanar MRI of the sellar region of the brain as the primary imaging modality. CT of the brain, with or without enhancement, may also be used if MRI is unavailable or contraindicated. Treatment includes hormone replacement therapy and in some cases in which a tumor is present, surgery and radiation therapy. Hypopituitarism is almost always permanent, requiring lifelong hormone and medication treatment.

Adrenal Gland Disorders

Cushing Syndrome

Cushing syndrome results from an excess of cortisol production by the adrenal cortex, or excessive use of glucocorticoid hormones. In some patients undergoing steroid therapy, this syndrome may have an iatrogenic cause and will generally recede once the steroids are discontinued. Individuals with this disorder tend to have round, "moon" faces, with excess fat deposits in the neck and trunk regions of the body. The patient's skin is thin and does not heal well after injury. Female patients tend to have male characteristics because of an increased production of androgens, and their menstrual cycles are usually quite irregular. An analysis of plasma and urinary cortisol is the most frequent form of diagnostic testing, but enhanced or unenhanced MRI of the head may be used to assess the presence of pituitary adenomas, which may increase ACTH secretion and is one cause of Cushing syndrome. Treatment of Cushing syndrome depends on the point of origin, adrenal cortex *versus* pituitary gland, and focuses on correcting the hyperfunction. In some cases, radiotherapy may be used to treat pituitary adenomas, or surgical resection of the adrenocortical tumor may be required. If the condition is not treated, over half of the individuals with Cushing syndrome die within 5 years.

Addison Disease

Addison disease is a rare disease of primary adrenal insufficiency. It most frequently affects women between ages 30 and 60 years and generally results from an autoimmune destruction of the adrenal cortex, which impairs both glucocorticoid and mineralocorticoid production. It may also be caused by infection, neoplastic disease, or adrenal hemorrhage. Addison disease is characterized by elevated ACTH accompanied by inadequate corticosteroid synthesis. Signs and symptoms include weight loss, fatigue, weakness, nausea, diarrhea, low blood sugar, and low blood pressure leading to orthostatic hypotension. The most common diagnosis involves laboratory tests for levels of plasma cortisol and ACTH. Treatment includes the use of lifelong HRT in combination with a special diet. If left untreated, this disorder may progress to a life-threatening adrenal crisis.

Adrenal Carcinomas

Adrenal carcinomas are rare and are typically an incidental finding during imaging for something unrelated. They are much less common than benign adrenal adenomas, with an estimated diagnosis of only 200 cases per year. Adrenal adenomas are found primarily in middle aged to elderly people, with the average age being 46 years. Adrenal carcinomas are often diagnosed earlier in children because they are more likely to be hormone secreting, and thus children will experience signs of excess hormone production. However, other types of cancers often metastasize to the adrenal glands. Lung cancers are the most common types of adrenal metastatic cancers, but cancers arising in the breast, kidney, pancreas, GI system, and lymphomas may also spread to the adrenal glands. Contrast-enhanced CT and MR studies are helpful in the diagnosis of adrenal masses. Sonography may also be employed. The risk of malignancy increases as the size of the tumor increases; therefore, most masses are surgically removed.

Pancreatic Disorders

Diabetes Mellitus

Diabetes mellitus is a syndrome that is associated with chronic hyperglycemia in combination with glucose intolerance and alterations in the metabolism of carbohydrates, fats, and proteins. Normal blood glucose levels range from 70 to 120 mg/dL, and fasting glucose levels greater than 126 mg/dL indicate the presence of this syndrome. According to the 2014 National Diabetes Statistics Report, approximately 9.3% of the United States population has diabetes. The most common

types of diabetes mellitus are type 1, caused by a defect in the primary β-cells, and type 2, resulting in insulin resistance (Table 11.2).

Type 1 diabetes mellitus appears to be a genetic disorder, and although it accounts for only about 5% of cases of diabetes mellitus in the United States, it is one of the most common diseases in childhood. Type 1 diabetes mellitus occurs when the body is unable to produce insulin, thus causing hyperglycemia. It can be further classified as type 1A and type 1B; type 1A is an autoimmune variation of the disease and is more common than type 1B. Type 1B is believed to be nonimmune in nature and generally occurs secondary to other pathologic processes. Type 1A diabetes mellitus is associated with a histocompatibility leukocyte antigen (HLA) marker that has also been linked to other autoimmune endocrine diseases such as Graves and Addison diseases. Additionally, environmental factors such as viruses have also been linked to the development of type 1 diabetes mellitus.

Type 1 diabetes mellitus is often referred to as *juvenile diabetes mellitus* because most cases manifest before the age of 30 years. These young individuals produce little to no insulin because of an autoimmune destruction of the pancreatic β-cells and are insulin dependent from a young age. Signs and symptoms of type 1 diabetes mellitus include weight loss, fluctuations in blood glucose level, increased urination, excessive thirst, and an increased appetite. Ketoacidosis or increased levels of circulating ketones in the bloodstream, which are caused by the absence of insulin, are a common complication associated with this disease. The goal of treatment is to adequately control glucose levels without causing hypoglycemia. Therefore treatment is varied and may include the use of immunosuppressive drugs, immunomodulation therapies, careful meal planning, exercise, and blood glucose checks multiple times per day in combination with daily insulin injections. Hypoglycemia is a common complication with daily insulin injections and can lead to mental confusion, loss of consciousness, seizure, and in severe cases, death. Current research is being conducted on the development of the artificial pancreas, using implanted continuous glucose monitoring systems and computer algorithms to dispense appropriate levels of insulin to the body.

Type 2 diabetes mellitus is characterized by high blood glucose levels, either from insulin-resistance or an inadequate secretion of insulin. It is much more common than type 1 in the United States, with over 90%

TABLE 11.2

Epidemiology and Etiology of Diabetes Mellitus

	Type 1 Diabetes: Primary β-Cell Defect or Failure	Type 2 Diabetes: Insulin Resistance with Inadequate Insulin Secretion
Incidence		
Frequency	One of the most common childhood diseases (5% of all cases of diabetes mellitus)	Accounts for most cases (>90%)
Change in incidence	Range from 29.5/100,000 (Finland) to 1.6/100,000 (Japan)	Prevalence rate in the United States (for age 18 years and older): 6.6%
	Increased incidence in British Isles, Finland, Norway, Denmark, Israel, Germany, and Poland; stable elsewhere	Prevalence for American Indian/Alaska Native; non-Hispanic black; Hispanic/Latino American; Asian American: 39.9%
		Incidence has risen in the United States since 1940
Characteristics		
Age at onset	Peak onset at age 11–13 years (slightly earlier for girls than for boys) Rare in children younger than 1 year and adults older than 30 years	Risk of developing diabetes mellitus increases after the age of 40 years; in general, incidence increases with age into the 70s; among Pima Indians, incidence peaks between ages 40 and 50 years, then falls
Gender	Similar in males and females	In the United States, more females than males
Racial distribution	Rates for Caucasians 1.5–2 times higher than for non-Caucasians	Certain racial groups may be more likely to develop type 2 diabetes mellitus when exposed to a particular environment
	Higher rates for those of Scandinavian descent than for those of central or southern European descent	Common in migrant groups encountering a different environment (e.g., Polynesians moving from traditional to Western lifestyle)
		In the United States, risk is highest for American Indians; rates are higher for Pacific Islanders, Japanese, Puerto Ricans, Hispanics, and African Americans than for Caucasian
Socioeconomic status	Conflicting data	A disease of the affluent in developing nations, but more common among those of lower income and less education in the United States
Seasonal distribution	More new cases documented during fall and winter in the northern hemisphere	No known association
Childbirth association	No association documented	Effect of parity on subsequent development of type 2 diabetes mellitus varies among different populations
Obesity	Generally normal or underweight	Frequent contributing factor to precipitate type 2 diabetes mellitus among those susceptible; a major factor in populations recently exposed to Westernized environment
		Increased risk related to duration, degree, and distribution of obesity

Continued

TABLE 11.2

Epidemiology and Etiology of Diabetes Mellitus—cont'd

	Type 1 Diabetes: Primary β-Cell Defect or Failure	Type 2 Diabetes: Insulin Resistance with Inadequate Insulin Secretion
Etiology		
Common theory	*Autoimmune:* genetic and environmental factors, resulting in gradual process of autoimmune destruction in genetically susceptible individuals	Disease results from genetic susceptibility (although the precise gene or genes have not been determined) combined with environmental determinants and other risk factors
	Nonautoimmune: Unknown	Associated with long-duration obesity
Heredity	Strong association with HLA-DQA and HLA-DQB genes	Risk to first-degree relative (child or sibling): 10%–15%
	Monogenic β-cell defect	
	Risk to sibling: 5%–10%; risk to offspring: 2%–5%	
Presence of antibody	Islet cell autoantibodies (ICA) and/or autoantibodies to insulin, and autoantibodies to glutamic acid decarboxylase (GAD_{65}) and tyrosine phosphatases IA-2 and IA-2β are present in 85%–90% of individuals when fasting hyperglycemia is initially detected	Islet cell antibodies not present
Insulin resistance	Insulin resistance rare	Insulin resistance is generally caused by altered cellular metabolism and an intracellular postreceptor defect
Insulin secretion	Severe insulin deficiency or no insulin secretion at all	Typically increased at time of diagnosis, but progressively declines over the course of the illness

Data from: American Diabetes Association: Diagnosis and classification of diabetes mellitus, *Diabetes Care* 28(Suppl 1):S-1, 2016. Available at http://care.diabetesjournals.org/content/39/Supplement_1/S13.short

of people diagnosed with diabetes mellitus presenting with type 2. The incidence of type 2 diabetes mellitus has doubled over the past 15 years. The risk of developing this type increases with age, especially after the age of 40 years. It is also more prevalent in women than in men and in African Americans, Native Americans, Pacific Islanders, and Hispanics than in Caucasians. Genetic susceptibility in combination with environmental factors is suspected to be the cause of this disease, as it is associated with obesity, smoking, hypertension, inactivity, and family history of the disease. Insulin resistance generally occurs as a result of altered cellular metabolism *versus* a defect in the primary β-cells of the pancreas.

Recently the medical community has identified **metabolic syndrome** as a precursor to type 2 diabetes mellitus. Metabolic syndrome is classified in individuals demonstrating three of the following five traits: (1) waist circumference greater than 40 inches in males and greater than 35 inches in females; (2) triglycerides 150 mg/dL or more; (3) high-density lipoprotein (HDL) cholesterol less than 40 mg/dL in males and less than 50 mg/dL in females; (4) blood pressure 130/85 mm Hg or greater; and (5) a fasting plasma glucose 100 mg/dL or greater. It is important to note that not all individuals with metabolic syndrome will develop type 2 diabetes mellitus, as individuals must also have genetic alterations that affect pancreatic β-cell function.

Individuals who have chronic type 2 diabetes mellitus for approximately 10 years also develop vascular complications. The risk for coronary artery disease (CAD), stroke, and peripheral vascular disease is increased for

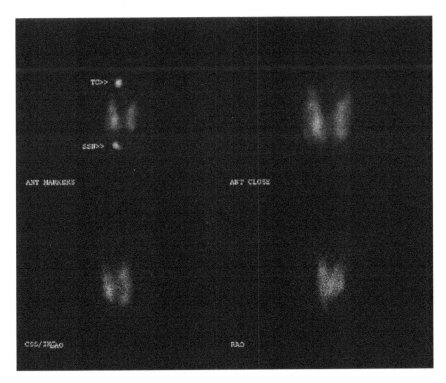

FIG. 11.13 A nuclear medicine ^{123}iodine thyroid uptake scan demonstrating elevated activity resulting from a goiter.

individuals with type 2 diabetes mellitus, and CAD is the most common cause of death for this patient population. The diagnosis and treatment of type 2 diabetes mellitus are similar to those for type 1.

Thyroid and Parathyroid Gland Disorders

Hyperthyroidism

Hyperthyroidism is most frequently caused by an autoimmune disorder termed Graves's disease. In this disorder, the body creates antibodies that attach to the thyroid TSH receptor and mimic TSH, causing the thyroid gland to secrete excess amounts of thyroid hormones. It is more common in females than in males, and a combination of genetic and environmental factors are linked to this disease. The normal hormonal regulatory mechanisms are inhibited by the production of thyroid-stimulating immunoglobulin antibodies leading to suppression of TSH.

Symptoms of this chronic disorder include an enlarged thyroid gland or goiter, fatigue, hair loss, increased sweating, and changes to the eyes and skin. Patients may also exhibit nervousness and hyperactivity. Left untreated, hyperthyroidism may result in a critical event termed a *thyroid storm*, which is a sudden worsening of symptoms resulting in a life-threatening situation that must be treated within 48 hours. It can also arise from infection or stress. Hyperthyroidism is diagnosed using laboratory tests to evaluate serum TSH, T3, and T4 levels in combination with a nuclear medicine ^{123}I thyroid uptake examination (Figs. 11.13 and 11.14). MRI of the brain, with or without contrast, with thin multiplanar sellar imaging may also be indicated, as well as a thyroid sonogram. Treatments include antithyroid drugs, surgical resection of the thyroid gland, and, most commonly, the administration of radioactive iodine (^{123}I).

Hypothyroidism

Hypothyroidism is a common disorder of the thyroid gland and results from a deficiency of TH. This disorder has many causes and can affect individuals of any age or gender. However, primary hypothyroidism most commonly affects women over the age of 60 years. The disorder is commonly seen in patients diagnosed

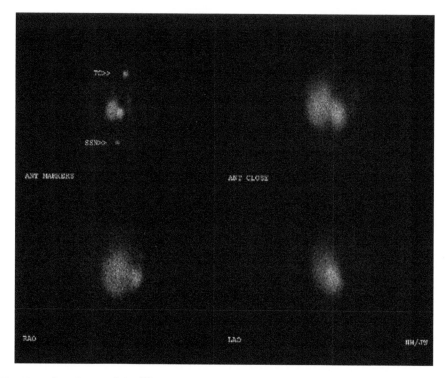

FIG. 11.14 A nuclear medicine ^{123}iodine thyroid uptake scan demonstrating a hyperactive hot nodule.

with autoimmune thyroiditis (Hashimoto disease). Deficiency of TH production results in an increase in TSH, which often results in a goiter. Hypothyroidism may also be iatrogenic in nature, resulting from treatment of a goiter through radioactive iodine therapy or surgical intervention, or from surgical resection of all or parts of the thyroid. Although rarely seen in the United States, it may also be caused by iodine deficiency. Signs and symptoms of hypothyroidism occur slowly over many months and include a decreased energy level, cold intolerance, personality changes, dry skin, constipation, and modest weight gain. This condition affects many organ systems throughout the body, including the neurologic, reproductive, hematologic, cardiopulmonary, renal, GI, and musculoskeletal systems, and the skin. Diagnosis is confirmed with a laboratory test for blood serum levels of TSH and T4. There is no cure for hyperthyroidism, but treatment generally involves HRT with synthetic hormones.

Thyroid Cancers

The majority of neoplasms of the thyroid gland are benign, with only two to three of every 20 being cancerous. Four types are malignant. These include (1) papillary, (2) follicular, (3) medullary, and (4) undifferentiated anaplastic cancers. Cancers of the thyroid are more common in younger individuals and in females. Approximately three out of four cases are found in women. Females are two to three times more likely to develop malignant neoplasms of the thyroid, especially papillary carcinomas. Although the exact cause remains unknown, a history of radiation exposure to the head, neck, or chest, especially in childhood, increases the incidence of malignant thyroid lesions, as well as certain inherited conditions. Signs and symptoms of thyroid cancers include changes in voice and symptoms resulting from compression of the esophagus such as dysphagia, or compression of the trachea. Thyroid nodules, benign or malignant, are often found on thyroid ultrasounds. The rate of thyroid cancer diagnosis has tripled in the past three decades, believed to be largely a result of increased usage of thyroid ultrasound. Diagnosis is made using a nuclear medicine ^{123}I thyroid uptake examination (Fig. 11.15) in combination with serum laboratory analysis, and the diagnosis is generally confirmed by histologic assessment of tissue samples obtained from a sonographic-guided fine-needle aspiration biopsy. The most common treatment is the

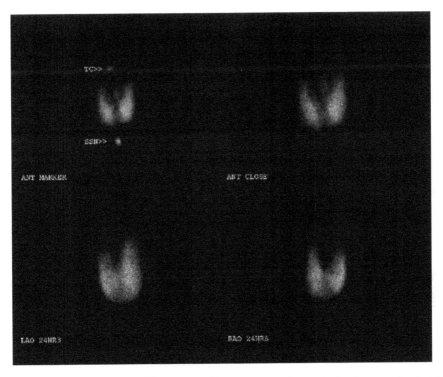

FIG. 11.15 A nuclear medicine ^{123}iodine thyroid uptake scan demonstrating increased radioactive iodine uptake.

surgical removal of the thyroid gland followed by the administration of radioactive iodine (^{123}I) to ablate any remaining thyroid tissue and medication to suppress production of TSH. The death rate from thyroid cancer has been steadily low for many years, and remains so compared with other types of cancers.

Hyperparathyroidism

Hyperparathyroidism is a fairly common disease of the endocrine system that affects the skeletal system. This disease is often very mild and may go undetected for a long time. As with all metabolic bone diseases, hyperparathyroidism affects the entire skeleton, with some sites more affected than others.

The skeletal system is involved in the balance of serum calcium and phosphorus levels, and the body strives to keep this ratio constant. Hyperparathyroidism applies to any disorder that disrupts the calcium–phosphate ratio and results in an elevated level of PTH. Excess PTH secretion overstimulates the osteoclasts responsible for bone removal, thus leading to bone destruction. This osteoclastic activity results in a decreased bone density, so a decrease in radiographic

exposure is necessary to produce a high-quality radiographic image.

The three types of hyperparathyroidism are (1) primary, (2) secondary, and (3) hyperparathyroidism caused by ectopic production of a parathyroid-like hormone. Treatment varies with each specific cause of hyperparathyroidism and is very complex.

Primary hyperparathyroidism most frequently affects adults over the age of 60 years and arises from an adenoma (Fig. 11.16), carcinoma, or hyperplasia of the parathyroid gland (Fig. 11.17). The excess production of PTH causes bone destruction, increased absorption of calcium by the intestines and kidneys, and an increase in urine calcium, which predisposes the individual to renal stones. The net effect of these reactions to the high level of PTH is an increase in serum calcium with a decrease in serum phosphate. Individuals affected by primary hyperparathyroidism commonly have symptoms associated with hypercalcemia, such as neuromuscular weakness and fatigue and may first demonstrate symptoms of renal colic as a result of renal stones or calcification of the kidneys (see later discussion of nephrocalcinosis). Radiographic investigation

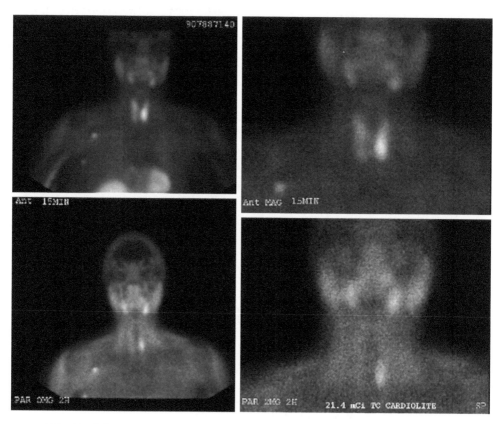

FIG. 11.16 A nuclear medicine sestamibi parathyroid scan demonstrating an adenoma.

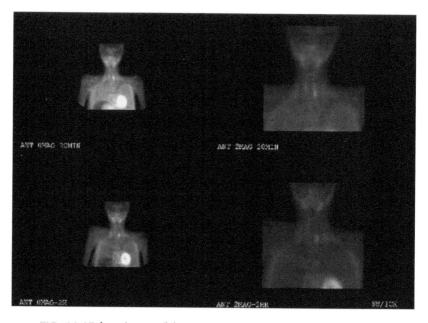

FIG. 11.17 A nuclear medicine scan demonstrating hyperparathyroidism.

demonstrates subperiosteal bone reabsorption or osteopenia, especially in the diaphyses of the phalanges and clavicles. Bone reabsorption is also radiographically evident in teeth. Pathologic fractures may be present as a consequence of the softened bone matrix.

Secondary hyperparathyroidism (Fig. 11.18) represents a response to hypocalcemia, hyperphosphatemia, or hypomagnesemia. It is caused by a very complex metabolic disorder that is beyond the scope of this text and is most commonly seen in individuals with chronic renal disease caused by failure of glomerular filtration. Decreased renal function leads to a loss of the kidneys' ability to produce vitamin D and compromises their ability to excrete phosphate.

CT, sonography, and sestamibi nuclear medicine studies may be used in evaluating adenomas. Treatment usually requires surgical intervention in combination with medications such as bisphosphonates, corticosteroids, and calcimimetics.

Nephrocalcinosis

Disturbances in calcium metabolism, as in hyperparathyroidism, may result in **nephrocalcinosis**, a condition that is characterized by tiny deposits of calcium phosphate dispersed throughout the renal parenchyma. These deposits are readily seen on radiographs of the abdomen. Ultrasound and CT may also be useful, with studies suggesting ultrasound is more sensitive for evaluation of nephrocalcinosis. Calcium may also be deposited throughout the parenchyma as a result of tissue damaged

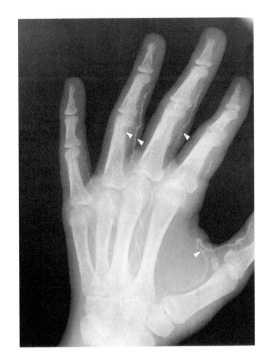

FIG. 11.18 Radiograph of the hand of an individual with secondary hyperparathyroidism. Note the subperiosteal reabsorption of bone and calcification of the arteries of the hand.

by some other disease process or injury. If a metabolic cause exists, treatment of the specific metabolic condition indirectly treats nephrocalcinosis. Treatment designed to lower serum calcium levels is also important.

Pathologic Summary of the Endocrine System

Pathology	Imaging Modality of Choice
Osteporosis	Bone mineral densitometry, radiography
Osteomalacia	Bone mineral densitometry, radiography
Paget Disease	Nuclear medicine bone scan, radiography
Acromegaly	MRI with and without contrast, radiography
Diabetes Insipidus, Diabetes Mellitus	MRI with and without contrast
Hypopituitarism	MRI with and without contrast, CT
Cushing Syndrome	MRI with and without contrast
Adrenal carcinoma	MRI with and without contrast, CT with contrast, sonography
Hyperthyroidism, Thyroid cancers	^{123}I thyroid uptake, MRI with or without contrast, sonography
Hyperparathyroidism	CT, sonography, and sestamibi nuclear medicine studies
Nephrocalcinosis	Sonography, CT, radiography

CT, Computed tomography; ^{123}I, iodine-123; MRI, magnetic resonance imaging.

1. Medical treatment designed to lower serum calcium levels is important in the management of:
   a. Cystitis
   b. Nephrocalcinosis
   c. Nephrosclerosis
   d. Polycystic kidney disease

2. *Osteopenia* is a term used to describe the radiographic appearance associated with a decrease in bone density and is associated with:
   a. Craniosynostoses
   b. Osteopetrosis
   c. Osteoporosis
   d. Scoliosis

3. Metabolic actions of the endocrine system in response to changes in blood chemistry best defines _____ stimuli.
   a. Hormonal
   b. Humoral
   c. Neural

4. Corticosteroid production occurs in the:
   a. Adrenal cortex
   b. Pancreas
   c. Pineal gland
   d. Thyroid gland

5. α-cells in the pancreas produce:
   a. Glucagon
   b. Gonadocorticosteroids
   c. Insulin
   d. Thyroxine

6. Acromegaly is a condition resulting from disorder of the _____ gland.
   a. Adrenal
   b. Pineal
   c. Pituitary
   d. Thymus

7. Grave's disease is associated with:
   a. Hyperthyroidism
   b. Hyperparathyroidism
   c. Hypothyroidism
   d. Hypoparathyroidism

8. Type 1 diabetes mellitus is most common in:
   a. Adults
   b. Children

9. Describe the mechanism behind the development of osteoporosis.

10. Compare and contrast T- and Z-scores obtained from bone mineral densitometry examinations.

CHAPTER 12

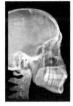
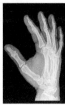
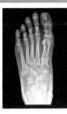

Traumatic Disease

ⓔ http://evolve.elsevier.com/Kowalczyk/pathology/

Legg-Calvé-Perthes disease

Level I trauma centers

Level II trauma centers

Level III trauma centers

Level IV trauma centers

Linear fractures

Luxation

Nonaccidental trauma

Noncomminuted fracture

Occult fracture

Open or compound fracture

Open reduction

Open reduction internal fixation

Pneumoperitoneum

Pneumothorax

Slipped capital femoral epiphysis

Stress fractures

Subluxation

Torus fracture

Traumatic brain injury

Whiplash injury

In the United States injury is one of the leading causes of death and disability. Trauma is the most common cause of death for individuals between the ages of 1 and 44 years, accounting for over 49,000 deaths in 2014. According to the CDC, the total U.S. medical costs associated with traumatic injury and violence in 2013 was $671 billion dollars. The magnitude of these costs demonstrates the importance of prevention strategies initiated by the CDC's National Center for Injury Prevention and Control. Annually, in the United States, traumatic injuries account for over three million hospitalizations, 27 million individual emergency department admissions with release, and over 192,000 deaths. Additional information can be obtained at the Centers for Disease Control and Prevention (CDC) National Center for Health Statistics website at www.cdc.gov/nchs/hus.htm.

The American College of Surgeons (ACS) Committee on Trauma periodically reviews its guidelines to ensure optimal patient care by classifying medical centers and hospitals according to their ability to treat various injuries and by publishing guidelines for trauma management. Trauma results primarily from motor vehicle accidents (MVAs), unintentional accidents at home or in the workplace, gunshot wounds, stab wounds, physical altercations, domestic violence, and physical abuse. According to the CDC, hospital emergency departments play a critical role in the U.S. health care system, from treatment of minor trauma to, more recently, the first-line defense against bioterrorism.

Deaths from traumatic injuries have a trimodal distribution (Fig. 12.1), with the first critical period occurring seconds after the injury. Death during this period results from lacerations of the brain and spinal cord or the heart and great vessels. The second critical period occurs during the first 4 hours after the injury, with death generally resulting from intracranial hemorrhage,

lacerations of the liver and spleen, or significant blood loss from multiple injuries. The third critical period occurs weeks after the injury, when death results from infection and multiple organ failure.

A well-designed emergency medical system (EMS) provides for prehospital care, acute hospital care, and rehabilitative care. Medical facilities are classified as level I, level II, or level III trauma centers based on the availability of specialized medical personnel and equipment. When patients are triaged (medically screened to determine their relative priority for treatment) at the site of an accident, their injuries are classified as life-threatening, urgent, or nonemergent. Multiple injuries most likely occur in conjunction with severe head injuries. These patients must be treated with utmost care. Before a trauma victim is transported, a clear airway must be established, acute bleeding must be controlled, and the patient must be immobilized to avoid displacing fractures of the skeletal system. Immobilization of the spine is paramount to avoiding further injury to the spinal cord, and this is accomplished with the use of splints, backboards with head blocks, cervical collars, and special air splint suits.

The EMS ensures that the trauma victim is taken to the closest appropriate medical facility to receive the proper medical care for their injuries, but not necessarily to the closest hospital. Once the patient arrives at the proper medical facility, another careful assessment is necessary. This secondary triage assessment includes evaluation of the patient's state of consciousness, vital signs (blood pressure, pulse, temperature, and respiration), pupil size and reaction to light, and motor activity of the extremities. Computed tomography (CT) of the cervical spine is the optimal modality to assess any damage to the cervical spine before the patient is moved. In addition, radiographs of the chest, abdomen, and

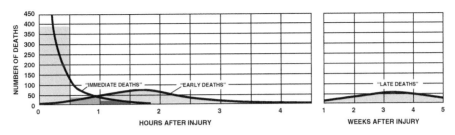

FIG. 12.1 Distribution of trauma deaths.

skeletal system must be obtained to evaluate the extent of injuries. Although national vital statistics show that only 5% of all trauma victims have life-threatening injuries, these types of injuries are responsible for 50% of all in-hospital trauma-related deaths.

Level I, II, and III Trauma Centers

The primary hospitals in the trauma system are **level I trauma centers**. Such medical centers can provide total care for all injuries. Key elements of a level I trauma center include 24-hour in-house coverage by general surgeons and prompt availability of care in specialties such as orthopedic surgery, neurosurgery, anesthesiology, emergency medicine, radiology, internal medicine, and critical care. Other capabilities include cardiac, hand, pediatric, and microvascular surgeries and hemodialysis. These guidelines are developed by the American College of Surgeons (ACS). The level I trauma center provides leadership in prevention, public education, and continuing education for the trauma team members, and serves as a research facility to help direct new innovations in trauma care. Level I trauma centers are generally located in large metropolitan areas and serve as both primary and tertiary care institutions. Another stipulation to being classified as a level I trauma center is that the institution must treat 1200 admissions or 240 major trauma patients per year with a response time of 15 minutes from patient arrival.

Level II trauma centers are the most common trauma facilities serving as community trauma centers. These institutions can handle the majority of trauma cases and transport patients to level I facilities only when necessary. Level II facilities include 24-hour immediate coverage by general surgeons, as well as coverage by the specialties of orthopedic surgery, neurosurgery,

anesthesiology, emergency medicine, radiology, and critical care. More critical patients with needs such as cardiac surgery, hemodialysis, or microvascular surgery may be referred to a level I trauma center. These medical centers are generally community hospitals located in smaller cities and towns and provide a valuable service.

Level III trauma centers are usually located in remote rural areas and serve communities that do not have a level II center. A level III trauma center has a demonstrated ability to provide prompt assessment, resuscitation, stabilization of injured patients, and emergency operations. The key components of a level III trauma center include 24-hour immediate coverage by emergency medicine physicians and the prompt availability of general surgeons and anesthesiologists, which is a 30-minute response time. The level III trauma center has formal transfer agreements for patients requiring more comprehensive care at a level I or II trauma center.

As determined by the ACS Committee on Trauma, a level IV trauma center has a demonstrated ability to provide advanced trauma life support (ATLS) before transfer of patients to a higher-level trauma center. A **level IV trauma centers** has basic emergency department facilities to implement ATLS protocols and 24-hour laboratory coverage. Transfer to higher-level trauma centers follows the guidelines outlined in formal transfer agreements.

Imaging Considerations

Radiography

Conventional radiography is one of the first imaging modalities required in the management of a trauma victim. A cross-table lateral cervical spine radiograph may be obtained to evaluate the presence or absence of a fracture before the patient is moved. Portable chest, abdominal, and pelvic radiographs are also generally obtained as soon as the patient arrives in the emergency department.

Conventional radiography is still the primary means of evaluating skeletal trauma. Additional information about damage to the muscle, tendons, ligaments, and soft tissue structures is obtained using magnetic resonance imaging (MRI). CT and nuclear medicine studies may also be employed to identify subtle skeletal fractures.

Computed Tomography

The high-energy impact associated with most MVAs often results in injury to the neck and head, so CT is an important tool in assessing the trauma victim. CT is excellent for imaging acute cerebral hemorrhage and fractures of the skull and facial bones. Guidelines governing the use of CT in the case of head trauma include the Canadian rule, which suggests that injuries with a Glasgow Coma Scale (GCS) score of 13 to 15 should be evaluated by CT, as well as the more comprehensive New Orleans helical computed tomography (HCT) rule. The New Orleans HCT rule mandates CT examination of patients with a GCS score of 15 in combination with any one of the following: headache, vomiting, above age 60 years, drug or alcohol intoxication, persistent amnesia, visible trauma above the clavicle, or seizure. In lieu of the increased awareness of radiation dose, patient protection, and public safety campaigns such as Image Gently and Image Wisely, the ACR Appropriateness Criteria now include a relative radiation level (RRL) for imaging procedures for both adult and pediatric patients.

With the prevalent use of multidetector CT (MDCT), CT evaluation of the cervical spine has become a standard procedure in evaluating trauma patients. The National Emergency X-radiography Utilization Study (NEXUS) and Canadian C-Spine Review (CCR) concluded that CT demonstrates 99.6% sensitivity for the identification of cervical spine fractures. CT has replaced conventional radiography as the first-line approach to imaging the cervical spine, with the meta-analysis of research studies performed in 2005 indicating that CT demonstrates a much higher specificity of 98% compared with a specificity of 52% for conventional radiography of the cervical spine. Axial CT of the cervical spine is performed in conjunction with

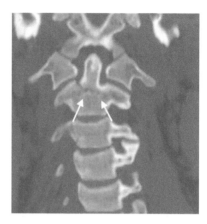

FIG. 12.2 A computed tomography scan of coronal reconstruction of a C2 fracture.

coronal and sagittal reconstruction to fully assess the areas of interest (Fig. 12.2). With more sensitive imaging techniques now available, CT and MRI have revealed a significant number of fractures and other injuries that are not diagnosed with radiography. CT evaluation can reduce hospital admission rates and results in more efficient surgical intervention by accurately identifying the presence and extent of injury in the trauma patient.

Blunt trauma to the abdomen is best evaluated with CT or abdominal sonography. Trauma to the urinary system occurs in about 10% to 15% of patients who experience blunt trauma to the lower abdomen and pelvis. In cases of hematuria, CT is preferred to conventional intravenous pyelography (IVP) or intravenous urography (IVU). Although the use of oral contrast agents for abdominal CT is debatable, intravenous contrast is routinely employed to allow evaluation of vascular injuries and to better visualize the spleen, pancreas, and kidneys. In addition, in cases of blunt abdominal trauma, CT is better able to visualize fractures of the transverse processes of the lumbar spine, often missed on conventional spine radiography. CT, in combination with a conventional anteroposterior (AP) pelvic radiography, is also used to assess pelvic fractures commonly associated with abdominal injury (Fig. 12.3, A). In cases of pelvic fractures, it is also imperative to identify any possible trauma to the urinary bladder and to perform CT (see Fig. 12.3, B) to determine the extent of injury. Occasionally, emergent cystography may be performed to visualize any injury to the urinary bladder. In cases of penetrating trauma to the abdomen, angiography may

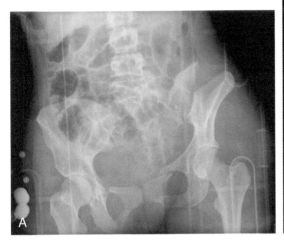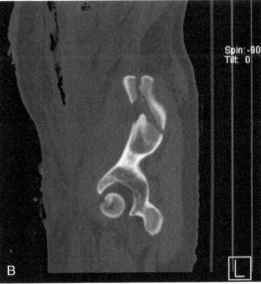

FIG. 12.3 A, Anteroposterior pelvic view from a motor vehicle accident trauma victim demonstrates multiple fractures. B, Computed tomography sagittal reconstruction of the same patient as in A, demonstrating multiple fractures of the ilium.

also be used to identify the extent of injury. Sonography plays little or no role in the evaluation of genitourinary trauma. Several studies have documented the inability of sonography to detect injuries of the kidney or bladder in trauma patients.

Trauma of the Vertebral Column and Head

The initial management of patients with head and spinal trauma is critical. Key items to assess at the scene of the accident include the mechanism of injury and changes in the patient's neurologic status. A neurologic assessment using the GCS should be conducted at the scene and cervical spine injury should be assumed to be present until it is ruled out by radiologic investigation. A cervical spine fracture can be present in up to 20% of patients with a severe head injury.

The head and neck should be immobilized, and care must be taken if intubation is necessary. Hyperextension injuries of the head and neck or direct trauma to the neck may injure the carotid arteries. Bleeding must be controlled to prevent shock, which may worsen the head injury. Once the patient arrives in the emergency department, cervical spine radiographs or a CT scan of the cervical spine must be obtained. CT of the head may also be indicated, especially if the patient is comatose.

Many studies have been conducted regarding the effectiveness of airbags and seatbelts in preventing head and neck fractures in the event of an MVA. By far, those who do not use any protective device sustain the most injuries. Those who depend only on the airbags sustain the second largest number of injuries to the head and face, followed by those who use only a seatbelt. The most effective protection results from the use of both protective devices. In addition, individuals using only a lap-type seatbelt have a high incidence of lumbar spine injuries, and individuals wearing only a shoulder belt without a lap belt sustain more cervical spine injuries.

Injuries to the Vertebral Column

The causes of vertebral column injuries include direct trauma and hyperextension–flexion injuries (whiplash injuries). Radiographic indications of spinal column injuries include the interruption of smooth, continuous lines formed by the vertebrae stacked on one another (Fig. 12.4). Either a dull or sharp pain in the posterior neck is the primary manifestation of a whiplash injury. The pain may radiate down the arms or back.

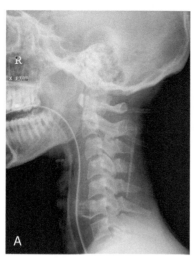
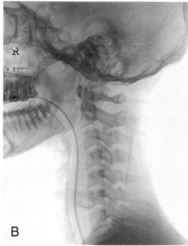

FIG. 12.4 A, A lateral cervical spine radiograph of an individual who was involved in a motor vehicle accident and has an endotracheal tube in place. B, The same radiograph as in A, but imaged in an inverted mode to assist with evaluation. This is one major advantage of digital imaging.

Muscle spasm as a result of trauma may cause a reversal or straightening of the normal spine curvatures. Imaging of whiplash injuries is limited to soft tissue studies, with the exclusion of fractures and dislocations being the first priority. The loss of lordosis is the most common finding on radiographs of patients with whiplash injuries (Fig. 12.5).

Perhaps the most common condition of the vertebral column is generalized back pain, typically in the lumbar area. This may result from injury to the area or from degenerative disease. Such back pain may not always result from bone involvement. Disk disease may cause muscle spasm, with pain referral throughout the back or down the legs. Finally, back pain may be secondary to referred pain from the hip.

Compression fractures are the most frequent type of injury involving a vertebral body. Usually, the damage is limited to the upper portion of the vertebral body, particularly to the anterior margin. Such fractures generally occur in the thoracic and lumbar vertebrae (Fig. 12.6), with the most common site being T11-T12 in the thoracic spine and T12-L1 at the thoracolumbar juncture. Compression fractures are also associated with osteoporosis and range from mild to severe. More severe fractures may cause significant pain, leading to inability to perform activities of daily living to life-threatening decline in the older patient. Cervical spine injuries may involve the odontoid process, usually at the junction of the odontoid and the body of the second

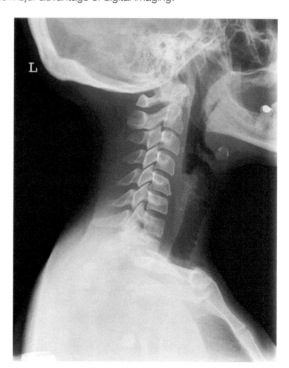

FIG. 12.5 A lateral cervical spine radiograph of a patient involved in motor vehicle accident. Note the loss of the normal lordotic curvature indicates a whiplash injury.

cervical vertebra (see Fig. 12.2). A **hangman's fracture** (Fig. 12.7) is a fracture of the arch of the second cervical vertebra and is usually accompanied by anterior subluxation of the second cervical vertebra on the third

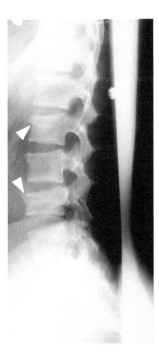

FIG. 12.6 A lateral lumbar radiograph demonstrating compression fractures of the second and fourth lumbar vertebral bodies with no apparent fracture of the posterior elements of the spine.

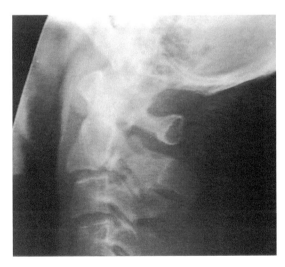

FIG. 12.7 A lateral cervical spine radiograph demonstrating a typical hangman's fracture with disruption of the spinal laminar line at C2 with the spinous process of C2 displaced posteriorly.

cervical vertebra. A hangman's fracture, sometimes referred to as *traumatic spondylosis*, results from acute hyperextension of the head.

Jefferson fracture was first described as a "burst fracture" of the first cervical vertebra (atlas). It generally occurs as a result of a severe axial force that causes compression, as in a diving accident. The vertebral arch literally bursts. Radiographically, particular attention needs to be paid to the transverse longitudinal ligament by reviewing the lateral masses on the open-mouth odontoid projection. MRI is the preferred imaging modality to best examine the transverse longitudinal ligament.

CT of the trauma patient with vertebral trauma is critical. Statistically, 5% to 10% of patients with one spinal fracture have another fracture elsewhere in the vertebral column. Fractures and dislocations of the spine are classified as stable or unstable. The spine may be visualized as two columns, with the anterior column composed of vertebral bodies and intervertebral disks and the posterior column composed of the posterior elements (e.g., spinous processes, lamina). If either the anterior column or the posterior column of the spine is fractured or dislocated, the injury is classified as stable. However, if both columns are involved in the injury, it is classified as unstable. In all cases, the patient should be immobilized until cross-table lateral radiographs or CT images have been obtained and cleared by a physician. To rule out possible fractures and dislocations, lateral cervical spine radiography must include all seven vertebrae in their entirety, including spinous processes and intervertebral disk spaces. At times this may require assistance with depressing the patient's shoulders or with the use of the specialized cervicothoracic lateral projection (Twining or swimmer's method) to clearly demonstrate the entire seventh cervical vertebra and the upper thoracic vertebra in a lateral projection. Additional trauma projections of the cervical spine such as the pillar projection or trauma oblique projection may be requested to better demonstrate the complex anatomy of the spine. Trauma cervical spine radiographs are analyzed to evaluate (1) the size, shape, and alignment of the vertebral bodies and spinous processes, (2) the position and integrity of the odontoid process of C2, (3) the orientation and clarity of the facet joints, (4) the relationship of C1 to the occipital bone, (5) the alignment of the spinolaminal lines, and (6) any prevertebral swelling.

Spinal injury often results in a loss of neurologic function that may be temporary or permanent, depending on the cause of the dysfunction. Compression of the spinal cord by contusion or hemorrhage leads to rapid swelling of the spinal cord. This causes a rise in intradural pressure and causes temporary neurologic dysfunction. This temporary loss of neurologic function usually resolves

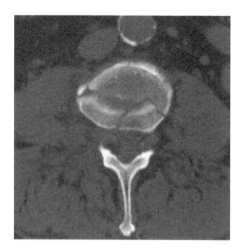

FIG. 12.8 An axial computed tomography scan demonstrating a comminuted fracture of a vertebral body and showing the location of each fragment.

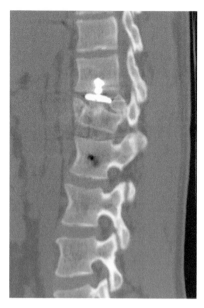

FIG. 12.9 A sagittal reconstruction computed tomography scan performed postoperatively after the repair of a comminuted fracture of L1.

in several days. However, lacerations of the spinal cord or transection of the cord results in permanent damage because the severed nerves do not regenerate. Laceration of the spinal cord above the fifth cervical vertebra is almost always fatal, and lacerations below this region result in permanent paralysis. Patients with lacerations or transection of the cord develop immediate flaccid paralysis with loss of all sensation and reflex activity, which gradually changes to spastic paraplegia within days.

Fractures or dislocations of the vertebrae may impinge on the spinal cord and cause significant damage. The responsibility of the radiographer in terms of proper patient handling and obtaining diagnostic-quality images cannot be overemphasized. CT plays a vital role in the diagnosis and treatment of vertebral fractures, dislocations, and associated problems (Fig. 12.8). In certain situations MRI may be used to evaluate the extent of ligamentous and soft tissue injury or injury to the spinal cord and is acceptable as a complementary procedure to CT, as designated by ACR Appropriateness Criteria.

Stable injuries to the spine are treated with complete bed rest and steroids until swelling and pain subside. Unstable injuries are immobilized with traction until bone and soft tissue structures have healed. Cervical radiographs are often obtained to demonstrate proper alignment while the patient is in traction. Surgery may also be necessary for internal fixation of the fractures or to remove displaced fragments and decompress the spinal cord. CT of the spine is used preoperatively to serve as a road map for the surgeon because this imaging

modality clearly demonstrates the size, number, and location of various fracture fragments. It may also be used postoperatively to demonstrate the success of the surgical procedure (Fig. 12.9).

Injuries to the Skull and Brain

The anatomy surrounding the delicate brain generally protects it well under normal conditions. The diploic arrangement of the calvaria, the mechanical buffering action of cerebrospinal fluid, and the tough dura mater all work to prevent brain injury. Despite this protection, sufficient force to the skull may cause injury to the brain. Head trauma is the major neurologic cause of mortality and morbidity in individuals under 50 years of age.

Head trauma may result in skull fractures, brain injury, or a combination of the two. The role of plain film radiography in evaluation of head trauma is rather limited, but CT allows rapid assessment of the nature of any brain injury. Assessment of the state of the brain after head injury is more crucial than that of the skull. For trauma victims, CT without IV contrast is the recommended imaging protocol. Skull fractures are often seen with accompanying hematomas. If patients sustain an open skull fracture, they are at risk for development of meningitis or brain abscesses. The technologist must constantly observe a patient with a head injury while

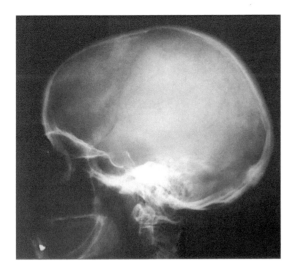

FIG. 12.10 A lateral skull radiograph demonstrating normal vascular markings within the cerebral cranium.

performing an examination. Any change noted in the patient's condition should be reported immediately.

Cerebral Cranial Fractures

The term *cerebral cranial fractures* usually refers to fractures in the calvaria of the skull. Vascular markings in the skull, either venous or arterial, are routinely demonstrated as linear translucencies and may occasionally be mistaken for cerebral cranial fractures (Fig. 12.10). In most cases, a fracture appears more translucent than a vascular marking because a fracture traverses the full thickness of the skull. Although the edges of the fractures may branch abruptly, they may be seen to fit together, whereas venous channels have irregular edges that cannot be fitted together. The sutures between the individual cranial bones remain visible radiographically, even after they become fused. To an untrained eye these sutures may also resemble a fracture.

In most cases, the location of the skull fracture is more important than the extent of the fracture. If the fracture crosses an artery, an arterial bleed may occur, resulting in an epidural hematoma. If an intracranial arterial injury is suspected, then CT angiography (CTA) or MR angiography (MRA) can be performed, depending on institutional preference. A fracture that enters the mastoid air cells or a sinus communicates with a potentially infected space and may lead to infection, possibly resulting in encephalitis or meningitis. Fractures visible after skull trauma are generally classified as linear, depressed, or basilar. **Linear fractures**

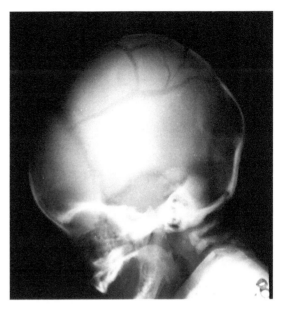

FIG. 12.11 A lateral skull radiograph of a 3-month-old infant with a history of striking his head on a bathtub. The radiograph reveals a linear skull fracture of the parietal bone.

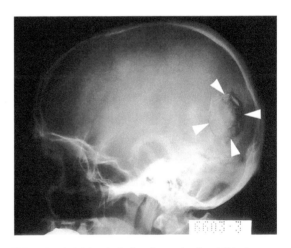

FIG. 12.12 A lateral skull radiograph of a child who was struck in the head with a baseball bat. The radiograph demonstrates a depressed fracture of the occipital bone.

appear as straight, sharply defined, nonbranching lines and are intensely radiolucent (Fig. 12.11). Up to 80% of all skull fractures are linear. A **depressed fracture** appears as a curvilinear density because the fracture edges overlap (Fig. 12.12). These fractures are caused by high-velocity impact by small objects. Injury to the cerebral cortex may result, causing bleeding into the subarachnoid space. A depressed fracture is best demonstrated when the x-ray beam is directed tangentially to the fracture.

Basilar skull fractures are very difficult to demonstrate radiographically. The presence of air–fluid levels in the sphenoid sinus or clouding of the mastoid air cells is often the only radiographic finding suggesting a fracture. Therefore it is important to include cross-table lateral skull radiography with the trauma skull radiographic series. CT and MRI are often used to better identify basilar area fractures and associated soft tissue damage within the skull (Fig. 12.13).

Brain Trauma

In addition to brain injury from a penetration wound (as could happen with a fracture), brain injury may also occur from acceleration and rapid deceleration of the head, which is termed a *closed head injury* or **traumatic brain injury** (TBI). With head trauma, the brain is traumatically shaken within the cranium and subjected to forces of compression, acceleration, and deceleration. Brain tissues are injured from compression, tension, and shearing, with the last perhaps most important (Fig. 12.14). The superficial cerebrum in the frontal, temporal, and occipital regions is most often affected.

TBI is a serious public health problem in the United States. Each year, traumatic brain injuries contribute to a substantial number of deaths and cases of permanent disability. Recent data from the CDC show that, on average, approximately 1.7 million people sustain a TBI annually and is a contributing factor in 30.5% of all injury related deaths in the United States. This incidence has increased significantly with athletic-related activities, and ongoing research is focusing on athletes from the junior high to professional levels.

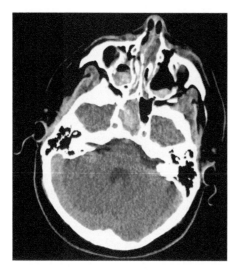

FIG. 12.13 A computed tomography scan demonstrating basilar skull fracture with air fluid levels in the sphenoid sinus.

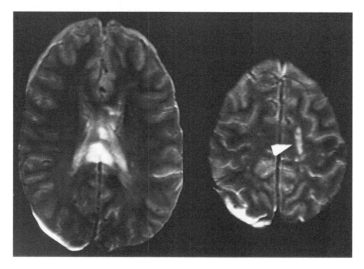

FIG. 12.14 A T2-weighted magnetic resonance imaging scan demonstrates a shearing injury of the corpus callosum (*arrow*) and a small subdural hematoma on the lateral margins of the brain in this young boy who had fallen and failed to regain consciousness.

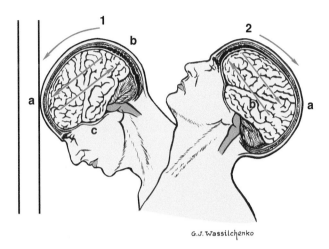

G.J.Wassilchenko

FIG. 12.15 Coup and contrecoup brain injury following blunt trauma. A, Coup injury: impact against object. B, Contrecoup injury: impact within skull. These injuries occur in one continuous motion—the head strikes the wall (coup) and then rebounds (contrecoup).

After a blow to the head, an individual may experience temporary loss of consciousness and reflexes. This widespread paralysis of brain function is known as a **concussion** and is characterized by headache, vertigo, and vomiting. Higher mental functions may be impaired for several hours, with the patient remembering little of the events surrounding the concussion. A strong tendency toward spontaneous and complete recovery exists because no structural damage to the brain occurs. Recovery generally takes place in less than 24 hours. Treatment is conservative once assessment (usually by CT) has ruled out any hemorrhage or fracture. Bed rest and possible admission to the hospital are the usual means of dealing with concussion.

A brain contusion may also result from a direct blow to the head. This bruising of brain parenchyma is more serious than a concussion. A contusion formed on the side of the head where the trauma occurs is called a **coup lesion**, and one formed on the opposite side of the skull in reference to the site of trauma is a **contrecoup lesion** (Fig. 12.15). **Contusions** are characterized by neuron damage, edema, and punctate (pinpoint punctures or depressions) hemorrhaging. During CT, contusions appear as small, ill-defined foci of increased density (Fig. 12.16). Subdural or epidural hematomas may occur in conjunction with a contusion and result in increased intracranial pressure that may be life-threatening. Signs seen in the patient with a contusion

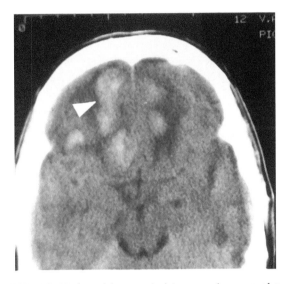

FIG. 12.16 An axial computed tomography scan of a young male patient demonstrates hemorrhagic contusions of the brain as a result of a car accident.

include drowsiness, confusion, and agitation. Hemiparesis and unequal pupil size may also be seen. CT plays a major role in the diagnosis of hematomas resulting from contusions, providing ready visualization of hemorrhagic blood, as described in the next section. Treatment is generally conservative, centering on prevention of shock, control of edema, and drainage of any hematoma present.

Persistence of loss of consciousness for more than 24 hours is known as a **coma**. This is usually a serious condition and may be fatal. Comas result from trauma to the head or from nontraumatic metabolic malfunctions or circulatory problems that prevent sufficient blood flow to the brain. Diagnosis related to a coma may involve use of CT, MRI, positron emission tomography (PET), or fusion imaging and focuses on determining, if possible, the cause of the coma. Advanced neuroimaging techniques (single-photon emission computed tomography [SPECT], positron emission tomography [PET], perfusion CT and MRI, diffusion tensor imaging [DTI], functional MRI, and magnetic resonance spectroscopy [MRS]) may have a role in assessing cognitive and neuropsychological disturbances, as well as their evolution following head trauma. Treatment then rests on success in treating and alleviating the cause of the coma.

Hematomas of the Brain

As noted earlier, brain trauma may result in hemorrhaging of blood from a ruptured artery or vein. Although venous bleeding occurs more slowly than arterial bleeding, both types of hemorrhaging and resultant edema of the brain cause an increase in intracranial pressure. Because the skull's structure does not allow expansion, the increased pressure displaces the brain toward its opening, the foramen magnum. This trauma to the brain results in serious neurologic consequences, and even death if not treated promptly. CT plays the major imaging role in diagnosis of hemorrhaging.

A **hematoma** is a collection of blood and four primary types of cerebral hematomas have been identified: epidural, subdural (Fig. 12.17), subarachnoid, and intracerebral. The highest mortality rate is associated with an *epidural (extradural) hematoma* (Fig. 12.18). Even when promptly recognized and treated, it has a mortality rate of up to 30%. An epidural hematoma results from a torn artery, usually the middle meningeal artery, with blood pooling between the bony skull and the dura mater. Most commonly, the artery or its branches are torn by a fracture of the thin, squamous portion of temporal bone. In more than 80% of cases, the skull fracture is visible radiographically. As an arterial bleed, it accumulates rapidly and quickly causes neurologic symptoms, including early coma. It is seen on CT scans as an increased density, generally occupying a small area with a sharply convex appearance. It is

often accompanied by a fracture of the skull or facial bones. If not diagnosed and surgically treated quickly, the outcome is fatal as a result of brain displacement and herniation.

A *subdural hematoma* is positioned between the dura mater and the arachnoid meningeal layers (Figs. 12.19 and 12.20). It usually follows blunt trauma to the frontal or occipital lobes of the skull and results from tearing of the subdural veins connecting the cerebral cortex and the dural sinuses. As a venous hemorrhage, it bleeds much more slowly than an epidural hematoma. In the acute stage, it is seen on CT as a curvilinear area of increased density on parts or all of the cerebral hemispheres. It pushes the brain away from the skull and causes a mass effect (i.e., brain shift across the midline), with an accompanying shift of the ventricles. In the subacute stage (up to several days old), it appears on CT as a decreased or isodense fluid collection. In the chronic state (2–3 weeks old), the surface of the hematoma becomes concave. Delayed coma may occur with a subdural hematoma.

A *subarachnoid hematoma* accumulates between the arachnoid layer and the thin pia mater that invests the brain. It occurs most frequently at the vertex, where the greatest brain movement occurs during trauma, and it results from tearing of small vessels. In most head trauma cases, a subarachnoid hemorrhage is usually limited to one or two sulci, where it has a dense appearance (Fig. 12.21). Less commonly, the rupture of a major cerebral vessel results in a subarachnoid hematoma.

An *intracerebral hematoma* may result from trauma or from nontraumatic causes such as a ruptured hemangioma or stroke (cerebrovascular accident [CVA]). Common sites after trauma are the frontal, temporal, and occipital lobes of the brain. Small parenchymal vessels tear as a result of coup and contrecoup forces. An intracerebral hematoma is seen by CT as an increased density within the brain causing significant mass effect (Fig. 12.22) and may have an accompanying subarachnoid component. These hematomas develop edema around them as time passes and are slowly reabsorbed if the patient survives.

Diagnosis of hematomas is made primarily through clinical history and neurologic signs and symptoms. As noted, CT and MRI play a major role in ready visualization of bleeding. Angiography may be used to visualize any defects in the cerebral vasculature. Treatment is

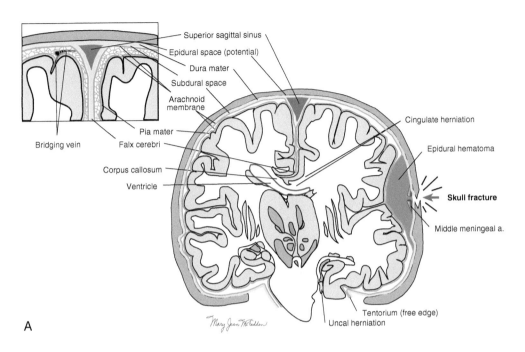

- Superior sagittal sinus
- Epidural space (potential)
- Dura mater
- Subdural space
- Arachnoid membrane
- Bridging vein
- Pia mater
- Falx cerebri
- Corpus callosum
- Ventricle
- Cingulate herniation
- Epidural hematoma
- **Skull fracture**
- Middle meningeal a.
- Tentorium (free edge)
- Uncal herniation

A

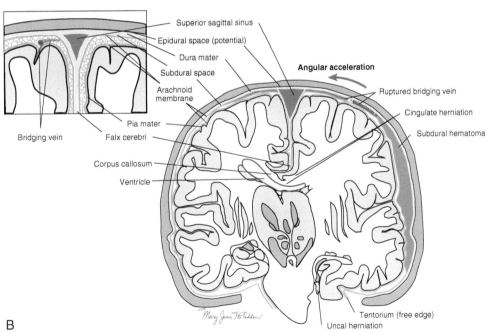

- Superior sagittal sinus
- Epidural space (potential)
- Dura mater
- Subdural space
- Arachnoid membrane
- Bridging vein
- Pia mater
- Falx cerebri
- Corpus callosum
- Ventricle
- **Angular acceleration**
- Ruptured bridging vein
- Cingulate herniation
- Subdural hematoma
- Tentorium (free edge)
- Uncal herniation

B

FIG. 12.17 A, Epidural hematoma and B, subdural hematoma.

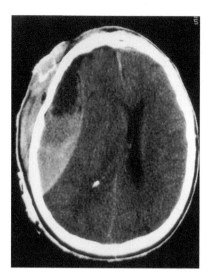

FIG. 12.18 A noncontrast axial computed tomography view of this young male patient injured in an motor vehicle accident readily demonstrates a large epidural hematoma.

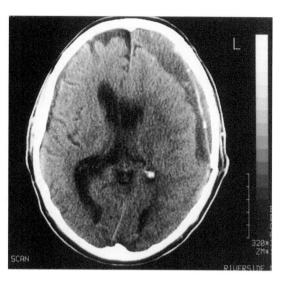

FIG. 12.19 Computed tomography demonstration of a large subdural hematoma outside of the brain tissue in the left frontoparietal area of this 76-year-old man.

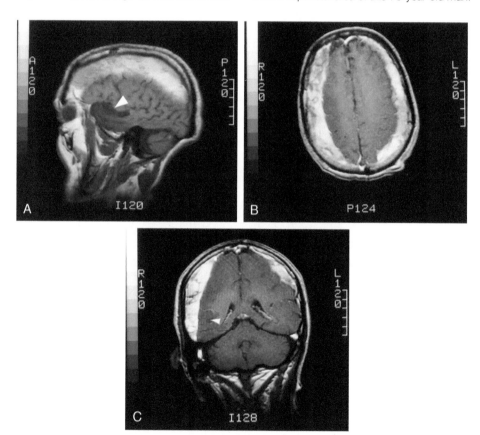

FIG. 12.20 A, A T1-weighted sagittal magnetic resonance imaging (MRI) view demonstrates a large subdural hematoma and a temporal lobe infarct (*arrow*). The white *versus* gray appearance of the hematoma distinguishes subacute (fresh) from older blood. B, A T1-weighted axial MRI view with gadolinium demonstrates a large, bilateral subdural hematoma in this 67-year-old man. C, A T1-weighted coronal MRI view with gadolinium demonstrates the same bilateral subdural hematoma. The arrow indicates the right-sided temporal lobe infarct.

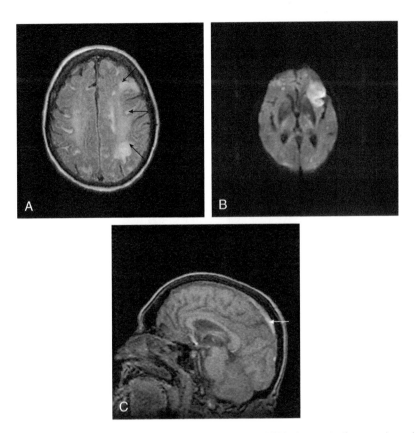

FIG. 12.21 A and B, Axial magnetic resonance imaging (MRI) demonstrating a subarachnoid hemorrhage as indicated by the sulci opacified by blood. C, Sagittal fluid-attenuated inversion recovery (FLAIR) MRI of the same patient.

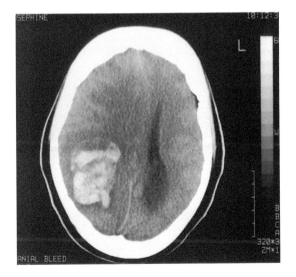

FIG. 12.22 A massive intracerebral hematoma that occurred spontaneously in this 63-year-old woman. The patient died within a few hours after the bleed began.

often conservative unless active bleeding or significant mass effect is present, in which case an opening in the skull may be created surgically to allow drainage of blood and prevent complications. Prevention of infection and meningitis is important in the case of a fractured skull.

Skeletal Trauma

Fractures

A fracture is a discontinuity of bone caused by mechanical forces either applied to the bone or transmitted directly along the line of a bone. When a fracture occurs, blood vessels are broken as a result of the break in the endosteum and periosteum. As blood, lymph, and tissue fluids infiltrate this area, swelling and pain result. Such soft tissue swelling is a major clue to diagnosis (Fig. 12.23). Digital imaging is an asset in evaluating the soft tissue structures

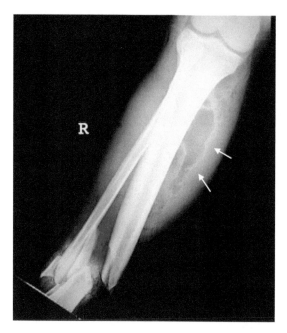

FIG. 12.23 A computed radiography image of a comminuted fracture of the tibia and fibula with associated soft tissue edema.

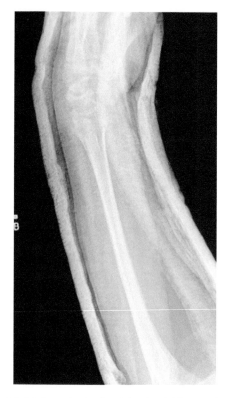

FIG. 12.24 A postreduction lateral wrist image showing proper alignment in the cast.

surrounding a skeletal fracture because one image can be manipulated to demonstrate details of both soft tissue and bone.

Radiography is extremely important in the evaluation of skeletal trauma and serves several purposes. The most obvious of these is to diagnose the presence of a fracture or dislocation. If a fracture is present, for example, a determination can be made as to whether underlying bone is normal or whether the fracture is pathologic in nature. Before the fracture is stabilized, radiographs are taken to show the position of the bone ends. Fractures are in "good alignment" when no perceptible angulation or displacement is present in frontal and lateral projections. Postreduction radiographs indicate the success of the fracture reduction (Fig. 12.24). If the fracture is placed in a cast, the exposure factors do not need to be altered to radiograph through a dry fiberglass cast but must be increased differently to penetrate the wet fiberglass or plaster cast. Finally, subsequent radiographs are taken to assess continued alignment, healing, and any possible complications of fractures.

In any case of trauma, it is essential to have at least two projections of the part, preferably taken at right angles, or 90 degrees to each other. A minimum of two projections is also necessary to adequately determine fracture alignment (Fig. 12.25). If long bones are involved, these radiographs should demonstrate the joint above and below the area of trauma because dislocation may be present and because the injury may transfer force to a point distal or proximal to the point of injury. An example is a fracture or dislocation of the fibular head concurrent with an ankle or distal tibial fracture, as in a Maisonneuve fracture.

Frequently, fractures are obvious during a clinical examination, but radiographic changes in appearance may be subtle. Fractures usually appear as radiolucent lines, but they may be thin and easily overlooked. Occasionally, a fracture appears as a radiopaque line if the fragments overlap. A step in the cortex, as

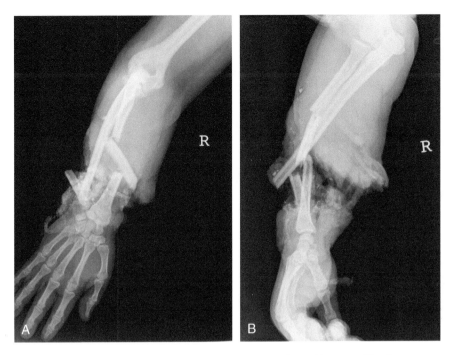

FIG. 12.25 A, An anteroposterior projection of an open comminuted fracture of the forearm caused by a machine injury. B, A lateral projection of the same forearm demonstrating anterior and posterior displacement of the fractured bones.

indicated by a break in the normal bone contour, is a second radiographic indication (Fig. 12.26). Other signs include interruption of the trabeculae, bulging or buckling of the cortex, soft tissue swelling, and joint effusion. Also, the relationship of the end of a bone to its shaft is an important sign, as in the loss of normal volar tilt to the distal radial articular surface with an impacted distal radial fracture. CT (Fig. 12.27) and nuclear medicine bone scan are often used in combination with conventional radiography to assess skeletal fractures. MRI is used as an adjunct to conventional radiography to assess soft tissues, muscles, ligaments, and tendons.

Skeletal trauma usually causes significant soft tissue injuries, including neurovascular damage, capsular and ligamentous tears, cartilage injury, and hemarthroses. Such injury may be assessed in several ways, but the primary modality for assessing damage is MRI. Stress radiography may also be used to determine ligamentous stability. Radiographs of both extremities are often used to compare epiphyseal appearance. Arteriography

is used to assess any vascular damage as a result of skeletal trauma.

When performing radiography of the skeletal system, it is critical for the technologist to choose the appropriate exposure factors to produce a radiograph that demonstrates good soft tissue definition in addition to achieving adequate penetration of the bony anatomy. It is often helpful to the interpreting physician if the radiographer notes areas of point tenderness with a detailed patient history. This may be a specific indication of a fracture that may be subtle radiographically. Larger body parts such as the hip, femur, and knee are less assessable for point tenderness; instead, inability to bear weight or significant decrease in range of motion may suggest a fracture. Again, an important role of the radiographer is to assess the patient with regard to symptoms, signs, range of motion, and mechanism of injury to provide the physician with as much information as possible, both on the radiographs and verbally, or in writing with the patient's clinical history.

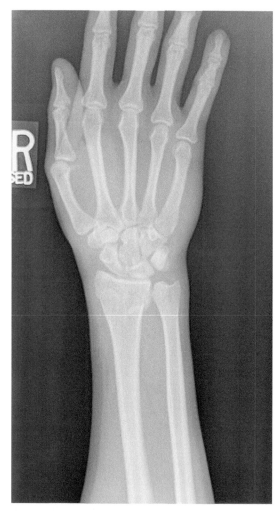

A posteroanterior projection of the wrist demonstrating a subtle fracture of the radius. Note the break in the bony cortex and discontinuity of the cortical bone.

Bone tissue is unique in its ability to repair itself, in that it reactivates processes that normally occur during embryogenesis (Fig. 12.28). Initially, the break in the bone is filled by a large clot that temporarily bridges the fracture. Within 2 to 3 days, osteoblasts slowly begin to appear around the injured bone. Immobilization of the injured site is critical because any unnatural movement interferes with the deposition of the calcified matrix necessary for permanent union of the fracture. Provisional callus is mainly composed of cartilage and begins to form approximately 1 week after the fracture. As calcium continues to be deposited within the provisional callus, it is replaced by bony callus (Fig. 12.29), which is responsible for rigidly uniting the fracture site. Although the break is rigidly united within 4 to 6 weeks, excess bone still encircles the external fracture site, and excess bone is still found within the marrow space at this time. Remodeling of the bone and total healing require months. Weight-bearing force on the fracture site tends to guide the modeling process, so in many cases, the patient may be instructed to begin using the affected limb in a limited fashion at this point in the healing process. If everything goes well during the healing process, the bone may repair to the point that the fracture site is no longer visible on subsequent radiographs. Proper healing greatly depends on the initial immobilization (casting, splinting, pinning, or plating), proper alignment or reduction of the fracture, and proper metabolic activity, which includes good vascularity and blood supply, proper nutrition, and normal hormone levels. Bacterial infections of the fracture site may inhibit callus formation, thus complicating the healing process.

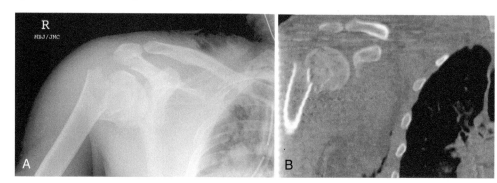

A, A conventional anteroposterior projection of a shoulder demonstrating a fracture of the humeral neck sustained in a motor vehicle accident. B, A computed tomography coronal reconstruction of the same patient.

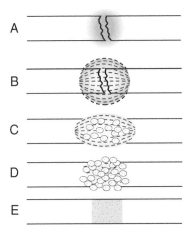

A schematic representation of the bone healing process. A, Bleeding at broken ends of the bone with subsequent hematoma formation. B, Organization of hematoma into fibrous network. C, Invasion of osteoblasts, lengthening of collagen strands, and deposition of calcium. D, Callus formation; new bone is built up as osteoclasts destroy dead bone. E, Remodeling is accomplished as excess callus is reabsorbed and trabecular bone is laid down.

Delayed union is a term referring to a fracture that does not heal within the usual time. If a fracture is not reduced properly or is not properly immobilized, malunion may occur. *Malunion* refers to a fracture that heals in a faulty position, thus impairing the normal function or cosmetic appearance of the affected body part (Fig. 12.30). The most serious complication is nonunion. *Nonunion* refers to a fracture in which healing does not occur and the fragments do not join (Fig. 12.31). This is often the result of lack of vascularization. Injuries to other soft tissue structures or organs can be associated with skeletal fractures such as a rib fracture that penetrates the lung and results in a pneumothorax. Additional complications of skeletal fractures include muscular ossification and fat emboli occurring in bones containing yellow bone marrow.

Fracture Classifications

Several means of classifying fractures exist (Fig. 12.32). One distinction is whether the fracture is open or closed. An **open or compound fracture** is one in which the bone has penetrated the skin (Fig. 12.33). This type of fracture leaves an open route for bacteria to enter from outside the body, which may lead to

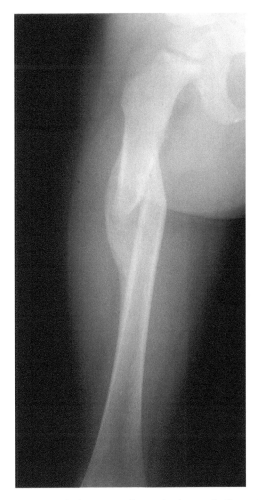

A femoral radiograph demonstrating advanced callus formation following a transverse fracture of the femur.

infection. As described earlier, the intrusion of bacteria may alter the healing process, so precautions must be taken to prevent infection from setting into bone or surrounding soft tissue structures. These fractures often require surgical intervention to irrigate and debride the area of interest. A **closed fracture** (formerly referred to as a *simple fracture*) is one in which the skin is not penetrated, which reduces the chance of infection (Fig. 12.34).

Fractures may be classified according to the mechanics of stress that produce the break or the appearance of the fracture line. Such classifications include torsion (twisting), transverse, linear, and spiral fractures.

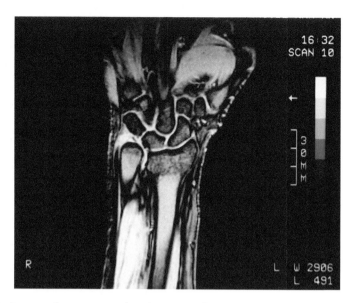

FIG. 12.30 A magnetic resonance imaging scan after fracture of the wrist of a 55-year-old woman with a 2-month history of increasing pain and disability. The scan shows malunion of the distal radial fracture with loss of palmar inclination and reversal with subsequent dorsal inclination.

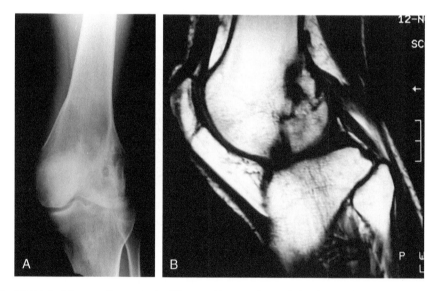

FIG. 12.31 A, A knee radiograph of a 32-year-old man who sustained a gunshot wound to the left knee 3 years previously. Nonunion of the lateral femoral condyle is demonstrated. B, A magnetic resonance imaging scan of the same patient demonstrating nonunion of the posterior lateral femoral condyle with large subchondral defects.

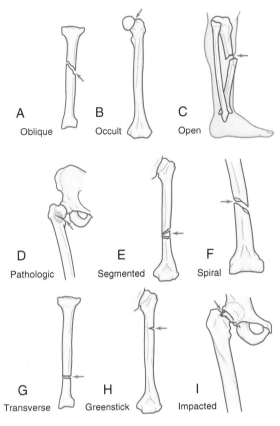

A
Oblique

B
Occult

C
Open

D
Pathologic

E
Segmented

F
Spiral

G
Transverse

H
Greenstick

I
Impacted

FIG. 12.32 Types of bone fractures.

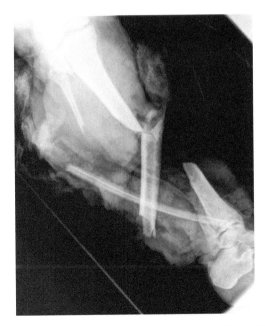

FIG. 12.33 An open, comminuted fracture of the tibia and fibula with amputation.

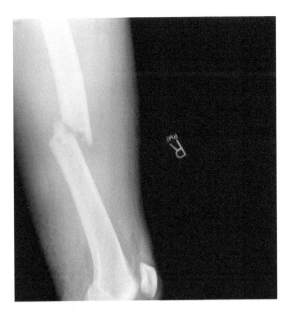

FIG. 12.34 A closed transverse fracture of the femur.

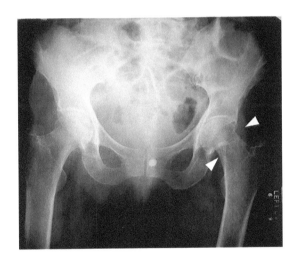

FIG. 12.35 A radiograph of the pelvis of an older woman with trauma to her left hip. The radiograph demonstrates an impacted fracture of the left hip.

When one of the fractured bone ends is jammed into the cancellous tissue of another fragment, it is called an **impacted fracture** (Fig. 12.35).

Fractures may also be classified according to their location, for example, intertrochanteric, transcervical (Fig. 12.36), supracondylar (Fig. 12.37), or transcondylar. Fractures often do not fit into a specific classification because they demonstrate mixed features.

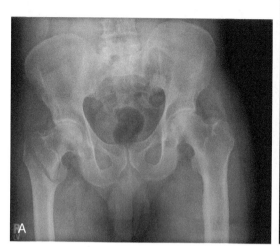

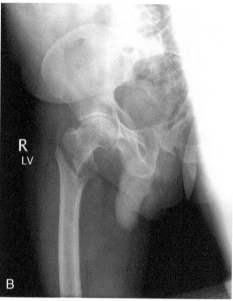

FIG. 12.36 A, An anteroposterior (AP) projection of the pelvis demonstrating an intertrochanteric fracture of the femur. B, An AP projection of the affected hip in A.

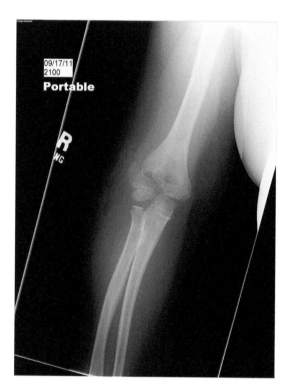

FIG. 12.37 Anteroposterior (AP) projection of a supracondylar fracture of the elbow.

Different types of treatments exist for skeletal fractures. The choice of treatment usually depends on the classification and severity of the fracture. For closed and nondisplaced fractures, the most common treatment is splinting, casting, or both (Fig. 12.38). For a displaced fracture, it is necessary to improve the alignment of the fracture. This reduction may be either closed or open. **Closed reduction** requires that a local or general anesthetic be given to the patient for pain management. A splint or cast is then applied. **Open reduction** is required when orthopedic hardware is needed to maintain fracture reduction or when an open fracture needs to be irrigated. Generally, this is referred to as **open reduction internal fixation** (ORIF) (Fig. 12.39). Again, immobilization devices are often applied after surgery. It is imperative when imaging a patient with orthopedic hardware to include it in its entirety on the radiographic images.

Comminuted Fractures

Sometimes, one or more fragments separate along the edges of the major fragment in addition to the major line of the fracture. Such fractures are said to be *comminuted* (Fig. 12.40). **Comminuted fractures** differ from multiple fractures as follows: in the case of a multiple

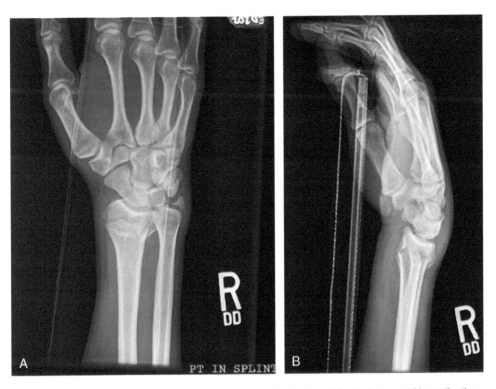

FIG. 12.38 A, Oblique and B, lateral views of a closed reduction of Colles fracture with application of a cast.

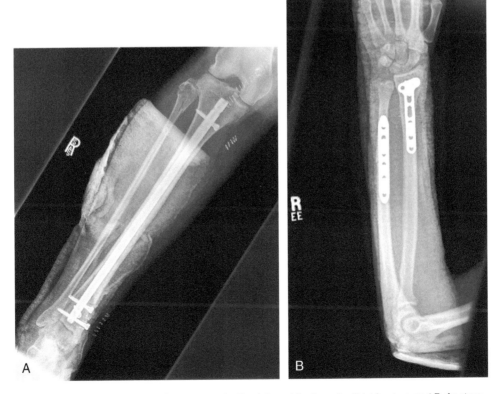

FIG. 12.39 A, A radiograph of an open reduction internal fixation of a tibial fracture and B, fracture of the radius and ulna (B).

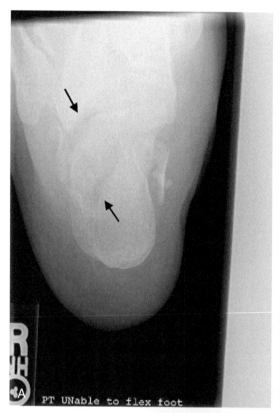

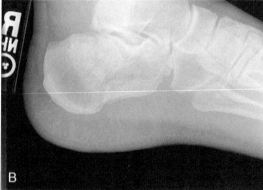

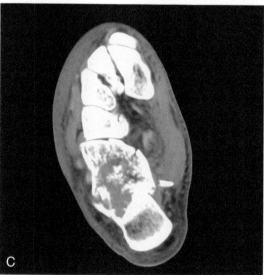

FIG. 12.40 A comminuted fracture of the calcaneus as depicted by conventional radiographs. A, An anteroposterior axial projection. B, A lateral projection. C, An axial computed tomography scan of the same patient.

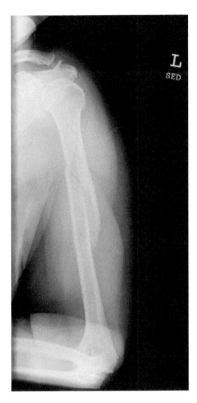

FIG. 12.41 A humerus radiograph of an individual who sustained a twisting injury of the humerus. The radiograph demonstrates a spiral fracture of the humerus.

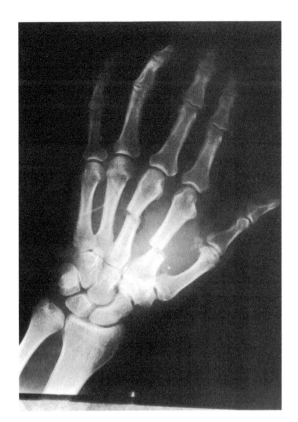

FIG. 12.42 A hand radiograph of a 32-year-old man involved in an industrial accident, demonstrating transverse fractures of the second and third metacarpals.

fracture, each fracture is complete, leaving a fragment of intact shaft between them. Comminuted fractures do not represent a complete thickness of bone as do multiple fractures. Occasionally, the bone involved in a comminuted fracture may be extensively shattered, as might occur from a gunshot wound. Such fractures are also particularly apt to be open fractures (see Figs. 12.25 and 12.33).

A *butterfly fracture* is a comminuted fracture in which one or two butterfly wing–shaped or wedge-shaped fragments split off from the main fragments. A *splintered fracture* is a comminuted fracture with long, sharp-pointed fragments.

Complete, Noncomminuted Fractures

A complete, **noncomminuted fracture** is one in which the bone has separated into two fragments. The fracture may be recognized according to the

direction of the fracture line. A *spiral* or *oblique fracture* is an example of this type. Such a fracture usually results from a rotary type of injury that twists the bone apart and is particularly common in the shafts of long bones (Fig. 12.41). A *transverse fracture* (Figs. 12.42, 12.43, and 12.44) is another type of complete, noncomminuted fracture. Demonstrated radiographically, such a fracture through normal bone is invariably ragged along the fracture line. A *pathologic fracture* is commonly a transverse fracture occurring in abnormal bone that is weakened by various diseases such as a bone cyst or metastatic bone neoplasm (Fig. 12.45). It may result from the disease process itself or from a relatively minor trauma. Often, pathologic fractures may be the first indication of the presence of pathology. *Multiple fractures* are another type of complete, noncomminuted fracture in which two or more

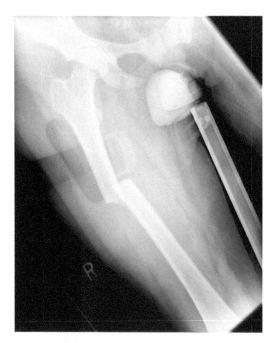

FIG. 12.43 An anteroposterior projection of a transverse fracture of the femur.

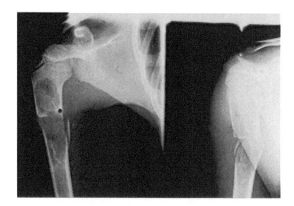

FIG. 12.45 A humerus radiograph demonstrating a pathologic fracture through a bone cyst. The patient had complained of pain and denied a history of trauma associated with this fracture.

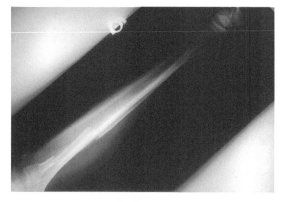

FIG. 12.46 A forearm radiograph of an individual involved in a motor vehicle accident. The radiograph revealed multiple fractures of the forearm.

complete fractures occur involving the shaft of a single bone (Fig. 12.46).

Avulsion Fractures

Avulsion fractures occur when a fragment of bone is pulled away from the shaft. Such fractures usually occur around joints because of ligament, tendon, and muscle tearing, as associated with a sprain or dislocation (Fig. 12.47), or may affect the spinous processes of the vertebral column. A *chip fracture* is an avulsion fracture of a small fragment or chip of bone from the corner of a phalanx or other long bone. These are very common in the fingers and are often tiny. A mallet finger is an example of this (Fig. 12.48).

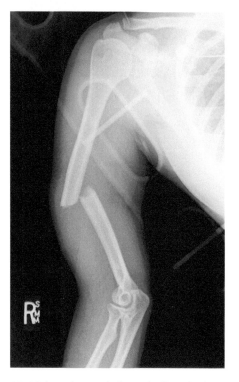

FIG. 12.44 An anteroposterior projection of a transverse fracture of the humerus sustained in a motor vehicle accident. Note the backboard visible on the image.

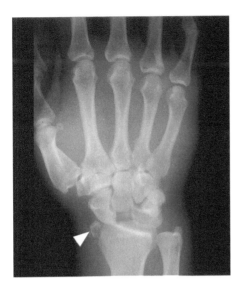

FIG. 12.47 A wrist radiograph obtained after trauma to the wrist that resulted in perilunate dislocation with an associated avulsion fracture of the distal radius.

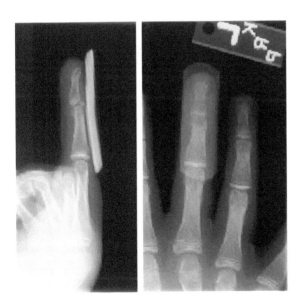

FIG. 12.48 A radiograph demonstrating an old mallet finger injury on the dorsal lip of the fifth distal phalanx associated with arthritic changes in the distal interphalangeal joint.

Incomplete Fractures

Incomplete fractures are those in which only part of the bony structure gives way, with little or no displacement. A common example is the **greenstick fracture**, in which the cortex breaks on one side without

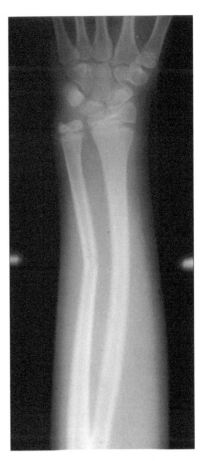

FIG. 12.49 A forearm radiograph of a child who sustained a fall. The radiograph demonstrates a greenstick fracture of the middle portion of the ulna. Note the incomplete break of the cortex of the ulna.

separation or breaking of the opposing cortex (Fig. 12.49). The effect is similar to that of trying to break a green twig, hence its name. Greenstick fractures are found almost exclusively in infants and children under the age of 10 years because of the softness of the cancellous bone. A **torus fracture**, commonly referred to as a *buckle fracture*, is a greenstick fracture in which the cortex bulges outward, usually in the metaphysis, producing only a slight irregularity (Fig. 12.50). Such fractures are commonly found in the distal forearm or tibia-fibula after a fall.

Incomplete fractures may also occur in demineralized bone, as occurs with osteoporosis. The bone in question breaks only part of the way through, resulting in a sharp angular deformity without displacement.

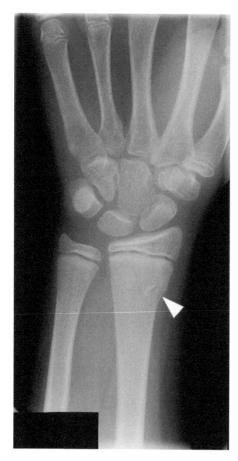

FIG. 12.50 A forearm radiograph of a 14-year-old girl who fell on her hand, resulting in a torus fracture of the distal radius.

Penetrating fractures are a type of incomplete fracture resulting from penetration by a sharp object such as a bullet or a knife. Frequently, a comminution exists at the site of the injury.

Growth Plate Fractures

Growth plate fractures involve the end of a long bone of a child (Fig. 12.51). The fracture may be limited to growth plate cartilage and is thus not directly visible unless displacement occurs, or it may extend into the metaphysis, epiphysis, or both. Crush injuries of the growth plate may also occur. These growth plate fractures are classified according to severity and involvement of the epiphysis. This system is known as the *Salter-Harris system;* fractures are numbered I through VI, with I being least severe and VI being most

severe. Comparison projections are often used with such fractures to compare growth plate appearances, and MRI may be used to further evaluate epiphyseal separations. Healed injuries of this type may result in an alteration of the length of the involved bone. Because of possible length discrepancies, frequent radiographic examinations may be required, often up to years after the injury.

Slipped capital femoral epiphysis (SCFE) is another example of a growth plate injury. SCFE is a posterior and inferior slippage of the proximal femoral epiphysis on the metaphysis through the physeal plate. It frequently affects adolescents, especially after a growth spurt. It is more common in obese children and more prevalent in boys than in girls. SCFE is generally idiopathic in nature and related to obesity, physeal orientation, and hormonal changes experienced during puberty, which may affect physeal strength. Physical examination usually yields intermittent limping and generalized groin, thigh, or knee pain. An injury is not necessarily associated with SCFE. Radiographic examination is the most common method of diagnosis. Bilateral AP and lateral hip projections or AP and frogleg pelvis projections are obtained so that comparisons can be made (Fig. 12.52). Severity of SCFE is classified according to stability and whether surgical intervention is required. The most widely accepted treatment is *in situ* fixation using a single central screw (Fig. 12.53). Unstable SCFE may require corrective osteotomy. Avascular necrosis is a complication that may occur as a result of SCFE.

Stress and Fatigue Fractures

Stress fractures usually occur as a result of an abnormal degree of repetitive trauma. They are generally found at the point of muscular attachments, as in the tibia or fibula of a runner. Stress fractures may not be clearly visible on plain radiographs, especially initially on injury, but may be diagnosed with a nuclear medicine bone scan or MRI of the affected area (Fig. 12.54). **Fatigue fractures** occur at sites of maximal strain on a bone, usually in connection with unaccustomed activity. Most frequently, fatigue fractures are found in the metatarsals, particularly the second metatarsal—the classic "march" fracture. Other common names for fatigue fractures include *stretch fractures* and *insufficiency fractures.*

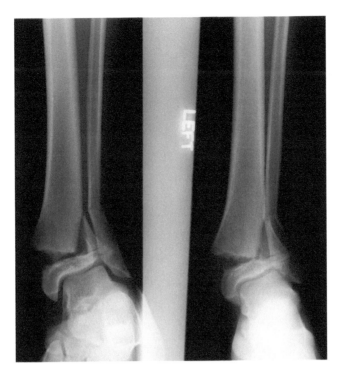

FIG. 12.51 A lower leg radiograph demonstrating an epiphyseal-metaphyseal fracture of the tibia with a transverse diaphyseal fracture of the distal fibula.

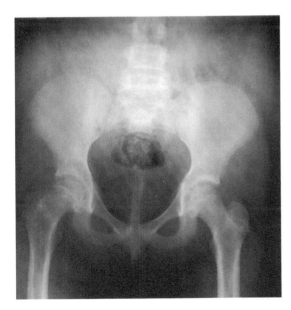

FIG. 12.52 Anteroposterior pelvic radiograph demonstrating slipped capital femoral epiphysis in the hip of an 11-year-old girl.

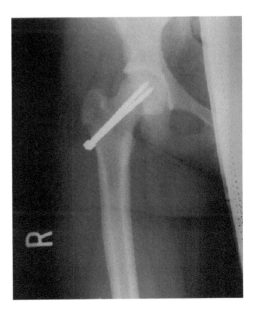

FIG. 12.53 Radiographs demonstrating postsurgical intervention with a single central screw to correct the slipped capital femoral epiphysis in the patient in Fig. 12.51.

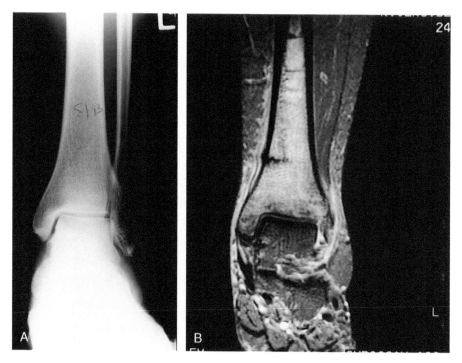

FIG. 12.54 A, An ankle radiograph of a 55-year-old woman complaining of pain in the medial aspect of the distal tibia. The radiograph appears normal, with no evidence of fracture. B, A magnetic resonance imaging scan of the same patient demonstrating a stress fracture of the distal tibia.

Occult Fractures and Bone Bruise

In an **occult fracture**, clinical signs are manifested without radiologic evidence. Follow-up examination within 10 days reveals bone reabsorption or displacement at the fracture site (Fig. 12.55). The most common sites for occult fractures are the carpal scaphoid and the ribs. A bruise to the bone may be revealed during MRI examination (Fig. 12.56) and is presumed to represent hemorrhage and edema, usually beneath an adjacent joint surface. A common area for a bone bruise is the distal femur with an associated knee injury such as a meniscal or ligamentous injury. Nuclear medicine bone scan may also be helpful in assessing subtle rib fractures.

Fractures in Specific Locations

Some fractures occur in selected areas and are usually easily recognized. One of these is *Colles' fracture* (Fig. 12.57), which is a fracture through the distal inch of the radius. The distal fragment is usually angled backward on the shaft, with impaction along the dorsal aspect. An avulsion fracture of the ulnar styloid process occurs in more than half of all Colles' fractures. This is the most common wrist fracture and it usually results from falling on an outstretched hand (FOOSH injury). The external skin contour in Colles' fracture displays a "dinner fork" deformity. *Smith fracture* is the opposite of Colles' fracture, with displacement of the distal fragment toward the palmar aspect of the hand. A direct blow or fall with the wrist in hyperflexion is the usual mechanism of injury.

A *boxer's fracture* occurs when the fifth metacarpal (and occasionally the fourth metacarpal) fractures as a result of a blow to or with the hand (Fig. 12.58). It is the most common type of metacarpal fracture and may be immobilized with or without reduction, as it is difficult to maintain the reduction in this type of fracture. *Bennett fracture* is a fracture and dislocation of the first carpometacarpal joint. This fracture results in an avulsion fracture of the base of the first metacarpal in association with a dislocation of the trapezium from the pulling action of the abductor pollicus longus tendon in

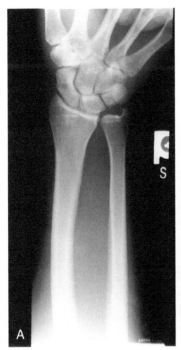

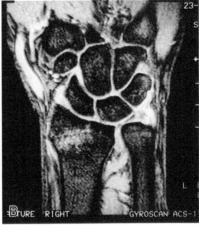

FIG. 12.55 A, A right wrist radiograph of a 31-year-old man who sustained an injury by falling while ice skating. No definite fracture or dislocation is demonstrated. B, A magnetic resonance imaging scan of the right wrist of the same patient as in *A,* demonstrating an occult, oblique, intraarticular distal radial fracture beginning just proximal to the styloid and extending to the middle third of the radius.

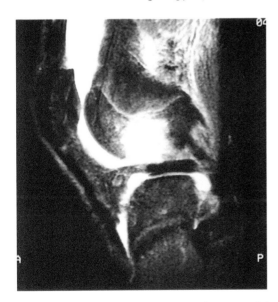

FIG. 12.56 A magnetic resonance imaging scan of the right knee of a 17-year-old boy who suffered a rotary injury while playing basketball. The image demonstrates extensive bone bruising of the lateral meniscocondylar notch and femoral condyles.

the hand. The injury occurs when the thumb is forced backward while in partial flexion and is commonly seen in basketball players and skiers. It may be repaired with a closed pinning technique if the fracture displacement is less than 3 mm or with an open reduction in cases of displacement greater than 3 mm. *Monteggia fracture* is a fracture of the proximal third of the ulnar shaft, with anterior dislocation of the radial head (Fig. 12.59). *Galeazzi fracture* occurs at the proximal radius, with a dislocation of the distal radial-ulnar joint (DRUJ). With both proximal and distal injuries to the forearm, it is important to ensure that both joints are included on the radiograph.

In the ankle, the most common injuries are to the malleoli. *Pott fracture* involves both malleoli, with dislocation of the ankle joint (Fig. 12.60). A trimalleolar fracture involves the medial and posterior malleoli of the tibia and the lateral malleolus of the fibula (Fig. 12.61). Less common fractures may seem more like minor sprains, requiring the radiologist to examine every aspect of the bone anatomy. *Maisonneuve fracture* (Fig. 12.62) is a less frequent ankle injury. It consists

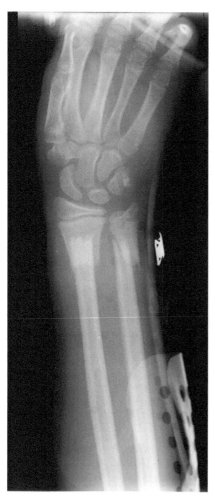

FIG. 12.57 A radiograph of the wrist of an older woman who fell on an outstretched hand. The radiograph demonstrates a classic Colles fracture.

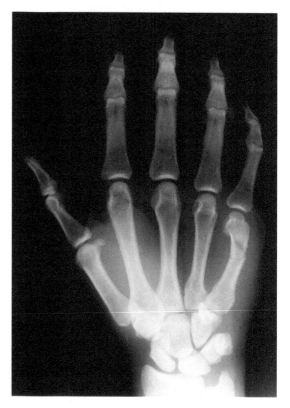

FIG. 12.58 A radiograph demonstrating a boxer's fracture of the fifth metacarpal head of the right hand.

of a severe ankle sprain or disruption of the syndesmosis between the distal tibia and fibula with a fracture of the proximal third of the fibula. This fracture may be easily overlooked because the more painful ankle injury may cause the proximal fibular injury to be missed. Most disruptions or ligamentous injuries involving the ankle syndesmosis require surgical intervention.

As mentioned earlier, radiographic signs of some fractures are subtle at best. Such is sometimes the case with the elbow. The elbow "fat pad sign" may be an indicator of a nonvisualized, underlying fracture of the bones of the elbow. In the elbow, normally a small accumulation of fat is present adjacent to the anterior surface of the distal humerus and the anterior surface of the proximal radius. These radiolucencies are normally visible radiographically on a lateral projection of the elbow. A similar pad is found along the posterior surface of the distal humerus but is normally not visualized radiographically. If the joint capsule is distended by fluid as a result of a fracture, the posterior fat pad becomes displaced from bone and is visible on the lateral projection of the elbow. Visualization of a posterior fat pad is considered a sign of a possible underlying fracture or dislocation. The anterior fat pad may also be displaced, giving a sail-shaped appearance (Fig. 12.63). This is a prime example of how soft tissue demonstration can assist in making a diagnosis. Fractures of the elbow may include supracondylar fractures (especially in children), radial head fractures from a fall on an outstretched hand, or an olecranon fracture. These may

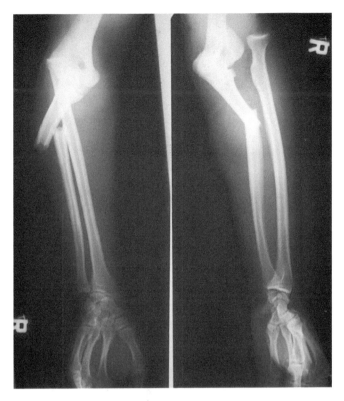

FIG. 12.59 A forearm radiograph of an individual who fell off a cliff, landing on an outstretched hand with the elbow partially flexed. The radiograph demonstrates a Monteggia fracture of the forearm.

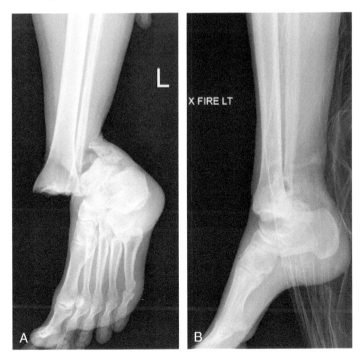

FIG. 12.60 Ankle radiographs (A, anteroposterior projection; B, lateral projection) depicting Pott fracture of the ankle. Note the bimalleolar fracture and dislocation of the joint. The injury was sustained in a motor vehicle accident between a car and semitruck.

Continued

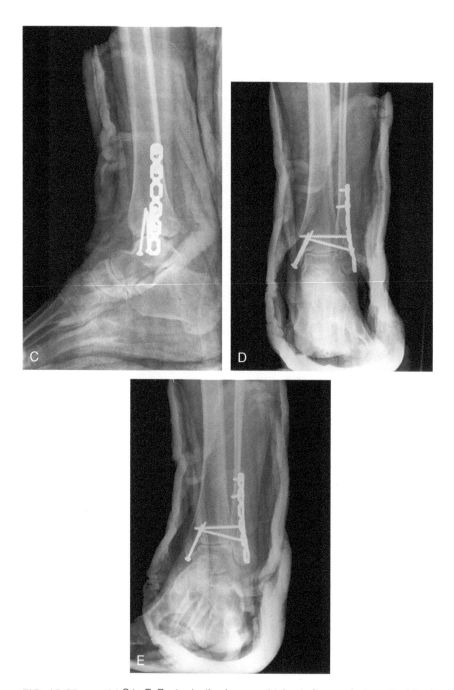

FIG. 12.60, cont'd C to E, Postreduction images obtained after surgical repair of the fracture.

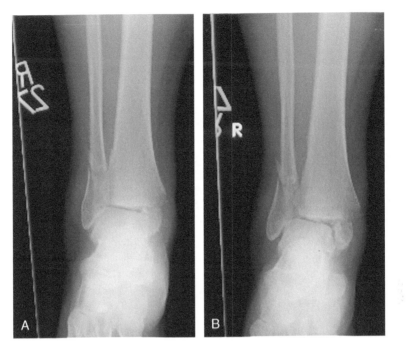

FIG. 12.61 A, Anteroposterior and B, internal/medial oblique projections of the ankle demonstrating a trimalleolar fracture.

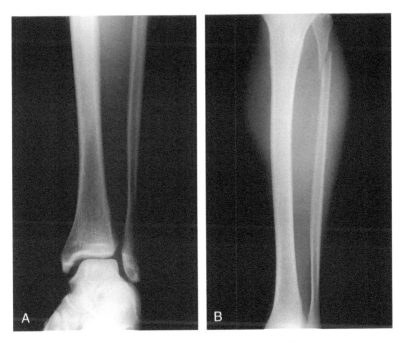

FIG. 12.62 A, A left ankle radiograph of a patient sustaining a twisting injury demonstrates a widening ankle mortise on the medial aspect with marked soft tissue swelling indicative of a Maisonneuve fracture. B, A left tibia–fibula radiograph of the same patient demonstrating a Maisonneuve fracture with minimal angulation and external rotation of the proximal fragment.

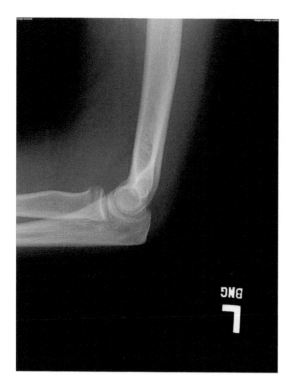

FIG. 12.63 Lateral elbow demonstrating a positive anterior fat pad sign.

require treatment from splinting to open reduction internal fixation (ORIF).

Visceral Cranial Fractures

Visceral cranial fractures are fractures of the facial bones and generally result from a blow to the face. As discussed earlier, facial or head trauma may also indicate a possible cervical spine fracture or injury. In addition, soft tissue injury of the eyes, nose, and mandible is often accompanied by bone fractures. CT has largely replaced the use of conventional radiographs in evaluating fractures of the maxillofacial bones and orbits (Fig. 12.64).

A *zygomatic arch fracture* may initially be difficult to recognize because of the edema. However, a fracture may be indicated by clinical signs, which include black eyes, flattening of the cheek, and a restriction of the movement of the mandible. Careful examination by palpation is performed by the physician because a fracture of the zygomatic arch may be present without accompanying facial fractures. A depressed fracture of the zygomatic arch may also be difficult to demonstrate radiographically (Fig. 12.65). If radiographs

are requested, an oblique submentovertical projection (tangential projection) may be used to best demonstrate the extent of the fracture. A parietoacanthial projection (Waters method) is also of value in examining the fractures of the zygomatic arch.

A *tripod fracture* occurs when the zygomatic or malar bone is fractured at all three sutures: frontal, temporal, and maxillary (Fig. 12.66). The patient with a tripod fracture complains of restricted jaw movement because the mandible's coronoid process is trapped by the zygoma. This fracture results in a free-floating zygoma and may cause facial disfigurement if not diagnosed and properly treated.

The mandible is highly prone to fracture because of the prominence of the chin; therefore, any patient who has sustained a head or facial injury should be clinically examined for a *mandibular fracture*. Anatomically, the mandible is strongest at the center and weakest at the ends, with the most common site for fracture at the angle, followed by the condyles. It is not uncommon for such fractures to be bilateral because of the transmitted force and shape of the mandible. Mandibular fractures (Fig. 12.67) are generally detected by the patient's inability to open the mouth and pain when moving the mandible. These fractures also cause a misalignment of the patient's teeth. Care must be taken to demonstrate all areas of the mandible (body, ramus, and symphysis) when ruling out mandibular fractures. The mandible is the slowest healing bone in the body and will show clinical union much sooner than radiographic union.

Fractures of the maxilla are serious because of the adjacent nasal cavity, paranasal sinuses, and orbit and the close proximity of the brain. The maxilla also transmits cranial nerves and major blood vessels. Maxillary fractures may be divided into three major classifications: horizontal, pyramidal, and transverse. A *horizontal* fracture of the maxilla (LeFort I) refers to a separation of the body of the maxilla from the base of the skull above the palate and below the zygomatic process. This type of fracture results in a freely movable jaw. A *pyramidal* fracture (LeFort II) involves vertical fractures through the maxilla at the malar and nasal bones, forming a triangular separation of the maxilla. A *transverse* fracture (LeFort III) is the most extensive and serious type of maxillary fracture; it extends across the orbits and results in separation of the visceral and cerebral cranium (Fig. 12.68).

A **blowout fracture** results from a direct blow to the front of the orbit that transfers the force to the

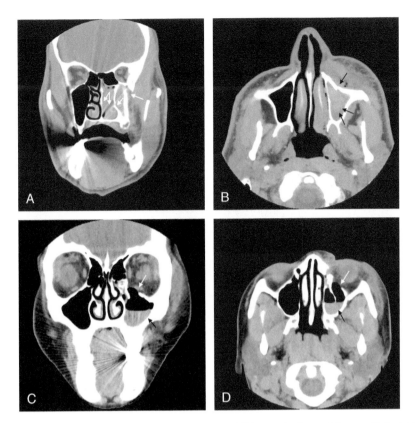

FIG. 12.64 Axial and coronal computed tomography (CT) examinations of the maxillofacial bones after trauma to the face. A, A coronal CT scan of a patient complaining of a nosebleed after being hit in the face. The CT scan demonstrates blood in the nasal and sinus cavities, with associated facial bone fractures and displacement of the nasal septum. B, An axial projection of the same patient as in A. C, A coronal CT scan of a patient sustaining a direct blow to the left orbit resulting in a blowout fracture of the floor of the left orbit. Note the blood in the maxillary sinus. D, An axial CT scan of the same patient as in C.

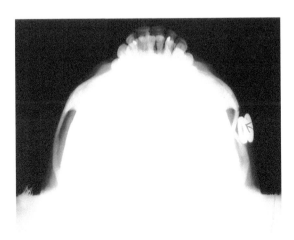

FIG. 12.65 A submentovertical projection of the zygomatic arch demonstrating a depressed fracture of the zygomatic arch resulting from a direct blow to the left cheek.

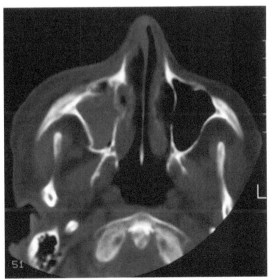

FIG. 12.66 A computed tomography image demonstrating a tripod fracture of the right zygomatic bone.

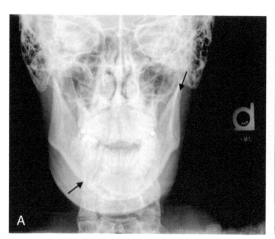
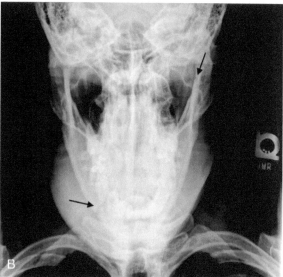

FIG. 12.67 A, Posteroanterior and anteroposterior axial and B, Towne method projections of the mandible demonstrating a mandibular fracture.

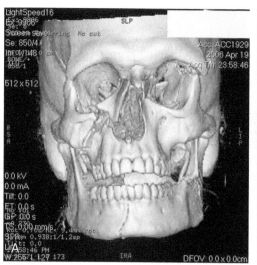
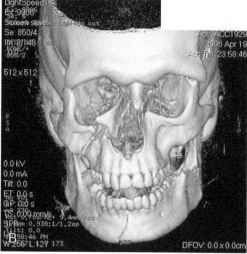

FIG. 12.68 Three-dimensional computed tomography reconstructions of a patient involved in a motor vehicle accident demonstrating bilateral zygomatic arch fractures, comminuted fracture of every wall of the right maxillary sinus, the medial and posterior walls of the maxillary sinus, bilateral orbital floor fractures, fractures of the lateral walls of both orbits, fracture of the left pterygoid plate, and both temporoparietal regions. Please note that three-dimensional CT creates a virtual image that can be rotated and viewed from any perspective.

orbital walls and floor. This fracture occurs in the thinnest, weakest portion of the orbit, the orbital floor just above the maxillary sinuses (see Fig. 12.64, C and D). If this condition is not diagnosed and treated, impairment of extraocular movements develops. A modified parietoacanthial projection (modified Waters method) provides the most information in terms of conventional radiographic diagnosis of blowout fractures because the petrous ridges are projected below the floor of the orbit. CT is the best modality for imaging the orbits.

The nasal bone is the most frequently fractured facial bone. The fracture is usually transverse and depresses the distal portion of the nasal bones. A *nasal bone fracture* may be accompanied by a fracture of the ascending process of the maxillae (anterior nasal spine) or of the nasal septum. The nasal septum is composed of the vomer and the perpendicular plate of the ethmoid bone. *Epistaxis*, or nosebleed, is usually present with a nasal bone fracture. As discussed earlier, CT is the best method for assessing fractures of the facial bones (see Fig. 12.64, *A* and *B*); however, radiographs of nasal bone fractures may be obtained in addition to a clinical examination to confirm a fracture or ascertain fracture displacement (Fig. 12.69).

Dislocations

A joint **dislocation**, or luxation, results when a bone is out of its joint and not in contact with its normal articulation (Fig. 12.70). Common sites for joint dislocations are the shoulder, hip, and acromioclavicular joints. A **subluxation** is a partial dislocation, often occurring with fracture (Fig. 12.71). The ankle and the vertebral column, especially the cervical spine, are common sites of subluxations.

Shoulder joints most commonly dislocate anteriorly (Fig. 12.72). Such dislocations are readily detectable

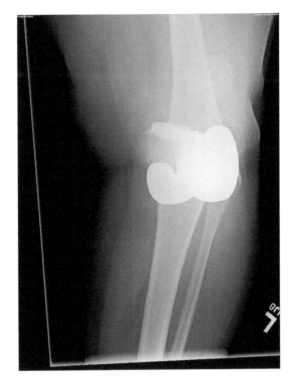

FIG. 12.70 An anteroposterior projection of a dislocated knee prosthesis.

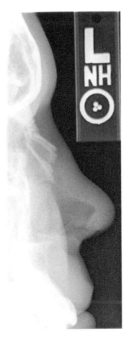

FIG. 12.69 A lateral nasal bone radiograph of a man who was struck in the face. The radiograph demonstrates nasal bone fracture.

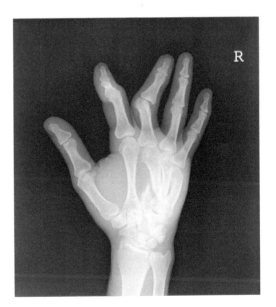

FIG. 12.71 An anteroposterior view of a hand demonstrating a metacarpal fracture and subluxation of the proximal interphalangeal joint, third digit.

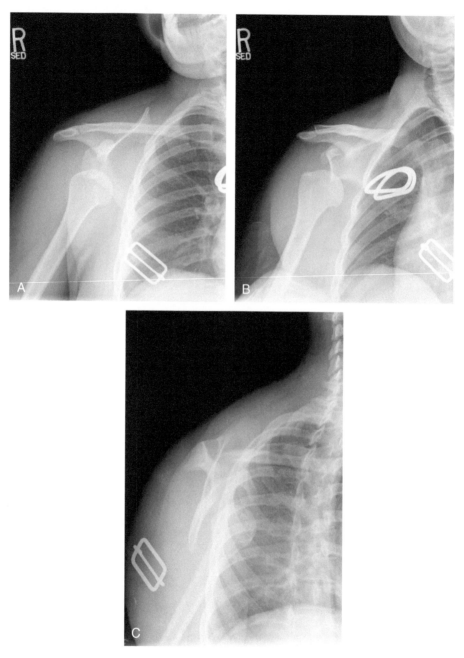

FIG. 12.72 A, Anteroposterior, B, oblique, and C, transscapular projections of the shoulder demonstrating an anterior dislocation of the humeral head. Note the location of the humeral head below the glenoid fossa and coracoid process of the scapula.

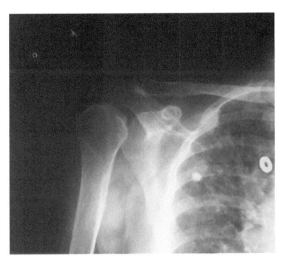

FIG. 12.73 A shoulder radiograph demonstrating a posterior dislocation of the humerus with the humeral head overlapping the rim of the glenoid fossa. The humeral head is also displaced slightly superolaterally.

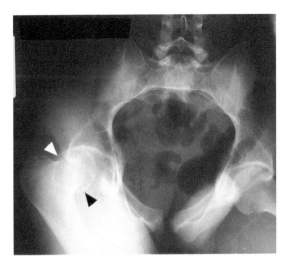

FIG. 12.74 A pelvic radiograph of a 25-year-old man whose right knee struck the dashboard in a motor vehicle accident, resulting in a posterior dislocation of the right femoral head.

radiographically because the humeral head usually locates below the glenoid fossa and coracoid process. Often an avulsed greater tuberosity is present with anterior dislocations. A Hills-Sachs deformity is a compression fracture of the humeral head. It occurs on the superior and posterior head of the humerus because of impaction of the humeral head against the glenoid labrum during dislocation. If undetected by the clinician, this defect may increase the risk of subsequent dislocations of the same shoulder. It is detected radiographically with the West Point method. Posterior dislocations of the shoulder (Fig. 12.73) are more difficult to diagnose, as they may appear normal on an AP radiograph. A transscapular (Y) and a posterior oblique projection are useful in locating the humeral head of a suspected posterior dislocation. Other than trauma, seizure disorders and electric shock are the major causes of shoulder dislocations. In fact, a posterior dislocation may be the first sign of a seizure disorder.

With traumatic dislocation of the hip, the femoral head is most commonly displaced posteriorly to lie against the sciatic notch (Fig. 12.74). It may also displace anteriorly and lie adjacent to the pubis or obturator foramen. Congenital hip dislocations are not caused by trauma, are usually unilateral, are more common in female patients, and are recognized by a shortening of the extremity. If the condition is not recognized until

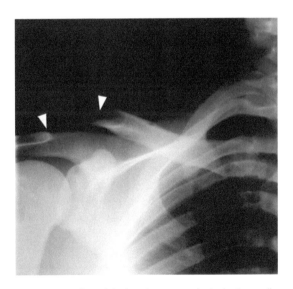

FIG. 12.75 A weight-bearing acromioclavicular radiograph demonstrating a dislocation as evidenced by uneven alignment of the acromial end of the clavicle and the acromion process of the scapula.

the child begins to walk, conservative therapies may be replaced by surgical intervention.

Acromioclavicular joint separations (Fig. 12.75) are more common in children than in adults. The typical imaging sequence for this diagnosis involves radiographs taken with or without weights with the patient in the upright position. Determining the alignment between the acromial end of the clavicle and the acromion process of the scapula allows for assessment of a joint separation. These radiographs are commonly performed bilaterally for comparison.

Battered Child Syndrome

Battered child syndrome is a term associated with a physical form of child abuse and was first described in 1860, but the term was not used until Henry Kempe did so in 1962. Battered child syndrome is also referred to as **nonaccidental trauma** (NAT). Physical child abuse often coexists with both emotional and sexual abuse. This syndrome affects boys and girls equally, generally under the age of 4 years. Approximately 16.1% of cases involve children under the age of 3 years. In addition, about 20% of the children who survive physical abuse suffer permanent injuries. An accurate incidence of child abuse is difficult to ascertain, but statistics from the National Child Abuse and Neglect Data System indicate that in the United States, approximately 1520 children died of neglect or abuse in 2013. It has been shown that family history is a strong predictor of child abuse because adults who were abused as children often abuse their own children, primarily because they do not know how to handle their anger. Statistics also indicate a higher incidence of abuse in homes with single parents, homes with young parents, families in which substance abuse is prevalent, or families living in poverty. Radiographs are often used as evidence in cases of suspected child abuse.

Physical signs of battered child syndrome include bruises, burns, abrasions, and fractures in various stages of healing. Active children who are not abused often have bruises over the bony areas of the body such as the knees and elbows. However, bruising or injury around the eyes, cheeks, mouth, buttocks, or thighs, bite marks, certain bone fractures, and cigarette burns are suspicious. In most cases, the explanation for the injury is inconsistent with the actual injury.

Radiographic skeletal surveys including the bones of the upper extremities, lower extremities, skull, spine, and ribs should be performed on initial inspection of the child if abuse is suspected. In some cases, the bone survey may be repeated 2 weeks later to better identify new fractures not visible during the initial series.

Radiographic signs of child abuse include hematomas and single or multiple fractures of varying ages, especially in areas where self-infliction of injury is difficult (Fig. 12.76). Often fractures may indicate that an extremity has been twisted or turned until it breaks, or multiple rib fractures indicate repeated traumatic injuries, generally inflicted by a parent or guardian.

Shaken baby syndrome is a severe type of physical abuse that affects the child's head and neck. Shaking of the child causes whiplash injury to the neck and brain trauma such as a subdural or subarachnoid hematoma, with no evidence of trauma to the external cranium. Shaken baby syndrome is associated with a high morbidity and mortality rate, with more than 25% of cases resulting in death. CT and MRI of the brain are excellent modalities for diagnosing this syndrome.

All emergency room personnel should be familiar with signs of child abuse and are legally and ethically required to report suspected cases of child abuse to the proper authorities. In addition, children may be admitted to the hospital or transferred to a specialized crisis intervention facility for further evaluation.

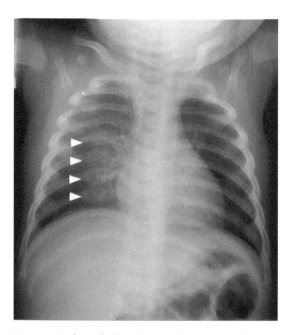

FIG. 12.76 A pediatric chest radiograph revealing numerous rib fractures with adjacent soft tissue masses resulting from hemorrhage surrounding the fracture sites.

Avascular Necrosis

Avascular necrosis is a term used to denote bone death resulting from inadequate blood supply. It frequently affects the hip, knee, shoulder, or carpal scaphoid and is most common in men between ages 30 and 60 years. It may occur idiopathically or may follow trauma to a joint (posttraumatic avascular necrosis), especially in cases of joint dislocation involving a tear of the joint capsule. The symptoms are nonspecific but may include pain up to 1 year or more after the trauma. If the lower extremity is affected, a limp may also be present.

MRI is the modality of choice for evaluating avascular necrosis of bone because it can demonstrate abnormalities associated with early-stage necrosis. Additional information is obtained with a nuclear medicine bone scan or CT. Conventional radiography is not sensitive enough to demonstrate early signs of avascular necrosis, but does demonstrate the later stages of the disease. The radiographic appearance of avascular necrosis at a later stage includes sclerosis in combination with a collapse of the affected bone and narrowing of the joint space. Treatment consists of analgesics for pain and exercise to maintain range of motion. If the condition is diagnosed early, surgical intervention to provide cortical bone grafts or core decompression may help provide support and relieve pressure to allow revascularization of the bone.

Legg-Calvé-Perthes Disease

Legg-Calvé-Perthes disease is a common form of avascular necrosis affecting the femoral head. The cause of this disorder is unknown, and the disease process is fairly quiet. *Perthes* refers specifically to ischemic necrosis of the head of the femur. It tends to occur in boys between ages 5 and 10 years. It may be idiopathic or may follow injury or trauma to the affected hip. Clinically, these patients have a limp that is accompanied by little or no pain.

Radiographically, the bone in the center of the epiphysis is fragmented, and the head of the femur is flattened (Fig. 12.77) and contains both areas of sclerotic bone and osteolytic regions. MRI images normally demonstrate low signal intensity from the affected hip in Legg-Calvé-Perthes disease (Fig. 12.78). In many cases, the patient develops a secondary degenerative osteoarthritis (see Chapter 2). This condition is treated with casting, traction, and bed rest or with surgical osteotomy and internal fixation.

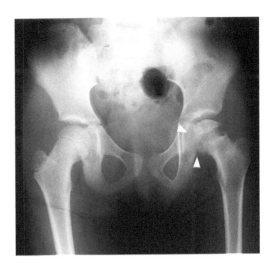

FIG. 12.77 An anteroposterior pelvic radiograph of a young man demonstrating Legg-Calvé-Perthes disease of the left femoral head. Note the asymmetry of the femoral heads.

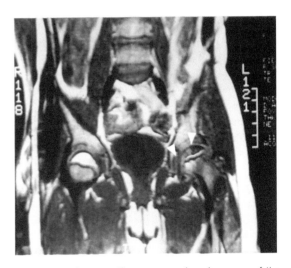

FIG. 12.78 A magnetic resonance imaging scan of the patient in Fig. 12.74. The image demonstrates low signal intensity in the left femoral epiphysis, consistent with Legg-Calvé-Perthes disease.

Trauma of the Chest and Thorax

Approximately 25% of all trauma deaths occurring annually result from chest injuries. Diagnosis of the cause of the respiratory distress and the extent of the injury must be made quickly. For patients with acute respiratory distress with suspected hemothorax or

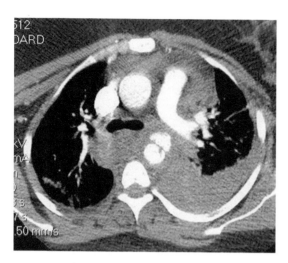

FIG. 12.79 A computed tomography scan demonstrating traumatic aortic injury at the level of the isthmus with an enlarged mediastinal hematoma displacing the trachea anteriorly. Right and left pleural effusions are also present.

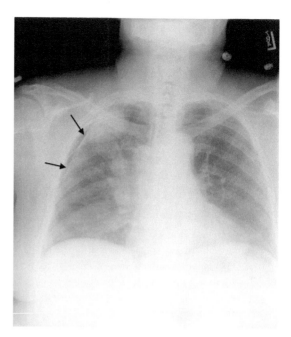

FIG. 12.80 An anteroposterior chest image obtained from mobile radiography equipment demonstrating a traumatic pneumothorax and atelectasis of the right upper lobe of the lung.

pneumothorax, a chest tube may be inserted in the fourth or fifth intercostal space without waiting for a chest radiograph. Portable chest radiography is then performed to further evaluate the thorax after placement of the "blind" chest tube. Bone injuries such as rib fractures, clavicular fractures, scapular fractures, and sternal fractures may result in penetration of the lungs and damage to the heart and the great vessels. Pulmonary contusion may also result from other penetrating, compressive, or decelerating trauma to the chest. Radiographically, changes in the lungs from contusion appear 4 to 6 hours after the trauma. The radiographic appearance changes frequently during the first 24 to 48 hours, so multiple chest radiographs may be necessary to assess the damage to the lung tissue because pulmonary contusions are usually much larger than apparent on the initial chest radiograph.

Blunt trauma to the chest may also result in injury to the descending thoracic aorta. Patients may have upper back pain, a cough or wheezing, and hemoptysis. A traumatic injury to the thoracic aorta may be visualized as a widened mediastinum during chest radiography, CT (Fig. 12.79), MRI, and transesophageal sonography.

Pneumothorax

A **pneumothorax** occurs when free air is trapped in the pleural space and compresses lung tissue. This air

may enter the pleural space from perforation of the visceral pleura, allowing gas to enter from the lung, from penetration of the chest wall, or by generation of gas by gas-forming organisms in an empyema.

Common causes of a pneumothorax (Fig. 12.80) include penetrating chest trauma such as stab wounds, gunshot wounds, fractured ribs, or a thoracocentesis needle, and a spontaneous blowout of a bleb (a flaccid vesicle such as a blister) resulting from some other pulmonary disease (Fig. 12.81). A pneumothorax may occur spontaneously from trauma or as the result of some pathologic process. The typical manifestation of a spontaneous pneumothorax is sudden, one-sided chest pain followed by dyspnea. This tends to occur more frequently with tall, hyposthenic male patients.

Radiographically, a pneumothorax appears as a strip of radiolucency devoid of vascular lung markings, with separation of the visceral and parietal pleura. It is best demonstrated on an erect expiration PA chest radiograph obtained in conjunction with routine PA and lateral inspiration chest radiographs. Occasionally, wrinkles in the patient's skin produce artifacts that may mimic a pneumothorax. Such an artifact is called a *pseudopneumothorax*.

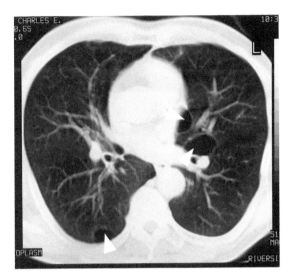

FIG. 12.81 Large emphysematous blebs as seen by computed tomography. Spontaneous blowout of these could result in a pneumothorax.

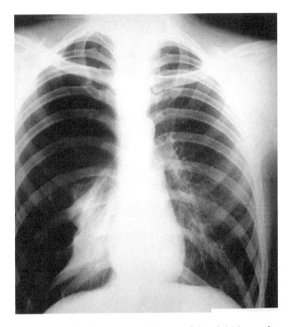

FIG. 12.82 Tension pneumothorax of the right lung after a stab wound in this 25-year-old man. The collapsed lung has almost no air in it and is seen as a soft tissue density adjacent to the heart.

A *tension pneumothorax* occurs when air enters the pleural space but cannot leave because of a check valve mechanism in the fistula. This results in a complete collapse of the lung and a shift of the mediastinum to the side opposite the pneumothorax (Fig. 12.82). A tension pneumothorax requires immediate medical attention to prevent life-threatening circulatory collapse.

Treatment of a pneumothorax depends on the amount of lung collapse and the type of pneumothorax. A collapse of 30% or less is usually treated by bed rest and needle aspiration. Immediate treatment of a tension pneumothorax might involve insertion of a needle into the chest wall to equalize air pressure. Otherwise, many pneumothoraces are treated with decompression by a closed-tube thoracostomy attached to a water-seal drain.

Atelectasis

Atelectasis means incomplete expansion of the lung as a result of partial or total collapse. In trauma situations, this often occurs in combination with a penetrating wound to the chest. Atelectasis itself is not a disease, but it is a sign of an abnormal process. One common manifestation is bibasilar atelectasis, which is also seen after trauma to the thorax occurs during surgical procedures. A chest radiograph reveals the airless area of the lung, which may be segmental or lobar. If an entire lobe is affected, the mediastinum shifts to the affected side because of loss of volume of the affected lung. The chest radiograph also demonstrates a decrease in the intercostal interspace, elevation of the hemidiaphragm of the affected side, and depression or elevation of the hilum, depending on which lobe is affected. If the atelectasis is segmental, the radiographic shadow is triangular, with the apex of the triangle pointing toward the hilum of the affected lung.

Compression atelectasis occurs when blood, pleural effusions, pneumothoraces, or other space-occupying lesions cause collapse (Fig. 12.83). Air that is completely absorbed from alveoli beyond an obstructed bronchus results in *absorption atelectasis*. *Plate-like atelectasis* describes the radiographic appearance of one or more linear opacities, usually at the lung bases and parallel to the diaphragm (Fig. 12.84).

Treatment of acute atelectasis is accomplished with appropriate respiratory therapy such as coughing and deep breathing. Bronchoscopy may also be used to allow suctioning of secretions that are causing an obstruction. Thoracocentesis is used to relieve the compression caused by an effusion.

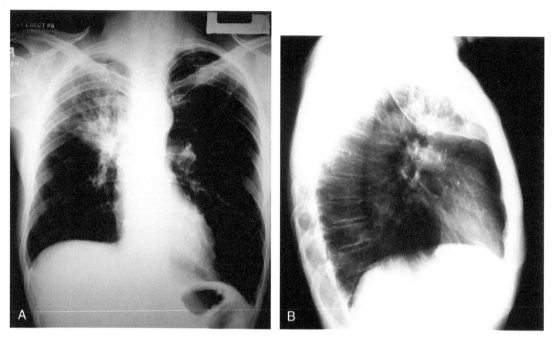

FIG. 12.83 A, Absorption atelectasis caused by the obstructive effects of carcinoma of the bronchus supplying the upper lobe of the right lung. B, The lateral projection of the same patient clearly demonstrates atelectasis of the right upper lobe secondary to bronchogenic carcinoma.

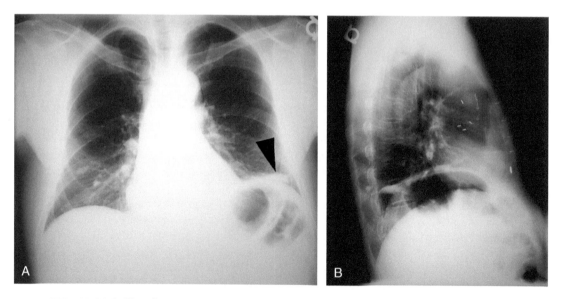

FIG. 12.84 A, Plate-like atelectasis (*arrow*) seen as a linear opacity in the base of the left lung in this posteroanterior projection. B, A lateral projection of same patient also clearly demonstrates plate-like atelectasis.

Abdominal Trauma

Traumatic injuries to the abdomen result from gunshot wounds, stab wounds, and blunt abdominal trauma. Although abdominal injuries account for only approximately 15% of trauma deaths, most occur more than 48 hours after trauma and usually result from sepsis. As mentioned earlier in this chapter, the severity of injuries sustained in an MVA are greatly reduced by wearing both shoulder and lap belts, whether the individual is in the front seat or back seat of a motor vehicle; however, chest and abdominal contusions and abdominal trauma may result from a rapid deceleration into the seatbelt, even when it is worn properly. Many patients with serious abdominal injuries from MVA initially have very minimal symptoms and physical findings. Abdominal trauma may cause serious injury not only to the gastrointestinal (GI) tract but also to abdominal organs such as the liver, spleen, kidneys, and pancreas; the retroperitoneum; the aorta; and the pelvic organs. Blunt trauma from steering wheel injuries often damages the liver and the spleen because the energy of deceleration and compression frequently damages the parenchyma of these structures (Fig. 12.85).

Supine and erect abdominal radiographs and erect chest radiographs are most desirable after abdominal injury. Chest radiography is important to assess diaphragmatic injury. In addition, free air is best demonstrated radiographically with the patient in the erect position. Often, free air is well demonstrated on a chest radiograph because of the proximity of the central ray to the diaphragm. Free air ascends and accumulates under the diaphragm on one or both sides, and as little as 1 cc of air can be demonstrated radiographically on the erect projection. Much larger amounts of air must be present to be visualized on a supine radiograph. However, placing the patient erect is not always possible because of the patient's condition. Left lateral decubitus radiographs of the abdomen may be substituted for the erect projection, with any free air present accumulating over the lateral aspect of the liver and the lateral aspect of the pelvis (Fig. 12.86). Optimally, the patient should remain on the left side for approximately 5 to 10 minutes before the exposure to allow sufficient time for the air to ascend. For unstable patients, radiography and focused assessment with sonography for trauma (FAST) are the preferred methods of imaging. For stable patients, CT is the most appropriate imaging modality.

Supine abdominal radiographs help identify foreign objects such as bullets, separation in the bowel loops, or loss of the psoas muscle shadow as a result of fluid or blood within the peritoneum and air around the right kidney or psoas muscle margins. The initial inspection of the abdominal trauma may be followed by specific studies involving the urinary

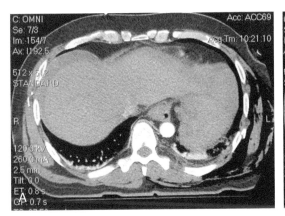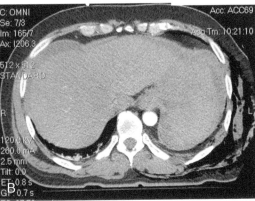

FIG. 12.85 Sequential axial computed tomographic images demonstrating a ruptured spleen resulting from blunt trauma from a motor vehicle accident. The patient was unrestrained and thrown from the vehicle.

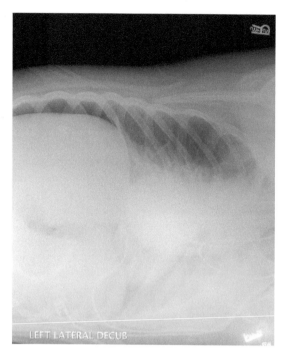

FIG. 12.86 Decubitus abdominal radiograph demonstrating free air over the dome of the liver.

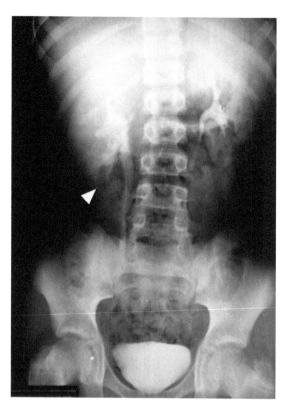

FIG. 12.87 An intravenous urogram demonstrating a right kidney fractured in a football injury.

tract (Fig. 12.87). IVUs may be indicated if injury to the urinary system is suspected; however, CT examination of the abdomen after an injection of an iodinated contrast agent provides a much clearer view of the renal anatomy and organ injury.

CT has also proven to be the best means of diagnosing GI trauma and is capable of visualizing lacerations, hematomas, and ruptures. Even small amounts of intraabdominal hemorrhage can be readily detected with CT. The duodenum is the portion of the GI tract most often damaged by blunt trauma. Because of its relationship to the spine, the duodenum may be compressed between the abdominal wall and the spine, resulting in a duodenal hematoma. Often CT evaluation of liver and spleen injuries helps in opting for surgical *versus* nonsurgical management of these injuries.

Penetrating abdominal wounds such as gunshot wounds may produce free air if the bowel has been injured. Some of the common conditions seen radiographically after trauma are fractures of the spine, pelvis, or ribs; subcutaneous emphysema; obliteration of normal fat planes and visceral margins; accumulation

of peritoneal fluid such as blood; and the presence of free peritoneal air (Fig. 12.88).

Intraperitoneal Air

In the normal person, the peritoneum is a closed cavity (except for the female reproductive system) containing only small amounts of serous fluid. The presence of free air in this cavity, a **pneumoperitoneum**, is usually abnormal and may indicate perforation of the GI tract. Large amounts of air likely indicate colon perforation, whereas small amounts of air are more indicative of duodenal perforation.

The common causes of a pneumoperitoneum (Fig. 12.89) include traumatic rupturing of the stomach or intestines or nontraumatic bowel perforations. In response to perforation, an intense inflammatory response develops and may eventually wall off the perforation into an abscess.

On an AP radiograph, with the patient in a supine position, the "football sign" may be demonstrated as an

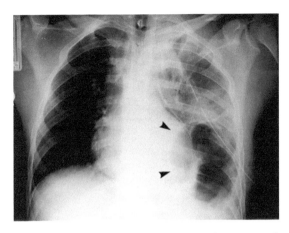

FIG. 12.88 A chest radiograph demonstrating a traumatic diaphragmatic hernia resulting from a motor vehicle accident.

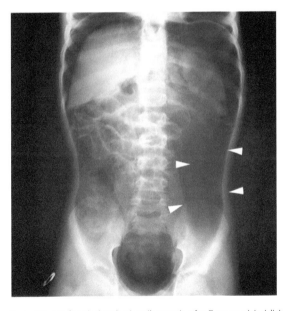

FIG. 12.89 An abdominal radiograph of a 5-year-old child with a passive pneumoperitoneum resulting from perforation of the stomach during anesthesia. Note how the free air outlines the outer border of the bowel, liver, and spleen.

indicator of a pneumoperitoneum. This is a lucent, oval gas collection that corresponds to the anterior peritoneal cavity. The pattern of gas resembles the shape of a football, with the seam of the football being the falciform ligament outlined by free air. Visualization of this sign requires a relatively large amount of free air to be present.

Pathologic Summary of *Traumatic Disease*

Pathology	Imaging Modality of Choice
Initial triage	Radiography, CT
Vertebral column—bony	CT, radiography
Vertebral column— soft tissue	MRI
Cerebral and visceral cranium	CT, MRI, radiography
Appendicular skeleton	Radiography, CT, MRI
Battered child syndrome	Radiography
Avascular necrosis	Radiography, MRI, CT
Legg-Calvé-Perthes disease	Radiography, MRI
Chest and thorax	Radiography, CT
Abdomen	Radiography, CT, sonography
Pelvis	Radiography, CT

CT, Computed tomography; *MRI,* magnetic resonance imaging.

Review Questions

1. A contusion formed on the side of the head where trauma occurs is called a:
   a. Concussion
   b. Contrecoup lesion
   c. Coup lesion
   d. Spondylosis
2. A fracture of the skeletal system in which the bone has penetrated the skin is termed:
   a. Closed
   b. Comminuted
   c. Noncomminuted
   d. Open
3. Fractures that occur at sites of maximal strain on a bone, usually in connection with unaccustomed activity, are classified as _____ fractures.
   a. Avulsion
   b. Fatigue
   c. Growth plate
   d. Stress

4. A fracture that heals in a faulty position is termed a:
   a. Callus
   b. Delayed union
   c. Malunion
   d. Nonunion
5. Shoulder dislocations are most commonly displaced:
   a. Anteriorly
   b. Posteriorly
   c. Interiorly
   d. Exteriorly
6. Avascular necrosis commonly affects the:
   1. Shoulder
   2. Hip
   3. Fingers
      a. 1 and 2
      b. 1 and 3
      c. 2 and 3
      d. 1, 2, and 3
7. "Incomplete expansion of a lung as a result of partial or total collapse" describes:
   a. Atelectasis
   b. Empyema
   c. Pleurisy
   d. Pneumothorax
8. Penetrating chest trauma could lead to a:
   a. Coma
   b. Coup lesion
   c. Pneumoperitoneum
   d. Pneumothorax
9. Demonstration of a pneumothorax is best accomplished by making the exposure with the patient in the:
   a. Erect, lateral position
   b. Lateral decubitus position

   c. Erect posteroanterior (PA) position during expiration
   d. Erect PA position on inspiration
10. Which portion of the gastrointestinal system is most frequently damaged by blunt trauma to the abdomen?
    a. Cecum
    b. Duodenum
    c. Ileum
    d. Jejunum
11. The "football sign" generally indicates which pathology?
    a. Pneumothorax
    b. Bowel obstruction
    c. Basilar skull fracture
    d. Pneumoperitoneum
12. Which imaging modality is recommended by the ACR for demonstration of a cervical spinal injury?
    a. Radiography
    b. CT
    c. MRI
    d. Nuclear medicine
13. Define the term *shaken baby syndrome*, and explain its effect on the central nervous system.
14. Spinal cord compression results in neurologic dysfunction that may be temporary or permanent. Explain the mechanism for each type of dysfunction described in the text.
15. Differentiate among the four types of hematomas to the brain, and specify which type has the highest mortality rate. Why?
16. What imaging modality or modalities best demonstrate stress or fatigue fractures? Why?
17. Describe the difference between comminuted and noncomminuted fractures of the skeletal system.

2-D Echocardiography Cross-sectional sonographic imaging of the heart demonstrating the heart chambers, valves, major vessels, and cardiac output

A

Achalasia A neuromuscular abnormality of the esophagus that results in failure of the lower esophageal sphincter to relax

Achondroplasia A hereditary, congenital disturbance that causes inadequate bone formation and results in a peculiar form of dwarfism

Acoustic neuroma A tumor of the peripheral nerve sheath

Acquired immunodeficiency syndrome (AIDS) An acquired viral infection that paralyzes normal human immune mechanisms

Acromegaly A disease marked by progressive enlargement of the head, hands, and feet caused by abnormal secretion of growth hormone

Acute Having a quick onset and lasting a short period of time with a relatively severe course

Acute glomerulonephritis An acute inflammation of the capillaries of the renal glomeruli

Acute lymphocytic leukemia A rapidly progressing form of leukemia in which there are too many very young (immature) white blood cells, called *lymphoblasts*, in the bloodstream and bone marrow

Acute monoblastic leukemia A type of acute myeloid leukemia

Acute myelocytic leukemia A cancer of the myeloid line of blood cells, characterized by the rapid growth of abnormal white blood cells that accumulate in bone marrow and interfere with the production of normal blood cells

Addison disease Deficiency in the secretion of adrenocortical hormones

Adenocarcinoma Carcinoma derived from glandular tissue

Adenocarcinoma of the prostate A cancer originating from glandular tissue in the prostate gland accounting for the majority of prostate cancers

Adrenal carcinoma A neoplastic disease of the adrenal gland, a small endocrine gland located above the kidney

Adrenal glands A pair of triangular-shaped endocrine glands located superior to the kidneys responsible for producing steroid hormones, epinephrine, and norepinephrine

Adventitia The outermost layer of connective tissue covering major organs and vessels within the body

Adynamic ileus A failure of bowel peristalsis, often seen after abdominal surgery, which may result in bowel obstruction

Agglutination Clumping that occurs when a specific immune serum is added to a bacterial culture

Albers-Schönberg disease A form of osteosclerotic osteopetrosis; a benign skeletal anomaly that involves increased bone density in conjunction with fairly normal bone contour

Alcohol-induced liver disease Liver damage caused by alcohol consumption resulting in hepatitis and cirrhosis of the liver

Alzheimer's disease A progressive degenerative disorder of neurons within the brain resulting in a common form of dementia including memory loss and cognitive, language, and behavioral changes

Anal agenesis Congenital disorder characterized by lack of an anal opening to the exterior

Anemia A condition in which level of hemoglobin in blood is less than 12 g per 100 mL

Anencephaly Congenital absence of the cranial vault

Aneurysm A localized ballooning or outpouching of a vessel wall as a result of weakening from atherosclerotic disease, trauma, infection, or congenital defects

Aneurysmal bone cyst A solitary benign osteoplastic serum or blood-filled lesion of the bone

Ankylosing spondylitis A form of rheumatoid arthritis of unknown cause that affects the spine in a progressive fashion, eventually fusing the spine into a rigid block of bone

Annulus fibrosus The outer layer of an intervertebral disk

Anomaly Any marked deviation from the norm, especially as a result of congenital or hereditary defects

Anthracosis Pneumoconiosis caused by inhalation and deposition of coal dust

Antibody The formation of protein substances by the human body in response to an antigen

Antigens Foreign substances introduced into the body, such as bacteria, or substances formed within the body that stimulate the formation of antibodies

Appendicitis An inflammation of the appendix

Arteries Blood vessels that carry blood away from the heart

Arthritis Inflammation in which lesions are confined to the joints

Asbestosis Pneumoconiosis caused by inhalation and deposition of asbestos dust

Ascites An accumulation of fluid in the peritoneal cavity

Aspiration pneumonia Pneumonia caused by entrance of foreign particles (e.g., vomitus) aspirated into the lower respiratory tract

Asthma Chronic inflammation of the bronchi resulting in hyper-responsiveness and airway obstruction

Astrocytoma A glioma composed of astrocytes, star-shaped neuroglial cells with many branching processes

Asymptomatic Showing or causing no identifiable symptoms

Atelectasis Loss of air in a lung resulting from a partial or total collapse of a lung

Atherosclerosis A common form of arteriosclerosis in which deposits of fibrofatty plaque or thickenings form within the intima or intermedia of large and medium-sized arteries

Atheroma A mass of plaque occurring in atherosclerosis

Atherothrombotic brain infarction An area of necrotic brain tissue resulting from an obstruction of blood circulation caused by a thrombus

Atresia Congenital absence or abnormal closure of a normal anatomic opening

Atrial septal defect An abnormal opening between the right and left atria of the heart which allows mixing of oxygenated and unoxygenated blood within the atria

Atrophy A reduction in size or wasting of cells, tissues, or organs as a result of poor nutrition or nonuse

Autoantibody Antibody acting against its own tissue or organism

Autoimmune disorder Disease in which antibodies form against and injure the patient's own tissues, in contrast to the normal process in which antibodies form in response to foreign antigens

Avulsion fracture A fracture in which a fragmented bone is pulled away from the shaft, usually occurring around a ligament or tendon and often with muscle tearing, as is associated with a sprain or dislocation

B

Basilar skull fracture A fracture of bones comprising the base of the skull and may include the occipital bone, sphenoid, ethmoid, and temporal bones

Benign neoplasm A localized tumor of well-differentiated cells that does not invade surrounding tissue or metastasize to distant areas within the body

Bicornuate uterus A uterus with paired uterine horns extending to the uterine tubes

Bladder carcinoma A malignant neoplasm originating from the epithelial lining of the bladder wall

Bladder diverticula A pouch in the wall of the urinary bladder

Bladder trabeculae Roughening of the normally smooth bladder wall

Blood-brain barrier The special functioning of the cerebral capillaries that prevents the passage of unwanted substances into the brain

Blowout fracture A fracture of the orbital floor resulting from a direct blow to the front of the orbit, with the force of the blow transferred to the orbital walls and floor

Brain abscess A collection of immune cells, pus, and fluid within the brain in response to a bacterial or fungal infection

Breast carcinoma A malignant neoplasm originating from the ductal or glandular tissue within the breast

Bright disease An inflammatory reaction of the renal parenchyma caused by an antigen–antibody reaction in the glomeruli

Bronchial carcinoid tumor A neuroendocrine malignant tumor situated in the submucosal tissues of large bronchi

Bronchiectasis Chronic dilation of the bronchi, with inflammation and destruction of bronchial walls and cilia

Bronchitis Inflammation of one or more bronchi

Bronchogenic carcinoma Carcinoma of the lung that arises from the epithelium of the bronchial tree

Bursitis Inflammation of the bursae of the tendons, with the subdeltoid bursa as the most common site

C

Callus An unorganized meshwork of woven bone

formed after a fracture, ultimately replaced by hard, adult bone

Cancellous bone Bone that has spongy, lattice-like structure filled by bone marrow

Capillaries Small blood vessels connecting venules and arterioles responsible for the exchange of water, gases, and nutrients within the blood

Carbohydrate intolerance The inability to digest and process sugars and starches into a source of energy because of an enzyme deficiency

Carcinoma A malignant growth composed of epithelial cells that tends to invade surrounding tissues and give rise to metastases

Carcinoma of the gallbladder A malignant neoplasm of the gallbladder of glandular origin

Cardiomegaly The appearance of an enlarged heart, as indicative of many cardiovascular disorders

Central venous pressure (CVP) line Specialized catheter inserted usually via the subclavian vein to the level of the right atrium to compensate for loss of peripheral infusion sites or to allow for fluid infusion in significant amounts

Cerebrovascular accident (CVA) A loss of blood supply to the brain from a cerebral bleed, a thrombus, or embolus

Cervical carcinoma A slow-growing, malignant neoplasm in the tissue within the neck of the uterus most commonly caused by human papillomavirus (HPV) infection

Cervical dysplasia Abnormal cellular changes within the epithelial cells of the cervix or uterine neck

Cervical spondylosis Degenerative joint disease affecting the cervical vertebrae, vertebral disks, and surrounding ligaments and connective tissue

Cholecystitis An acute inflammation of the gallbladder most frequently caused by obstruction

Cholelithiasis The presence of gallstones

Chondrosarcoma A malignant bone tumor composed of atypical cartilage

Chronic Presenting slowly and persisting over a long period of time

Chronic bronchitis A chronic inflammation of the bronchi

Chronic lymphocytic leukemia A type of B-cell lymphoma that occurs primarily in the lymph nodes

Chronic myelocytic leukemia A form of leukemia characterized by the increased and unregulated growth of predominantly myeloid cells in the bone marrow and the accumulation of these cells in the blood

Chronic obstructive pulmonary disease (COPD) Designation applied to conditions that result in pulmonary obstruction, most commonly chronic bronchitis and pulmonary emphysema

Cirrhosis Liver condition in which the parenchyma and architecture are destroyed and replaced by fibrous tissue and regenerative nodules

Closed fracture A fracture that does not produce an open wound

Closed reduction Manipulation of bone fragments to reduce a dislocation or fracture without surgical intervention

Clubfoot Deformity of the foot involving the talus

Coarctation of the aorta A narrowing or compression of the aorta

Coccidioidomycosis Systemic fungal infection caused by a fungus that thrives in semiarid soil and is particularly endemic in the southwestern United States and northern Mexico

Coin lesion Small solitary round nodules in the lung tissue

Colostomy An opening from the colon to the exterior abdomen created by a surgical procedure to allow for excretion of feces

Coma A state of unconsciousness from which the patient cannot be aroused

Comminuted fracture A fracture in which the bone is splintered or crushed

Compact bone Dense, outer portion of bone

Complete noncomminuted fracture A fracture in which the bone separates into two fragments

Compression fracture A fracture produced by compression

Concussion Brief loss of consciousness as a result of a blow to the head

Congenital Existing at, and usually before, birth and resulting from genetic or environmental factors

Congestive heart failure Condition existing when the heart is unable to propel blood at a sufficient rate and volume to prevent congestion of circulatory subsystems

Contrecoup lesion A contusion formed on the opposite side of the skull in reference to a trauma site

Contusion An injury in which the tissue is bruised but not broken

Cor pulmonale Hypertension in the pulmonary artery and an enlargement of the right ventricle of the heart

Coronary artery disease (CAD) Disease of the arteries of the heart often resulting from deposition of atheromas in the arteries supplying blood to the heart muscle

Corpus luteum ovarian cyst A cyst that develops in the yellow endocrine body formed in the ovary at the site of a ruptured ovarian follicle

Coup lesion A contusion formed on the side of the head on which trauma occurs

Craniopharyngioma A cystic, benign tumor that usually grows above the sella and upward into the third ventricle of the brain

Craniosynostosis Premature or early closure of the sutures of the skull

Craniotubular dysplasia An overgrowth of bone of the face and skull resulting in sclerosis and major skeletal deformities

Crohn's disease A chronic granulomatous inflammatory disease of unknown cause involving any part of the gastrointestinal tract, but commonly involving the terminal ileum; also known as *regional enteritis*

Crossed ectopy A condition in which one kidney lies across the body midline and is fused to the other kidney

Cryoablation A process that uses extreme cold to remove tissue

Cryptorchidism Failure of one or both testes to descend into the scroum

Cushing syndrome A syndrome resulting from excessive production of glucocorticoids

Cystadenocarcinoma Malignant neoplasm of the ovary; generally occurs in women over the age of 40 years

Cystic fibrosis Congenital disorder affecting exocrine gland function, with respiratory effects, including excessive secretions, obstruction of the bronchial system, infection, and tissue damage

Cystic teratomas (dermoid cysts) Cystic masses arising from unfertilized ova, containing hair, fat, or bone, and located in an ovary

Cystitis Inflammation of the bladder as a result of its infection

D

Degenerative Refers to deterioration of the body usually associated with the aging process

Depressed fracture A fracture of the skull in which a fragment is depressed inward

Developmental dysplasia of the hip An abnormal development of the hip joint that results in a misalignment of the femoral head and the acetabulum of the pelvis

Diabetes insipidus Increased urination and thirst resulting from inadequate secretion of the antidiuretic hormone

Diabetes mellitus A carbohydrate metabolism disorder caused by inadequate production or use of insulin

Diagnosis The name of a disease an individual is believed to have

Diaphysis Shaft of a long bone

Diastole The phase of the heart cycle in which the myocardium is relaxing

Diffusion The exchange of oxygen and carbon dioxide within the alveoli of the lungs

Diploë The spongy bone tissue found between the two tables of the cranial bones

Disease Any abnormal disturbance of the normal function or structure of a body part, organ, or system; may display a variety of manifestations

Dislocation The displacement of any part out of contact with its normal articulation

Dissecting aneurysm An aneurysm resulting from hemorrhage that causes longitudinal splitting of the arterial wall

Diverticulitis Inflammation of a diverticulum

Diverticulosis The presence of diverticula in the absence of inflammation

Diverticulum A pouch or sac of variable size occurring normally or created by herniation of a mucous membrane through a defect in its muscular coat

Ductal adenocarcinoma A malignant tumor originating in the ductal epithelium

Ductus arteriosus The blood vessel connecting the pulmonary artery to the proximal descending aorta in the fetus which should normally close at birth

Dysphagia Difficulty in swallowing

Dysplasia Abnormal tissue development

E

Ectopic kidney A kidney that is out of its normal position, usually lower than normal

Ectopic pregnancy A pregnancy in which the fertilized ovum is implanted outside of the uterus

Embolization Interventional angiography procedure in which devices such as coils are used to intentionally clot off vessels, often before surgery to prevent excessive bleeding

Emphysema A lung condition characterized by an increase in the air spaces distal to the terminal bronchioles and with destruction of alveolar walls

Encephalitis Inflammation of the brain

Endemic Term describing disease of high prevalence in an area where the causative organism is commonly found

Endochondroma A benign growth of cartilage arising in the metaphysis of a bone

Endocardium The inner membrane layer of tissue lining the heart

Endometrial carcinoma A malignant neoplasm arising from the inner lining of the uterus

Endometriosis A condition in which endometrial tissue implants in aberrant pelvic locations

Endoscopy The use of lighted instruments with optic connections to visualize disease of the esophagus and stomach, or rectum and distal colon (e.g., sigmoidoscopy)

Ependymoma A glial tumor that is firm and whitish and arises from the ependyma, the ventricle lining

Epicardium The inner layer of pericardium surrounding the heart which forms an outer layer of connective tissue covering the heart

Epidemiology The investigation of disease in large groups

Epididymo-orchitis A testicular condition that may result in benign masses of the testes

Epiphysis An ossification or growth center in the bones of children

Erythrocytes Red blood cells

Escherichia coli A gram-negative bacterium found in the large intestine that may produce a toxin causing intestinal illness

Esophageal varices Varicose veins of the esophagus that occur in patients with portal hypertension

Etiology The study of the cause and origin of disease

Ewing sarcoma A primary malignant bone tumor arising in medullary tissue, occurring more often in cylindric bones

Exostosis A benign bone growth, projecting outward from the bony cortex

Expectoration Expulsion of mucus or phlegm from the throat

Exudate Pus, celluar debris, or clear fluid that leaks out of the blood vessels into the surrounding tissues

F

Fatigue fracture A fracture that occurs at a site of maximal strain on a bone, usually connected with some unaccustomed activity (also known as a march, stress, or insufficiency fracture)

Fatty liver disease A buildup of lipids that are deposited in liver tissue

Fibroadenoma Adenoma containing fibrous tissue

Fibrocystic breast A benign, generally bilateral breast condition characterized by various-sized cysts located throughout the breasts

Foley catheter A catheter that is placed through the urethra and retained in the urinary bladder by a balloon that is inflated with air or fluid

Follicular ovarian cyst A cyst arising from the ovum

Foramen ovale An opening between the right and left atria

of the fetal heart that should normally close at birth

Fracture The breaking or rupturing of bone caused by mechanical forces either applied to the bone or transmitted directly along the line of a bone

Fusiform aneurysm An arterial aneurysm in which the entire circumference of the vessel wall is affected

G

Gallstone ileus A condition in which gallstones erode from the gallbladder, creating a fistula to the small bowel that may cause a bowel obstruction

Ganglion Cystic swelling that develops in connection with a tendon sheath, usually on the back of the wrist

Gastroenteritis General grouping of a number of inflammatory disorders of the stomach and intestines

Gastroesophageal reflux disease An incompetent cardiac sphincter allowing the backward flow of gastric acid and contents into the esophagus

Gated cardiac blood pool scan A gated nuclear medicine procedure of the heart that demonstrates heart motion and the ejection of blood from the heart

Genetic mapping A map assigning deoxyribonucleic acid (DNA) fragments to chromosomes

Genome The entirety of an organism's hereditary information, including both the genes and the noncoding sequences of DNA and ribonucleic acid (RNA)

Giant cell tumor A neoplastic growth of the skeletal system consisting of numerous multinucleated osteoclastic giant cells; also called an *osteoclastoma*

Glioblastoma multiforme The highest grade glioblastoma, a malignant brain neoplasm arising from the astrocytes (glial cells)

Glioma A tumor composed of tissue that represents neuroglia, commonly occurring in the cerebral hemispheres of the posterior fossa

Glucagon Secretion of the alpha cells of the pancreas to break down glycogen and increase sugar in the bloodstream

Gluten-sensitive enteropathy An autoimmune hereditary disorder involving increased sensitivity to the gliadin fraction of gluten, an agent found in wheat, barley, and rye products

Gouty arthritis An inherited, metabolic disorder with excess amounts of uric acid produced and deposited in the joint and adjacent bone, most commonly in the metatarsophalangeal joint of the great toe

Granulomatous colitis Chronic inflammation of the colon characterized by granulations associated with an infective process

Graves disease An autoimmune disease affecting the thyroid gland and the most common cause of hyperthyroidism

Greenstick fracture A fracture in which the cortex breaks on one side without separation or breaking of the opposing cortex

Growth plate fracture A fracture that involves the end of a long bone of a child and that may be limited to growth plate cartilage or extend into the metaphysis, epiphysis, or both

Gynecomastia Abnormal breast tissue development in males as a result of a hormone imbalance

H

Hangman's fracture A fracture of the arch of the second cervical vertebra, usually accompanied by anterior subluxation of the second cervical vertebra on the third cervical vertebra; also known as *atraumatic spondylosis*; such fractures usually result from acute hyperextension of the head

Haplotype A combination of DNA sequences at adjacent locations on the chromosome that are transmitted together

Hemangioma A benign tumor of dilated blood vessels

Hematocrit A common laboratory test that determines the body's total number of red blood cells

Hematogenous spread Spread through the blood

Hematoma A localized collection of blood in an organ, space, or tissue as a result of a break in the wall of a blood vessel

Hemocytoblast The stem cell for blood cell formation

Hemophilia (A, B, C) A genetic mutation disorder that inhibits proper blood clotting as a result of a variety of factors

Hemorrhagic stroke A stroke in which a blood vessel in the brain breaks or ruptures

Hemothorax Pleural effusion containing blood

Hepatitis An inflammation of the liver resulting from a variety of causes

Hepatocellular adenoma A benign tumor of the liver most frequently associated with oral contraceptives

Hepatocellular carcinoma A primary malignant tumor of the liver

Hepatomegaly Enlargement of the liver as might be seen with viral hepatitis

Hereditary Genetically transferred from either parent to child and derived from ancestors

Hernia The protrusion of a part of an organ (e.g., bowel loop) through a small opening in the wall of a cavity

Herniated nucleus pulposus Herniation of the nucleus pulposus of the disk through a rupture in the annulus fibrosus

Hiatal hernia Protrusion of any structure, especially some portion of the stomach, into the thoracic cavity through the esophageal hiatus of the diaphragm

Hirschsprung disease Absence of neurons in the bowel wall, typically in the sigmoid, preventing relaxation of the colon and normal peristalsis; congenital megacolon

Hodgkin lymphoma A malignant condition of lymphoid tissue associated with Reed-Sternberg cells

Hormonal stimuli A hormonal agent that directly influences the activity of the body

Horseshoe kidney A condition in which the lower poles of the kidney are joined across midline by a band of soft tissues, resulting in a rotation anomaly on one or both sides

Hospital-acquired infection Refers to diseases acquired in, or from a, health care environment

Human immunodeficiency retrovirus (HIV) The virus associated with acquired immunodeficiency syndrome (AIDS)

Human immunodeficiency retrovirus (HIV) protease An enzyme that converts immature, noninfectious HIV to its infectious state within the cell

Humoral stimuli Hormone release by endocrine glands as a result of changing levels of certain ions in body fluids such as blood or bile

Hydatidiform mole Represents an abnormal conception in which the fetus is absent and the uterus is filled with cystically dilated chorionic villi that resemble a bunch of grapes

Hydrocele A benign testicular mass consisting of a collection of fluid in the testis or along the spermatic cord

Hydrocephalus A congenital or acquired condition resulting from accumulation of cerebrospinal fluid in the ventricles of the brain and leading to ventricular enlargement, compression of brain tissue, and increased intracranial pressure

Hydronephrosis An obstructive disease of the urinary system that causes a dilation of the renal pelvis and calyces with urine

Hypercapnia A condition of high carbon dioxide blood levels usually associated with hypoventilation or lung disease

Hyperostosis frontalis interna A thickening of the inner side of the frontal bone as a result of a benign tumor

Hyperparathyroidism Abnormally increased activity of the parathyroid glands, causing excess hormone production; this overstimulates osteoclasts, which are responsible for bone removal

Hyperplasia Overdevelopment

Hyperthyroidism Excessive secretion of hormones by the thyroid glands that increases metabolism

Hypertrophic pyloric stenosis A congenital anomaly of the stomach in which the pyloric canal is greatly narrowed because of hypertrophy of the pyloric sphincter

Hypertrophy Increase in number of cells and tissue resulting in an increased organ size without the presence of a tumor

Hypopituitarism Decreased secretion of pituitary hormones

Hypoplasia Less than normal development

Hypothyroidism Diminished secretion of hormones by the thyroid glands that decreases metabolism

Hypoxemia A condition in which arterial blood is insufficiently oxygenated

Hysterosalpingography A radiographic examination for screening of the nongravid woman; injection of contrast into the uterus and the flow into the uterine tubes reveals their patency, which may affect the ability to become pregnant

I

Iatrogenic Pertains to any adverse condition that occurs in a patient as a result of medical treatment

Idiopathic Having no identifiable causative factor

Ileostomy An opening from the ileum to the exterior abdomen created by a surgical procedure to allow for excretion of intestinal waste

Impacted fracture A fracture in which fragments of one end of a broken bone are wedged or driven into the other end of the bone

Imperforate anus Congenital disorder characterized by the absence of the anal opening to the exterior

Incidence A statistical measure that refers to the number of new cases of a disease found in a given time period

Incomplete fracture A fracture in which only part of the bony structure gives way, with little or no displacement

Infarct An area of ischemic necrosis

Infection An inflammatory process caused by exposure to some disease-causing organism

Inflammatory Refers to the body process of destroying, diluting, or walling off a localized injurious agent

Insulin A hormone secreted by the β-cells of the pancreas to help maintain proper blood sugar levels

Intima The spread and multiplication of pathogenic organisms or malignant cells

Intussusception The prolapse of a segment of bowel into a distal segment

Invasion The prolapse of a segment of bowel into a distal segment

Involucrum A shell or sheath of new supporting bone laid down by periosteum around a sequestrum of necrosed bone

Ischemia A local and temporary impairment of circulation caused by obstruction of circulation

Ischemic stroke A stroke in which a blood clot blocks a blood vessel in the brain

J

Jaundice Yellowish discoloration of the skin and whites of the eyes caused by bilirubin accumulation in the tissues

Jefferson fracture A burst fracture of the vertebral arch resulting from a severe axial force that causes compression, as in a diving accident

Juvenile rheumatoid arthritis A form of rheumatoid arthritis that affects children

K

Kaposi sarcoma A sarcoma present in the connective tissue of about one fourth of all patients with acquired immunodeficiency syndrome (AIDS)

L

Lacunar infarction Small vessel disease that results in a thrombotic stroke

Left ventricular failure Congestive heart failure that results when the left ventricle cannot pump an amount of blood equal to the venous return in the right ventricle

Legg-Calvé-Perthes disease Osteonecrosis of the head of the femur caused by poor blood supply

Legionnaire's disease Severe bacterial pneumonia named for its outbreak at an American Legion convention in Pennsylvania in 1976

Leiomyoma A benign tumor derived from smooth muscle

Lesion General term used to describe the various types of cellular changes that can occur in response to a disease

Leukemia A malignant disease of the leukocytes and their precursor cells in blood and bone marrow

Leukocytes White blood cells

Level 1 trauma center The primary hospitals in the trauma system capable of providing total care for all injuries

Level 2 trauma center Hospitals that provide care for all but the most critical patients who may need cardiac surgery, microvascular surgery, or hemodialysis

Level 3 trauma center Hospitals that provide quick assessment, resuscitation, and stabilizations of patients before transferring them to a higher level trauma center

Level 4 trauma center Hospitals that offer basic emergency department facilities

Lewy body Abnormal aggregates of α-synuclein protein that develop inside nerve cells in individuals with Parkinson's disease

Linear fracture A fracture that extends lengthwise through a bone

Luxation A dislocation of vertebrae

Lymphatic spread Spread through the lymphatic system

Lymphocytes White blood cells important in building immunity

Lymphoma Neoplastic growth in the lymphatic system

M

Malignant neoplasm A lesion that grows, spreads, and invades other tissues

Malrotation Unnatural position of the intestines caused by failure of normal rotation during embryologic development

Manifestation Observable changes resulting from cellular changes in the disease process

Mastalgia Breast pain

Mastitis Inflammation of the breast, most often caused by *Staphylococcus* bacteria

Mechanical bowel obstruction Refers to a bowel obstruction that occurs as a result of blockage of the bowel lumen

Media The middle, muscular layer of a vessel wall

Mediastinal emphysema (pneumomediastinum) The presence of air or gas in the mediastinum as a result of leakage of air from the bronchial tree

Medical jaundice Jaundice resulting from a hemolytic disease in which excessive amounts of red blood cells are destroyed, or when the liver is damaged as a result of cirrhosis or hepatitis

Medullary canal Inner spongy or cancellous portion of a long bone where bone marrow is produced

Medullary sponge kidney A congenital anomaly of the urinary system in which the only visible abnormality is the dilation of the medullary and papillary portions of the collecting ducts, usually bilaterally

Medulloblastoma Soft, infiltrating tumors of neuroepithelial tissue that are highly malignant

Meningioma A hard, usually vascular tumor that occurs mainly along meningeal vessels and the superior longitudinal sinus

Meningitis Inflammation of the meninges caused by a bacterial or viral agent

Meningocele Hernial protrusion of the meninges through a defect of the skull or vertebral column

Meningomyelocele Protrusion of the spinal cord and meninges through a defect of the vertebral column, as is commonly associated with spina bifida

Metabolic syndrome A combination of medical disorders that, when occurring together, increase the risk of developing cardiovascular disease and diabetes

Metabolism The normal physiologic function of the body

Metaphysis The growing portion of bone

Metaplasia Conversion of a specific type of tissue into a different kind of tissue

Metastatic spread The spread of cancer cells

Metastatic liver disease The spread of another primary cancer to the liver

Miliary tuberculosis Type of tuberculosis caused by hematogenous spread of the disease, with a characteristic appearance similar to millet seeds, which are small, white grains

M-mode echocardiography Dynamic, one-dimensional sonographic images of the heart

Morbidity rate The incidence in the population of illness sufficient to interfere with an individual's normal daily routine

Morphology The form and structure of disease

Mortality rate The number of deaths from a particular disease averaged over a population

Multiple myeloma A malignant neoplasm of plasma cells characterized by skeletal destruction, pathologic fractures, and bone pain

Multiple sclerosis A chronic, slowly progressive disease of the central nervous system, characterized by demyelination of the nerve sheath

Murmur An abnormal extra heart sound indicating a structural or functional defect of the heart

Mycoplasma **pneumonia** The most common form of primary atypical pneumonia, occurring most frequently in young adults

Myelocele Protrusion of the spinal cord through the normally closed bony neural arch of the spine

Myeloid tissue Tissue within the bone marrow

Myocardium The muscular layer of the heart

N

Neoplastic Pertaining to new, abnormal tissue growth

Nephroblastoma (Wilms tumor) A rapidly developing malignancy of the kidneys, usually affecting children before the age of 5 years

Nephrocalcinosis A condition characterized by precipitation of calcium in the tubules of the kidney, resulting in renal deficiency

Nephroptosis Prolapse of a kidney

Nephrosclerosis Intimal thickening of predominantly the small vessels of the kidney as a result of reduced blood flow through arteriosclerotic renal vasculature

Nephrostomy tube A tube inserted through the abdominal wall into the renal pelvis to drain urine

Neural stimuli The release of hormones as a result of nerve stimulation of an endocrine gland

Neurofibroma A tumor of peripheral nerves caused by abnormal proliferation of Schwann cells

Neurogenic bladder A bladder dysfunction caused by interference with the nerve impulses concerned with urination

Noncomminuted fracture A fracture in which the bones do not break into multiple pieces or fragments

Nongravid Not pregnant

Non-Hodgkin lymphoma A malignancy of the lymphoid cells found in the lymph nodes, bone marrow, spleen, liver, and gastrointestinal system

Nucleus pulposus The inner soft portion of an intervertebral disk

O

Occult fracture A fracture that gives clinical signs of its presence without radiologic evidence; follow-up within 10 days reveals bone reabsorption or displacement at the fracture site

Oligodendroglioma A glioma, which is a slow-growing astrocytic tumor that is usually relatively benign

Oligohydramnios The presence of too little (less than 300 mL) amniotic fluid at term, generally associated with renal disorders in the fetus

Open or compound fracture A fracture in which the bone ends penetrate the soft tissue and skin, creating an opening to the exterior of the body

Open reduction Manipulation of bone fragments to reduce a dislocation or fracture with surgical intervention

Open reduction internal fixation The surgical placement of orthopedic hardware to repair a skeletal fracture

Osteoarthritis Noninflammatory degenerative joint disease occurring mainly in older persons, producing gradual deterioration of the joint cartilage

Osteoblastoma Tumors of the bone arising from osteoblasts

Osteoblasts The bone-forming cells responsible for bone growth, ossification, and regeneration

Osteochondroma A benign tumor of adult bone capped by cartilage

Osteoclastoma A tumor that is usually benign and characterized by osteolytic areas, most commonly found around the knee and wrist of young adults and composed of numerous, multinucleated osteoclasts; also called a *giant cell tumor*

Osteoclasts Cells that are associated with absorption and the removal of bone

Osteogenesis imperfect A congenital disease in which the bones are abnormally brittle and subject to fractures

Osteoid osteoma A benign tumor of bone-like structure that develops on a bone and sometimes on other structures

Osteoma A benign neoplasm of the bone

Osteomalacia A condition marked by softening of the bones, caused by a lack of calcium in tissues and failure of bone tissue to calcify

Osteomyelitis Infection of bone, most often caused by *Staphylococcus*, which may localize or spread to bone to involve marrow and other bone tissues

Osteopenia A softening of bone demonstrated radiographically as a decreased bone density, as in osteoporosis or osteomalacia

Osteopetrosis A hereditary disease characterized by abnormally dense bone, likely resulting from faulty bone reabsorption

Osteophytes Osseous outgrowths (spurs)

Osteoporosis Metabolic bone disorder resulting in demineralization of bone, most commonly seen in women after menopause

Osteosarcoma A primary malignancy of bone usually arising in the metaphysis, most commonly around the knee

P

Paget disease A metabolic disorder of unknown cause, most common in the elderly, characterized by an early, osteolytic stage and a late, osteoblastic stage

Palliative Treatment designed to relieve pain without the goal of cure

Pancreatic cancer A disease in which malignant cells grow from the epithelial cells of the pancreas

Pancreatitis Acute or chronic, asymptomatic or symptomatic inflammation of the pancreas caused by autodigestion by pancreatic enzymes

Paralytic ileus A failure of bowel peristalsis, often seen after abdominal surgery, which may result in bowel obstruction

Parkinson's disease A progressive neurologic disorder affecting movement resulting in muscular rigidity, tremors, and slow, imprecise movement

Patent ductus arteriosus Abnormal persistence of an open ductus arteriosus after birth, resulting in recirculation of arterial blood through the lungs

Pathogenesis Development of disease

Pathologic fracture A fracture that occurs in abnormal bone weakened by a disease process

Pathology The study of structural and functional manifestations of disease

Peau d'orange Orange-peel appearance of multiple small depressions on the skin surface as a result of hair follicles becoming visible from skin edema, as might occur with breast cancer

Pelvic inflammatory disease (PID) A bacterial infection of the female genital system, most often caused by bacteria

Peptic ulcer Ulceration of the mucous membrane of the esophagus, stomach, or duodenum

Percutaneous transluminal angioplasty (PTA) Use of a specialized catheter, typically equipped with an inflatable balloon, to perform vessel repair from within the artery or vein during angiography

Permanent catheterization Interventional angiography procedure, in which a catheter is placed in the subclavian or jugular vein and tunneled under skin to allow for improved dialysis access

Pessary A device inserted into the vagina to provide proper support to a uterus that lacks proper support

Phlebitis Inflammation of a vein, often associated with venous thrombosis

Physical mapping A form of genetic mapping based on direct analysis of DNA, in which the physical distance between DNA fragments are measured; this is used to assign DNA fragments to specific chromosomes

Pituitary adenoma A benign tumor of the pituitary gland

Placenta accrete Abnormal adhesion of the placenta to the uterine wall

Placenta previa The condition in which the placenta develops in the lower half of the uterus, on or encroaching on, and completely or partially covering, the internal cervical os

Plate-like atelectasis Radiographic appearance seen in atelectasis, in which one or more linear opacities are seen, usually at the lung bases and parallel to the diaphragm

Pleural effusion A collection of excess fluid in the pleural cavity

Placental abruption Condition in which a normally implanted placenta prematurely separates from the uterus

Placental percreta A condition in which the placenta extends into the myometrium

Pleural effusion An accumulation of fluid in the pleural cavity or space

Pleurisy Inflammation of the pleura with exudation into the pleural cavity and on its surface

Pneumococcal pneumonia The most common bacterial pneumonia, generally affecting an entire lobe of a lung

Pneumoconiosis A group of occupational diseases characterized by permanent deposits of particulate matter in the lungs and by resultant pulmonary fibrosis

Pneumocystis carinii **pneumonia** Life-threatening infection of the lungs most commonly associated with AIDS

Pneumonia The most frequent type of lung infection, resulting in an inflammation of the lung with compromised pulmonary function

Pneumoperitoneum The presence of air or gas in the peritoneal cavity

Pneumothorax An accumulation of free air or gas in the pleural space that compresses the lung tissue

Polycystic kidney disease A familial kidney disorder in which innumerable tiny cysts that are present congenitally gradually enlarge during aging to compress

and eventually destroy normal tissues

Polycystic ovaries Ovaries that contain multiple small cysts

Polydactyly The presence of more than five digits

Polyhydramnios An excess of amniotic fluid; it may be associated with anencephaly or gastrointestinal disturbances in the fetus

Polyp A small mass of tissue arising from the mucous membrane to project inward into the lumen of the bowel

Pott disease Tuberculosis of the spine

Prevalence A statistical measure that refers to the number of cases of a disease found in a given population

Prognosis The prediction of course and outcome for a given disease

Progressive disseminated histoplasmosis A respiratory disease endemic in the Mississippi and Ohio river valleys caused by a fungal infection

Prostatic calculi Stones within the prostate gland

Prostatic hyperplasia Abnormal benign cell growth within the prostate gland

Pseudocyst An abnormal or displaced space resembling a cyst

Pseudofracture A band of bone material of decreased density may form alongside the surface of the bone

Psoriatic arthritis An inflammatory arthritis associated with psoriasis of the skin

Pulmonary embolus A mass of foreign matter present in a pulmonary artery or one of its branches

Pulmonary tuberculosis A contagious bacterial infection

of the lungs caused by *Mycobacterium tuberculosis*

Pyelonephritis Bacterial infection of the kidney and its pelvis

Pyuria The presence of pus in urine, created by its drainage from renal abscesses into the kidney's collecting tubules

R

Radiofrequency ablation A process that uses radiofrequency waves to remove tissue

Reed-Sternberg cells A specific type of cells that help differentiate Hodgkin lymphomas from other types of lymphatic diseases

Reflux esophagitis The backward flow of gastric acids into the esophagus

Regional enteritis A chronic granulomatous inflammatory disease of unknown cause involving any part of the gastrointestinal tract, but commonly involving the terminal ileum

Reiter syndrome A group of symptoms associated with complications of urethritis

Renal agenesis The absence of the kidney on one side, with an unusually large kidney on the other side

Renal calculi Kidney stone

Renal colic Severe, agonizing pain that refers along the course of a ureter toward the genital and loin regions in response to the movement of a renal calculus

Renal cyst A fluid-filled growth within the kidney

Renal failure The end result of a chronic process that gradually results in lost kidney function

Respiratory distress syndrome (RDS) A respiratory disorder of infants born at less than a 37-week gestation caused by incomplete maturation of the surfactant-producing system

Respiratory failure Failure of the lungs to ventilate

Reticuloendothelial system Specialized cells found in the liver, bone marrow, and spleen whose function is phagocytosis

Reverse transcriptase An enzyme that converts viral RNA into a DNA copy that becomes integrated into the host cell DNA

Rh factor The factor first discovered in the blood of the rhesus monkey; contained by approximately 85% of the population who are said to be "Rh-positive"

Rheumatic fever An illness that results from an untreated strep throat condition

Rheumatoid arthritis A chronic, systemic disease primarily of joints, characterized by an overgrowth of synovial tissues and articular structures and progressive destruction of cartilage, bone, and supporting structures

Rh-negative Blood type that does not include the Rh (Rhesus) antigen factor

Rh-positive Blood type that does include the Rh (Rhesus) antigen factor

Rickets Osteomalacia that occurs before growth plate closure, caused by deficiency of vitamin D, especially in infants and children

S

Saccular aneurysm A localized sac affecting only a part of the circumference of an arterial wall

Sarcoma A type of tumor, often highly malignant, composed of a substance similar to embryonic connective tissue

Schwannoma A benign nerve sheath neoplasm or tumor

Scoliosis Abnormal lateral curvature of the spine

Seeding Traveling of cancerous cells to a distant site or distant organ

Sequelae Conditions resulting from a disease

Sequestrum A piece of dead, devascularized bone that separates from living bone during the process of necrosis

Sickle cell anemia An inherited blood disorder in which the red blood cells are distorted to a crescent shape, resulting in anemia and other manifestations

Sign An objective manifestation of disease perceptible to the managing physician, as opposed to subjective symptoms perceived by the patient

Silicosis Pneumoconiosis caused by inhalation of silica dust, as is common among miners, grinders, and sand blasters

Simple unicameral bone cyst A benign, fluid-filled bone neoplasm

Single-nucleotide polymorphisms A DNA sequence variation occurring when a single nucleotide in the genome differs between members of a biologic species or paired chromosomes in an individual

Sinoatrial (SA) node The heart's "pacemaker"; this is a bundle of nerve fibers located in the upper portion of the right atrium near the superior vena cava; from this node an electrical current is transmitted through the myocardium, resulting in a heartbeat

Sinusitis Inflammation of a sinus, which may be purulent or nonpurulent and acute or chronic

Situs inversus Complete reversal of the viscera of the thorax and the abdomen

Slipped capital femoral epiphysis A separation of the femoral head and shaft occurring through the epiphyseal plate

Sonohysterography A sonographic examination of the uterus and fallopian tubes in which normal saline is injected into the uterus

Spermatocele A cystic dilatation of the epididymis

Spina bifida A developmental anomaly characterized by incomplete closure of the vertebral canal, through which the choriomeninges may or may not protrude

Spondylolisthesis Forward displacement of one vertebra over another (commonly occurring at the L5–S1 junction), usually caused by a developmental defect in the pars interarticularis

Spondylolysis A condition marked by a cleft or breaking down of the body of a vertebra between the superior and inferior articular processes

Staghorn calculus A large renal calculus that assumes the shape of the pelvicalyceal junction, resembling the horn of a stag

Staphylococcus aureus Gram-positive micrococcaceae commonly present on skin and mucous membranes

Steatosis An excess of fatty acids within the liver leading to fatty infiltration of the liver

Stent A specialized device placed to provide patency, usually in a vessel or duct

Stress fracture A fracture that occurs as a result of due to repeated or unusual stress

Subarachnoid hematoma A hematoma that accumulates between the brain's arachnoid layer and its pia mater

Subcutaneous emphysema The presence of air or gas in the subcutaneous tissues of the body

Subdural empyema A collection of pus below the dura layer of the meninges

Subdural hematoma A hematoma positioned between the dura mater and the arachnoid meningeal layer

Subluxation An incomplete or partial dislocation

Supernumerary kidney A relatively rare anomaly consisting of the presence of a third, small rudimentary kidney

Suprapubic catheter A urinary catheter that is placed into the urinary bladder through the skin in the suprapubic area to allow drainage of urine

Surgical jaundice Jaundice that occurs as a result of biliary system blockage, which prevents bile from entering the duodenum

Sylvian triangle An anatomic landmark in cerebral angiography, created by the middle cerebral artery and its branches

Symptom Any subjective evidence of a disease as perceived by a patient

Syndactyly A webbing or fusion of digits

Syndrome A group of signs and symptoms that occur together and characterize a specific abnormal disturbance

Systole The phase of the heart cycle during which the myocardium is contracting

T

Tendonitis Inflammation of a tendon

Tenosynovitis Inflammation of a tendon and its sheath

Testicular choriocarcinoma A malignant germ cell tumor of the testicle

Testicular embryonal carcinoma A malignant germ cell tumor of the testicle

Testicular seminoma A malignant germ cell tumor of the testicle

Testicular teratoma A malignant germ cell tumor of the testicle

Tetralogy of Fallot A combination of four congenital cardiac defects: pulmonary stenosis, ventricular central defect, overriding aorta, and hypertrophy of the right ventricle

Thalassemia A genetic disorder resulting in abnormal hemoglobin molecules within blood, resulting in severe anemia

Thrombocytes Platelets

Thrombolysis An interventional angiography procedure in which urokinase, a high-intensity anticoagulant, is dripped over a period of hours directly onto a clot to dissolve it

Thrombophlebitis The presence of inflammation and blood clots within a vein

Thrombus A blood clot that obstructs a blood vessel

Torus fracture A fracture in which the cortex folds back on itself, with little or no displacement of the lower end of the bone

Trabecula The spongy substance found within a bone; it gives a characteristic appearance to bone details

Trabecular pattern The arrangement of supportive strands of connective tissue of the alveolar bone in relation to the bone marrow spaces within the cancellous bone

Transesophageal echocardiography (TEE) A type of echocardiographic procedure in which the patient swallows a mobile, flexible probe. The heart's structure can then be readily visualized without having structures such as the skin, rib cage, and chest muscles interfere

Transient ischemic attack (TIA) A temporary episode of neurologic dysfunction that can precede a cerebrovascular accident

Transitional vertebra A vertebra that assumes the characteristics of the vertebrae on each side of a major spine division

Transjugular intrahepatic portosystemic stent (TIPSS) An interventional angiography procedure in which a catheter is used to connect the jugular vein to the portal vein to reduce the flow of blood through a diseased liver

Transposition of great vessels Congenital malformation of the cardiovascular system, in which the aorta arises from the right ventricle and the pulmonary artery from the left ventricle

Transudates Fluid substances that pass through a tissue membrane

Transurethral resection of the prostate A cystoscopic surgical procedure in which a portion of the prostate is removed

Traumatic Pertaining to the effects of a wound or injury, whether physical or psychological

Traumatic brain injury Damage to the brain from an external mechanical force such as rapid acceleration or deceleration associated with neurologic deficits

Tuberculosis Any of the infectious diseases of man and animals caused by *Mycobacterium tuberculosis*, generally affecting the lungs

Type 1 diabetes mellitus A childhood autoimmune disease in which T-cells destroy β-cells in the pancreas, inhibiting the production of insulin

Type 2 diabetes mellitus A metabolic disease resulting in a hyperglycemia as a result of insulin resistance usually occurring in adults

U

Ulcerative colitis A chronic, recurrent ulceration of the colon mucosa of unknown cause

Unicornuate uterus A uterus whose uterine cavity is elongated and has a single uterine tube emerging from it

Uremia The retention of urea in blood, as characteristic of renal failure

Ureteral diverticula An outpouching in the ureteral wall

Ureteral stent A tube used to maintain patency of the ureter, with the proximal end placed in the renal pelvis and the distal end placed in the urinary bladder

Ureterocele Cyst-like dilation of the terminal portion of the ureter as a result of stenosis of the ureteral meatus

Urethral valves Congenital presence of mucosal folds that protrude into the posterior urethra, which may cause significant obstruction to urine flow

Urinary tract infection (UTI) The most common of all bacterial infections, a UTI is an infection in the urinary tract usually caused by a gram-negative bacillus, which invades by an ascending route through the urethra to the bladder to the kidney

Uterine fibroids Benign growths within the muscle layer of the uterus

Uterus didelphys Complete duplication of the uterus, cervix, and vagina

V

Valvular stenosis Narrowing of a valve

Venous thrombosis The formation of blood clots within a vein

Ventilation The process of air movement into and out of the lungs

Ventricular septal defects An abnormal opening between the right and left ventricles of the heart allowing for the mixing of oxygenated and deoxygenated blood

Vesicoureteral reflux The backward flow of urine out of the bladder and into the ureters

Viral pneumonia Pneumonia caused by a virus, spread by an infected person to a nonimmune individual

Virulence The ease with which an organism overcomes body defenses

Volvulus An intestinal obstruction caused by a twisting of the bowel about its mesenteric base

von Willebrand disease An inherited blood disorder resulting in a tendency to hemorrhage

W

Whiplash Hyperextension–flexion injury of the spine

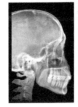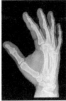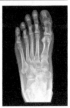

Image Credits and Courtesies

American College of Radiology, Reston, Virginia

Figs. 2.9, 2.11, 2.14, 2.18, 2.22, 2.23, 2.26A, 2.28, 2.38, 2.41, 2.44, 2.47, 2.48, 2.50, 2.51, 3.7, 3.11, 3.27, 3.30, 3.31, 3.34, 3.36A, 3.38, 3.40, 3.42, 3.48, 4.2, 4.3, 4.6, 4.7, 4.38, 4.41, 5.30, 5.34, 5.35, 5.38, 5.39, 5.40, 5.41, 5.44, 5.45, 5.48, 5.53, 5.55, 5.59, 5.60, 5.62, 5.64, 5.66, 5.67, 5.70, 5.71, 5.80, 5.81, 5.82, 6.37, 7.17, 7.22, 7.47, 7.76, 7.77, 8.20, 9.7, 9.8, 11.8, 11.10 to 11.12, 11.18, 12.4, 12.5, 12.6, 12.9, 12.34, 12.46, 12.49, 12.50, 12.72, 12.73, 12.75, 12.77, 12.81, 12.82, 12.88, 12.89

American College of Surgeons Committee on Trauma, Chicago, Illinois

Fig. 12.1

American Hospital Association: TrendWatch

Figs. 1.3, 1.4

Bontrager KL: *Textbook of Radiographic Positioning and Related Anatomy,* ed 6, St. Louis, 2005, Mosby.

Figs. 1.3, 1.4, 2.4, 5.7, 5.9

Bontrager & Lampignano: *Textbook of Radiographic Positioning and Related Anatomy,* ed 8, St. Louis, 2014, Mosby.

Figs. 2.1, 2.2, 2.3, 3.1A, 3.1B, 5.1, 5.2, 5.3A, 5.3B, 5.4, 5.5

Centers for Disease Control and Prevention (CDC)

Figs. 1.1, 1.2

Centers for Disease Control and Prevention (CDC), National Health Interview Survey, 1997-2014, Family Core Component)

Fig. 1.6

Cutter MG, Drexler E, McCullough LB, McInerney JD, Murray JC, Rossiter B, Zola J: *Mapping and Sequencing the Human Genome: Science, Ethics, and Public Policy,* Colorado Springs, Colorado: BSCS and the American Medical Association, 1992

Fig. 1.7

Nationwide Children's Hospital, Columbus, Ohio

Figs. 4.32, 4.34, 4.36, 5.31A, 5.31B, 5.32, 8.21, 8.22

Crowley LV: *Introductory Concepts in Pathology,* Chicago, 1972, Mosby.

Fig. 1.9

Damjanov I: *Anderson's Pathology,* vol 2, ed 10, St. Louis, 1996, Mosby.

Figs. 8.19, 10.27, 12.16

Drake R, Vogl AW, Mitchell AW: *Gray's Anatomy for Students,* ed 3, Philadelphia, 2014, Churchill Livingstone.

Figs. 8.4, 8.5, 10.1, 10.3, 10.34

Eisenberg RL, Johnson NM, *Comprehensive Radiographic Pathology,* ed 5, St. Louis, 2012, Mosby.

Fig. 11.4

Frank ED, Long BW, Smith BJ: *Merrill's Atlas of Radiographic Positioning and Procedures,* ed 11, St. Louis, 1994, Mosby.

Figs. 8.1, 8.3A, 8.3B, 8.3C

Haines DE: *Fundamental Neuroscience,* Philadelphia, 1997, Churchill Livingstone.

Fig. 8.23

Huether SE, McCance K: **Understanding Pathophysiology,** ed 3, St. Louis, 2004, Mosby

Fig. 11.1

Huether SE, McCance KL: **Understanding Pathophysiology,** ed 6, St. Louis, 2016, Mosby.

Figs. 8.37, 9.1, 9.2, 9.9, 9.14, 12.28, 12.32

Standring S: *Gray's Anatomy,* ed 4, Philadelphia, 2009, Churchill Livingstone.

Fig. 3.10

McCance KL, Huether SE: *Pathophysiology: the Biologic Basis for Disease in Adults and Children,* ed 5, St. Louis, Mosby.

Figs. 1.8, 1.9, 5.29, 5.33, 5.37, 5.83, 9.5, 11.7, 12.5

McCance KL, Huether SE: *Pathophysiology: the Biologic Basis for Disease in Adults and Children,* ed 6, St. Louis, 2010, Mosby.

Figs. 1.11, 4.35, 4.37, 4.42, 4.50, 5.43, 5.54, 5.65, 6.23

McCance KL, Huether SE: *Pathophysiology: the Biologic Basis for Disease in Adults and Children,* ed 7, St. Louis, 2014, Mosby.

Figs. 2.20, 2.21, 2.33, 2.34, 4.27, 4.29A, 4.30, 4.31, 4.33

Northcentral Technical College, Wausau, Wisconsin

Figs. 3.2, 3.16, 3.22, 3.24

Perkins DG: *Mosby's Color Atlas and Text of Neurology,* London, 1998, Mosby-Wolfe.

Fig. 8.52

The Ohio State University Wexner Medical Center, Columbus, Ohio

Figs. 2.4, 2.5, 2.6, 2.7, 2.8, 2.10, 2.12, 2.15, 2.24, 2.25, 2.26B, 2.27, 2.29, 2.30, 2.31, 2.36, 2.37, 2.39, 2.40, 2.42, 2.43, 2.45, 2.46, 2.52, 2.53, 3.3, 3.5, 3.8, 3.9, 3.12 to 3.15, 3.17 to 3.21, 3.23, 3.25, 3.26, 3.28, 3.29, 3.32, 3.33, 3.35, 3.36, 3.39, 3.40, 3.41, 3.43 to 3.47, 3.49, 3.50, 3.51, 3.53, 4.8, 4.15 to 4.26, 4.28, 4.29B, 4.39, 4.43, 4.44, 4.47, 4.53 to 4.56, 4.59, 5.6, 5.10, 5.11, 5.12, 5.14, 5.15, 5.16, 5.17, 5.18, 5.19, 5.20, 5.21, 5.22, 5.25, 5.28, 5.36, 5.42, 5.46, 5.47, 5.49, 5.51, 5.52, 5.57, 5.61, 5.72, 5.73, 5.74, 5.75, 5.76, 5.77, 5.79, 5.84, 6.3, 6.4, 6.5, 6.6, 6.7, 6.9, 6.10, 6.11, 6.12, 6.13, 6.14, 6.15, 6.18, 6.21, 6.22, 6.25, 6.26, 6.27, 6.28, 6.29, 6.31, 6.32, 6.35, 6.39, 6.41, 7.5, 7.6, 7.7, 7.8, 7.9, 7.10, 7.11, 7.12, 7.13, 7.14, 7.16, 7.18, 7.19, 7.20, 7.21, 7.23, 7.24, 7.25, 7.26, 7.27, 7.28, 7.30, 7.31, 7.33, 7.34, 7.35, 7.37, 7.43 , 7.44, 7.45, 7.48, 7.49, 7.50,7.51, 7.52, 7.53, 7.54, 7.55, 7.57, 7.58, 7.60, 7.61, 7.62, 7.63, 7.64, 7.65, 7.66, 7.68, 4.69, 7.70, 7.71, 7.79, 7.80, 8.7, 8.9 to 8.18, 8.24, 8.27, 8.28, 8.29, 8.32, 8.34, 9.3, 9.6, 9.10, 9.11, 9.12, 9.13, 10.4, 10.6, 10.10 to 10.14, 10.16 to 10.23, 10.25, 10.27 to 10.31, 10.33, 11.6, 11.9, 11.13 to 11.17, 12.2, 12.3, 12.7, 12.8, 12.12, 12.20, 12.22 to 12.26, 12.29, 12.33, 12.35 to 12.39, 12.41, 12.42, 12.43, 12.47, 12.51, 12.52, 12.58, 12.59, 12.60, 12.62 to 12.64, 12.66 to 12.71, 12.74, 12.76, 12.78, 12.79, 12.84, 12.85, 12.86, 12.87

Riverside Methodist Hospital, Columbus, Ohio

Figs. 2.16, 2.17, 2.19, 2.24A, 2.32, 2.41, 2.49, 2.50, 3.4, 3.6, 3.37, 3.52, 3.54, 3.55, 4.4, 4.9 to 4.14, 4., 4.40, 4.45, 4.46, 4.48, 4.49, 4.51, 4.52, 4.57, 4.58, 5.13, 5.18, 5.23, 5.24, 5.26, 5.27, 5.50, 5.56, 5.58, 5.63, 5.68, 5.69, 5.78, 5.85, 6.8, 6.16, 6.17, 6.19, 6.20, 6.24, 6.30, 6.33, 6.34, 6.36, 6.38, 6.40, 7.15, 7.29, 7.32, 7.36, 7.38, 7.39, 7.40, 7.41 7.42, 7.46, 7.56, 7.59, 7.67, 7.72, 7.73, 7.74, 7.75, 7.78, 8.8, 8.25, 8.26, 8.30, 8.31, 8.33, 8.35, 8.36, 8.38, 8.39, 8.40, 8.41, 8.42, 8.43, 8.44, 8.45, 8.46, 8.47, 8.48, 8.49, 8.50, 8.51, 8.53, 8.54, 9.4, 10.2, 10.5, 10.7, 10.8, 10.9, 10.10, 10.13, 10.24, 10.26, 10.32, 10.35, 10.36, 10.37, 10.38, 10.39, 10.40, 10.41, 10.42, 10.43, 10.44, 12.10, 12.11, 12.13, 12.14, 12.17 to 12.19, 12.21, 12.27, 12.30, 12.40, 12.44, 12.45, 12.48, 12.53 to 12.57, 12.61, 12.65, 12.80, 12.83

Thibodeau GA, Patton KT: *Anatomy & Physiology,* ed. 5, St. Louis, 2003, Mosby.

Fig. 11.5

Thibodeau GA, Patton KT: *Anatomy & Physiology,* ed. 7, St. Louis, 2009, Mosby.

Figs. 4.1, 4.5, 5.7, 6.1, 6.2, 8.2, 8.6, 11.2, 11.3

Thibodeau GA, Patton KT: *Anatomy & Physiology,* ed 8, St. Louis, 2008, Mosby.

Figs. 7.1, 7.4

Acholonu UC, Silberzweig J, Stein DE, et al.: Hysterosalpingography versus sonohysterography for intrauterine abnormalities, *JSLS* 15(4):471–474, 2011.

Adrenal cancer detailed guide. American Cancer Society website. http://www.cancer.org/. (Accessed April 10, 2016).

Aletaha D, Neogi T, Silman AJ, et al.: 2010 rheumatoid arthritis classification criteria: arthritis and rheumatism, *Am Coll Rheumatol* 62(9):2569–2581, 2010.

American Cancer Society: breast cancer detailed guide: http://www.cancer.org. (Accessed January 31, 2016).

American Cancer Society: guidelines for the early detection of cancer: http://www.cancer.org/. (Accessed January 31, 2016).

American Cancer Society: testicular cancer detailed guide: http://www.cancer.org. (Accessed January 31, 2016).

American Cancer Society Textbook of Clinical Oncology, ed 2, 1995. New York.

American Cancer Society: thyroid cancer detailed guide: www.cancer.org. (Accessed April 10, 2016).

American College of Radiology: appropriateness criteria: http://www.acr.org/SecondaryMainMenuCategories/quality_safety/app_criteria/pd/. (Accessed March 6, 2016).

American College of Radiology: *Manual on contrast media*. Available at www.acr.org, 2015. (Accessed May 20, 2016).

American College of Radiology: practice guideline for the performance of HSG: http://www.acr.org/~/media/b96d79998651431a8bd263017de707a5.pdf. (Accessed January 15, 2016).

American College of Surgeons: american College of Surgeons consultation/verification program reference guide of suggested classification: http://www.facs.org/trauma/vrc1.pdf. (Accessed May 25, 2012).

American Diabetes Association: diagnosis and classification of diabetes mellitus: http://care.diabetesjournals.org/content/39/Supplement_1/S13.short. (Accessed April 24, 2016).

American Diabetes Association: type 1 diabetes: www.diabetes.org. (Accessed April 10, 2016).

American Hospital Association: *TrendWatch Chartbook*. Washington D.C. http://www.aha.org/research/reports/tw/chartbook/ch3.shtml, 2015. (Accessed March 31, 2016).

American Thyroid Association: hypothyroidism: www.thyroid.org. (Accessed April 10, 2016).

Barnhart KT: ectopic pregnancy. N Engl J Med 07(4):379–387.

Boyce AM, Shawker TH, Hill SC, et al.: Ultrasound is superior to computed tomography for assessment of medullary nephrocalcinosis in hypoparathyroidism, *J Clin Endocrinol Metab* 98(3):989–994, 2013.

Brunetti JC: imaging in Gallstones (Cholelithiasis), 2015. Available online at: http://emedicine.medscape.com/article/366246-overview. (Accessed April 1, 2016).

Campion EW, Brunham RC, Gottlieb SL, et al.: Pelvic inflammatory disease, *N Engl J Med* 372(21):2039–2048, 2015.

Centers for Disease Control and Prevention, Division of Health Interview Statistics. U.S. Department of Health and Human Services: early release of selected estimates based on data from the 2014 national health interview survey: http://www.cdc.gov/nchs/data/nhis/earlyrelease/earlyrelease201506.pdf. (Accessed March 31, 2016).

Centers for Disease Control and Prevention. U.S. Department of Health and Human Services: injury prevention and control: Traumatic brain injury.

Centers for Disease Control and Prevention, National Center for Health Statistics. U.S. Department of Health and Human Services: http://www.cdc.gov/nchs/data/hus/hus14.pdf#024. (Accessed March 31, 2016).

Centers for Disease Control and Prevention. U.S. Department of Health and Human Services: national vital statistics reports, vol. 64, No 2: http://www.cdc.gov/nchs/data/nvsr/nvsr64/nvsr64_02.pdf. (Accessed March 31, 2016).

Centers for Disease Control and Prevention: HIV in the United States, 2012: http://www.cdc.gov/hiv/resources/factsheets/PDF/HIV_at_a_glance.pdf. (Accessed May 15, 2012).

Centers for Disease Control and Prevention: *Trends in tuberculosis*, www.cdc.gov/tb/publications/factsheets/statistics/tbtrends.htm, 2014.

Center for Disease Control and Prevention: *Tuberculosis Data and Statistics*, http://www.cdc.gov/tb/statistics/default.htm, 2015.

Center for Disease Control and Prevention: *National Center for Health Statistics*, http://www.cdc.gov/nchs/fastats/asthma.htm, 2015.

Centers for Disease Control and Prevention: National Diabetes Statistics Report. www.cdc.gov, 2014. (Accessed April 10, 2016).

Center for Disease Control and Prevention: *Lung cancer*, http://www.cdc.gov/cancer/lung/basic_info/index.htm, 2014.

Center for Disease Control and Prevention: press Release - Injuries cost the US $671 billion dollars in 2013. Available online at: http://www.cdc.gov/media/releases/2015/p0930-injury-costs.html. (Accessed June 16, 2016).

Centers for Disease Control and Prevention: get the stats on traumatic brain injury in the United States. Available online at: https://www.cdc.gov/traumaticbraininjury/pdf/bluebook_factsheet-a.pdf. (Accessed June 16, 2016).

Centers for Medicare and Medicaid Services: National Health Expenditure Data. https://www.cms.gov/research-statistics-data-and-systems/statistics-trends-and-reports/nationalhealthexpenddata/downloads/highlights.pdf, 2014. (Accessed March 31, 2016).

Chan YY, Jayaprakasan K, Zamora J, et al.: The prevalence of congenital uterine anomalies in unselected and high-risk populations: a systematic review, *Human Reproduction Update* 17(6):761–771, 2011.

Clarke RC: Small Intestinal Diverticulosis. http://emedicine.medscape.com/article/185356-overview#a4, (Accessed January 30, 2016).

Darwin PE: Cholangiocarcinoma. http://emedicine.medscape.com/article/277393-overview, 2015. (Accessed April 3, 2016).

Fernando RJ, Thakar R, Sultan AH, et al.: Effect of vaginal pessaries on symptoms associated with pelvic organ prolapse, *Obstet Gynecol* 108(1):93–99, 2016.

Gaillard F: Rickets. Radiopaedia.org: http://radiopaedia.org/. (Accessed April 10, 2016).

Gill BC: Bladder Anatomy. WebMD. http://emedicine.medscape.com/article/1949017-overview. (Accessed 5/13/16).

Gilsanz V, Ratib O: *Hand bone age: a digital atlas of bone maturity*, Berlin, 2012, Springer-Verlag.

Golatta M, Harcos A, Pavlista D, et al.: Ultrasound-guided cryoablation of breast fibroadenoma: a pilot trial, *Arch Gynecol Obstet* 291(6):1355–1360, 2015.

Heuman DM: Gallstones (Cholelithiasis) Workup. Available online at: http://emedicine.medscape.com/article/175667-workup, 2015. (Accessed March 25, 2016).

Hogg S, Vyas S: Endometriosis, *Obstet, Gynaecol, Reprod Med* 25(5):133–141, 2015.

Hope WW: Gastric Volvulus. http://emedicine.medscape.com/article/2054271-overview. (Accessed January 1, 2016).

Hubble W: Something old, something new: skeletal imaging with F[18]-sodium fluoride PET/CT, *Adv Med Imag Radiat Oncol*, 2011.

Joura EA, Giuliano AR, Iversen OE, et al.: A 9-valent HPV vaccine against infection and intraepithelial neoplasia in women, *N Engl J Med* 372(8):711–723, 2015.

Juranek J, Salmon M: Anomalous development of brain structure and function in spina bifida myleomeningocele, *Dev Disab Res Rev* 16:23–30, 2010.

Karavitka N, Cudlip S, Adams C, et al.: Craniopharyngiomas, *Endocrine Rev* 27(4):371–397, 2006.

Kolon TF, Herndon CD, Baker LA, et al.: Evaluation and treatment of cryptorchidism: AUA guideline, *J Urol* 192(2):337–345, 2014.

Kosuga K1, Hattori R, Eizawa H, et al.: Long-term prognosis after thrombolytic therapy for acute myocardial infarction, *Int J Cardiol Sep* 51(2):149–156, 1995.

Kumar V, Gupta J: Tubal ectopic pregnancy, *BMJ Clin Evid* 2015, 2015.

Levine MS, Rubesin SE, Laufer I: Pattern approach for diseases of mesenteric small bowel on barium studies, *Radiology* 249(2):445–460, 2008.

Lovig KO, Ward BA: Benign breast diseases in elderly women and men. In Rosenthal RA, editor: *Principles and practice of geriatric surgery*, Springer Sciences and Business Media, LLC, 2011, pp 469–478.

McCance KL, Huether SE, Brashers VL, et al.: *Pathophysiology: the biologic basis for disease in adults and children*, ed 7, St. Louis, MO, 2014, Mosby.

McVary KT, Roehrborn CG, Avins AL, et al.: Update on AUA guideline on the management of benign prostatic hyperplasia, *J Urol* 185(5):1793–1803, 2011.

Merck Co: *Merck manual of diagnosis and therapy*, ed 19, NJ, 2011, Whitehouse Station.

Merck Manual of diagnosis and therapy, 2016. Merck Sharp & Dohme Corp., a subsidiary of Merck & Co., Inc., Kenilworth, NJ, USA. Available online at: http://www.merckmanuals.com/professional/. (Accessed June 5, 2016).

Milne S, King GC: Advanced imaging in COPD: insights into pulmonary pathophysiology, *J Thorac Dis* 6(11):1570–1585, 2014.

National Cancer Institute: A snapshot of lung cancer. http://www.cancer.gov/research/progress/snapshots/lung, 2014.

National Cancer Institute: PDQ® Endometrial Cancer Treatment. Bethesda, MD: National Cancer Institute: http://www.cancer.gov/types/uterine/patient/endometrial-treatment-pdq. (Accessed January 31, 2016).

National Cancer Institute: PDQ® Breast Cancer Treatment. Bethesda, MD: national Cancer Institute: http://www.cancer.gov/types/breast/patient/breast-treatment-pdq. (Accessed December 31 2016).

National Institute of Health, National Institute of Diabetes, and Digestive and Kidney Diseases: acromegaly: http://www.niddk.nih.gov/. Published April 2012. Updated 2012. (Accessed April 10, 2016).

National Institute of Health, National Institute on Aging: the Basics of Lewy Body Dementia: https://www.nia.nih.gov/alzheimers/publication/lewy-body-dementia/basics-lewy-body-dementia. (Accessed June 5, 2016).

National Institute of Health National Institute of Diabetes and Digestive and Kidney Diseases: diabetes insipidus: http://www.niddk.nih.gov/. (Accessed April 10, 2016).

National Institutes of Health, National Cancer Institute: human papillomavirus (HPV) vaccines: www.cancer.gov. (Accessed January 31, 2016).

National Institute of Health, U.S. National Library of Medicine: MedlinePlus: Hyperthyroidism: https://www.nlm.nih.gov.libproxy.lib.unc.edu/medlineplus. (Accessed April 10, 2016).

National Institute of Health, U.S. National Library of Medicine: Medline Plus: Hypopituitarism: https://www.nlm.nih.gov. Updated 2013. (Accessed April 10, 2016).

National Institute of Health, U.S. National Library of Medicine: MedlinePlus: Osteomalacia: https://www.nlm.nih.gov/medlineplus/. (Accessed April 10, 2016).

National Institutes of Health: SEER stat fact sheets: cervix uteri cancer: seer.cancer.gov. (Accessed January 31, 2016).

National Cancer Institute, Survellance, Epidemiology, and End Results Program: SEER stat fact sheets: prostate cancer: http://seer.cancer.gov. (Accessed January 31, 2016).

National Institute of Health, U.S. National Library of Medicine: Testicular torsion: https://www.nlm.nih.gov/medlineplus/. (Accessed January 31, 2016).

Ojesina AI, Lichtenstein L, Freeman SS, et al.: Landscape of genomic alterations in cervical carcinomas, *Nature* 506(7488):371–375, 2014.

Ostrom QT, Gittleman H, Stetson L, et al.: Epidemiology of gliomas, *Cancer Treat Res* 163:1–14, 2015.

Park C-H, Jung M-H, Ji Y-I: Risk factors for malignant transformation of mature cystic teratoma, *Obstet Gynecol Sci.* 58(6):475–480, 2015.

Peterson CM, Anderson JS, et al.: Volvulus of the gastrointestinal tract: appearance at multimodality imaging, *Radiographics*, 2009. http://pubs.rsna.org/doi/pdf/10.1148/rg.295095011. (Accessed January 30, 2016).

Porth CM: *Essentials of pathophysiology*, ed 3, Philadelphia, PA, 2011, Lippincott Williams & Wilkins.

Rabinowitz SS: Pediatric Meckel Diverticulum Workup. http://emedicine.medscape.com/article/931229-workup#c6. (Accessed January 29, 2016).

Roberts A: Magnetic resonance-guided focused ultrasound for uterine fibroids, *Seminars in Interventional Radiology* 25(4):394–405, 2008.

Saloner D, Uzelac A, Hetts S, et al.: Modern meningioma imaging techniques, *J Neuro-Oncol*, 2010.

Sanders R: *Clinical sonography: a practical guide*, ed 3, Philadelphia, PA, 2011, Lippincott.

Schilz A, Kornak U: CLCN7-related osteopetrosis. NIH October 14, 2010: www.ncbi.nlm.nih.gov/books/NBK1127. (Accessed).

Singer FR, Bone HG, Hosking DJ, et al.: Paget's disease of bone: an endocrine society clinical practice guideline, *J Clin Endocrinol Metab* 99(12):4408–4422, 2014.

Society of Nuclear Medicine: Guidelines for sodium 18F-fluoride PET/CT bone scans. www.snm.org/docs/Practice%20Guideline%20NaF%20PET%20V1.pdf, 2011. (Accessed).

Solomon CG, Stewart EA: Uterine fibroids, *N Engl J Med* 372(17):1646–1655, 2015.

Type 2 diabetes: overview. PubMed Health: http://www.ncbi.nlm.nih.gov.libproxy.lib.unc.edu/pubmedhealth. (Accessed April 10, 2016).

U.S. Department of Health and Human Services, Administration on Children, Youth and Families: child maltreatment 2010: http://www.acf.hhs.gov/programs/cb/pubs/cm10/cm10.pdf#page = 70. (Accessed).

WebMD LLC: Developmental dysplasia of the hip. 2011 emedicine.medscape.com/article/1248135, 2011. (Accessed).

Weerakkody Y, Pant HP: Osteoporosis. Radiopaedia.org: http://radiopaedia.org/. (Accessed April 10, 2016).

Wright NC, Looker AC, Saag KG, et al.: The recent prevalence of osteoporosis and low bone mass in the United States based on bone mineral density at the femoral neck or lumbar spine, *J Bone Mineral Res* 29(11):2520–2526, 2014.

Note: Page numbers followed by *f, t,* or *b* indicate figures, tables, or boxes, respectively.

Alzheimer's disease, 4–5, 276–277, 277t, 278f
Ambulatory care centers, 5
Amenorrhea–galactorrhea syndrome, 287
American College of Radiology (ACR)
  chest radiography guidelines of, 61
  hepatobiliary system imaging guidelines of, 195
  JRA classification criteria of, 32
  RA classification criteria of, 32
American College of Surgeons (ACS), 368–369
American Heart Association (AHA), 281
American Joint Committee on Cancer (AJCC), 15
AML. *See* Acute myelocytic leukemia
Amniotic fluid, pregnancy disorders and, 335–336
AMOL. *See* Acute monoblastic leukemia
Amoxicillin, 153–154
Amphiarthrodial joints (cartilaginous joints), 19–20
Ampulla of Vater (hepatopancreatic ampulla), 186, 190
Amylase, 186
Anal agenesis, 145
Anaplasia, 9t
Anemia, 298
Anencephaly, 27–28, 28f
Aneurysmal bone cysts (ABCs), 43–44
Aneurysms
  abdominal aortic, 116–117, 116f–117f
  of cardiovascular system, 115–118
  dissecting, 115–116, 115f–116f
  fusiform, 115–116, 115f
  saccular, 115–116, 115f
  thoracic aortic, 117–118, 117f
  types of, 115–116, 115f
Angiocardiography, 98–99
Angiography
  arterial stents and, 99–102, 102f
  cardiovascular, for atherosclerosis diagnosis, 112, 113f
  cardiovascular system imaging considerations with, 98–102
  cerebral, for head and neck vasculature, 265, 265f
  CO_2 as contrast agent in, 99–102, 103f
  diagnostic, 98–99
  embolization and, 99–102, 101f
  magnetic resonance, 97, 100f
  permanent catheterization and, 99–102
  PTA and, 99–102, 102f

Angiography *(Continued)*
  PTCA and, 99–102
  renal, 224, 225f
  therapeutic, 99–102
  thrombolysis and, 99–102, 100f
  TIPS and, 99–102, 101f
Ankles
  Maisonneuve fractures and, 397–398, 401f
  Pott fractures and, 397–398, 399f–400f
  trimalleolar fractures and, 397–398, 401f
Ankylosing spondylitis (Marie-Strümpell disease), 34–35, 34f
Annulus fibrosus, 259, 260f
Antacids, for GERD, 152
Anterior lobe, 348
Anteroposterior pelvis, 26
Anterospondylolisthesis, 38–39, 38f
Anthracosis (black lung disease), 77, 77f
Antibiotics, 29
  for peptic ulcers, 153–154
  for PID, 324
Antibodies, 301
Antidiuretic hormone (ADH), 348
  DI and disrupted secretion of, 357
Antiretroviral therapy (ART), 305
Anus, 127–128
  imperforate, 145
Aorta, coarctation of, 105, 105f
Apert syndrome, 25, 27
Appendicitis, 158–159, 158f–159f
Appendicular skeleton, 18, 19f
Appendix
  appendicitis and, 158–159, 158f–159f
  surgical removal of, 159
Arachnoid mater, 256–257, 257f
ARO. *See* Autosomal recessive osteopetrosis
ART. *See* Antiretroviral therapy
Arterial blood gas (ABG) measurement, 67
Arterial oxygen level (Po_2), 67
Arteries, 90
  hardening of, 111
Arthritis
  acute, 31
  ankylosing spondylitis and, 34–35, 34f
  chronic, 31
  gouty, 36, 36f
  infectious, 31
  joint inflammation and, 31
  osteoarthritis, 12, 35, 35f
  psoriatic, 31
  rheumatoid, 31–34

Arthropathies, 31–38
Asbestos, 77
Asbestosis, 77
Ascending colon, 127–128
Ascites, 197–198, 197f
Aspiration (chemical) pneumonia, 71–72, 71f
Aspirin, 179–180
Asthma, COPD and, 76
Astrocytes, functions of, 260t
Astrocytomas
  of brain, 283–284, 285f
  of spinal cord, 292
Asymptomatic, 2
Atelectasis, 67, 411, 412f
Atheroma formations (fibrofatty plaques), 111–112
Atherosclerosis, 12, 111–113
  cardiovascular angiography for diagnosis of, 112, 113f
  carotid artery occlusion and, 111f
  CRP for, 112–113
  development of, 111–112, 112f
  Doppler sonography for diagnosis of, 112, 113f
  femoral artery occlusion in, 111f
  incidence of, 111
  MRI for diagnosis of, 112, 113f
  risk factors with, 111
Atherothrombotic brain infarction (ABI), 279
ATLS. *See* Advanced trauma life support
Atresia
  bowel, 143–145, 144f–145f
  colonic, 144–145, 144f–145f
  definition of, 141–143
  duodenal, 143–144, 144f
  esophageal, 141–143, 142f–143f
  ileal, 143
  TE fistula associated with, 143, 143f
Atrial septal defects, 106, 106f
Atrophy, 8–9
Autoantibodies, 10
Autoimmune disorders, 10
Automatic exposure control (AEC), 55
Autosomal dominant osteopetrosis type II (ADOII), 24
Autosomal recessive osteopetrosis (ARO), 24
Avascular necrosis, 409
Avulsion fractures, 373f–374f, 392
Axial skeleton, 18, 19f
Axons, 258–259

B

β-cells. *See* Beta cells
Back pain, 372
Bacteria, 10
Bacterial meningitis, 270–271, 270f
Barium enema, 133, 133f
    air-contrast, diverticulosis
        demonstrated with, 173, 175f
    via colostomy, 134f
    double-contrast
        for colon cancer diagnosis, 181, 182f
        for colonic polyps, 179–180
    Hirschsprung disease (congenital
        aganglionic megacolon)
        demonstrated with, 148, 148f
    intussusception demonstrated with,
        169f
    for UC, 159–160, 160f
Barium studies, on esophageal varices,
    161, 162f
Barium sulfate, 130–131
Barrett esophagus, 177
Basilar skull fractures, 376, 376f
Battered child syndrome, 408, 408f
Benign neoplasms, 12–14, 13t
Benign prostatic hyperplasia (BPH),
    339–344, 340f
Bennett fractures, 396–397
Beta cells (β-cells), 186
Bicornuate uterus, 322–323, 323f
Bilateral agenesis, 229
Bilateral lumbar ribs, 27f
Bilevel positive airway pressure (BiPAP), 67
Biliary tree
    anatomy and physiology of, 186, 188f
    operative cholangiography for,
        190–191, 190f
    PTC for, 189–190, 189f–190f
    radiography showing pneumobilia in,
        188–189, 189f
    T-tube cholangiography for, 191, 191f
Bilirubin, 203
BiPAP. *See* Bilevel positive airway pressure
Birth, life expectancy at, 3–4, 3f
Bismuth citrate, 153–154
Black lung disease (anthracosis), 77, 77f
Bladder. *See also* Kidneys, ureters, and
    bladder radiography
    anatomy and physiology of, 213–214,
        214f
    carcinoma of, 249–250, 249f–251f
    cystitis of, 239–240, 240f
    cystography demonstrating diverticula
        of, 218, 220f

Bladder *(Continued)*
    diverticula of, 234, 234f
    IVU demonstrating ureter entrance
        into wall of, 217, 220f
    nephrostomy tube for neobladder,
        225–226, 227f
    neurogenic, 239–240
    trabeculae, 239–240, 240f
Blood cells, types of, 298, 299t
Blood clotting
    cascade, ischemic stroke and, 279
    mechanism of, 300, 300f
Blood types, cross-matching, 298, 300t
Blood urea nitrogen (BUN), 214–215,
    242
Blood-brain barrier, 257–258
Blowout fractures, 402–404
Bone marrow
    MRI for evaluation of, 302, 302f
    red, 18, 301
    yellow, 301
Bone mineral densitometry, 351. *See also*
    Dual x-ray absorptiometry
Bone spurs, 35, 35f
Bones. *See also* Skeletal system
    abnormalities of, diagnosis of, 40
    bruise to, 396, 397f
    composition of, 18, 19f
    healing process of, following skeletal
        fractures, 384, 385f
    malignant tumors of, 40
    of skeletal system, 18–20
    "worm-eaten," 30–31
Botulinum toxin, 171
Bouchard nodes, 35
Bowel. *See also* Large bowel; Small bowel
    atresia, 143–145, 144f–145f
    gallstone ileus and, 168–169, 169f, 202
    intussusceptions, 167–168, 168f–169f
    malrotation of, 146, 147f
    obstruction of, 166–170, 167t
        mechanical, 167–170, 167f–168f
        paralytic ileus and, 166, 170, 170f
    volvulus, 167, 168f
Bowman's capsule, 212–213, 213f
Boxer's fracture, 396–397, 398f
BPH. *See* Benign prostatic hyperplasia
Brain
    abscesses, 271–273, 272f
    anatomy and physiology of, 256, 256f
        blood-brain barrier, 257–258
        Circle of Willis, 257, 259f
        dura mater sinuses and venous
            drainage, 257, 259f

Brain *(Continued)*
        lateral ventricles, 257, 258f
        meninges, 256–257, 257f
    CT for
        tissue density, 263–264, 264f
        white and gray matter
            differentiation, 263–264, 263f
    DWI for conditions of, 261, 263f
    encephalitis and, 271, 272f
    MRI for posterior fossa region of,
        260–261, 262f
    PET scans for, 264, 265f
    PWI for, 261–263, 263f
    radionuclide scans of, 264, 265f
    sonography for neonate, 264, 264f
    traumatic injuries to, 374–381
        coma, 378
        concussions, 377
        contusions, 377, 377f
        coup and contrecoup lesions, 377,
            377f
        hematomas, 378–381, 379f–381f
        MRI for, 376f
    tumors of
        acoustic neuromas, 290–292, 291f
        astrocytomas, 283–284, 285f
        central nerve sheath tumors,
            290–292, 291f
        characteristics of, 281–282
        craniopharyngiomas, 288–290, 290f
        CT for, 282
        ependymomas, 283–284, 286f
        glial and nonglial, 282
        glioblastoma multiforme, 283–284
        gliomas, 282–285, 283f–286f
        medulloblastomas, 285–287, 286f
        meningiomas, 287, 288f
        MRI for, 282–283
        oligodendrogliomas, 283–284, 285f
        pituitary adenomas, 287–288, 289f
        schwannomas, 290–292, 291f
        secondary, 292, 292f
        sites of, 282f
Brainstem, 256, 256f
Breasts
    anatomy of, 317–318, 318f
    cancer of
        male, 344
        sonography for, 321
    mammography for, 319–320
    masses of, 331–335
        carcinoma, 333–335, 334f–335f
        fibroadenomas, 331–332, 331f–332f
        fibrocystic, 332, 332f–333f

Hydroceles, 342, 342f
Hydrocephalus, 268, 269f–270f
Hydronephrosis, 217
  causes of, 244–245
  CT for kidney, 244–245, 244f–245f
  pyelonephritis causing, 244f
  sonography for kidney, 223f
  urinary system and, 244–245
Hypercapnia, 67
Hyperextension injuries, of spine, 38–39, 38f
Hyperflexion injuries, of spine, 38–39, 38f
Hyperostosis frontalis interna, 42
Hyperparathyroidism, 363–365, 364f–365f
Hyperplasia, 8–9
  benign prostatic, 339–344, 340f
  kidneys and, 229–230
Hyperthyroidism, 350
Hypertrophic pyloric stenosis (HPS), 145–146, 145f
Hypertrophy, 8–9
  compensatory, 229
Hypoglycemia, 348–350, 358
Hypopituitarism, 357
Hypoplasia, of kidneys, 229–230, 230f
Hypothalamus, 348
  anatomy and physiology of, 348, 349f
Hypothyroidism, 350, 361–362
Hypoventilation, 67
Hypoxemia, 67
Hysterosalpingography (HSG)
  for bicornuate uterus, 323f
  female reproductive system considerations with, 318–319, 318f–319f
  for HPV, 328f
  for unicornuate uterus, 323f
  for uterine leiomyomas, 329f–330f

I

IABP catheter. *See* Intraaortic balloon pump catheter
IAO. *See* Intermediate autosomal osteopetrosis
Iatrogenic reactions, 2
IBD. *See* Inflammatory bowel disease
Idiopathic disease, 2
Ileal pouch-anal anastomosis (IPAA), 160–161
Ileostomy, 133

Ileum, 126–127
  atresia, 143
  CD and string sign in diseased, 155–156, 156f
  Meckel's diverticulum of, 148–149
Ilizarov procedure, 23–24
Immunoglobulins, 298
  types of, 301
Impacted fractures, 385–387, 387f
Incarcerated hernias, 162, 164f
Incidence, 3
Incomplete fractures, 393–394, 393f–394f
Infants
  HPS and, 145–146
  malrotation and, 146–147
  mediastinum appearance in, 59, 60f
Infarcts, 113, 279
Infection, 11
Infectious arthritis, 31
Infectious diseases, of CNS, 270–273
Inferior vena cava (IVC), 99–102, 103f
Inflammatory bowel disease (IBD), 132. *See also* Crohn's disease
Inflammatory diseases, 10–11
  of abdomen, 150–161
  of CNS, 270–273
  of female reproductive system, 323–324
  of GI system, 150–161
  of hepatobiliary system, 196–204
  of respiratory system, 69–77
  of skeletal system, 28–38
  of urinary system, 237–240
Inflammatory reaction, 10
Inguinal hernia, 162, 162f–163f
Insulin, 186, 350–351, 358
Intermediate autosomal osteopetrosis (IAO), 24
Intermediate lobe, 348
Interphalangeal (IP) joints, 31
Interstitial (viral) pneumonia, 72
Intertrochanteric fractures, 387, 388f
Intervertebral disks, 259, 260f
Intima, 90
Intraaortic balloon pump (IABP) catheter, 65–66, 66f
Intraarterial thrombolysis, 265–266
Intracerebral hematomas, 378, 381f
Intraperitoneal organs, 125
Intravascular ultrasound (IVUS), 94
Intravenous pyelography (IVP), 215. *See also* Intravenous urography

Intravenous urography (IVU)
  adverse reactions to, 215–216
  for bladder carcinoma, 249, 249f
  calyces examination with, 217, 219f
  collecting system sequence in, 216–217, 217f
  indications for performing, 215
  nephrogram phase of, 216, 216f
  for PKD, 235–236, 235f
  postvoid, 216–217, 219f
  prone positioning in, 216–217, 219f
  for pyelonephritis, 237f–238f
  RCC confirmed with, 246
  for renal failure, 242–244, 244f
  of UPJ and UVJ, 216–217, 218f
  for ureter entrance into bladder wall, 217, 220f
  for urinary system, 215–217
Intussusceptions, 167–168, 168f–169f
Invasion, 14
Involucrum, 29, 30f
Involutional change, 317
Iodine thyroid uptake scan
  hyperthyroidism demonstrated with, 361, 361f–362f
  for thyroid cancer diagnosis, 362–363, 363f
IP joints. *See* interphalangeal joints
IPAA. *See* Ileal pouch-anal anastomosis
Ischemia, 113
Ischemic strokes, 278–281, 280f
Islets of Langerhans, 186, 350–351, 351f
IVC. *See* Inferior vena cava
IVP. *See* Intravenous pyelography
IVU. *See* Intravenous urography
IVUS. *See* Intravascular ultrasound

J

Jaundice
  CBD and, 204, 204f
  hepatobiliary system and, 203–204, 204f
  medical (nonobstructive), 189–190, 203
  surgical (obstructive), 189–190, 203–204
Jefferson fractures, 373
Jejunum, 126–127
Joints
  distal interphalangeal, 31
  inflammation and arthritis, 31
  interphalangeal, 31
  peripheral, RA and, 32
  types of, 19–20
JRA. *See* Juvenile rheumatoid arthritis

Luteinizing hormone (LH), 348
Lymph, 300–301
Lymph nodes, 300–301
Lymphatic spread, 14
Lymphatic system, 300–301
Lymphocytes, 301
Lymphoid system, 300
Lymphoma, 14–15
    CT for, 301–302, 301f
    Hodgkin, 301–302, 311–312, 312f
    non-Hodgkin, 310–311, 311f

M

Magnetic resonance angiography (MRA), 97, 100f
    for CNS evaluation, 265–266
    contrast-enhanced, 278–279
    for head and neck vasculature, 261, 262f
    for renovascular hypertension, 224–225, 225f
Magnetic resonance cholangiopancreatography (MRCP), 194–195, 195f
Magnetic resonance colonography (MRC), 181
Magnetic resonance enterography (MRE), 136
Magnetic resonance imaging (MRI), 14–15. *See also* Diffusion-weighted imaging
    for ABCs, 43–44
    for abdomen, 135–136, 136f
    for acoustic neuromas, 290–292, 291f
    for Alzheimer's disease, 278, 278f
    for appendicitis, 159
    for atherosclerosis diagnosis, 112, 113f
    for avascular necrosis, 409
    for bone marrow evaluation, 302, 302f
    brain abscess demonstrated with, 272, 272f
    for brain posterior fossa region, 260–261, 262f
    for brain tumors, 282–283
    for breast evaluation, 321, 322f
    for bronchogenic carcinoma, 82–83, 84f
    for CAD, 114
    cardiovascular system considerations with, 97, 99f–100f
    for CD, 157
    for cervical carcinoma, 328
    for cervical spondylosis, 273–275, 275f
    CNS considerations with, 260–263, 262f

Magnetic resonance imaging (MRI) *(Continued)*
    for colon cancer diagnosis, 181
    for craniopharyngiomas, 288–290, 290f
    for CVA, 278, 279f
    for degenerative disk disease, 273, 274f
    for dementia, 278, 278f
    for encephalitis, 271
    for endocrine system, 352
    for female reproductive system, 320f–322f, 321
    functional, 261
    for GI system, 135–136
    for gliomas, 283, 283f–285f, 285
    for hepatobiliary system, 194–195, 195f
    for hydrocephalus visualization, 268, 269f
    for ischemic strokes, 280f
    for Legg-Calvé-Perthes disease, 409, 409f
    for liver hemangioma, 204, 205f
    for male reproductive system, 338, 339f
    for medulloblastomas, 286f
    for meningiomas, 287, 288f, 293f
    for meningitis, 270f, 271
    for meningomyelocele, 267f–268f
    for MS evaluation, 260–261, 275–276, 276f
    for neoplastic diseases, 41
    for neurofibromas, 293f
    for osteoid osteomas, 44, 45f
    for osteosarcomas, 46, 46f–47f
    for ovarian cysts, 324–325, 325f
    for pituitary adenoma diagnosis, 287–288, 289f
    for prostate gland carcinoma, 340f–341f
    RCC demonstrated with, 246, 247f
    for renal cysts, 245, 246f
    for schwannomas, 290–292, 291f
    skeletal system considerations using, 20–21, 20f–21f
    for subarachnoid hematomas, 381f
    for subdural hematomas, 380f
    for TBI, 376f
    for urinary system, 224–225, 225f
    for uterine leiomyomas, 329f
    for uterus, 320f–322f, 321
    for vertebral column injuries, 39, 40f
Magnetic resonance venography (MRV), 261

Maisonneuve fractures, 397–398, 401f
Male reproductive system, 338
    anatomy and physiology of, 338, 339f
    congenital diseases of, 338–339
        cryptorchidism, 338–339
    imaging considerations for, 338
    MRI for, 338, 339f
    neoplastic diseases of, 339–344
        BPH, 339–344, 340f
        breast cancer, 344
        gynecomastia, 344
        prostate gland carcinoma, 340, 340f–341f
        testicular masses, 342–344
        testicular torsion, 341, 342f
Malignant neoplasms, 12–14, 13t
Mallet finger, 392, 393f
Maloney dilator, 150–151
Malrotation
    of bowel, 146, 147f
    GI system and, 146–147
    infants and, 146–147
    of kidneys, 231–232
    sonography for, 147
    UGI series for, 146–147, 147f
Malunion, of fractures, 385, 386f
Mammography
    for breast carcinoma, 334, 334f–335f
    for breasts, 319–320
    for fibroadenoma examination, 331–332
    for fibrocystic breasts, 332f
Mandibular fractures, 402, 404f
Manifestations, 2
Mantoux test, 73
Marble bone, 24
Marie-Strümpell disease (ankylosing spondylitis), 34–35, 34f
Mastalgia, 317
Mastitis, 324
Maxillary fractures, 402, 404f
Maxillary sinuses, 54–55
MBS. *See* Modified barium swallow
MDCT. *See* Multidetector computed tomography
Mechanical bowel obstruction, 167–170, 167f–168f
Meckel scans, 137
Meckel's diverticulum, 148–149
Media, 90
Mediastinum, 59–61
    chest radiography and penetration of, 92
    division of, 54
    radiographic, 59

Mediastinum *(Continued)*
  emphysema, 60–61, 60f
  infant appearance of, 59, 60f
  sagittal view of, 59f
  subcutaneous emphysema and, 60–61, 61f
Medicaid, 5–7
Medical (nonobstructive) jaundice, 189–190, 203
Medulla oblongata, 256, 256f
Medullary canal, 18
Medullary sponge kidney, 236, 236f
Medulloblastomas, 285–287, 286f
Melanocyte-stimulating hormone (MSH), 348
Melatonin, 348
Meninges, 256–257, 257f
Meningiomas
  of brain, 287, 288f
  of spinal cord, 292, 293f
Meningitis, 270–271, 270f
Meningocele, newborns and, 266–267, 267f
Meningococcal meningitis, 270–271
Meningomyelocele (spina bifida), 27, 28f, 266–267, 266f–268f
Mesenteroaxial volvulus, 166
Mesentry, 124–125, 125f
Metabolic diseases, 12
Metabolic syndrome, 360
Metabolism, 12
Metaphysis, 18, 41–42
Metaplasia, 8–9, 9t
Metastasis (metastases)
  brain and, secondary, 292, 292f
  respiratory system sites, 84–85, 85f
Metastatic disease, from carcinoma in skeletal system, 48–50, 49f
Metastatic liver disease, 205–206, 206f
Metastatic spread, 14
Metatarsophalangeal joint, 36
Methotrexate, 32
Metoclopramide, 136–137
Metronidazole, 153–154
MHE. *See* Multiple hereditary exostoses
MI. *See* Myocardial infarction
Microglia, functions of, 260t
Miliary tuberculosis, 73–74, 74f
Miller-Abbott tube, 141
Mineralocorticosteroids, 348–350
Mitral valve
  prolapse, 108
  stenosis, 108–109

MM. *See* Multiple myeloma
M-mode echocardiography, 93–94
Modified barium swallow (MBS), 130–131, 130f
Molar pregnancy (hydatidiform mole), 336–337, 338f
Monocytic leukemias, 309–310
Monteggia fractures, 396–397, 399f
Morbidity rate, 5
Morphology, 3
Mortality rate. *See also* Death
  definition of, 4
  fluctuation of, 5
Motor vehicle accidents (MVAs), 368, 370
  abdomen trauma from, CT for, 370–371, 371f
  blunt trauma from, CT for, 413, 413f
  whiplash injury from, 371–372, 372f
MRA. *See* Magnetic resonance angiography
MRC. *See* Magnetic resonance colonography
MRCP. *See* Magnetic resonance cholangiopancreatography
MRE. *See* Magnetic resonance enterography
MRI. *See* Magnetic resonance imaging
MRV. *See* Magnetic resonance venography
MS. *See* Multiple sclerosis
MSH. *See* Melanocyte-stimulating hormone
MUGA. *See* Multiple gate acquisition scans
Multidetector computed tomography (MDCT), 135, 370
Multiple fractures, 391–392, 392f
Multiple gate acquisition scans (MUGA), 96
Multiple hereditary exostoses (MHE), 41–42
Multiple myeloma (MM), 40, 308–309, 309f
Multiple sclerosis (MS)
  CNS and, 275–276
  MRI for evaluation of, 260–261, 275–276, 276f
  plaques, 275–276
Murmurs, heart, 104
MVAs. *See* Motor vehicle accidents
Mycobacterium avium, 303–304
Mycobacterium tuberculosis infection, 30–31, 73, 270–271
Mycoplasma pneumoniae, 69, 71

Myelin, 258–259
Myelocele, 266–267
Myelocytic leukemias, 309–310
Myelography, 39
Myeloid tissue, 301
Myocardial infarction (MI), 114–115, 115f
Myocardial perfusion scan, 95–96, 96f
Myocardium, 88

N

NAFLD. *See* Nonalcoholic fatty liver disease
Nasal bone fractures, 404–405, 405f
Nasoenteric decompression tubes, 141
Nasogastric (NG) tubes, 140–143, 141f
NAT. *See* Nonaccidental trauma
National Center for Health Statistics (NCHS), 2, 4–5
National Emergency X-radiography Utilization Study (NEXUS), 370
National Human Genome Institute, 8
National Institutes of Health, 7
NCHS. *See* National Center for Health Statistics
Neck
  cerebral angiography for vasculature of, 265, 265f
  cervical spondylosis and, 273–275, 275f
  MRA for vasculature of, 261, 262f
Needle guidewire localization, breasts and, 320
Neobladder, nephrostomy tube for, 225–226, 227f
Neonatal intensive care unit (NICU), 264
Neoplasms
  benign, 12–14, 13t
  classification of, 12, 13t
  malignant, 12–14, 13t
  origination of, 12–14, 14f, 14b
Neoplastic diseases, 12–15
  of abdomen, 176–183
  of CNS, 281–294, 282f
  CT usage for, 41
  of female reproductive system, 324–328
  of GI system, 176–183
  of hematopoietic system, 308–312
  of hepatobiliary system, 204–209
  of male reproductive system, 339–344
  MRI for, 41
  nuclear medicine for, 41
  of respiratory system, 81–85

Prosthetic hip and shoulder replacements, 32, 33f
Proton pump inhibitors (PPIs), 152–154
PSA. *See* Prostate-specific antigen
Pseudocyst, CT of pancreatitis and, 202, 202f
Pseudofactors (Looser zones), 353–354
Pseudopneumothorax, 410
Psoriatic arthritis, 31
PTA. *See* Percutaneous transluminal angioplasty
PTC. *See* Percutaneous transhepatic cholangiography
PTCA. *See* Percutaneous transluminal coronary angioplasty
PTH. *See* Parathyroid hormone
Pulmonary artery catheter (Swan-Ganz), 65, 66f
Pulmonary circulation, 88
Pulmonary embolism (PE)
 cardiovascular system and, 119–120, 119f
 CTA for, 119, 119f
 SPECT for evaluation of, 63–64
 from thrombus, 119
Pulmonary emphysema, 93
 symptoms and characteristics of, 75, 75f–76f
 treatment for, 76
Pulmonary fibrosis, 76–77
Pulmonary tuberculosis, 73–74, 73f–74f
Pulsion diverticulum, 171–172
PWI. *See* Perfusion-weighted imaging
Pyelonephritis, 237–239
 diagnostic medical sonography for, 238–239, 238f
 hydronephrosis caused by, 244f
 IVU for, 237f–238f
 KUB radiography for, 237f
Pyloromyotomy, 146
Pyramidal fractures (Le Fort II), 402
Pyuria, 237–238

Q
Quantitative computed tomography (QCT), 21

R
RA. *See* rheumatoid arthritis
Race, life expectancy by, 3f
Radiography, 14–15. *See* Kidneys, ureters, and bladder radiography

Radiography *(Continued)*
 for abdomen, 128–129, 129f–130f
 ascites considerations in, 197–198, 197f
 for acromegaly, 356f–357f
 for avulsion fractures, 373f–374f
 for battered child syndrome signs, 408, 408f
 for biliary tree showing pneumobilia, 188–189, 189f
 for boxer's fracture, 398f
 for CD, 156–157, 156f
 for cerebral cranial fractures, 375f
 for CF, 68, 69f
 chest
  ACR guidelines for, 61
  for anthracosis, 77, 77f
  for bronchiectasis, 72, 72f
  for bronchogenic carcinoma, 82, 82f–83f
  for cardiovascular system, 91–93, 92f–93f
  for CF, 68, 69f
  CHF causing cardiomegaly demonstrated with, 110f
  for histoplasmosis, 78, 78f
  for HIV/AIDS, 305, 306f
  mediastinum penetration in, 92
  OID and SID for heart, 92
  for patent ductus arteriosus, 104–105
  for pleural effusion, 79–80, 79f–80f
  for pulmonary emphysema, 75, 75f–76f
  RDS and, 69, 69f
  respiratory system imaging considerations for, 55–57, 56f–57f
  for Valvular disease, of cardiovascular system, 108–109, 109f
  for ventricular septal defect, 106, 107f
 for cholelithiasis, 201f
 for CNS, 260
 for Colles' fractures, 398f
 for compression fractures, 372–373, 373f
 for duodenal atresia, "double bubble sign" and, 143–144, 144f
 for endocrine system, 351
 for esophagus, 131
 gallstones demonstrated with, 201f
 for gastric volvulus, 166

Radiography *(Continued)*
 for GI system, 129–130
 for gluten-sensitivity enteropathy, 149, 149f
 for growth plate fractures, 375f–376f
 for hangman's fractures, 372–373, 373f
 for hepatitis and hepatomegaly, 200
 for hepatobiliary system, 188–189, 189f
 for hyperparathyroidism, 365f
 for incomplete fractures, 393f–394f
 for Jefferson fractures, 373
 for large bowel, 132–133, 133f, 135–136
 for Legg-Calvé-Perthes disease, 409, 409f
 for Maisonneuve fractures, 397–398, 401f
 for Meckel's diverticulum, 148–149
 of mediastinum division, 59
 for MM, 308–309, 309f
 for Monteggia fractures, 396–397, 399f
 for multiple fractures, 392f
 for nasal bone fractures, 404–405, 405f
 for oropharynx, 130–131, 130f
 for osteoporosis, 354f
 for osteosarcomas, 46, 47f
 of Paget's disease and, 354–356, 355f
 for paralytic ileus, 170, 170f
 for pathologic fractures, 391–392, 392f
 for pneumoperitoneum, 414–415, 415f
 for pneumothorax, 410, 410f
 for Pott fractures, 397–398
 for renal cysts, 245, 246f
 respiratory system imaging considerations with, 55
 of rickets, 355f
 for SCFE, 394, 395f
 for scoliosis, 26–27
 for shoulder dislocations, 405–407, 406f–407f
 for sinusitis, 80, 81f
 skeletal system considerations using, 20
 for skeletal trauma fracture evaluation, 382–383, 382f–383f, 398–402, 402f
 for small bowel, 132, 134–135
 for spinal cord conditions, 260, 261f
 for spiral fractures, 391–392, 391f
 for stomach, 131–134

Type 1 diabetes mellitus (juvenile diabetes mellitus), 358
Type 2 diabetes mellitus, 358–360

U

UBCs. *See* Unicameral bone cysts
UC. *See* Ulcerative colitis
UGI series. *See* Upper gastrointestinal tract series
Ulcerative colitis (UC), 159–161, 160f–161f
Ultrasonography, 14–15
Unicameral bone cysts (UBCs), 43, 43f
Unicornuate uterus, 322–323, 323f
United States (US)
  health expenditures in, 5–7, 6f, 7t
  morbidity rates in, 5
  uninsured rate in, 5–7, 7f
UPJ. *See* Ureteropelvic junction
Upper gastrointestinal tract (UGI) series
  for malrotation, 146–147, 147f
  procedure for, 131–132
Urea breath tests, 137
Uremia, 242–244
Ureteral stents, 226, 229f
Ureterocele, 234, 234f
Ureteropelvic junction (UPJ), 216–217, 218f
Ureterovesical junction (UVJ), 216–217, 218f
Ureters. *See* Kidneys, ureters, and bladder radiography
  anatomy and physiology of, 213, 214f
  diverticula of, 234, 234f
  double, 232, 233f
  IVU demonstrating bladder wall entrance of, 217, 220f
  ureterocele of, 234, 234f
Urethra, 338
  anatomy and physiology of, 214
  RUG and, 220, 221f–222f
Urethral valves, 234, 235f
Urinary meatus, 214
Urinary system
  anatomy and physiology of, 212–214, 212f–214f
  calcifications of, 240–242
    common sites of lodging, 241–242, 242f
    CT for, 241f
    gender and development of, 240–241
    noncalcified defects, 240–241, 240f
    pain from, 241–242

Urinary system *(Continued)*
    pancreatic calcifications, 242, 243f
    prostate gland calcifications, 242, 243f
    sonography for, 241f
    staghorn calculus, 240–241, 241f
  congenital and hereditary diseases of, 227–236
    kidney fusion anomalies, 230–231, 230f–231f
    kidney number and size anomalies, 229–230, 229f–230f
    kidney position anomalies, 231–232, 232f
    lower urinary tract anomalies, 234, 234f–235f
    medullary sponge kidney, 236, 236f
    PKD, 235–236, 235f
    renal pelvis and ureter anomalies, 232, 233f
  CT for, 223–224, 224f
  cystography for, 218–220
  degenerative diseases of, 242–245
    hydronephrosis, 244–245
    nephrosclerosis, 242
    renal failure, 242–244, 244f
  imaging considerations for, 214–215
  inflammatory diseases of, 237–240
    acute glomerulonephritis, 239
    cystitis, 239–240, 240f
    pyelonephritis, 237–239, 237f–238f
    UTI, 237
  IVU for, 215–217
  KUB radiography for, 215–227, 215f
  MRI for, 224–225, 225f
  neoplastic diseases of, 245–250
    bladder carcinoma, 249–250, 249f–251f
    nephroblastoma, 248, 248f, 249t
    RCC, 246–248
    renal cysts, 245
  pathologic summary of, 250t
  percutaneous nephrostography for, 225–226, 226f
  renal angiography for, 224, 225f
  retrograde pyelography for, 220, 222f
  sonography for, 223
  tubes and catheters for, 226–227
Urinary tract anomalies, lower, 234, 234f–235f
Urinary tract infection (UTI), 226–227, 235–237
US. *See* United States

U.S. Department of Health and Human Services (USDHHS), 4
Uterine fibroids, 328–330
Uterus
  anatomy of, 316–317
  bicornuate, 322–323, 323f
  didelphys, 322–323
  masses of, 328–331
    endometrial carcinoma, 330–331
    leiomyomas, 328–330, 329f–331f
  MRI for evaluation of, 320f–322f, 321
  pessary for support of, 317, 317f
  sonography for pregnant, 321, 335
  unicornuate, 322–323, 323f
UTI. *See* Urinary tract infection
UVJ. *See* Ureterovesical junction

V

Vagina. *See also* Female reproductive system
  anatomy of, 316
  pessary insertion into, 317, 317f
Valsalva maneuver, 59
Valves of Houston, 127–128
Valvular disease, of cardiovascular system, 108–109, 109f
Valvular stenosis, 108, 109f
Vasa deferentia, 338
Vascular access lines, 64–66
Vascular dementia, 277, 277t
Vascular diseases, of CNS, 278–281
Vasopressin, 357
VCUG. *See* Voiding cystourethrography
Veins, 90
Venous thrombosis, 118, 118f
Ventilation, 54
Ventricles, lateral, 257, 258f
Ventricular pacing electrodes, 66, 67f
Ventricular septal defects, 106, 106f–107f
Ventriculojugular shunts, 268, 270f
Vertebra (vertebrae)
  anomalies of, 26–27, 27f–28f
  lower lumbar, 28f
  transitional, 27
Vertebral column injuries
  CT demonstrating, 39, 40f
  MRI demonstrating, 39, 40f
  skeletal system and, 38–39
  traumatic, 371–374
    back pain, 372
    compression fractures, 372–373, 373f
    CT for, 373–374, 374f
    hangman's fractures, 372–373, 373f